Undoing Perpetual Stress

Undoing Perpetual Stress

*The Missing Connection
Between Depression, Anxiety, and
21st Century Illness*

RICHARD O'CONNOR, PH.D.

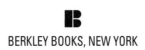

BERKLEY BOOKS, NEW YORK

THE BERKLEY PUBLISHING GROUP
Published by the Penguin Group
Penguin Group (USA) Inc.
375 Hudson Street, New York, New York 10014, USA
Penguin Group (Canada), 10 Alcorn Avenue, Toronto, Ontario M4V 3B2, Canada
(a division of Pearson Penguin Canada Inc.)
Penguin Books Ltd., 80 Strand, London WC2R 0RL, England
Penguin Group Ireland, 25 St. Stephen's Green, Dublin 2, Ireland (a division of Penguin Books Ltd.)
Penguin Group (Australia), 250 Camberwell Road, Camberwell, Victoria 3124, Australia
(a division of Pearson Australia Group Pty. Ltd.)
Penguin Books India Pvt. Ltd., 11 Community Centre, Panchsheel Park, New Delhi—110 017, India
Penguin Group (NZ), cnr Airborne and Rosedale Roads, Albany, Auckland 1310, New Zealand
(a division of Pearson New Zealand Ltd.)
Penguin Books (South Africa) (Pty.) Ltd., 24 Sturdee Avenue, Rosebank, Johannesburg 2196,
South Africa

Penguin Books Ltd., Registered Offices: 80 Strand, London WC2R 0RL, England

This book is an original publication of The Berkley Publishing Group.

Neither the publisher nor the author is engaged in rendering professional advice or services to the individual reader. The ideas, procedures, and suggestions contained in this book are not intended as a substitute for consulting with your physician. All matters regarding your health require medical supervision. Neither the author nor the publisher shall be liable or responsible for any loss or damage allegedly arising from any information or suggestion in this book.

First edition: March 2005

Library of Congress Cataloging-in-Publication Data

O'Connor, Richard, Ph.D.
    Undoing perpetual stress : the missing connection between depression, anxiety, and 21st century illness / by Richard O'Connor.
        p. cm.
    Includes bibliographical references and index.
    ISBN 0-425-19826-X (alk. paper)
    1. Stress management.   2. Stress (Psychology)   3. Anxiety.   4. Civilization, Modern—21st century—Health aspects.   I. Title.

RA785.O296 2005
155.9'042—dc22   2004057081

PRINTED IN THE UNITED STATES OF AMERICA

10   9   8   7   6   5   4   3   2   1

To my children and their generation, who I fear will need this even more than my generation.

Contents

Acknowledgments

I owe a very real debt to two very good friends and skilled therapists—Hope Payson and Helen Bray-Garretson—who read early versions of the manuscript and gave me valuable encouragement and direction. In fact, many of the ideas in this book were initially hatched during case discussions with them, and they deserve more credit than I can really give here. I also owe a great deal to Irwin Hoffman and Paul Lippmann, who, at different times in my life, helped me keep going through dark periods but did it in such a way that it stimulated my own search for answers.

My agent, Jim Levine, has become a friend, critic, and independent source of valuable ideas; not bad for one guy. Christine Zika, my editor at Berkley, has been very patient and helpful; once she finally saw the manuscript, her evident and sincere liking for the book has helped sustain me through the last dreary stages of cutting and polishing; and her editorial advice was good too. Sheila Moody, the copyeditor, did an outstanding job on a complicated book.

My biggest source of inspiration is my patients. You'll meet some of them in these pages, in disguised form. Their stories—and those of all my patients—are profoundly moving. It's not that I attract a rare breed, but that the process of therapy brings two people close in such a way that they can't help but be moved. Most of my patients these days suffer from depression; I find these people so courageous, so generous, so kind and loving that I truly wish they could see themselves through my eyes. Writing a book like this is an attempt.

Since the time of my first book and this one the Internet has arrived, making the unaffiliated author's life a lot simpler; so I would like to express my gratitude to PubMed and MedLine, the American Psychological Association's online database, Amazon, and the United Parcel Service.

I'm not a neurologist, nor even a biological scientist, so there may be some mistakes in the way I present the brain, nervous system, and stress response system. I've relied on some new giants in these fields—Robert Sapolsky, Allan Schore, Antonio Damasio, Joseph LeDoux, Bruce McEwen, Daniel Siegel, Jeffrey Schwartz—for the best information I could obtain. If there are errors they are mine alone, and I hope they are not fatal to the points I'm trying to establish here. I feel slightly more confident of my skills as a social scientist, but of course my ideas are based on or influenced by many—Philip Cushman, David Buss, Martin Seligman, Daniel Goleman, Mihalyi Csikszentmihalyi, Judith Herman, David Myers, Deborah Tannen—to name only the most prominent influences. I don't expect that all these individuals will agree with every idea of mine in relation to their work but I sincerely hope that I have understood their positions and treated them fairly. Finally, I should be most confident of my skills as a therapist, but here again I feel that I'm standing on the shoulders of giants: Irwin Hoffman, Marsha Linehan, Stephen Mitchell, Zindel Segal, Jeremy Safran, Barry Magid, James Mann, Jerome Frank, Paul Wachtel, Mark Epstein are some. I think I've stated their ideas clearly, but some of the conclusions I've drawn are, again, strictly my own.

My wife, Robin, has been my biggest cheerleader, source of support and structure, and skilled editor and wordsmith. She's been extremely patient as I spent long winter nights shut up in the study. In our earlier days together, when it was necessary, she literally kept me alive. What more can you say?

Introduction

THIS is a long book, and some parts of it are complex, but the major ideas are simple. Let me state them first, explain them a little, and then give the reader some orientation about how this book is organized.

There are two major ideas.

The first major idea is that our nervous systems are not built for the stresses of the twenty-first century. This is a result of exponential change in both the nature of the stresses we face and how we are trained (by parents, schools, mass media, popular culture) to face them. At the same time, there are powerful influences that keep telling us this is a wonderful world and we ought to be happy and healthy. The result is a conflict between how we really feel and how we think we should feel—which is another major stress. In an effort to cope, we develop what I call the Perpetual Stress Response—the fight-or-flight response stuck in the "on" position. We become caught in a vicious circle in which the effects of stress on our minds damage our bodies and brains in a measurable, physical way; and these physical changes further affect our minds—the way we think, feel, and relate—in an invisible, unconscious way. Physical and mental, observable and unconscious—these injuries reinforce each other, trapping us in a cycle from which there seems to be no escape. We feel the effects of perpetual stress in many different ways: as depression and anxiety; as physical symptoms; as motivations for addictions; as dysfunctional relationships; and as empty, unhappy lives.

The second major idea is that, just as our brains and nervous systems are vulnerable to the damage of stress, we have the power to heal that damage by making deliberate choices about how we live. The new neuroscience is showing that the brain is constantly changing in reaction to experience; thus, *we can literally rewire our own brains*. The brain—and the mind—are both much more subject to influence than we ever imagined, and that influence can hurt us or heal us. We can reverse the vicious circle that traps us, and create what I call an *adaptive spiral*—a progressive cycle in which the changes we make in how we think, feel, act, and treat ourselves all reinforce each other, making change easier, more effective, and more permanent. We can get the observable and the unconscious, the mind, brain, and body, all working together in synchrony, to help us recover from what ails us now and to protect us from future stress.

In order to get that adaptive spiral started, we have to do a number of things:

- Recognize the effects of the Perpetual Stress Response; develop mindful awareness of the factors at work in our lives that make us feel out of control, empty, and frightened—and the forces that make us pretend we're doing just fine.
- Stop blaming ourselves. No one can survive today without substantial emotional scars. It's not our fault if we're depressed or scared or ill or addicted. But it is our responsibility to do something about it.
- Recognize that most of our conventional responses to stress only make matters worse by playing into the circularity of our problems.
- Cultivate a *mindful* attitude toward ourselves, our stresses, and the world. Mindfulness means paying more attention yet at the same time being a little detached. It means watching and noticing what is happening without judging our experience, without our habitual thoughtless categorizing of things instantaneously so we can move on to the next thing. It means being open to subtlety. It means creativity.
- Identify our own defenses: the assumptive world we create to explain our experience, with all its distortions, blind spots, and excuses.
- Learn to experience our emotions more fully at the same time as we control their expression more deliberately.
- Build self-control and will power by developing greater awareness of how we make—and avoid making—decisions.
- Understand the nature of the stories we have about ourselves—how they predict and control our experience of the world—and learn how to rewrite those stories.
- Learn to appreciate real joy, which is much more plentiful than we think, as opposed to fake joy, the kind we think we should be having (and feel inadequate because we don't).

- *Practice* mindful living by taking time for ourselves, cultivating healthy relationships, taking care of our bodies, facing our fears, developing creativity.

Together, these activities rewire our brains in the same way that good psychotherapy—or good parenting—does. We can repair a disconnect in the prefrontal cortex, the home of the self in the brain, that's been damaged by trauma and stress. We can clear up the guilts, shames, inadequacies, and pains that have tortured us since childhood. We can develop a new self that is resilient, creative, competent, and hopeful, capable of taking what life throws at us and finding joy and peace within it.

That is an ambitious message—"develop a new self." But I know there are hundreds of self-help books on the shelves making similar claims. "How to stop worrying and start living." "Doing what works, doing what matters." "A practical guide to personal fulfillment." "Harnessing the infinite power of your mind." Let me say here why I can make these claims, and why you should, if not believe me, at least listen to me. First, I'm an experienced therapist. I'm not a media creation or a self-appointed guru; I've been working with people for twenty-five years, all kinds of people, all kinds of settings. Nor am I a head-in-the-clouds theorist with a lot of big words; whenever possible, I prefer common sense. Second, I was trained as a skeptic. Where I was educated, we learned to think critically, examine the evidence, not jump to conclusions, not argue beyond the facts. I've never been able to find a comprehensive theory of human behavior I can sign off on, although it certainly is tempting to wish for a prophet who can explain it all for us. So I look for the best, the wisest, the most proven, in a whole lot of theories, and keep trying to put it all together in a way that works—that is actually helpful to people. Third, I've been where you are. My first book, *Undoing Depression,* described my own struggle with depression, along with a different way of thinking about depression and a lot of practical advice. Many readers have commented that my openness made it easy to connect with me. I don't think that having struggled myself gives me much special status, but it does make me want to focus on what's practical and useful for the reader. In that book and this, I've taken what is known as the "practice wisdom" of my profession—the knowledge won from experience of what works with people, what gets them moving—and tried to put it into advice you can use, skills you can practice.

Since that book came out, I've continued to work with patients and continued to educate myself by reading and attending workshops, and some facts have been dawning on me. One is that depression is not the isolated disease I thought it was; it is intimately related to most other mental health disorders and many physical health problems, as well as addictions and so-called personality disorders. Another is that the line between mental illness and mental health is getting increasingly blurred, as so many people seek help for problems that are hard to pin a label on. A third is that everyone is burning out. The strain on our nervous systems of living in today's overstimulated world is too much for anyone to handle without a deliberate effort to counter it; our natural responses to stress—good for avoiding predators and healing from physical trauma—don't work so well when the stress is constant.

At the same time I've been learning the facts that support the message of hope that I promise here. We can learn new ways of reacting to stress that will be much more helpful and healthy, and will lead to a richer and more serene life. In learning these things we are actually changing the structure of our brains, reorganizing the circuits so that responses that seem awkward and forced at first begin to seem like second nature to us.

So those are the main ideas, and a little about why you should listen to me. Let's go on now to flesh out these ideas.

At first, this was going to be a modest book about the links between depression, anxiety, and some unexplained contemporary illnesses, but it wasn't long before I saw that my subject had grown far beyond those original aims. It's not just my patients, but almost everyone I know, who's in trouble now—unsure, worried, feeling cut off from life, uncertain how to parent or how to be in relationships with other adults, looking for something but not sure what. I think we're in uniquely troubled times, for several reasons:

- The *rate* of social change we're experiencing is unprecedented in history and has enormous impact, much of it negative, on our minds and bodies.
- Our parents and generations going back to the Industrial Revolution also experienced cataclysmic social change, and that has had cumulative impact, again most of it negative, on the way we were parented and how we parent today.
- The *direction* of social change has had a largely negative impact on our minds and our nervous systems—the breakdown of the family, the loss of

faith in institutions like government and the church, the development of a consumer culture, revolutions in health care and aging, our loss of contact with the natural world.

And all that change has led to where we are now, with grim and growing rates of depression, anxiety, psychosomatic illness, violence, and addictions— and for the lucky few without a formal diagnosis, still a lack of confidence, an inability to find love, a life without much meaning.

Not everyone will agree with my gloomy outlook. That's fine with me, and I secretly hope that I'm being overly pessimistic about our culture. But it's beside the point here because I don't have to prove that things are horrible in order to accomplish the main goal of this book, which is to help those who are affected by twenty-first-century stress. We can all certainly agree that life is difficult, even if it's not as bad as I believe, and that all of us can use some help in how to control our problems so that we can find joy and meaning in life.

Although I'm going to be talking a lot about the negative impact of change, there are unquestioned benefits as well. One of the greatest benefits of all the social and technological change we've been experiencing is that we are making tremendous strides in understanding how the brain works. This is thanks to new imaging systems like PET scans and MRI scans that allow researchers to see in detail what is happening in the brain in real time as we think, feel, solve problems, and make decisions. We are now able to combine new understanding of how the brain works with new knowledge from social science and psychotherapy in order to help ourselves deal with some of our most troubling personal problems. Since completing my first book, *Undoing Depression*, a few years ago, I've been thrilled to see that my basic hunch—that life events, including psychotherapy, have a discernible effect on the brain, its structure, chemistry, and network of connections—has been validated by new scientific data. But I've been dismayed to see how little effect that news has had on how we view ourselves. To me, this discovery is more revolutionary than finding life on Mars, because it disproves what science has been telling us about the nature of man for the past two hundred years. Still, the belief that we are powerless against forces like faulty brain chemistry, our genetic endowment, our unconscious minds, our miserable childhoods, has a deep grasp upon us.

Because if life affects the brain, we have the power to choose how we live; thus we have some control over our own brains, how they develop and grow. *If we want to be well, we have to* do *well.* And we have to *learn* how to do well, perhaps even unlearn much of what we've come to take for granted about ourselves and the world.

Let me give you a brief preview of what's to come in this book. The first three chapters are meant to help you understand more clearly why I think stress is so damaging to us in these times—where the Perpetual Stress Response comes from and how it affects us in brain, body, and mind. We'll review the social and cultural changes that have put us in this fix, and discuss the need for a new scientific model that recognizes the circularity of our problems to help us understand the effects of stress. We'll apply this model to organize some of the new discoveries about the interaction of the brain and our everyday experience, and we'll talk about the effects of stress on our emotional lives. Emotions like anxiety and anger, hopelessness and guilt, are our early-warning system about the impact of stress, but we're woefully inept about what these signals mean and what we should do in response.

Chapter 4 begins the second part of the book, what to do about perpetual stress. Here we discuss the role of emotions in our lives, especially the painful emotions of anger, fear, guilt, and shame. We'll talk about the essential paradox of emotions for humans at this time in history—to experience our emotions more deeply at the same time as we control their expression more effectively. Chapter 5 focuses on *mindfulness* as a core skill necessary to help us begin to escape the vicious circle of stress. Then we'll go on in Chapter 6 to talk about how stress distorts our perception of the world in various unnoticed ways, and learn how we can apply mindfulness skills to help us see things as they are. Chapter 7 looks at depression, anxiety, addictions, and personality disorders as manifestations of the Perpetual Stress Response, and discusses what that changed perspective means about recovery. Then in Chapter 8 we'll go on to explore how stress affects our thought processes; how our judgment and decision-making skills are directly impaired, and our consequent bad decisions just perpetuate the vicious circle that we're in. We'll learn how to put the two halves of the brain, the rational and the emotional, together so that we can repair the damage to our thinking skills. Chapter 9 focuses on the impact of perpetual stress on our bodies, resulting in our current epidemic of nonspecific illness, and what we need to do to reverse the process and get on an adaptive spiral of health. In Chapter 10 we'll look at relationships—our lovers, our families, our friends and careers and co-workers—and see how our impaired skills have created the obstacles that keep us from attaining intimacy and success.

The last chapter lays out a simple program for healing, with practical guidelines for how to stay out of future trouble. Be prepared for the fact that I'm go-ing to ask you to give an hour a day to your recovery. That may seem like a lot to ask of busy people—but if you will give it an honest try for two or three months you'll see the benefits and wonder how you ever got along without it—and you'll have more time for the other important things in your life. I have some specific recommendations—which, in themselves, are not hard to follow—that can result in great relief from our most troubling symptoms and a tremendous improvement in health and happiness. But as we all know, we are our own worst enemies, and we won't implement these changes without a lot of self-discipline. We'll discuss why it is that we keep getting in our own ways and what we can do (it is not difficult!) to learn the discipline we need to keep us on the adaptive spiral. It's not lack of will, but lack of skill, that keeps us stuck in the Perpetual Stress Response.

Part One

What's Wrong

1

The Big Picture

THANKS to the new tools that allow scientists to observe the brain as it works, we're in the midst of a revolution in mind-body medicine. Recent discoveries are opening up minds to reconsider old assumptions. Researchers are demonstrating that stress gets into our DNA. Childhood trauma programs us for autoimmune disease and other conditions once thought to be exclusively physical. Depression and anxiety make physical wounds heal more slowly. Social isolation is as great a mortality risk as smoking. Stress increases susceptibility to the common cold. Chronic stress results in atrophy of certain parts of the brain; big spaces appear on MRIs where there used to be brain tissue. Psychotherapy results in brain changes visible on PET scans. When placebos work, they do so by changing brain chemistry. The brains of London cabdrivers, whose knowledge of the city is legendary, are enlarged and enriched in the areas associated with navigation and spatial orientation. Serotonin levels in baboons vary with social status; the top baboon has the highest serotonin. If you take him out of his tribe, his serotonin drops and someone else's rises; if you restore him to the tribe and he's able to regain his status, his serotonin rises again. Stroke victims can be taught to literally reprogram their brains so that they can control limbs and speech with other parts of their brains that do not normally control those functions. Science is beginning to demonstrate how the forces of everyday life affect our brains and rewire our circuitry. There is fundamental new knowledge being discovered every day, which is teaching us a lot about the damage of stress and its relationship to emotional disorders. But it's also pointing the way to the optimistic news, about how our brains adapt to difficulties and grow and change with experience.

When I studied psychology in college, I was taught a basic truth: adults don't grow new brain cells; after we reach a relatively young age in childhood, neuron "die-off" begins, and it's physically impossible to replace the dead cells with new ones. In the last days of the twentieth century, that truth was proved false. Deep in the adult brain, in memory centers like the hippocampus, there are colonies of rapidly dividing cells—stem cells, which have the potential to replace any specialized cell in the brain. These new cells can migrate outward to areas like the higher cortex. Learning stimulates this cell division. Learning takes place by growing and enriching the connections between nerve cells. Practicing a task seals the connections between the new cells and the existing ones. *Experience changes the physical structure of the brain.* And if this is so, we have some ability to choose the kinds of experiences we will have, and some ability to affect the structures and connections of our own brains, both for good and for ill.

This news changes the paradigm for science and the nature of man that we've held for over 350 years—the idea that mind and body are separate and distinct, which in philosophy is known as Cartesian dualism (see "Descartes' Error, Skinner's Fumble" on page 499 in the endnotes). This assumption, and its opposite extreme, materialism, which held that there is no such thing as mind, have dominated science so completely that it's very difficult for us to stand back and get an unbiased perspective on the extent of their influence. One specific result: they've encouraged Western medicine to ignore the role of mental processes in health and disease, which is one reason why so many people are now interested in alternative medicine. Another result: they've contributed to the stigma of mental illness, because we've never understood that mental illnesses are "real." Now we are beginning to understand the interconnections between the mind and the physical world, which may lead us to wonderful new discoveries—perhaps just in time to save us from ourselves.

Because at the same time as there is so much new understanding of our brains and our emotional lives, there is also much to be concerned about. Depression is now ten times as prevalent as it was just a generation ago, and the average age of onset has gone from thirty to fifteen years old. Besides depression, another 17 percent of us suffer from debilitating anxiety. Ninety million Americans live with a chronic health problem, many of them still not understood by Western medicine. For 25 million, their condition is stressful enough to disrupt their lives and cause them persistent pain; a growing percentage of these are coping with stress-related illnesses like chronic fatigue syndrome, back pain, or autoimmune disease. Unknown numbers struggle with addictions to alcohol, street drugs, or prescription medicines. And "personality disorders"—narcissistic, borderline, and others—are increasingly popular diagnoses for people who can't seem to get out of their own way, and suffer greatly in the process. Although contemporary medicine and psychiatry have some powerful tools for us, their promise falls short: very few people make a complete recovery from any of these problems; instead, the quality of their life is permanently diminished.

Then there are those without a diagnosis: I can't estimate the number who feel their lives are out of control because they can't lose weight, they can't stop procrastinating, they can't get out of debt, they can't speak up for themselves—"soft addictions," bad habits that make them feel miserable and ashamed. There are still others who are like the living dead—numb to their own existence, busy working, buying, doing—feeling vaguely empty but compelled to continue, too busy even to sit and look at their lives. Their depression has grown on them so insidiously that it feels normal; they just believe life stinks, and there's nothing they can do about it. And finally there are the rest of us, who still have to find confidence, connection, love, who have to raise children without guidance in a crazy world, often watch our parents lose their minds if they live long enough, and wonder about the meaning and importance of our lives. Even for those of us supposedly without emotional problems, there is still the nagging fear that we're faking it, just making it up as we go along, and praying we don't stumble.

Freud had hoped that psychoanalysis would eventually be able to treat all mental illness, while what he referred to as "common human misery" would remain an inevitable and untreatable fact of life. As we begin a new century, scientists are recognizing that the line between psychopathology and ordinary suffering is not so distinct at all. With the exception of some rare conditions like schizophrenia and manic depression,[1] most "mental illness" is the result of stress acting on a vulnerable individual—the effect of a lifetime of common human misery. And despite all the new medications, which often provide real relief from some of the most distressing symptoms, people seek psychotherapy just as much as they ever did. They are finding that their symptoms are only half the story—they still seem to keep fighting the same battles over and over,

---

1 Even these "biologically based" mental illnesses seem to develop in response to stress. Most first episodes can be traced to a specific event. The individual may be so vulnerable that it takes only a little stress to push him or her over the threshold; but the stress is there and real.

often getting in their own way, rarely able to feel good. Although we can't hope to eliminate sorrow from life, most of us understand very well that a great deal of our suffering is caused by our own self-destructive habits.

While researching my last book on clinical depression, I was surprised to see how much overlap there is between depression and other states of distress. I probably should not have been so surprised to see the overlap between depression and anxiety—after all, most of the patients I've treated for depression have been worried and frightened by their condition. But I was a little shocked to find that more than half of patients with major depression also meet the formal diagnostic criteria for an anxiety disorder. My training as a therapist had taught me to classify patients according to their distress; and certainly the push toward medication in psychiatry has emphasized the necessity of classification. After all, the conventional wisdom until very recently has been that the pill that helps with anxiety is not so good for depression, and vice versa; the ideal patient should have one or the other, never both.

I was more surprised to see how many patients who are treated by their physicians for conditions that we generally consider to be physical in nature— chronic pain or illness—also suffer from anxiety or depression. I don't refer to people who have a debilitating illness like stroke or cancer and suffer an expectable episode of grief or worry in reaction to their disability. I mean people who have a vague or recalcitrant illness—chronic fatigue syndrome, chronic back pain, irritable bowel syndrome—these are what I call "nonspecific" illnesses.[2] No one understands their cause and no one knows how to treat them successfully. Modern medicine has gotten a lot better at understanding the

---

2 "Nonspecific" is the best term I can come up with to describe a range of illnesses that have three things in common: their causes are mysterious, they are resistant to treatment, and often they are of relatively recent discovery or attention. Chronic fatigue syndrome, fibromyalgia, irritable bowel syndrome, Epstein-Barr syndrome, multiple chemical sensitivity, silicone-associated rheumatic disease, sick building syndrome, multiple food allergies, chronic candidiasis, and Gulf War syndrome are among those that have only recently become the subject of medical attention. But bad backs and other chronic pain conditions, as well as ulcers, colitis, and other digestive problems, fit the picture and have been known since history began. In addition to being difficult to explain and to treat, these conditions are also often referred to as psychosomatic, in that they seem to be related to psychological stress. "Psychosomatic" is considered an offensive term by many of the sufferers of these conditions, who feel they are being told the disease is only imaginary, so I avoid it here; we'll discuss these illnesses in detail in Chapter 9.

mechanisms involved—for instance, how stomach ulcers are caused by a bacterial infection—but can't explain why some people get ulcers and others don't, when almost everyone has the guilty bacteria in their stomach. People who suffer from nonspecific illnesses almost inevitably have problems with depression or anxiety as well. Their emotional symptoms usually predate the physical symptoms, but often have never been treated. Since I've always worked in outpatient mental health settings, it's been unusual for me to receive a referral from an MD treating a patient with a nonspecific illness. Most doctors, unfortunately, are so conditioned to the stigma of mental illness that they don't like to suggest that their patients get psychological help. So I did not realize, for instance, that the vast majority of patients with depression first contact their physicians because of physical symptoms, pain, or sleep disturbance, or that anxiety/depression is one of the most common reasons why people visit their MDs.

Yet I had known all along that the patients I saw in my office were much more complicated than their diagnoses suggested. It's very rare for people in my business to see a patient with a circumscribed problem. Most of my patients seek me out for help with depression now, but all of them also have problems with anxiety, with their bodies, with relationships, with bad habits. Depression is not merely an illness; it doesn't select its victims for no reason. Most of my depressed patients also want to talk about loneliness, about their difficulties with relationships, about what constitutes success and happiness. These issues are not simply manifestations of depression; they are problems that we all share, and finding the right pill or correcting depressed thinking patterns doesn't make them go away.

Addictions too seem to be much more common than we realize. Alcohol has been with us since the earliest civilization. Coca, opium, marijuana, psychedelics, caffeine, and tobacco also go back a long way. There's a natural desire for us to use something to make us feel better when we're down or anxious, to numb pain, to give us a high for a while, a vacation for the mind. Now technology has added many new chemicals that create the same kinds of effects. It might be nice if we could use some of these things occasionally, purely for recreation. But most of them are highly addictive, in the sense that they create a physical dependence, an intense need for more, and an uncomfortable withdrawal reaction. And all of them can be psychologically addictive in the sense that we want more, and are apt to let that wanting impair our judgment: to choose to go on a mind trip for a while when we really need to be taking care of business. Despite all our education about the addictive power of drugs, and all our new approaches to treating addictions, the overall rate of addictions remains about the same as it has always been. The only change has been a trend away from the stimulating drugs like cocaine and speed to an increase in use of opiates—painkillers. Does this mean we have an increased need to escape, to insulate ourselves from life? I know a lot of fathers of my generation who vigorously defend their daily marijuana or alcohol use; they don't understand why their wives and children resent that they choose to be in an altered state rather than being genuinely present with the family. And there are what some call the "soft" addictions—overeating, overspending, web surfing, procrastinating—there is an effort to fill up a vague emptiness, a mild depression. But it just makes things worse, because the individual is only likely to feel out of control and ashamed, more empty still. There is an awful lot of self-destructive behavior out there.

There's another ugly fact your doctor probably hasn't told you: each of these conditions makes the others worse. If you're diagnosed with anxiety but also have physical problems, your chances of recovery nosedive. If you have a bad back and also have depression, doctors don't consider you a good candidate for back treatment. If you have a personality disorder, nobody wants to treat you at all. And if you have an addiction, everyone agrees that you can't get over your depression or other illnesses until you've brought your addiction "under control." In a way, this makes intuitive sense; if you're depressed you're less likely to have the kind of energy and dedication it takes to rehabilitate your back. If you're anxious and have physical symptoms you're likely to just worry more about your symptoms and not get to the bottom of your anxiety. If you have an addiction, it takes up too much space in your brain for much else to happen at all. But it also seems to be more than that: there is a synergy between illness, anxiety, addiction, and depression so that all are both cause and symptom of each other. Yet conventional medicine likes clean, uncomplicated diagnoses. You can be an apple, a pear, or a peach, but you can't be a hybrid. Unfortunately, most of us are hybrids, and that makes it almost impossible for us to recover by relying on the American medical system. Bottom line: instead of treating one symptom at a time, we have to change our approach so that we treat the whole person instead.

As we get to know more about how the brain functions, we learn that the old distinction between the mind and the body doesn't make sense anymore. We know, for instance, that stressful life events in childhood cause changes in the brain that appear to be related in adulthood to autoimmune diseases like lupus, to chronic pain conditions, and to not-yet-understood illnesses like fibromyalgia. New technology is demonstrating that the brain and the mind are intimately involved in many illnesses that we used to consider purely physical: diabetes, heart disease, chronic pain conditions. A whole new science, psychoneuroimmunology, has been developed in the past twenty years, to explore the connections between mind, body, and health. What we're learning gives us new hope that if we can generate for ourselves the right kinds of life experience we can affect not only the state of our mind but the state of our bodies as well; but first we have to understand what our minds are doing to our bodies.

We'd better move quickly, because each of the conditions I've been describing seems to be on the increase in Western society. According to the World Health Organization, depression is the second biggest public health problem in the world, just behind heart conditions but ahead of cancer, AIDS, and anything else you can name. Anxiety disorders are equally crippling, and the most severe, post-traumatic stress disorder, is increasingly common. No one keeps reliable data on the incidence of personality disorders, but consider just one, antisocial personality, in relation to the growth in the U.S. prison population (from 800,000 in 1985 to over 2 million in 2002; earning for us the distinction of matching Russia as the country with the highest rate of incarceration). Nonspecific illness is too new a concept for us to have reliable data on, but any doctor will tell you that patients with these illnesses are most troubling. Addiction is too politicized for us to have objective data, but ask any teen if we're winning the war on drugs.

Doing Well

My thesis is that all these problems—anxiety, depression, addiction, nonspecific illness, personality extremes, and much of the worry that besets all of us— are *all tips of the same iceberg,* all manifestations of our response to the stresses of contemporary life, all connected beneath the surface, all reinforcing and buttressing each other. Contemporary research shows that *you can't fully recover from any of these conditions by focusing on the symptoms. You have to change the way you live.* Scientists who have been investigating these problems separately have all been discovering the same essential truth—that merely attacking the symptoms of depression, anxiety, illness, or addiction just makes us feel more victimized by the disease. There is much more than a little bit of self-destructive behavior involved in all of them: behavior that we learned long ago in an effort to adapt to difficult circumstances, behavior that made sense then, behavior that has worked its way into our brains so that it is natural and unconscious, but still self-destructive. Lasting recovery requires a deliberate and thoughtful effort to change the way we have been living. *Being well requires that we do well; that we practice emotionally healthy behavior until it becomes natural.*

This may be hard news to some. It's natural to wish for easy solutions, for Santa to slide down the chimney or God in a machine to descend from the heavens and take our troubles away. Besides, we have a strong emotional desire to believe in simple causes, single causes. They are neat and clean. Our left brains have been working since we were three years old to find the relationships between events: *If A, then B.* Advertising depends on this wish of ours: *If you drink our beer, you'll have friends. If you take our pill, you won't be depressed.* Unfortunately we're a lot more complicated than that. Single causes imply simple solutions; solutions for the twenty-first century are going to take some work on our part.

These problems are all signals to us that we are out of sync with ourselves. Each is an example of a vicious circle in action. We respond to stress by doing what we know how to do; but those responses don't help the stress, they only make it worse. Depression actually creates failure and disappointment. Anxiety feeds on itself; by worrying, we find more things to worry about. Addiction creates a physical dependency (for alcohol and drugs) or a psychological dependency (on self-destructive habits); either can mean climbing the walls while we try to control ourselves. Nonspecific illness makes us avoid the activities that would lead to recovery. Personality disorders are vicious circles personified, looking for love in ways that guarantee rejection, for success in ways doomed to failure.

For decades, psychiatry and medicine have been flummoxed by people caught in vicious circles. Freudians saw us as "fixated" at some primitive point in development, doomed to pursue the same self-defeating strategy over and over, making others out to be the parents who neglected us, trying to get care by being sick, trying to get attention through self-destructive behavior, mad at the world but unable to express our anger directly. Behaviorists viewed us as controlled by our environment, shaped by reward-punishment contingencies like Pavlov's dogs. Psychiatry now has found another dehumanizing direction—to paint us as victims of our own brains, our distresses caused by inadequate serotonin levels or faulty circuitry that can only be repaired by finding the right pill or administering electroshock or applying magnets to the brain. The more I learn about the brain the more scared I get about this kind of tinkering; the brain is a very finely tuned instrument, which we don't understand very well yet, and all our current ways of intervening directly with it seem to me like trying to plant petunias with a bulldozer.

Vicious Circles

The Freudian, behavioral, and biochemical views of man are all materialistic, fundamentally degrading views of the human condition, ignoring our ability to change ourselves. We're not stuck in the past, and we don't have personalities that perversely cause us misery. Our brains, if they are out of whack, got that way through the circumstances of our lives, and circumstances can put them right again. What's going on right now in our everyday lives is making us miserable. Our problem is that we don't know how to respond any differently to stress. When we get upset, we can only do more of the same of what we've always done—and that just leads to more disappointment, pain, hopelessness. We try desperately to control our experience, but that desperation guarantees failure. We're caught in a vicious circle, and we simply don't know how to escape.

The essence of a vicious circle is that the problem creates conditions that tend to perpetuate the problem. If I have an infection, my immune system goes into effect to isolate and kill the pathogens—no vicious circle. If I am disappointed—say I get turned down for a promotion—my psychological defensive system goes into effect. I may "forget" the disappointment for a while, but later on talk out my hurt feelings with my wife, who will comfort and reassure me, then help me figure out what to do to get the promotion next time around—no vicious circle. But other defenses may not be so effective. I may rationalize, tell myself I'm really the best person for the promotion and my boss is a fool. This is likely to make me isolate myself from my boss, go over his head, look for another job, begin trashing him behind his back—all strategies that don't have me looking at why I didn't get the promotion. I don't learn from the experience, but my defenses just get more brittle. I may be beginning a vicious circle of isolation and rationalization that will leave me less worthy of promotion.

Current practice overemphasizes control of symptoms: take an antidepressant; learn self-hypnosis for anxiety; take a pill to overcome your addiction to alcohol; find a doctor to give you drugs to make you feel less pain or discomfort. *By focusing on symptoms like this, we play into the vicious circle of disease.* We waste our lives trying to control our experience, trying to avoid discomfort. We spend so much time and attention tending to ourselves that we forget that we are more than our symptoms. A *person* sits in the middle of the vicious circle, a unique individual who must be empowered to step forward and reclaim his or her life.

The Perpetual Stress Response

There is one immense vicious circle that affects all of us today, everyone who lives in contemporary culture and doesn't mindfully try to resist its effects:

- Because there is constant stress, largely unrecognized, we're caught in fight-or-flight mode, unable to turn it off. This has various nasty effects on various body and brain systems.
- Our minds try to deny both the reality and the effects of perpetual stress. But the effects keep building until they become impossible to ignore.
- Emotionally, we rely on psychological defenses to keep our subjective distress out of awareness. But all defenses distort reality to some extent. We become less able to look at our problems objectively.
- We blame ourselves, and get sick. Or we blame others, and get in trouble. Either way, we only add to our stress load.
- Because we keep trying to live in unreality, our understanding of reality becomes increasingly constricted, fragile, and out of touch. Again, we add to our stress load because it gets harder and harder for us to see things as they really are.

After enough time in the vicious circle, time spent in pain, anxiety, and frustration, we can lose hope that we can do anything to help ourselves, and we may adopt a new identity—a *victim,* cheated of what life has to offer, powerless to change (or else bitter, begrudging, out for ourselves, blaming everyone else). When this happens, we stop preparing for joy and only work to try to protect ourselves from misery. This new identity pervades our entire being, like a metastatic cancer. It affects not only how we feel, but what we see, how we think, how we act, how we love. And because it affects how we see, we become blind to the changes taking place in ourselves. Only rarely do we remember that at one time we were happy, confident, active.

Even if we're not ready for the victim role yet, the vicious circle of stress pervades our bodies right down to the cellular level. Overwhelmed by too many stress hormones in the system, our cells close down receptor sites to try to compensate; but that just makes the endocrine system pump out even more stress hormones. Continually bathed in neurotransmitters telling us there is constant danger, our immune systems, muscles, bones, guts, and hearts wear out. And our brains become rewired by stress, our neural circuitry restricted to firing along preconditioned pathways, so that we are literally unable to think of new solutions, unable to come up with creative responses.

For an overwhelming number of people today, the result is a state of permanent malfunction—dissatisfied, irritable, overwhelmed and hopeless, out of control, frightened, physically run down and in pain. For want of a better term, this is what I call the "Perpetual Stress Response." The many other labels for this state depend on how the victim perceives the condition or which healer the patient consults for it. Is it depression, anxiety, chronic fatigue? Is it a neurological, endocrine, mental, emotional, spiritual problem? My answer is yes— it's all of these, and more.

Eight out of ten of the most commonly used medications in the United States treat conditions directly related to stress: antidepressants, antianxiety medications and sleeping pills, medications for gastric problems and high blood pressure. We have all kinds of pills that address one or another manifestation of stress. But taking the pills too often is like taking painkillers so we can continue to play football with a broken leg. We need to pay attention to what our bodies and minds are telling us: back off, give ourselves time to heal, then learn how to protect ourselves from stress and how to cope with it effectively. If we don't, we take on the sick role, we think of ourselves as victims, and we keep searching fruitlessly for the next new pill or procedure that's magically supposed to heal us.

The new responses that we have to learn in order to cope effectively with stress will feel awkward and difficult at first, but we're rewiring our brains and bodies to learn new behavior, much like we do when learning to type or ride a bicycle. After some practice, we don't have to think, consciously, about where the keys are or how to maintain our balance; we've developed a neural network that does those things without our awareness.[3] We can do the same with new emotional, cognitive, and interpersonal skills. Gradually we can integrate ways of dealing with stress that actually relieve the problem rather than making it worse. As these new responses become part of ourselves we can set that adaptive spiral in motion. An *adaptive spiral* is the opposite of a vicious circle. An adaptive spiral can start when something good happens to us, and as a result we feel more confident about ourselves, which leads us to take a chance we might not otherwise have taken, which leads to another good event, and so on in a potentially endless upward spiral of mental and physical health. Instead of continuing only to perform more of the same responses to stress that have never worked before, we become open to new and creative solutions and experiences. Though these won't work all the time, they work often enough that we can sustain our optimism and flexibility. After a little time on the upward spiral we start to believe in ourselves again. *Little things lead to big changes.* Our bodies begin to relax from their state of hypervigilance. Our brains lay down new connections so that our more effective responses begin to feel natural. We become fluid, responsive, adaptable, instead of frozen into position. We experience relief from our perpetual stress. *Doing well comes to feel natural and rewarding.*

The good news is that psychology knows a great deal about principles for recovery that we can apply to getting on and staying on an adaptive spiral. Although vicious circles are tough to break, there is one very important and hopeful implication of circularity: we don't have to waste time looking for the "true" cause of our distress. When we think in terms of what scientists call *linear causality*—every phenomenon has one and only one true cause—we also assume that if we don't find that one true cause (the childhood trauma, the disturbed brain chemistry, the hidden viral infection) all our efforts are doomed to failure because we're only treating symptoms and not the "real" disease. But *circular causality* implies that we can start to change things anywhere and everywhere without worrying that our efforts are in vain. We can learn to manage our symptoms at the same time as we prioritize our lives, learn to live with emotions, de-stress our relationships, and take care of our

---

3 A study new in 2004 (Draganski et al., 2004) shows that learning to juggle results in changes in brain structure that are *visible to observers* (using high-tech brain-imaging techniques). The analogy to exercising a muscle is maybe more apt than we think.

bodies—all with confidence that our efforts will not only pay off but reinforce each other. Please look at the Browns' case (pages 61–65) to see how openness to circular causality can change our perspective.

A truly complete recovery from any of these conditions is likely to resound in every aspect of our lives. We will have to question our values and priorities, we'll have to accept our limitations, and we'll have to understand our own emotions. Then we must learn how to take care of ourselves and how to communicate with others. Finally, we must begin to see ourselves as centers of creativity, as active agents in creating our own lives, not merely passive victims. Through conscious self-direction we can recapture the ability to experience joy and meaning.

Twenty-First-Century Stress

We do not ride on the railroad; it rides on us.
—Henry David Thoreau

"STRESS" has become one of the most overworked words in English. Everyone complains about being stressed, but I think very few are truly aware of the nature of the stress people in developed economies face today. It may feel a little whiny to complain, when we are so much better off than the rest of the world, have so much more freedom and so many more options than people have had at any other time in history. But it's important to recognize that it is just because the world has changed so much (while our nervous systems haven't) that we're under stress. One meaning of stress is being subjected to conditions you weren't designed for, and that's exactly where we are today. From the point of view of stress, it doesn't matter that the changed conditions are supposed to be in our best interests; it's the change itself that we may have trouble adapting to.

It surprised me to learn that our conventional meaning of stress—too much to do, too much worry—wasn't part of the vocabulary fifty years ago. We owe it to Hans Selye, the father of all stress research, for taking an engineering concept and applying it to humans. Stress in general refers to force exerted on a system. When I try to run the coffeepot and microwave in my kitchen at the same time, I'm forcing the system to do more than it can handle. The wires are literally too weak for that much electricity, so they heat up within the walls; fortunately, I have circuit breakers that are designed to fail before the wires get so hot that I start a fire. Too much snow on the roof, too much speed for a car's tires on a slick road, too many passengers in an airplane—stress can lead to catastrophic system failure. But houses, tires, and planes are designed to withstand expectable stresses, so catastrophes are thankfully rare.

Animals—including humans—have highly developed responses to stress. Two systems—nervous and endocrine—are involved in our first reactions, and they activate the rest of our body's responses; muscular, circulatory, digestive, sensory, and reproductive systems all get involved. Imagine an impala being chased by a cheetah. The impala's nervous and endocrine systems send electrical and chemical signals throughout the body that increase heart rate, redirect energy to the muscular and sensory systems, shut down digestion and reproduction, send immune cells into storage depots, deploy steroids to help it heal from wounds. This is the fear, or stress, or fight-or-flight response; everything going on within the animal is designed to help it deal with danger more effectively. Once the impala is safe, systems return to normal. Heart rate slows, and the animal once again gets interested in things like food, sex, and comfort, items that were low priorities while danger loomed.

Now imagine a cruel experiment. Chain the impala and cheetah to the ground so that the antelope is just out of reach. It's in no danger, but it doesn't know that, and it can't escape from the danger it thinks it's in. Its stress response will continue without relief. Its brain and endocrine system will keep on pumping out the neurotransmitters and hormones associated with high arousal, which eventually will lead to all kinds of bad outcomes—exhaustion, cardiac strain, kidney stress, muscle fatigue, damage to the digestive and circulatory system. It won't be able to eat, so eventually it will starve. Its immune system will be impaired, so it will be more vulnerable to infection. It won't be interested in reproduction; a herd of impalas under chronic stress will have a dramatic decrease in birthrate. It may "learn helplessness," a condition in which animals exposed to one inescapable stress seem to adopt the attitude that it's pointless to try to avoid any danger at all.

Humanity in the twenty-first century is in the position of the chained impala. Our natural responses to stress are good for helping us escape from cheetahs, but not so helpful for dealing with stresses that are more chronic: traffic, difficult career choices, money troubles, family conflict. And our more advanced brains can make things worse for ourselves. "There is nothing either good or bad, but thinking makes it so," says Hamlet. While that may be a slight exaggeration, we can certainly increase our stress level by magnifying dangers, thinking pessimistically, ruminating over the past, and all the other fiendish tricks our magnificent brain can play on us when its power is turned in the wrong direction. We can create imaginary cheetahs behind every rock, which can turn out to be as deadly in the long run as the real thing. Many of us de-

velop "automatic negative thoughts" that accompany the stress response—
Everybody is watching me. I can't handle this. I'm going to faint. I'm such a loser.
These mental habits can make the stress response last longer and make it much
more punishing than it needs to be.

We have to live with the fact that our nervous systems have not changed
much for 160,000 years, since the first modern human appeared. We're not
wired for the kinds of stress we face today. There is an essential conflict between what our bodies and brains were naturally designed for and what life
makes us put up with now—the breakdown of the family and community; the
lack of meaningful work, of contact with nature, of natural sleep, physical intimacy, exercise; the intrusion of ambiguous dangers like traffic jams, cell
phones, mortgages, commercials, HMOs. We can't run fast to escape these
problems, or call on friends and pick up big sticks to beat them to death—but
that's what our bodies were designed for. Under chronic stress, our neurotransmitters, hormones, and other "information substances"—basic constituents of
our animal selves—go haywire, affecting our immune, nervous, and endocrine
systems and causing emotional distress and physical illness—like the trapped
impala. We develop that Perpetual Stress Response. Bruce McEwen, a leading
stress researcher, calls it "allostatic load," but I'll stick with my term.

Whenever we face stress there are both physical and mental responses,
which interact with each other. The interactions can make things worse.
Chronic stress acts on the body to put us in a constant state of arousal, which
restricts our perception and thoughts, interferes with concentration and decision making, and makes us feel afraid. In the mind, we add content to those
fears based on our memories of similar experiences. We also create explanations for our fears, which may or may not be accurate representations of reality
and may or may not be helpful in addressing the immediate problem. When
we've crossed over into depression, anxiety, addiction, or illness, those explanations by definition have become part of the problem.

Stress is not a bad thing in itself. We need challenge. We feel our best when
the activities we're engaged in require us to stretch our abilities. Both physical
and mental exercise are good for us. It's constant stress that wears us down,
problems that can't be resolved by quick action. With longer life spans, higher
expectations, and more decisions to make, the kinds of pressure we experience
today seem perfectly designed to keep us in a constant state of stress. But from
an evolutionary perspective, the damaging effects of long-term stress make
sense. Mother Nature is only interested in keeping us alive long enough to re-

produce and pass along our genetic material. So now that our life span is pushing eighty-five, it might seem that our stress response systems have evolved in a very shortsighted way. But 100,000 years ago, when a human was lucky to live to thirty, it didn't matter that there might be long-term negative consequences built into our stress response system. Be alert for the big predators, and don't worry about ulcers or cardiovascular disease.

Overwhelmed and Demoralized: The Postmodern Condition

Here is where I leave trying to explain physiology and turn to something I know about—life as it's lived today in the USA. I get to hear all about it from my patients, a wonderful cross-section—aging Yankees, rising Yuppies, farm and factory workers, teens and seniors. They're not even all from the East Coast, because I do some telephone therapy, too. The issues discussed here match what I hear them telling me about in their own lives.

Most people are living with, I think, a fear of fear. There is a sense that something is fundamentally wrong with the way we are living our lives, but a reluctance to look closely at that. We *know* deeply that we're in serious trouble, but we live our daily lives as if everything is fine, whistling past the graveyard. We try to purchase inner peace, knowing perfectly well that's impossible, but not seeing an alternative. Or we tell ourselves that someone will figure out what's wrong someday, and until then we'll just have to wait. Or we'll simplify our lives later. Or we may believe for a while in the latest fad—a political leader, a spiritual leader, a self-help guru. We try to follow what the fad tells us, but it usually doesn't do much for our troubles, so we give up and try to forget again.

I think our sense that something is wrong comes from two losses that seem to be an inevitable fact of contemporary life. One is our loss of a sense of meaning and purpose in our lives, which used to be sustained by a connectedness with each other, with other generations, with a community in which we felt a part, with a belief in a God that gave our lives a purpose even if we could not understand the purpose ourselves. The other is our loss of a sense of being in a relationship with the natural world, the feeling that humanity is just one thread of the fabric of life, a part of a constant flow of birth—fruition—death—rebirth. It's not that we have lost Eden and need to recapture it; our lives in former times were much more difficult. But the sense of connection with each other,

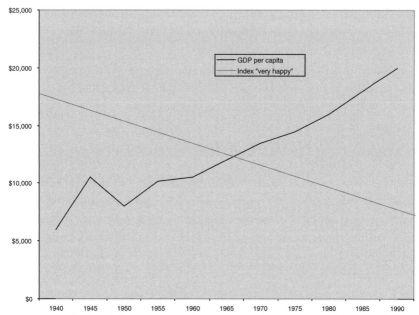

Percentage of Americans who rate themselves "very happy," compared to growth in gross domestic product, 1940–1990. (SOURCE: LANE, 2000.)

Figure 1

with God, and with nature gave us some insulation from stress—it protected our brains and nervous systems and gave them the opportunity and resources to regroup and recover.

I'm not the only one who's saying these things. Psychologists and psychiatrists are worried about the continuing increase in depression and anxiety disorders. Some philosophers are calling this the "age of depression." Social scientists who study what is called "subjective well-being" have noticed how it seems to begin to decline in each country as it becomes Westernized. Robert E. Lane's massive *Loss of Happiness in Market Democracies* lays out a chilling case for growing anomie, alienation, and loss of satisfaction as economic conditions improve. Look at his graph (Figure 1) comparing the growth in U.S. gross domestic product with the associated decline in numbers of Americans who say they are "very happy" over the last fifty years. There is a vast and growing body of literature out there now trying to explain these trends. I've read enough of this to know something about the major ideas, but I'm going to base my discussion here largely on my clinical experience, because I think it puts these trends in a much more human light.

Loss of Meaning

When I refer to a loss of meaning and purpose in our lives, I am talking about the results of immense social change over the last two centuries. This has led to, among other things, the treatment of the individual worker as a commodity to be used up, and the concomitant disjointing of the individual from his or her daily activities—so, except for a few specialized careers, what we make or what we do gives us little sense of pride, accomplishment, or contribution. Social change has contributed to the breakup of the family as an institution, so that we think it's perfectly acceptable for the new young couple to move across country, away from extended family, in pursuit of "opportunity"—meaning the chance to make more money. Housing patterns have contributed to the loss of sense of community; the ideal of the "single-family home" has isolated and estranged us from neighbors. Parenting, at least in the United States, has broken down; the one thing most parents know is that they don't want to raise their kids the way *they* were raised. But without a knowledge base they are extremely insecure about how to parent their children—or else too busy, preoccupied, or estranged. There is no reference to the past, to the old way of doing things, that once gave people a sense of safety and identity. Now our identity comes from mass culture.

One of the worst aspects of the problem is that we are being trained to doubt our own experience and common sense, which automatically puts us in a state of anxiety. I am referring to the disparity between how we imagine our lives should be and how we actually experience them. Much of this disparity comes from stereotypes of culture as portrayed in mass media. Unfortunately, this doesn't apply only to entertainment media, which everyone knows is distorted, but supposedly objective media like the network news and even respected outlets like the *New York Times* and NPR. All tend to focus on the scandal of the hour—and then, in an apparent effort to counterbalance the negative news, they relay stories that portray how well our society is working fundamentally. There is no thoughtful discussion that things might be gravely wrong.

For instance, the image portrayed of the economic growth of the 1990s was that everyone in America was benefiting from the expanding economy, when in fact only the wealthiest were seeing any growth in real income. Virtually all income growth went to the richest fifth of the population, while real wages for the bottom three-fifths had stagnated or fallen. *In 1976, the richest 10 percent of Americans controlled 49 percent of all wealth; in 1999, they controlled 73 percent of the wealth*—not much left over for the rest of us. Now, after a recession, we're told we're in recovery; but it can't create jobs, because all manufacturing is now done overseas. This is a recovery that benefits the wealthy exclusively, and creates only McJobs for the shrinking middle class. Just watch the news: every time unemployment increases, the stock market goes up; when unemployment decreases, and workers might be in a position to demand better wages and working conditions, the stock market goes down. It's not class warfare to point out that the interests of the workers and the interests of the shareholders are in conflict. Of course, the American dream has been to turn each worker into a shareholder, and many of us have our little retirement accounts with Vanguard or Magellan, but the growing disparity between the wealthy and the middle class has made a mockery of that dream. CEOs in the United States in 2004 were earning approximately 500 times what their average worker makes; in 1980 it was only 40 times.

Another example of the media's reinforcement of false positive stereotypes: although you will see the occasional horror story about managed care, the effects of the breakdown of the health-care system on the average person in terms of expense, inconvenience, and poorer health are not documented—the myth is still that America has the best health-care system in the world. In fact by most measures, our national health ranks seventeenth among developed countries, despite our spending $4,180 per person annually on health, compared to $2,172 in Belgium, the healthiest country.

One more quick example: most thinking Americans are aware that our national anti-drug policy has been a dismal failure, causing great damage to minority communities and making us all feel like hypocrites; but serious discussion of a sane drug policy is nowhere to be seen.

Experiences like these, where, like the Emperor's new clothes, the truth we perceive is not acknowledged, cause a disconnect between how we feel (confused and anxious) and how we think we should feel (happy and content). When this kind of disconnect happens to children, researchers now have enough evidence to show that it leads to mental health problems in adulthood. When it happens to us as adults, we may be so used to it—so distorted by all our previous experience—that we don't notice it; we discount our own perception of reality, even though the anxiety and confusion is still there under the surface, and it continues to be damaging.

Workplace Stress

If you sense that you're working too hard, you're not alone. See Figure 2. In the past twenty-five years, the average American workweek has increased from slightly over forty hours per week to slightly over fifty; and the amount of time we have left over for leisure has declined from over twenty-six hours per week to under twenty. People have to work much harder nowadays—a 25 percent increase in the workweek, and a corresponding 25 percent decrease in leisure time—to maintain the standard of living we expected twenty-five years ago. As of Labor Day 2003, Americans were working more hours than the workforce in any European country, and equal to the Japanese (where suicide of "salarymen" from overwork is a common phenomenon). Alan Greenspan and the Bureau of Labor Statistics don't like to talk about it very much, but the vaunted growth in American productivity is illusory. We're not more efficient, except at squeezing the employee. People are working longer hours, and usually not getting paid for it.

When the Soviet Union broke up, and workers were no longer guaranteed jobs for life, the average life expectancy for men dropped from sixty-four to fifty-nine years—a reversal never experienced in any country in peacetime. While it's doubtless true that most of this effect was due to the stress of sudden instability, disruption of the health-care system, and other factors, it is interesting to speculate about just how much wear and tear on health is inherent in a capitalist society where it's taken for granted that everyone competes for scarce resources and that your job could disappear tomorrow and there's not much you can do about it. In 2004 it was estimated that workplace stress costs the U.S. economy more than $300 billion each year.

Changes in working hours have made things exponentially worse for families. The two-career family is now the norm and the stay-at-home wife is the exception. Four out of ten Americans work largely at evenings, weekends, night shifts, or other nontraditional schedules. Our social institutions, like schools, are still stuck in *Leave It to Beaver*–land: schools still dismiss at 2:30 every day and take summers off, as if Mom is going to be there to supervise the kids; but Mom isn't. However, she gets to feel guilty about it.

In fact, we all get to feel more guilty now, because so much more seems expected of us; and that's a major cause of burnout. Americans take less vacation time than workers in any other industrialized nation—and they actually take less vacation time off than they earn, because they have been conditioned to believe that they owe their company something; or they fear that someone else will take their job while they're gone or that the boss will see that the organization gets along fine without them. Unemployment is so institutionalized by now that the workplace is full of fear. Employers have replaced as many salaried workers as they can with contract employees, or freelancers, who earn no vacation and no benefits.

Nowhere is the inherent insanity of our system more evident than in our breezy acceptance of debt. Despite the fact that people are afraid for their jobs, Americans have built up more indebtedness now than at any time in our history. In 1952, household indebtedness (mortgages, bank loans, etc.) was equal to 36 percent of after-tax income. That fraction has steadily grown to the point where, in 1997, indebtedness equaled 95 percent of income; households were spending 17 percent of their income for debt service (interest and principal).

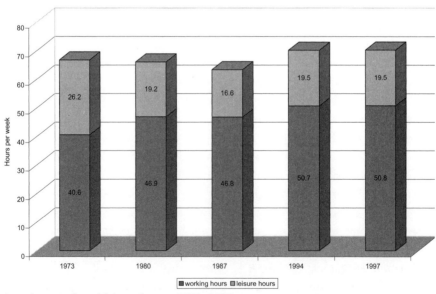

American work and leisure hours, 1973–1997. (SOURCE: GOOZNER, 1998)

Figure 2

Much of the increase is due to the easy availability of personal credit cards (though borrowing for college has also added to the problem as tuitions have skyrocketed). Many Americans feel they are managing their money well if they are merely making the minimum monthly payment on their charge cards. It seems to me that a capitalist couldn't ask for a better labor market: everyone in debt, deathly afraid of losing their jobs, willing to work longer and longer hours for less and less money, very little job protection—yet unable to mobilize against the unfairness of such a system because we have been so conditioned to believe it's the only way and we really can be happy after all if we only buy more. We're such perfect consumers that we're killing ourselves as producers.

Another reason why the work world is so insane is that, for the past twenty years or so, business schools have been teaching (*teaching!*) that management's only responsibility is to produce a profit for stockholders. This means that other priorities like keeping a skilled and happy labor force, reinvestment of capital in plants and equipment, and product quality, fall by the wayside. Stockholders have been spoiled by this trend; the stock market is seen as a way to get rich quick, instead of as a way for companies to raise capital. And management is scared because they know they'll be replaced by the stockholders if they don't show a profit at the end of every fiscal year; there's always someone out there who can figure out how to cut costs even more. It's this kind of pressure that led Enron and WorldCom management to start lying to their accountants and present a distorted picture to the public. We may have reforms now that will lead to greater scrutiny and less distortion, but as far as I know no one is questioning the ultimate wisdom of this business model.[1]

Splitting the Nuclear Family

Besides our extended working hours and two- and three-job families, we haven't even mentioned divorce. That *Leave It to Beaver* family, where it's the first and only marriage for both parents, Dad is the sole breadwinner, and

---

1 I'm not much of an economist, so I don't really know where I might be stepping on toes, and I am concerned that the reader will conclude that I think there is something inherently wrong with capitalism. Not so; but I believe there have to be checks on capitalism, and that our current laissez-faire attitude is inherently exploitative of the individual. As far as I'm concerned, Karl Polanyi proved in the 1940s that the unchecked market economy requires turning both people and natural resources into commodities, assuring the destruction of both society and the environment unless the economy is closely regulated (Polanyi, 2001).

Mom stays home to care for the children, is now down to about 5 percent of the total population. The divorce rate is currently about 49 percent. It seems to have leveled off at that point after rising for the last twenty years, but shows no sign of declining. Of children today, about 45 percent will go through a parental divorce. More than twice as many children of divorce compared to those from intact families will see a mental health professional during their lifetime. And the effects of divorce on the divorcing parents aren't that great either; though some tend to jump into divorce as impulsively as they jumped into marriage, they usually find that they're poorer, more stressed, and feel guiltier after the divorce. Despite these findings, divorce is increasingly accepted as normal. Mass culture plays a role here: in lab studies, both men and women who are bombarded with images of highly attractive members of the opposite sex report decreased commitment and love for their current partner. But what do we get each day from television, movies, and magazines? It certainly isn't a celebration of the way everyday people look.

Suburban living has its own deleterious effects on the family. Suburban sprawl leaves everyone dependent on automobile travel, adds to obesity and health problems, and leads to isolation. Look at Figure 3, which charts the trend in frequent visiting with neighbors over the past forty years. Parents don't have neighbors or grandparents to help them with parenting. It used to be that the whole community was involved in child rearing; now there is no community. The task falls solely on parents and professionals, who seem to be more and more at odds. If a neighbor takes it on herself to reprimand a child for misbehavior on the street, she fears a lawsuit. School administrators are being driven crazy by the need to protect against gender discrimination, bullying, violence, and the possibility of mass murder, at the same time that they are expected to show continuous improvement in standardized test scores, all without any budget increase. Parents and children alike are overwhelmed by mass culture, without a support system to reinforce any alternatives.

We can see how our children are suffering. We drop them off at day care, pick them up from the babysitter, and feel like we have almost no time for them. Their little lives have to be programmed with a Palm Pilot. Mom and Dad don't get to spend time *with* the kids; they spend all their free time on the phone arranging activities *for* the kids. Worst of all, children today grow up in a world of fear. In kindergarten they are taught about stranger danger; in fourth grade they are taught about the dangers of drugs; in junior high, the

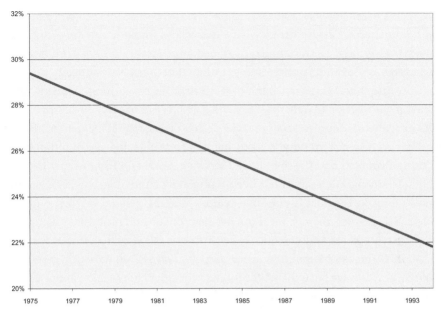

Percentage of Americans reporting frequent visiting with neighbors, 1975–1993.
(SOURCE: NATIONAL OPINION RESEARCH CENTER, CITED IN LANE, 2000.)

Figure 3

subject is AIDS. Have you noticed that you don't see children playing outside anymore? Increasingly, children are inside, in the air-conditioning, playing alone. Part of it is our paranoia about child abduction; most of it has to do with TV and video games as the electronic babysitter. But on television, politicians disgrace themselves, sports heroes become murderers, and no one takes responsibility. No one is to be trusted. And Mom and Dad aren't home to comfort their confused and frightened children.

At my office, and in the schools and day-care centers, we see the effect on kids. Something's going haywire with them. A third of the boys are on Ritalin, a third of the girls on Prozac. Kids go to school literally unable to sit still and attend; their brains aren't wired up correctly. Television is partly to blame: according to the American Academy of Pediatrics, each hour per day of television watching increases a child's risk of ADHD by 9 percent. These disaffected and disconnected kids are especially vulnerable to drugs. The Department of Health and Human Services estimates that there are about 2.6 million new marijuana users per year, the vast majority of them teens; and 25 percent of all high school students got drunk in the two weeks immediately preceding the DHHS survey. The DARE antidrug education program doesn't work, according to the GAO, but it continues to get funded because it's politically popular and because it gives us the feeling that we're doing something. Affluent teens have higher rates of anxiety disorder and substance abuse than inner-city kids. The incidence of depression among children is on the rise: 10 percent of all kids will have a major depressive episode before age twelve; the age of initial onset is getting younger and the severity of the first episode is getting worse. The suicide rate among adolescents has been rising at a frightening pace, and no one knows why. In the past twenty-five years, while the general incidence of suicide has decreased, the rate for those between fifteen and nineteen has quadrupled. Sixty percent of adolescents know someone who has made an attempt.

As if all this isn't enough to cause perpetual stress, we have our parents to take care of, and we have the whole industry of elder care to learn about. I hope that I will lead a healthy and independent life until I'm about eighty, at which point I will die suddenly and painlessly, preferably while water-skiing. Everyone hopes for an end like that. But you know that kind of death is for the lucky few. Advances in medicine have given us longer, but not more meaningful, lives. Seniors have to worry about spending their last years in nursing homes, using up what savings they'd hoped to leave for the kids, living with strangers, being treated like babies, and losing their minds. My skin crawls when I go into some of these places, and we have some very nice ones in my part of New England. Most of the residents are on antidepressants, and no wonder: they've been forgotten about and they have nothing to look forward to. It's different in other societies where seniors are revered for their wisdom and perspective, where it's a family's duty to take care of grandparents. It's very hard on the younger generation emotionally and physically to have our roles reversed, to see our parents reduced to dependency, pain, depression, and incompetence—and to foresee the same future for ourselves. Yet our culture tells us this is the way we do things now.

The Hedonic Treadmill
We're being trained to believe that consumerism is the path to happiness, but in fact it only adds to stress. It seems like the brass ring is always a little out of reach. Last year's luxury becomes this year's necessity. Last year you couldn't afford a flat-screen TV; this year you can't get by without it. If you ask Ameri-

cans what it takes to have a comfortable income, they always say it's just a little more than whatever they have right now (see Figure 4). And when we work harder and start making that much more, of course it's no longer enough. No wonder we always feel stressed out and inadequate; we never make enough money to afford what we tell ourselves we need.

This is partly due to a phenomenon called the "Hedonic Treadmill." Studies of human response to positive and negative events have shown that we are highly adaptable. When our living conditions change, we get used to it pretty quickly, and return to near our individual baseline of happiness. This has its good side—it helps us get through difficult experiences like concentration camps, disability, and grief. But we also return to baseline pretty quickly after good things happen to us, too—*which means we always want more.* That raise that we wanted, that we thought would make the difference between feeling poor and feeling rich?—guess what, we got it, and we still don't feel rich. The Hedonic Treadmill was first described in a famous article entitled "Lottery

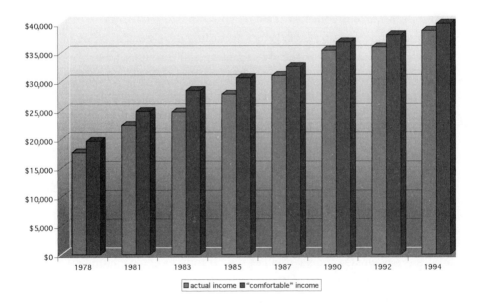

Chasing comfort: Actual versus perceived "comfortable" income for a family of four.
(SOURCE: SCHOR, 1998.)

Figure 4

Winners and Accident Victims: Is Happiness Relative?" The authors studied both groups in the title, and found that lottery winners, as a rule, were only a little happier a year after their winnings, while disabled accident victims were only a little unhappier—the change in either group was much less than the variation you routinely observe between one individual and another. Later research has tended to confirm these findings. What we once found thrilling we now take for granted—exotic foods, illicit drugs, attractive sex partners. The more you get, the more you want. Worse yet, *the pain of losing outweighs the joy of acquiring;* some studies suggest that losses have more than twice the impact of equivalent gains. You love your new BMW at first, then you take it for granted. But if you lose your job and have to sell the Beemer, you'll *really* miss it. Losing it will make you feel like a bigger failure than getting it made you feel a success. The Hedonic Treadmill suggests that we are not only voracious consumers of the new and improved, but also very jealous and protective of our prizes, even though they don't bring us much happiness.

Barry Schwartz gives another example. I give you a choice between a sure $100 right now, or a coin toss: Heads, you win $200; tails, you win nothing. Most people take the sure $100. Why? According to Schwartz, the joy of getting $200 isn't twice as great as the joy of getting $100. To tempt most people, I'd have to offer the chance to win about $240. But reverse the conditions: I'm going to take away from you $100 right now, or you can have a coin toss in which I'll take away either $200, or nothing. Under this condition, most people opt for the coin toss. Why the discrepancy? Losing the first $100 hurts more than losing the second $100. And losing the first $100 produces negative feelings that are more intense than the positive feelings produced by a gain of $100. So taking a chance to lose nothing seems like a good bet to us; but taking a chance when you might win nothing doesn't seem like a smart choice.

The Tyranny of Choice

Then there is what some have called the tyranny of choice. Humans seem to have been designed to live in an extended family group, perhaps a small village of two hundred or so in the savannas of Africa or rural China or medieval Europe. Under those circumstances, life was in many respects predictable and foreordained. We knew almost everyone we were likely to ever meet, and the occasional traveler was a big deal. We knew what we were going to be when we grew up, because we were going to be whatever our father or mother was.

Exercise 1. **Needs and Wants**

These are simply questions designed to get you thinking:

- Think about yesterday. Try to remember three things that made you feel good. Did any of them involve material goods? Watching television?
- Think back over the past year. What were your major purchases? How much joy are they bringing you? How many do you regret now?
- Try to think of two or three occasions in the past year when you felt very happy or content. Did any of these involve purchases? Money? Work?
- Did you take a vacation last year? How long?
- How do you know if you're relaxing? How do you know if you're enjoying yourself?
- Who's the happiest person (adult) you know? What's their secret?
- Are you optimistic about the way the country's going?
- Are you drinking more alcohol than you feel right about?
- How many hours are you working? How many hours do you have for reading, hobbies, exercise, socializing?
- What's your workplace atmosphere like? Are people there friendly and supportive?
- Does what you do for a living make a contribution to people's lives?
- How much time do you spend with your significant other, just talking?
- How much debt are you carrying? Over the past few years, has it increased or decreased?
- Has your take-home pay increased, stayed flat, or declined relative to inflation?
- Have your benefits (health insurance, sick time, vacation pay, comp time) increased or diminished over the past five years?
- How much time of your day goes into television? The research suggests that heavy viewers (four or more hours per day) actually enjoy their TV watching *less* than light viewers (under two hours per day).
- Are you concerned about changing values in American life—e.g., more vulgarity, less respect for others, deeper political divisions?
- How many pills are you taking regularly?

(Continued)

- Compared to ten years ago, how's your medical care?
- Do you think you and your contemporaries are happier than your grandparents when they were your age?
- Do you think your children will have less, more, or the same amount of stress in their lives as you do?

We were pretty sure about whom we'd marry, because there were only two or three choices. We went to bed when it was dark and got up when it was light. We lived in harmony with the cycles of the seasons. I don't mean to paint an overly idyllic picture; our world is safer and much more interesting now. Within limits, we can go where we want, do what we want, within a much wider range of choices than was available to our grandparents, let alone our medieval ancestors. But sometimes it's good to have things taken care of for us. There are an awful lot of single young women out there who didn't get married in their early twenties and are now desperate, depressed, and blaming themselves. There are a lot of young people flipping burgers because the factory where their fathers worked has closed up and moved to Mexico. And sometimes the range of choices itself can seem like a burden. Do we really need to have seventy-two varieties of yogurt available at the grocery? In the last thirty years, the varieties of Pop-Tarts available have increased from 3 to 29, Frito-Lay chips from 10 to 78, running shoe styles from 5 to 285. Does all this make us feel like Masters of the Universe? I know a woman, severely depressed, who managed every morning to get herself up, bathed, and breakfasted on autopilot; but she would routinely burst into tears when she looked into her closet and tried to figure out what to wear. Her first decision of the day was overwhelming. I think her situation is a microcosm for how many of us feel.

It takes a lot of advertising to teach us what kind of running shoes to buy. But advertising has been a potent force in society only for the past hundred years. Advertising is meant to convince us to purchase goods and services that we don't need, because we're going to buy the necessities anyway. Since its beginning the industry has realized that the most effective way to disguise this problem is to associate their products with desirable personal qualities—beauty, financial success, social acceptance, status, good taste, personal satisfaction. Of necessity these are low-end values. You can't sell a product that promises wisdom, generosity, or the ability to be a good citizen[2]—advertising is meant to appeal to our insecurities and vanities, our doubts about ourselves, our basest values. And since we are bombarded with it day and night, we are continually debased. Philip Cushman writes:

> Consumers "know," without being told or convinced, that they are not adequate as they are. They appear to be fully aware that they are inadequate, unattractive, incompetent, or inconsequential and must be transformed into different people in order to be happy, loved, and fulfilled.

Perhaps the greatest triumph of advertising has been selling clothing by printing the logo of the designer prominently on the article—so prominently that often this is the only distinctive feature of the clothing: Nike, Reebok, Polo, Louis Vuitton, Donna Karan.[3] As if wearing a shirt with a designer's name means you belong to something, a club of people with good taste. In fact it does the opposite, advertising to the world your insecurity and gullibility. But we have come to believe in personality, rather than character—personality being something we can build by learning charm and wearing the right clothes. Celebrities embody personality. Celebrities are famous not for anything they've accomplished, rather just for being who they are (or are portrayed to be). Celebrities appear to embody the qualities we want—self-confidence, popularity, beauty. If we mimic their outward appearance, we can be like them, confident and popular. We don't stop to think that confidence is acquired through learning how to do things, that friendship is won by listening and caring.

---

2 Occasionally advertisers try to sell products based on more transcendent values, but their efforts usually look ludicrous. A commercial for Land Rover a few years ago showed an early-middle-aged couple using their $65,000 SUV to rescue a dog lost on a busy highway on a rainy night. The screen fades to black with the single word "Courage" illuminated. We hope that people who are smart enough to have $65,000 available for a car are smart enough to laugh at this message—but if they're that smart, would they spend it on a car?

3 Evidence for the universal appeal of irony: the garbagemen in New York have taken to wearing T-shirts with "DSNY" (Department of Sanitation New York) looking exactly like the familiar DKNY logo.

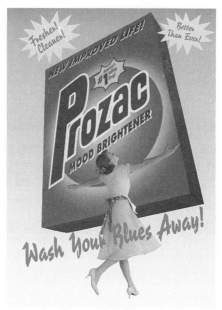

SOURCE: ADBUSTERS MEDIA FOUNDATION

Advertising and the media try to provide us with pseudo-intimacy, a sense of belonging to something that is inherently shallow. Sports fandom is one great example. While there is some truth in the perception that males have a hard time talking to each other and that talking sports gives them something they can connect around, television portrays it as something much more than it is. As if being a fan brings you into a special community, a world where athletes, commentators, cheerleaders, and fans are all part of one glorious club. Beer commercials do the same. In beer commercials there are always groups of Good Friends (healthy, attractive, and thin) sharing stories, laughing at each other's jokes, obviously having a Good Time. If we buy that brand we can join in. Mass culture in general, television in particular, and commercials above all, give us the idea that life should be easy. The unspoken corollary is that if it's not, it's our fault. My grandparents, and I'll bet yours, knew that life wasn't supposed to be easy. My grandfathers worked in factories and considered themselves lucky to have jobs that provided for their families. My grandmothers worked from dawn to dusk. They knew how to enjoy themselves, but they didn't *expect* to be enjoying themselves all the time; they didn't feel like there was something wrong with them if they weren't grabbing for the gusto every second.

The latest wrinkle is the advertising of prescription drugs. This DTC (direct-to-consumer) advertising has only flourished in the last ten years (and is still prohibited in the European Union). In 2000 alone, $2.5 billion (twice as much as our proposed new venture to the moon) was spent on DTC advertising—at the same time as drug costs were soaring and taking drug companies' profits up along with them. You can't watch the nightly news without being bombarded with commercials promising to cure your athlete's foot, depression, yeast infection, constipation, and whatever it is that "today's purple pill" is supposed to do.[4] You can't read a newsmagazine without finding ten-page "advertorials" (in the exact format and typeface of the legitimate news pages) promoting the same medicines, and more. I was astounded to see an electronic display, at the Hartford mall in the middle of Christmas season, promoting Effexor. Perhaps Wyeth, Effexor's manufacturer, recognizes that buying and consuming really doesn't cure depression.[5] On the other hand, a competing antidepressant, Celexa, is being touted as an effective treatment for what is called "compulsive shopping disorder." I guess we need both.

Imagine if drug manufacturers tried to sell you a new prescription with the slogan "Take this medicine; it's better than nothing." It seems like a weak premise to get you to put some unfamiliar chemical into your system. Yet that is all that manufacturers have to demonstrate in order to get FDA approval for a new drug—that it outperforms a sugar pill, and sometimes not by very much, as became public in the case of the newer antidepressants. The pill doesn't have

---

4 Actually, "today's purple pill," Nexium, addresses exactly the same thing that yesterday's purple pill, Prilosec, did—stomach acid reflux. But because Prilosec's patent ran out and generic equivalents became available, the manufacturer, AstraZeneca, tweaked the formula a little and is trying to convince everyone now that Nexium is a great improvement. Eli Lilly tried the same strategy with Prozac, changing the name to SeraFem and promoting it for use in PMS. But apparently female consumers were offended by the commercial that had a woman with PMS running other shoppers down with her shopping cart, and the campaign was pulled.

5 On its website Wyeth asks, "Are these symptoms of depression interfering with your life?: Not involved with family and friends the way you used to be? Low on energy? Not motivated to do the things you once looked forward to doing? Not feeling as good as you used to?"

Of course these "symptoms" are so vague they are likely to fit anyone who has bothered to look up the website; and so mild that they fit half the population. There is no mention of suicidality, the terrible guilt and shame that accompanies depression, the fear that you're growing crazy. They don't want to scare anyone into thinking that depression is a serious disease.

to show that it's as effective as getting more exercise, meditating, changing your diet, or reducing your stress level. It's a very low standard, yet we go on popping pills, often before we try any other alternative.

The effect of all this DTC advertising is to put doctors in the position of having to explain to patients why a different medication, or a generic equivalent, might be preferable or why the patient doesn't need a medication at all. Often they don't argue, and just give the customer what he or she wants. The power of the American pharmaceutical industry is difficult to overstate. It reaches into the FDA, which published a report in 2003 distorting its own research to suggest that doctors agreed that DTC advertising resulted in health benefits to patients when, in fact, they didn't. It's no coincidence that depression has become big news only after there was money to be made from it. The older generation of antidepressants had gone generic; when Prozac and its cousins came along, the drug companies spent billions "educating the public" about depression. This wasn't all bad, by any means; I'm glad awareness of the reality of depression has increased. But the myth has been sold that, if you take the right pill, you'll be just fine, and that's not so. Recovery from depression, or any emotional problem, takes skilled treatment and hard work; but nobody will say so.

Feeling good has become an end in itself, perhaps the only worthwhile goal. We've lost sight of the fact that feeling good is a by-product of how we live. Self-esteem is not an attribute we can gain by parroting catchphrases, wearing the right clothes, even by climbing the corporate ladder, but an accomplishment we earn by working hard and making difficult choices. Feeling good is not a right, but an achievement. My own profession has contributed to these misconceptions by suggesting that, if you don't feel good, it's because you're sick, and we can cure you. There are, in fact, plenty of people who should feel good but don't, or can't, and it's good that we can help them. But there are many more people who are trying to feel good without facing the fact that life is hard work, that we're constantly faced with difficult decisions, that we're responsible for how we treat others.

When we had a more cohesive society, it may have been easier to feel good because the rules were clear. Philip Cushman observes that a fundamental change of focus in our culture has come about because a sense of well-being has become our only goal, rather than a by-product of pursuing a superior common goal. "Individuals ceased to be thought of as public citizens whose behavior was evaluated according to an external moral standard; instead citizens began to be thought of as individual patients whose behavior was an uncontrollable manifestation of medical illness." In other words, we used to feel good or bad about ourselves because we were comparing ourselves to the standards of our society; now we see feeling bad about ourselves as a disease, feeling good as a fundamental right. In the old days, if we felt bad we changed our behavior; now if we feel bad we take a pill. There were of course dangers and disadvantages inherent in evaluating ourselves by social standards, but it was a system that had generally served humanity well enough for all of recorded history. Now we're in completely uncharted territory.

No More Heroes
It seems that our most trusted social institutions are breaking down right and left. Public education doesn't work anymore; we need school vouchers to give parents the freedom to move their children to private schools. American business practices have been shown to be a disgrace; what companies tell their shareholders, what brokers tell their customers, has been exposed as routinely fraudulent. Most politicians base their campaigns on reducing the role of government in our lives, as if we take it for granted that government is an evil that has to be curbed (and apparently we do; see Figure 6 for the trend in percentage of Americans who say they trust the government). And nothing is worse than what's happened to the Catholic Church, when those who were once revered have been unmasked as abusers.

We can't even trust our doctors any longer. American medicine has become so corrupted by the marketplace that our physicians and hospitals have to balance taking good care of us with pleasing the managed care companies. Pharmaceutical manufacturers reap unconscionable profits while promoting a drug culture and manipulating our physicians' prescribing habits. Doctors are paid, and earn continuing education credits, for attending industry-sponsored promotions of their drugs that are held at flashy events and venues like Yankees games and yacht cruises. We're still constantly told we have the best health care in the world, yet we all know people who have experienced medical errors and neglect that have seriously compromised their health. And what about the—at last count—43.6 million uninsured? These contradictions set up a cognitive dissonance: *If things are so good, why am I so worried?* Far too many people then jump to the self-blaming conclusion: *There must be something wrong with me for feeling the way I do.*

My profession, psychotherapy, has been a big part of the problem. Problems in living, problems we have developed because we are lonely or scared or our life lacks meaning, have been medicalized—turned into illnesses that, suppos-

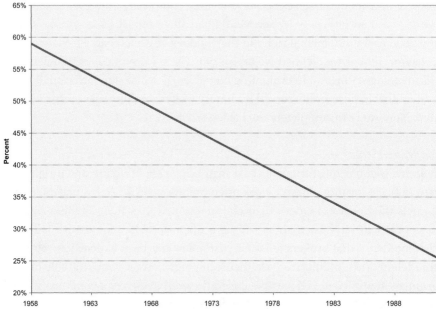

Percentage of Americans who say they trust the government "most of the time."
(SOURCE: NATIONAL OPINION RESEARCH CENTER, CITED IN LANE, 2000.)

Figure 6

edly, we can cure through therapy or with a pill. There's a lot of money to be made by medicalizing a problem. Say you come to me because you're mildly depressed after being passed over for a promotion at work and a string of bad luck trying to find a girlfriend. I can't collect from your insurance company if I say your problem is bad luck or shyness or loneliness or lack of interpersonal skills. But I can collect if I say your problem is social anxiety or depression. Giving you an illness is also an attractive solution because it seems to absolve you of blame. But by doing so it also subtly deprives you of the power to do something about your situation—say, by helping you see how the way you express your needs drives others away; or by changing your job or profession so that your lack of assertiveness won't be such a liability. Medicalizing your condition in this way also supports the idea that all's right with the world as it is, rather than challenging us to look carefully at what society is telling you about what's appropriate for you.

We have trouble recognizing that the times we live in are historically unique;

that the way things are is not the only way for things to be. We believe that "success" is the highest value, and success is measured in terms of individual achievement and money. But in the years before the Industrial Revolution, people were expected to fit into the community, control their desires and impulses, and work for the common good. "The ideal man, then, was pleasant, mild-mannered, and devoted to the good of the community. He performed his duties faithfully, governed his passions rationally, submitted to his fate and to his place in society, and treated his dependents with firm but affectionate wisdom," writes E. Anthony Rotundo in *American Manhood*. But after the opening of the American West and the rise of capitalism, self-interest and individual initiative came to be more respected as manly virtues. The individual, not the community, was seen as the basic unit of society, and each individual was expected to find his proper place in the world through his own efforts. Our current emphasis on competition for individual achievement by amassing wealth through work, which in itself is competitive, is something new in history. These values over-emphasize material success and make those who are not rich consider themselves to be failures. They also define relationships in terms of competition rather than mutual aid, and teach us to keep vulnerabilities hidden and to resolve conflict through intimidation. Such attitudes promote social isolation and denial of one's own interpersonal needs, further increasing vulnerability to stress.

Philip Cushman's book, *Constructing the Self, Constructing America*, is a wonderful, comprehensive, and chilling cultural history of America seen through the lens of psychotherapy. One of his major theses is that psychiatry and psychotherapy have let down their patients by accepting bourgeois values—assuming that our patients have an illness when they may be suffering because society's expectations are unhealthy. Cushman writes: "Victorian-era doctors, especially psychiatrists, explained [the] psychological disorders . . . of their female patients . . . through biologically based theories. The social conditions of women's lives, their lack of legal standing, their economic dependence on men, the numerous sociopolitical restrictions on female behavior, dress, and speech, and the lack of personal autonomy—all were thought to be the natural order of things and thus could not be sources of female distress." So women were made to feel that they were naturally second-class, weak, overemotional, not to be trusted with responsibility, not to be ambitious, not to desire an education—and their therapists supported this. Even Freud himself, when his female patients revealed memories of childhood sexual abuse, eventually decided that he was hearing their own repressed incestuous wishes.

Suppose we are in the same position now. The new "natural order of things" suggests that we cut ourselves off from family and community to follow employment, that both adults in a household are expected to work full-time jobs or more, that relationships are innately disposable, that we derive meaning in our lives from the things we buy, that we permanently indebt ourselves so that we can buy more things, that we can only exercise our political voice through choosing the lesser of two evils, that we have no faith in any institution (church, government, education, medicine), that we deny the existence of homelessness or poverty, that we fear dying insane and alone in a nursing home—*but we don't consider that these facts could be the sources of our troubled minds.* For the past century we have been taught to look inside ourselves for our discontent. We have developed a self that experiences the loss of family connection, natural structure, and social meaning in our lives as a lack of self-worth, an absence of self-esteem, a vague anxiety, an empty depression, "a self that embodies the absences, loneliness, and disappointments of life as a chronic, undifferentiated emotional hunger." "On the eve of the third millennium, depression has become the psychical epidemic of democratic societies, even as treatments offering every consumer an honorable solution proliferate." Why? *Looking inward rather than outward protects the cultural status quo. We won't try to give our society the radical reconstruction it needs as long as we believe the emptiness is within ourselves.*

It *is* much more difficult to develop our awareness of that cultural status quo and try to examine it objectively. It surrounds and envelops us so pervasively that for us to be fully aware is like expecting a fish to discover water. I certainly can't do it myself all the time. When I'm feeling down, I long for a new pill. I have trouble not buying new toys. I want to wave the flag, especially when we face such hatred around the world. It's easier and tempting to go along with things as they are, but to do so is truly unhealthy. I hope that my attempts to look objectively at things here don't come across as shrill reactionaryism. We have to know how we stand before we can help ourselves.

On the other hand, I write as a white male who can pass for WASP, the most privileged position in our culture. The situation for women and minorities is of course worse yet. The myth that we live in a free society in which opportunity is open to all results by necessity in a lot of blaming the victim. Because after all, if our society is the meritocracy it wants to be, if you can't make it, then it must be your own fault. Again, my own profession participates in the process, by pathologizing behavior that might be better considered appropriate for a nonwhite nonmale, or at least appropriate to the social environment. I'm refer-ring to the antifeminine bias in the diagnosis of depression, for example, where behaviors that are natural to women, like crying, are considered symp-toms of disease, while male behaviors like withdrawal and irritability are not. And I'm referring to the pathologizing of behavior like the restlessness of schoolchildren in a boring classroom where they don't feel at ease, or the drug use and violence that are natural responses to a world where minority youth feel they don't have a chance.

I'm aware that I haven't mentioned terrorism yet. I'm writing as we ap-proach another anniversary of 9/11, and I still find it an extremely difficult subject. Our world has changed dramatically. Every American suffered some degree of vicarious traumatization as the towers fell, and for many the effect was devastating. Images are seared in my mind: the clouds of ash and dust rolling down the streets, people diving under parked cars in panic; the "Miss-ing" flyers, poured out from Kinko's, with youthful, smiling faces, taped to every bus shelter and fence in lower Manhattan; the fire station near my office on Fifty-ninth Street, which lost six of its crew. Our culture does a great deal to deny the presence of death, but here it was in our faces.[6] Those who lost loved ones, those who had a narrow escape, those who participated in the rescue and cleanup efforts, are likely to bear permanent emotional scars. Our oceans have always protected us from the horror of war, but now we know we're not so safe. And to know that you're hated so deeply is also an extremely disturbing feeling. But the response of our government has been to reflexively protect all our old ways of doing things, often at great expense, without questioning why we are so hated, and to look for a scapegoat, someone we could beat up on, to make us all feel more powerful—at the expense of building more hatred. A "war" on terrorism is like a "war" on drugs, trying to solve a complex social problem with brute force. It can't be done.[7]

We don't know what effects we are likely to see from living under threat. It certainly adds stress to the system. Tom Ridge's words are chilling: "To defeat

---

6 There is evidence that television made the trauma worse. Ahern et al., 2002, found that, among a random sample of Manhattan residents, those who repeatedly watched the most graphic coverage had the greatest likelihood of post-traumatic stress disorder.

7 And what happened to the war on poverty? Did we declare victory and leave? Did we win? I sus-pect that we won by denial.

an enemy that lurks in the shadows and seeks relentlessly for some small crack through which to slip their evil designs—such a victory requires the vigilance of every American." Each of us is supposed to watch for suspicious people or activities, to have a home emergency preparedness kit (including duct tape), and to have a family evacuation plan. You don't know whether to laugh or cry. Ridge's clichés evoke Fu Manchu and Dr. Moriarty, but there really are lurking enemies with evil designs. We joke about the duct tape and the color-coded system, but when they announce a rise in threat level, who doesn't worry a little more? We know that all it takes to damage the immune systems of rats and stop the production of nerve cells in their brains is a few weeks of confinement at certain times during the day. What does living under threat do to humans?

If you think that the foregoing is a jaundiced view of Western, especially American, culture, you may be right. I am constitutionally a depressive, and I have more than my share of what's called "depressive realism." In my opinion, that's the uncomfortable tendency of depressives to see the truth when most people are kidding themselves. It's true, things have been worse for people in the past. Lives are longer now, health is better, we (most of us) have greater affluence and more choices. The United States is still, in many ways, the most opportunity-rich culture in the world. But it's not my job here to discuss the positives, rather to point out that there are hidden costs associated with these benefits.

A Way Out?

We're seeing movement on both the right and left ends of the sociopolitical spectrum that seeks to undo some of the damage that's being done to us. There are a great many people, some of whom I've had the pleasure to work with, who build their response around their religion. They homeschool their children or place them in private schools. They place great emphasis on family time; often, there's no television at all. They seek to insulate their children from mass culture not only by restricting their access, but also by emphasizing the role of parents as arbiters of standards. They actively seek to practice what they preach, both by donating their own time and talents in the service of social justice and by conscientious self-examination. Their fuel seems to come primarily from concern about how children are affected by contemporary life.

On the other end of the spectrum, we have the whole "New Age" movement, so difficult to define. Alternative medicine, a desire to enrich the self spiritually, a turning away from mass culture—these are elements. There are many leaders—Herbert Benson, Andrew Weil, John Sarno, Pema Chödrön, Dean Ornish, Joan Borysenko, Gary Zukav, Jon Kabat-Zinn, and Deepak Chopra are just a few of the respectable ones, those who have something serious to contribute. They advocate a holistic approach to health, an emphasis on the mind-body connection, an interest in Eastern religion, meditation, or mysticism. Much of the fuel for this movement seems to come from a dissatisfaction with Western medicine, a sense that health is much more than the absence of disease. At the same time as there are valuable contributions here, there are also many frauds who manage to attract desperate though educated people. "In Western societies we are seeing an unbelievable growth in the little world of bonesetters, wizards, clairvoyants, and mesmerists," observes the French social critic Elisabeth Roudinesco, commenting on what she calls the Depressive Society.

Different as these responses are, they both are attempts at addressing the emptiness of contemporary culture, that which the media seems to portray as the natural order of things. A culture of buying and consuming, where identity is expected to come from the clothes you wear, the music you listen to, and the teams you cheer for, where we think feeling good is a right and feeling bad a disease—this is something to be really worried about.

Loss of Nature

One of the most pervasive losses for mankind in the twenty-first century is our relationship with nature. I don't necessarily mean backpacking into the woods and living in a tent, though that can be worthwhile. I mean the real world intruding into our everyday lives. Until recently in history, most of us went to bed when it was dark and got up when it was light. Few people had clocks or watches, so time was told by the sun. We worked until we were tired, or until the job was done. We lived in intimate contact with other species, either domesticated, hunted, or just observed as neighbors in the wild. We were surrounded with reminders to be humble—that earth and the universe were much bigger than us, that birth and death were all around us, that hunger was always just around the corner. Most of our day was spent making sure we had enough to eat. We had a lot of quiet time when we could let our minds shift into a contemplative state—watching the sun rise, waiting for the fish to bite, hauling water, making bread.

We still have a powerful desire to connect with nature—witness vacations, hiking, gardening, cycling; our relationship with pets; our fascination with the distant universe and with how life works. With the exception of the slightly mystical views of Carl Jung, psychology has not paid a lot of attention to these desires. They've been dismissed as childish or else assumed to be merely healthy recreation, but the effects on us of the loss of opportunity to be part of nature haven't been taken seriously. Harold Searles first pointed this out in 1960, but no one has followed his lead very far. Searles proposed that we have a need for a sense of *relatedness* with the world outside us—separate but connected, in harmony or in conflict, still connected. I agree completely: relatedness with the world outside gives us the sense of being a part of a larger whole, not a separate creature who's immune from the world. This keeps us humble. Relatedness to nature also, ironically, assuages our fear of death by reminding us that birth and death happen all the time. It makes us feel more *real*— grounded, substantial. It quiets the noise in the head. It makes us part of a common humanity. As with interpersonal relations, the more we can see nature "objectively," the healthier our relationship to it will be.

But look at what we're doing to the world we live in. We've corrupted much of the environment, so that air is dangerous to breathe and water is dangerous to swim in or drink. We've overfished the oceans, so that many species are in danger of dying out. We've filled much of our lives with constant noise, interfering with our ability to think and relax. We've damaged the ozone layer so that it's become dangerous for us to get a suntan, the glaciers are receding, plant and animal habitats are changing. Our diets have become full of fats, carbohydrates, sugars, and meats, making us obese, vulnerable to all sorts of health problems, and taking much more than our rightful share of the world's food supply. We're eating genetically modified food, and we don't know what it will do to us. Allergies are out of control because we've both damaged our own immune systems and polluted the air. We squander oil and gas supplies, supplies that once used can never be restored. We go everywhere nowadays, scattering our trash behind us, in our SUVs and ATVs, leaving nothing pristine. Our work has become monotonous and sedentary, depriving us of the opportunity to have regular exercising and stretching as a natural part of the day. Yet we don't have time to just be still—to rest on the hoe while we look at the sunset, smell and listen and taste the world—essential to nourish the right brain, the creative side of our natures. We don't have the opportunity for transcendent experiences when we can be in touch with something larger than ourselves—the sea, the sky, the mountains, the grass growing, the wind blowing, the leaves falling.

Remember what we said about adaptation and the Hedonic Treadmill. It's easy for us to get used to all this, to accept this loss as the natural order of things and not be aware of the damage it does to us and the rest of the world. It's wonderful that we are so adaptable, *but there are some things we should not adapt to.* Some things we can't let happen. These are losses that are so profound that we must heighten our awareness of what is happening to us as a result. Our brains and nervous systems were designed by nature to be part of nature. To live in an artificial world makes us exotic, fragile, easily damaged. It puts enormous strain on our systems; strain that gets expressed as emotional disturbance, physical symptoms, a reliance on pills, a calcification of the self into something ugly and brittle.

Science and Medicine: Part of the Problem

So there is a great deal going on in our society that has us trying to cope with stress of a kind we are not biologically prepared for—stress that seems to have no escape, so that we live in a perpetual state of helplessness, which we may experience as anxiety, depression, or illness.

But stress is only half the picture. If we want to understand why Jim, Joe, and Jack go through roughly the same difficult experience, and Jim gets depressed, Joe gets an ulcer, and Jack seems perfectly fine, we have to talk about individual differences—what traits make them respond differently to stress. *Illness is the result of the combination of stress and a vulnerable individual.* Unfortunately for all of us, this is a subject where contemporary science has contributed more heat than light.

The debate over how much of any human characteristic is "genetic" (meaning inevitable, programmed into our cellular structure) versus how much is "learned" (meaning taught or learned from experience) is actually a lot more complicated than anyone realized twenty years ago. It turns out that genes, with a few exceptions like that for cystic fibrosis, are far from inevitable. Genes control much more of our being than we generally imagine, but they do it by being "turned on" by experience. We develop our individuality through a highly complex interaction between genetics and learning.

Genes manufacture the basic cellular material that, when turned on in a nerve cell, makes the cell adapt *and change.* A nerve cell that has repeatedly sent an alarm signal on to the next nerve cell has been changed by this experience; it has adapted itself to make it more ready and easy to send the alarm signal next time. The same process of change occurs in the cell if it repeatedly sends "chill out" signals. This is the process known as *long-term potentiation* of cells. It's how the brain gets changed by experience. Every event that registers in the brain has an impact on gene expression (chemistry and structure) in the brain that lasts for hours or days, not mere seconds; and the more stressful the event, the greater the impact. A neuron on the receiving end of a transmission from another neuron will turn on its little genetic factory in the nucleus and change itself. Not only does each neuron transmit a message to the next, but the neuron itself is changed a little in the process. That's just the way genes work; it's the genes in the nucleus that prepare the neuron to transmit its message, and as they do so they change the neuron itself a little bit. *Every future stressor affects a brain that has been changed by previous stressors.* Animal studies focusing on the immediate effects of stressors like injection of chemicals have taught us this much, and that is a great deal. But it will take years of long, valuable lab time for us to learn about the effects of chronic stress like learned helplessness or psychosocial stress like isolation.

Researchers have also been demonstrating that there are considerable innate differences among us at birth. We are not "blank slates" who would all have the same personality if we were all raised exactly the same. This is not going to be news to most mothers. But it's more than a matter of gross differences like energy level. Some babies are inquisitive, others shy; some are cuddly, others are stiff; some are expressive, others stolid; some cranky, some placid. There are "developmental lines"—of perception, thinking, coordination, and attachment—along which children mature at different rates. The interaction of the infant's continually unfolding temperament and the mother's personality—and the mother's emotional state and availability during the child's infancy, which can vary greatly from one child to another, so that no siblings ever have the same mother—yields a dynamic, always changing dance in which both the mother and the child are programming each other. By first grade, much of the child's personality is formed already, and some of those individual vulnerabilities to stress can be identified. Others will develop later during childhood and adolescence, as the child and the world interact with each other.

Vulnerabilities aside, there is reliable research now to show that many personality variables are greatly determined by our genes. These include:

- Introversion (shyness)—slightly over 50 percent genetic
- Positive affectivity (bubbliness)—about 50 percent genetic

- General intelligence—also about 50 percent genetic
- The so-called Big Five character traits: openness, conscientiousness, extroversion (sociability, liveliness), agreeableness, and neuroticism (moodiness, anxiety, irritability)—all about 40 percent genetic
- Activity level—about 25 percent genetic
- Conservatism (conformity, following the rules, obeying authority)—about 30 percent genetic

We have to keep in mind that when these data say that, for instance, general intelligence is about 50 percent heritable, that means that half *at most* of anyone's intelligence is due to hereditary factors. And those genes have to be turned on by experience—Mozart was clearly a musical genius at birth but might have died perhaps as nothing other than a great whistler if his father had not pushed him to learn. We need to think about the interplay of inherited characteristics and environment over time: a baby who is high on the bubbliness factor is likely to attract a lot of positive attention from adults, while one who is more introverted will not. Each will have their character traits reinforced by their experience in a complicated developmental dance that will last their lifetimes. The more introverted, less agreeable, more anxious child will likely have more negative interactions with people, and will likely become more vulnerable to stressors as time goes on because of the continuing damage of those negative interactions.

There are things that parents can do to help their children, and things that adults with vulnerabilities can learn to help themselves; we'll get to those in later chapters. For now let's just keep in mind that illness, suffering, and difficulty adapting to life result from the interaction of stress and individual vulnerabilities, both genetic and learned. It's a highly complicated interaction, and that's where science has gotten us in trouble.

It's important to recognize that *the scientific method was developed to isolate and identify single causes; it's not so useful when many forces are in play.* The experimental method requires us to control all the variables in a situation; we then allow one variable to change, and if we find that permitting change in that one variable leads to change in the outcome of our experiment, we know with nearly absolute certainty that the variable in question is responsible for the outcome (*Penicillin kills the spirochete. Radiation causes genes to mutate. Animals can be trained to salivate at the sound of a bell*). The scientific method doesn't work, however, when we can't control the variables.

We can't take people with depression and put them in a sterile lab while we test medications; not only would it be inhumane, their individual personalities, beliefs, histories, and expectancies will all have an impact on the way the medication affects them. We can't study teenage drug use by considering separately the effects of poverty, divorce, childhood trauma, discrimination, and exposure to violence, because each of those variables is inextricably intertwined with the others. *When it comes to people, heredity versus environment is a false dichotomy.* Children program their parents in how to parent; biological siblings separated at birth demand certain responses from their adoptive parents, so that they end up being parented more alike than adopted siblings in the same household do. And the kind of parenting we receive in turn influences how our genetic endowment will be expressed; thus although there appears to be a genetic vulnerability to depression, children with that vulnerability who are raised by uninvolved or critical parents are more likely to develop the illness than children raised by supportive and interested parents. When it comes to understanding people, we're reduced to looking at correlations, interactions from which we may infer causation. Sophisticated statistical analysis, which is beyond the ability of anyone to grasp intuitively, allows us to estimate the relative influence of multiple causes. The science is clumsy, arcane, and aesthetically unsatisfactory, but it's the best we can do in studying people.

The elegance of the scientific method has become a modern myth partly because it reinforces our emotional desire to find single causes. Freud, for very good reasons of his own, was desperate to be seen as "scientific," and modeled his conception of the mind on the mechanical explanations of his day (*Depression is a punitive superego.*). Contemporary research proceeds with the same biases (*Depression is an imbalance in serotonin.*). *People are much too complicated for the scientific method, at least at our current level of knowledge.* Besides, we are just beginning to develop the tools that will allow us to understand how the brain, mind, and body interconnect. Thirty years ago, researchers had identified perhaps 50 connections between the hypothalamus, a center of emotions in the brain, and the cerebral cortex, the thinking part of the brain. Today, we've identified over twenty-five hundred connections, and no one knows what they all mean. Nevertheless, we *want* so strongly to believe in simple solutions—the pill, the light wavelength, the cognitive errors, the magic bullet, the single thing that will uncomplicate our lives—that we pour billions of research dollars, tons of newsprint, and hours of TV news blurbs into the chase.

One recent soundbite-of-the-month was that scientists have "isolated the gene for aggression in mice." What this means is vastly more complicated: mice who have been bred so that they lack a specific gene that prompts the brain to manufacture serotonin show an increased tendency to attack other mice, and a reluctance to explore new environments. It's quite likely that these mice have an abnormally high anxiety level that causes them to see threats where other mice don't; thus they respond aggressively. But there are thousands of other genes, even in the mouse, that influence the expression of aggression and anxiety, and human brains are much more complex than mouse brains. The implication that if we could control the expression of this gene in humans we'd be able to control aggression, or that overly aggressive humans are perhaps damaged somehow in this particular gene, is ridiculous—but it grabs our attention on TV.

We no longer believe in witches or voodoo but when we can't do what we want we use our understanding—often our misunderstanding—of science to supply an explanation. If we can't shake our sad mood, or calm down, or sit still, our brain chemistry must be responsible. We don't ask what changed our brain chemistry; we assume it's immutable except by adding more chemicals. If we wake up with nightmares, experience overwhelming fear for no clear reason, keep getting into dangerous situations despite our best conscious efforts, we look back at past traumas and assume we are reliving them. We don't think about the interaction between trauma and brain chemistry. If we are in pain and there is no wound or disease, we create one—with the enthusiastic cooperation of the medical/pharmaceutical system—and seek the medication for it. We don't think about the connections between our brains and our bodies. If we find ourselves as adults still doomed to live out or struggle with our parents' opinion of us—*unworthy of love and care; dangerous; incompetent; never good enough*—we may find a therapist to help us escape this curse. But neither we nor the therapist is likely to look at where, exactly, in our brains and bodies, this curse exists.

Illness is complicated and personal; recovery is the same. It's the easy way out to medicalize our problems and look for pills to help us adapt better to the way things are. It's our wish for a simple answer in action. Unfortunately the simple answers just make us sicker. Remember that we're already perhaps too adaptable to bad situations.

Systems Thinking

Marsha Linehan has a wonderful book with a forbidding title, *Cognitive-Behavioral Treatment of Borderline Personality Disorder*, which, despite its specialized subject, has had considerable impact on the way all psychotherapy is conducted. Linehan's approach, to which this book owes a great deal, is much more radical than the title suggests; it involves trying to look as objectively as possible, with as few assumptions as possible, at everything that's going on in the patient's life. When you do this unflinchingly, you find that even the most bizarre behaviors make sense in the patient's own little world. Like Linehan, I am unwilling to accept the idea that any one system can be totally responsible for causing illness. People can be understood in many ways—as bundles of chemical messengers; as simple machines that react to external stimuli; as thinking machines whose thoughts guide our behavior and sometimes cause our problems; as a set of drives in conflict with reality and with our conscience; as conscious, self-directed organisms responsible for our own conditions; as an interactional self only manifested in relation to others. All of these have been popular, and very useful, ways of understanding us. But each of these is only one arbitrary viewpoint we have created for our own convenience, to help us in organizing our observations. None is inherently more "true" or complete than any other. All human behavior involves all systems at the same time. Accordingly, if we want a complete understanding of ourselves, we should take each into account, and be open to more viewpoints besides. This requires what is called a "systems" point of view. This way of thinking accepts the complexity of human beings, the idea that many factors may be involved in any illness, and the necessity of considering sometimes conflicting theories if we want to change.

Systems thinking doesn't see a conflict between the fact that depression can be lifted both by medication and by psychotherapy; thoughts, emotions, and motivations—the stuff of the mind—are carried by neural pathways—the stuff of the brain. What happens in neural pathways can certainly be affected by medication, but apparently it can also be affected by thoughts, emotions, and behavior. Systems thinking views the addict's need for his or her drug not only as an effect of the drug on the brain, but also as a result of social and personality variables that made drug use an attractive alternative to life as it is. It views an illness like atrial fibrillation not only as an electrical problem in the heart, but also as a result of social, genetic, and environmental variables that affect how the individual person with the heart deals with stressful situations. In *Active Treatment of Depression* I presented a detailed systems-based model for how depression works. I'm not going to try to repeat that for all the conditions addressed in this book, but rather apply the systems viewpoint, which is simply a way of organizing any number of variables when each of them can interact with the others in a complex relationship in which all can be both cause and effect. With this goes the assumption that the patient's symptoms—physical, emotional, relational—make sense in some way, perhaps not consciously accessible to the patient, but still a logical response to a distorted perception of the world.

We live in a vast system that involves stresses unprecedented in human history, our ability (for both good and ill) to adapt to those stresses, our individual vulnerabilities, and our interactions with each other and with the culture in which we swim. An effect of those stresses is to make many of us sick: we "burn out," in the vivid common metaphor. The concept of the vicious circle is an intuitive attempt to portray a systems approach. Individual and interpersonal variables influence the form our sickness will take: depression, anxiety, fibromyalgia, hard or soft addiction, a difficult personality; or a combination of any or all of those manifestations.

Out of that vast system each of us develops a mental model to help us make sense of our experience. We'll talk more of those mental models, variously called schemas, character types, and lifetraps, later, in Chapter 6. For now, consider one aspect of how we can conceptualize our burnout: that we have an illness. If we have an illness, we are ushered into what sociologists call the sick role. The sick role has its advantages: it gets us to the attention of medical professionals who can perhaps help us, and at the same time we are excused from many ordinary responsibilities. But it also has disadvantages: we can come to think of ourselves as weak, unable to take it, a failure. I've known a number of patients who worked hard to convince the Social Security Administration that they were disabled enough to qualify for psychiatric disability payments, who now view it as the greatest mistake of their lives, because a new, damaged and defective, identity has gotten into their bones. And I think of my patient from the 1970s who feigned paranoia to get out of Vietnam, only to develop the delusion that agents from Military Intelligence were following him around. The sick role is majestically ironic, and contemporary medicine plays right into the irony.

The late George Engel and his followers have been calling for a general reform of Western medicine for almost twenty-five years now. They have achieved great respect, and a significant following in specialized medical fields like psychoneuroimmunology and in health psychology, but their viewpoint has had little influence on everyday medical or hospital practice. Engel proposed a *biopsychosocial* approach to illness, emphasizing that a symptom involves not only the biomechanics of the patient, but his or her individual psychology and the meaning of the symptom in society. Thus, for instance, there is no such thing as depression in China, where patients never complain of it (because of shame) and doctors aren't trained to recognize it. But there is a great deal of neurasthenia in China. Neurasthenia has exactly the physical symptoms of depression—fatigue, poor appetite, disturbed sleep—the same thing that Freud was treating in Vienna as "nervous exhaustion" or what we call burnout now—but it is more respectable than depression because it implies that you have simply worn yourself out dealing with a very difficult situation. So when a lonely, isolated, older patient in the United States visits her MD complaining of aches and pains, weakness and fatigue, the MD should of course run all the medical tests to detect a disease process at work; and when they come back negative perhaps the MD should not try to treat chronic fatigue syndrome but try to find a way to help the patient deal with her isolation and loneliness. And if the MD does consider that this might be depression rather than a "physical" illness, and prescribe an antidepressant in response, that's still not good enough.

Antidepressants don't work unless we can change our lives. Physicians have generally been trained only in the *biomedical* model, assuming that "science" means focusing on disease processes, forgetting that there are other sciences, nonlaboratory sciences, that deal with human relations. Doctors have generally been taught a reductionist science that encourages them to look for single causes; to find a cure that involves reversing a disease process; to focus on the disease, not on the patient. The common medical practice of first "ruling out organic disease" exemplifies this process; it's based on a hierarchical conception of the primary importance of organic disease, and the belief that the mental and the physical realms can be neatly divided. When there is a simple "physical" disease, this is great. But most of those diseases can be treated rather easily now, and we bring more complex problems to our doctors. Two-thirds of patients in primary care now have unexplained physical symptoms, but doctors have been trained to dismiss them as functional. Or to blame the patient for being noncompliant.

David Mechanic, a respected sociologist of medicine, relates how a distinguished physician could find no help from the medical community for his advancing macular degeneration (causing progressive blindness); because it couldn't be cured, no one was interested in helping him learn how to live with it. Mechanic also talks about how his own aging mother's depression was dismissed as inevitable until a physical therapist showed her some simple strategies that improved her independence. As the population ages, as more and more of us cope with chronic stress, we look in vain to medicine for practical help; not to cure us, but to arrest or reverse disability. The same is true in psychiatry; if the pill can't help you, if your problems aren't caused by repressed conflict, too many practitioners will dismiss you as resistant when you could really use some support and realistic advice for coping.

The solution for medicine is not to blindly incorporate half-baked New Age methods like aromatherapy, nor to switch to "alternative medicine"—some of which may be simply substituting a new dogma—but to rigorously apply a systems approach to illness, the biopsychosocial model. Until that happens, we have to take better care of ourselves—recognize the effects of stress, accept it, and respond accordingly. The next chapter will focus on how stress affects our brain and nervous system, and take a quick look at the immune and endocrine systems, also deeply involved in how we respond to stress. Then we'll go on and figure out what to do about it all.

But first look at the story of Mr. and Mrs. Brown, to see how a systems viewpoint changes the practice of psychotherapy.

The Browns: Systems at Work

When Mary Alice first came to see me, she was in desperate shape. Only a month out of the hospital following a suicide attempt, she was on three medications that didn't seem to be working. She still had suicidal impulses and felt that she'd lost her mind. She had three young children whom she loved dearly, but was afraid they weren't safe with her. She couldn't stop being angry at her husband over what she felt were little things, even though he was trying to be patient with her. She couldn't sleep, couldn't relax, couldn't stop crying, couldn't stop yelling at the kids, and was tortured by recurring thoughts that she was a failure, a weakling, defective.

She had a family history made for depression and low self-esteem for women. Her father had left the family when she was a child. As the only girl, Mary Alice was expected to stay home and help her mother while the boys had fun. When her mother became gravely ill while Mary Alice was in high school, she was not supposed to tell anyone. She kept the secret for two years, nursing her mother alone. Her mother died just before Mary Alice left for college, and Mary Alice had no home to go back to. In the first month of college, she met her husband-to-be, James.

I wanted to understand what led to the suicide attempt, and Mary Alice was able to hold off on any further attempts for a few weeks while we figured this out. It seemed that her desperation had been building for a while, largely fueled by fights with her husband. The fights were always about money or his drinking. Mary Alice felt they were living beyond their means and that James's regular weekend alcohol use was excessive. They had been in couples counseling, but it hadn't done any good. Mary Alice admitted that her own temper was part of the problem. The angrier she got, the more calm and quiet her husband got. When couples counseling ended, Mary Alice felt she was the problem. Her mental state went downhill from there, culminating in her suicide attempt and hospitalization.

As we talked through this story, Mary Alice calmed down somewhat. I told her how frequently mothers of young children had to struggle with depression, especially those without a mother of their own, and urged her to get together with other mothers as often as possible. I used other arguments as much as I could to normalize her problems and rebuild her self-esteem. I gave her concrete advice about how to stop yelling at the kids and get them to listen to her. She seemed to be feeling so much better that we ended therapy after a few months. In her more positive frame of mind, she thought she and her husband could work things out.

But later on Mary Alice called again. She continued to feel better and function better with the children, but she wasn't getting anywhere with her husband, and she worried that her mental state was slipping.

When they came in together, I started to get James's side of the story. He was an ambitious young man who was clearly on his way up in his business. Still, he seemed to be very devoted to his wife and children; he knew the marriage was in big trouble and he wanted to make it work. He understood that Mary Alice needed his support, but he also felt that he worked very hard and did a lot around the house besides, and he needed some support also. He agreed that their fights were always about money or his drinking. They had been overextended financially, he agreed, but things were getting better (Mary Alice rolled her eyes). As for his drinking, it was only on weekends, and he had actually cut back on quantity quite a bit. Mary Alice jumped in: maybe he had cut back a little, but there were still far too many times when he had a few with the boys and drove home drunk. On other occasions he would tell her he would be home or call at a certain time, then would not show up and couldn't be reached.

Our first agreement in couples counseling was that James would not come home drunk or late again. When he broke that pledge, the real work began. As we hashed and rehashed these things over many weeks I understood why Mary Alice had been made to feel it was all her fault. Her anger was truly something fierce, and she could often sound unreasonable. In fact there were many times when it seemed that she just didn't hear what was being said to her, by James or me, and I had to be careful not to sound as if I was talking down to her. On the other hand James couldn't seem to fulfill his commitments, despite all his sincere talk. One or the other was always just on the verge of walking out. I began to dread their sessions, and often developed a headache during them.

Gradually—over months—James began to understand that his drinking was a serious issue, and he really did cut back greatly, and he started to keep his commitments. Mary Alice began to feel better and went off most of her medication. As she developed more trust that we might get somewhere, she went back to the subject of money. It turned out that, while James made upwards of $150,000 in his Wall Street job, more than a third of that was in the form of bonuses, which really couldn't be counted on. Meanwhile they lived in a $500,000 + house, with two mortgages, and were carrying almost $50,000 in credit card and other debt. They had seen a financial counselor, who had them on short rations to pay off their debt. The house was a big bone of contention. It had been their dream home, built according to their own design, but they had run out of money before they could furnish, decorate, or landscape it. Mary Alice was sick of it; she wanted to move and downsize so that they wouldn't be in debt and have to worry each time one of the kids had to go to the dentist. James wanted to hang on. He was convinced he would be making more money soon. We talked about these, and other, issues over many sessions, me trying to support Mary Alice's belief in her own sanity while at the same time trying to get her to listen better, and reminding James that her feelings had merit even if he didn't like how she expressed them.

Another crisis again took months to play out. James's company merged with another. He was promised a promotion, and a substantial salary bump. He didn't want to sell the house while all this was up in the air. Mary Alice was still for getting out from under as soon as possible. I was torn. Though I thought Mary Alice was making a lot of sense in terms of the stress they were under and the values they wanted to practice, I could sympathize with James's difficulty giving up his dream house. I suggested a compromise: put the house on the market to see what happens, but don't make any decisions until James's job offer comes through. They did this, but James's company kept him dangling for six months; meanwhile Mary Alice found the patience to keep a lid on her desire to get a decision made. We put couples counseling on hold until James got his news.

When it came, James's job offer didn't point clearly in one direction or another. His salary increase was less than what he'd hoped for, but his bonus potential was even greater yet. As we talked through the numbers, I felt that it was possible for them to *stay in the house if they wanted, though it would be risky. I felt I really couldn't advise them—they would have to agree somehow. But things looked bleak for that. Mary Alice was very angry, tearful, and short-fused. She wouldn't let James talk without attacking him, and he was fed up with her. I left the session very discouraged. That night Mary Alice called my answering machine; they had just gotten an offer on their house. We scheduled a Saturday session, and I was not looking forward to it at all.*

I should trust my clients more. In the intervening three days, Mary Alice had continued to follow my advice about talking to friends. One knew a real estate agent. Mary Alice met the agent and found a house in a moderate price range she thought James would like. She took him there that night and he loved it. Though not nearly as big or pretentious, it was in a settled neighborhood, and he liked that very much—kids playing on the street, walking distance to town, feeling a part of a community— things that Mary Alice had wanted all along. They could finally get out of debt and start to save. He could look forward to the day when the idea of losing his job might not terrify him so much. Our final session together was a celebration of their patience with and commitment to each other, their individual resourcefulness, and their finding a way to live that enabled them to reduce their stress and pursue the values they really believed in.

I don't know why I was so successful at refusing to pathologize either one of them. There was a lot to support the idea that Mary Alice really was seriously depressed and needed help adapting to life as is. There was a lot to support the idea that James really did have an alcohol, as well as a responsibility, problem. But when I listened to them, they just kept making sense to me. Their problems seemed to be first of all reactions to each other, then to be reactions to the stresses they both shared. A stay-at-home wife with young children and no support system. A driven husband working too many hours and constantly in fear about his position. A mountain of debt, and the feeling that there's no way out. They needed, most of all, the sense that they could rely on each other to pull in the same direction.

Though the specifics are different, the same dynamics apply to millions of couples. When you think about it, it's inevitable that one person in a pair is going to be more anxious, more conservative, less inclined to take risks than the other. Depending on where you stand on these things, you may be likely to consider the anxious one weak, or the confident one unrealistic. As they work on each other over time, their roles can get into their brains, the self-fulfilling prophecy at work. The anxious one develops depression; the confident one becomes impulsive, thoughtless, perhaps increasing alcohol use as a way of getting relief from the tension in the home. The more rigid their posi-

tions, the more they approach what we consider mental illness. Couples can drive each other crazy. How our loved ones feel about us gets into our brains and into our bones. But couples, if they truly make an effort to listen to each other and be considerate of each other's feelings, can also produce mental health.

3

Brain and Body

The brain does not mechanically store the information that it acquires. It is changed forever each time it interacts with the world. Each time, it *becomes* the information.

—John J. Ratey

LET me warn you here. This is a long and difficult chapter. You can skip over it if you want, though I hope you don't. This is partly because I want you to share my fascination with what we're learning about the brain, the mind, and their relationship with the body; and partly because I think that understanding why things are the way they are really does help us understand what we have to do in order to recover. If you do skip this chapter now, I hope you'll at least dip back into it later, when you run into concepts you'd like to know more about. The way I would do this would be to read this chapter lightly now, just introducing myself to these ideas without trying to integrate them. The integration should come in later chapters as we apply this knowledge.

We ended the last chapter having introduced the concept of systems. There are always systems within systems. The brain itself is a vastly complex system, which interacts with the immune, endocrine, and other systems in the body to control how we respond to stress. Scientists now have the tools and knowledge base to understand much more completely than ever before how the brain works. We can see how it is damaged by such things as child abuse and neglect, and emotional trauma in adult life. We are beginning to see how it is affected by chronic stress. There are fascinating hints that we can identify the small part of the brain that is the home of the self, where consciousness and self-awareness reside. We are also learning how emotions are expressed by the brain and how they affect our thoughts and our bodies. Stress-related damage in these areas results in vulnerability to depression, anxiety, nonspecific illness, damaged personality structure, and susceptibility to addiction. Understanding how the child's brain ideally develops—without overwhelming stress—into a confident, resilient, loving, expressive adult brain points us to understanding how we can recover from the damage of the Perpetual Stress Response.

Brain Structure

The human brain is composed of billions of neurons, the basic nerve cell that transmits energy and information to other cells. Each neuron has a nucleus, which maintains the cell's viability and contains genetic material. The neuron cell builds a network of dendrites, branches that receive transmissions from other cells. At one end of the neuron is a single long axon, the transmitting portion of the cell, which may branch many times before it ends. The axon works by releasing small packets of chemicals known as *neurotransmitters,* which flow across the tiny spaces (synaptic gaps) between the axon and the dendrites of other cells, where they will affect the action of those other cells. (See Figure 7.)

It used to be thought that neurotransmitters simply activate or inhibit the action of the receiving neuron, but the picture is really much more complex than that. There are currently fifty-three known neurotransmitters, each of which can have a different impact on the genetic factory in the nucleus of the receiving cell, modifying how the genes respond, and determining what kind of signal the cell sends on to other cells in the chain. Axons also release other molecules known as *neuromodulators*, which seem to have more long-term effects on the growth of neuronal networks and the likelihood of other neurons firing. Endorphins, the endogenous opiates of the body that are associated with pleasure and relief from pain, are considered neuromodulators. Serotonin, dopamine, epinephrine (adrenaline), and norepinephrine are called variously neuromodulators or neurotransmitters, depending on who's doing the talking. The axon-dendritic network is so complex that, on average, each neuron connects with about ten thousand others. Since there are about 10 billion neurons in the adult brain, with over 2 million miles of axons, and at least fifty-three neurotransmitters, the number of possible firing patterns is close enough to infinity that we should never worry about filling up the brain with too much information.

Besides that, the brain is always changing. The question of how exactly the brain learns new information has bedeviled scientists for generations. Fifty

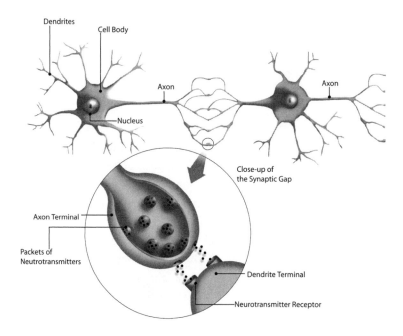

One nerve cell communicates with another by sending chemical signals from its axon to the dendrites of the receiving cell at the synapse, the minuscule gap between the neurons. The sending cell releases packets of neurotransmitters across the synaptic gap, which bind with specialized receptors in the receiving cell's dendrites. Currently there are fifty-three known neurotransmitters, each of which can have a different effect on the receiving cell. (Credit: Kerry Gavin Studio)

Figure 7

years ago, Canadian psychologist Donald Hebb proposed a simple principle: "Neurons that fire together, wire together." In other words, whenever we practice a skill or learn a new fact or associate a person with a feeling, our brains are somehow strengthening the physical connections between neurons. But Hebb was ahead of the science that could prove his principle. Finally, Eric Kandel was awarded the 2000 Nobel Prize for showing exactly how that happens in the lowly sea slug *Aplysia* (which has very large neurons): when neurons fire repeatedly, new synaptic connections are formed and existing ones are strengthened, through that long-term potentiation (LTP) process. Scientists have since gone on to show that this same principle works in higher animals.

Practicing new behavior, or learning new information, results in the formation of new connections between nerve cells.

Now we have evidence that this is so in humans too. In a delightful recent study, researchers taught twelve volunteers to juggle, then compared their brains to a matched group of nonjugglers at three intervals: before they began learning to juggle, after three months of practice, and again after three months without any practice. After three months of practice, there were visible (though tiny) expansions in gray matter in two separate areas of the brain. After three months without practicing the differences disappeared. It makes me wonder what is the effect of all the mental juggling that we have to do, and if that can be measured somehow. But the bottom line is we're constantly forming new connections in our brains; *our experience of life changes our brain structure.*

The adult brain is a complex system of interconnected structures, groups of specialized neurons that perform different functions (many of which are still not well understood). But at birth, the infant brain is remarkably undifferentiated. It develops through an intricate dance between the genes in the cells, which contain the instructions for what the cell can and cannot do, and the child's experience. All adult brain functions exist as potential in the infant's brain, and many are preprogrammed to develop at certain times in childhood and adolescence (in the same way that cicadas are programmed to emerge after seventeen years), but the environment must provide the opportunity at the appropriate time in order for that development to take place. Thus children born with cataracts who don't have them removed before the correct developmental window in life closes forever never can "learn" to see depth or shape later. The same seems true of language; children like Genie, kept confined in silence by disturbed parents until she was thirteen, can learn to use words but can't learn to string them together to express thoughts. Most importantly from our point of view, scientists are now gathering evidence that the same interplay between genetics and experience at critical times in development is equally important for emotional "skills," like identifying and modulating emotions, development of a stable self-concept, and empathy. Genie many years later still has trouble differentiating between people and objects; children raised in an environment that doesn't teach them about feelings may never learn to recognize or control them. Recent studies showing that the brain continues developing new cells, circuits, *and structures*—perhaps throughout our lives—emphasize the critical role of experience in determining how we think, feel, and see the world.

Daniel Siegel makes it easy to visualize much of the structure of the adult brain. Make a fist, with your thumb under your closed fingers. Imagine that your wrist is the spinal cord. Now the palm is the base animal brain, the brain stem. It is the part that keeps us breathing, that reacts automatically to stimuli like light and sound, the part that we're usually completely unconscious of but which regulates body functions, including the immune system. The thumb (it helps if you imagine you have two thumbs, as these structures appear on both sides of the brain) is the limbic system, the center of emotions in the brain. The limbic system is made up of substructures like the amygdala and hippocampus, which we'll discuss in more detail, just above the pituitary, the master gland (imagine that you are holding a small olive just under your thumb pad). The limbic system differentiates between pleasure and pain; it tells us what we want, and what we fear. The fingers are the cerebral cortex or neocortex, the thinking brain, the part with many folds and fissures and that is overdeveloped in humans. The fingertips, curled under so that they are in close connection with all the other parts of the brain, represent the prefrontal cortex, an area thought to be very important to identity, self-concept, and self-esteem. The tips of the two middle fingers are the orbitofrontal cortex (*orbit* meaning eye socket), the center of consciousness and the self.

The Emotional Brain

For many years scientists have conceived of the limbic system as the source of emotions in the brain. Now it's becoming clear that the picture is a lot more complex than that: emotions are the result of the interaction of many brain and other physical systems that are distributed over the whole body. Nor can we say neatly and cleanly that the neocortex is the center of logical thinking, divorced from the emotionality of the limbic system. Instead, the two parts of the brain are intimately connected, as they are also with the endocrine and immune systems; emotions and cognitions are all mixed up together. New studies using brain-imaging technology suggest that the different basic emotional responses (fear, anger, joy, sadness, and perhaps others) are due to the activation of characteristic pathways—connections between structures—rather than structures themselves.

Nevertheless, it's true that the limbic system is the Grand Central Station of emotions and motivation. It's the structure that we share with other mammals, which often seem to display many of the same emotions we do. Mammals are also social creatures and are able to communicate their feelings to each other. Since the young are born immature, the mother-infant bond is extremely

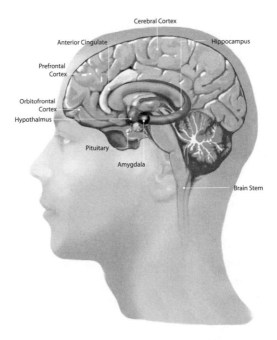

A cross section of the human brain, emphasizing the limbic system and the prefrontal regions. The limbic system components include the amygdala (the fear-processing center) and the hippocampus and anterior cingulate. (The left hippocampus is shown in shadow, as if in three dimensions.) The prefrontal cortex, at the forehead, includes the orbitofrontal cortex, just behind the eyes. The orbitofrontal cortex is in a position to link directly the three major parts of the brain: the cortex (thinking), the limbic system (emotions), and the brain stem (body functions, including the immune response).
(Credit: Kerry Gavin Studio)

Figure 8

important. Mother mammals have some ability to recognize their infants' needs, through communication with heavy emotional content that gets processed in the limbic system. By studying the effects of life experience on its structures, scientists in the past ten years or so have made some truly revolutionary discoveries, discoveries that are both disturbing and hopeful. So let's talk briefly about what constitutes the limbic system and the emotional brain.

The *hippocampus,* a string bean–shaped structure in the limbic system, seems to play an important role in consolidation of memory. (There are actually two hippocampi, one on each side of the brain.) Memories are in flux in the brain for several weeks after the event. Damage to the hippocampus can mean the loss of recent memories, but beyond that time memories seem to be consolidated in other areas of the brain. The hippocampus has been described as placing the individual in the context of space and time (it's what gets enlarged in the brains of London taxi drivers), reminding us where we are physically and where we are in the context of the present and past; it also plays a role in linking emotional memories with events. Because of the hippocampus, we have especially strong memories for highly emotional events; for instance, remembering exactly where we were and what we were doing when we first learned of 9/11. Prolonged or severe stress means excess production of cortisol, a neurotransmitter that can damage neurons in the hippocampus, interfering with our ability to consolidate memory of an event. For these reasons, the hippocampus seems especially implicated in dissociative disorders like posttraumatic stress disorder (PTSD). Several studies have found that the hippocampus is significantly reduced in size in people with PTSD, but recent work has shown that administration of some of the new antidepressants apparently helps the hippocampus reverse the process and increase in size, and improve its memory function. It's also speculated that placebos, which are often very effective with stress-related conditions, derive their benefit from their calming effect in the hippocampus. The patient feels relieved by medical attention, an explanation for his condition, and a plausible treatment plan. Relief means less cortisol production, allowing the hippocampus to function normally again.

The hippocampus is one area where we know that new neuronal stem cells are formed, even in adulthood and old age. There appears to be a great deal of neuronal turnover in the hippocampus, neurons frequently dying off only to be replaced by new cells. Interestingly, exercise appears to stimulate the growth of new neurons. There is also a fascinating finding that infant rats who are raised by mothers who lick and groom them frequently have better memories and have more densely branched neurons in the hippocampus. It appears that the mother's attentiveness means that more neurons survive. These findings in rats suggest ways in which humans can take better care of their hippocampi.

The *amygdala*, an almond-shaped structure at the front of the hippocampus, is a center for emotional responses, especially the fear response (again, there are actually two amygdalae, on each side of the brain). The amygdala connects through the hypothalamus directly to the rest of the body to generate the fight-or-flight response without a detour through the thinking part of the brain. So we jump out of the way of the oncoming bus before we are aware we feel afraid. The amygdala also contains centers that are important for emotional communication like face recognition. It seems to contribute to our ability to evaluate a stranger's face in a split second, unconsciously, as friendly or threatening, pleasant or unpleasant. (In depression and bipolar disorder, there is evidence that face evaluation is disrupted, with a bias toward interpreting others' expressions as sad.)

Recent research has shown that, under repeated stress, the neurons in the amygdala sprout new branches, resulting in new connections with other nerve cells, which may account for the generalization of a specific fear into free-floating anxiety.

Although I just said that the amygdala sends its fear signals directly to the body without the thinking brain being involved, that is an oversimplification. Besides the direct connection, there is a scenic route for these fear signals through the higher cortex, specifically that *orbitofrontal cortex* (OFC) that seems to be so important for self-concept. The orbitofrontal cortex is able to engage the neocortex to get us to think about the situation before we respond automatically; the executive functioning of the brain that permits us to override the impulses of the limbic system. The OFC then may send out signals that inhibit the fear response in the rest of the body—which is what happens when we perceive that what we first took to be a threat is not real. Some have called this the "high road," and the direct amygdala-body connection the "low road." It is the low road that permits what Daniel Goleman in *Emotional Intelligence* calls an "emotional hijacking"—when our emotions control our actions without input from the thinking brain. Vietnam veterans with PTSD, shown movies of wartime, are hijacked down the low road—they experience a severe fear response and want to get out of the room. Those without PTSD are able to sit and see that the movies are not a real threat. The difference is that part of that orbitofrontal cortex does not work properly in the vets with PTSD. The hippocampus is also part of the problem—it's essential in transmitting messages from the amygdala to the OFC so that the higher road is possible. But too much adrenaline and norepinephrine interfere with, in fact damage, the hippocampus, so it's less likely to engage the OFC.

The emotional brain is highly subject to conditioning of the Pavlovian variety. You remember Pavlov: Give a dog food while you ring a bell, and pretty soon the dog will start to salivate, as he would at seeing food, merely at the sound of the bell (my dog starts to drool when he hears the dog-food cabinet door being opened). The bell (or the door) has become a *conditioned stimulus* for salivation. Salivation is an endocrine response triggered by messages from the unconscious part of the brain; it's involuntary. We can't control it, but it does turn off when we see there is no food. In the same way, we can easily associate the fear response (adrenaline coursing throughout the body, increased heart rate, sweating palms, dilating pupils, blood to the large muscles, etc.) with any circumstances that happened to be going on when something happened to make us fearful. We can't control the fear response either, but we can learn to discriminate better between real and false threats. When the emotion is powerful enough, we can make the connection through what psychologists call one-trial learning; we don't need the repetitions that Pavlov's dogs did. That's why the Vietnam vet may experience fear at the sound of helicopters; or why a panic attack in a particular place (say a tall building) makes us fearful whenever we go into a tall building from that point on. It's also why we get a warm glow when we think of our sweetie, or feel our stomach churning when we smell something that made us sick once (for me, it's shrimp). This phenomenon will be important to keep in mind later when we discuss unconscious defense mechanisms; experiences of stress in the past may lead us to avoid, deny, or dissociate from those experiences in the present, without being aware of what we're doing, which can often just make things worse for us. But the fact that the emotional brain is subject to conditioning is also cause for hope; it means that we are capable of learning new emotional connections and better ways of regulating old ones.

Neocortex: The "Logical" Brain

"Logical" is in quotes above because, as we've said, new research is showing that the neocortex, or cerebral cortex (the outer layer of the brain with all the folds and wrinkles), is intimately connected with the "emotional" brain, so much so that the distinction is hardly valid anymore. But let's maintain it for the time being, just to help us keep organized. It is true that it is the neocortex that is vastly more complicated in man than in other species. It seems to endow us with the special human qualities of abstract reasoning, induction and deduction, mathematical calculation, and so on.

A complication of the cerebral cortex is that the right and left sides of the brain differ slightly in function. Generally, the right side of the brain controls movement and sensory input from the left side of the body, while the left side of the brain controls the right side of the body. But more important is that the two hemispheres seem to think differently. These differences are somewhat subtle and subject to debate, but the popular conception that (for most people) the left side of the brain is "logical" and remembers facts, while the right side is more emotional and creative, is generally correct. For right-handed people,[1] the left brain is involved in logical and analytic thinking, especially in verbal and mathematical functions. It processes information in a linear and sequential manner, organizing information historically: this happened, then that happened, then the other thing. The right brain seems more holistic. It is specialized for taking in visual and spatial information. It's involved with spatial orientation, creative and artistic thinking, body image, and facial recognition. It processes information more impressionistically and globally than the left brain. It's responsible for social intelligence and the capacity to distinguish rapidly between safety and danger. The right side of the cortex is dominant during the first three years of life; it cues into the nonverbal aspects of communication, being responsible for emotional perception, body awareness, and social cognition. The left side comes into dominance later and is responsible for children's remarkable ability to absorb information during their educational years. The left side uses logical processes of the "if A then B" sort, and makes linear connections between events. It tells us when things seem right (expectable according to our understanding of the laws of nature) and seem wrong (unexplainable, paradoxical, curious). But there are some surprising findings about how the two hemispheres process emotion. The left side, the rational and logical side, seems to be involved in positive emotions, while the right side processes negative feelings like fear, anger, and disgust. It may be that the right, impressionistic side is activated in situations of danger, which we associate with those negative feelings.

Damage to the left hemisphere, as from a stroke, often results in language impairment; damage to the right may leave language alone, but interfere with the ability to remember faces or to have a clear perception of one's own body in relation to objects around it. Some people with right hemisphere damage can speak perfectly well but cannot dress themselves. But for most of us, most of the time, the two hemispheres work well together, complementing each other in ways we don't understand yet, but allowing us to perform complex tasks unconsciously once the left brain has learned the sequence. These left-right brain

---

1 These observations are true for most right-handers. Lefties have the same differentiation between the hemispheres, but are inconsistent. Some have the same pattern as right-handers, some just the opposite.

distinctions have been confirmed in animals other than man; birdsong, for instance, like man's speech, is dominated by the left hemisphere. Rats, like humans, do their sequential processing in the left brain, their spatial processing in the right.

Allan Schore, whose work we will be describing soon, suggests that it is the right hemisphere that is the seat of the unconscious, and specifically of the unconscious early representations of the self in relationship with the primary caregiver—the attachment relationship. This hypothesis makes sense given the dominance of the right side of the brain during the first three years of life. The right brain stores an "internal working model" of the attachment relationship, which becomes the basis for how we regulate emotion throughout our life. Schore offers evidence to suggest that the right brain mediates unconscious emotional responses, while the left is occupied with conscious awareness of emotions.[2] I have a strong suspicion, which I share with many others though we can't yet back it up with research, that part of our problem dealing with twenty-first-century stress is that, for the last two hundred years or so, culture has made us overuse the left brain and neglect the right. We're driven by schedules and we have to remember a lot of stuff. Our left brains must be busy as hell trying to sort and classify all the sensory experience we receive just driving down the highway, watching television, or going to the mall. We don't have the opportunity for some of the "brainless" (read right-brain) daydreaming or woolgathering that we enjoyed as children. As they say, to the man with a hammer everything looks like a nail. Perhaps we get so habituated to using the left brain that it becomes difficult for us to back off from analyzing and calculating to consider the larger picture. And I think that one of the ways an activity like mindfulness meditation helps us is to put us in touch with the right brain, allowing us to distance ourselves from all our frenetic left-brain activity by viewing things from the more impressionistic perspective of the right.

The neocortex is responsible for the "top-down" executive functioning of the brain: observing, monitoring, investigating, and planning: the "high road"

---

2 You may not be aware of unconscious emotional processes because they are, after all, unconscious. We will discuss this concept in more detail later when we talk about psychodynamics, but anyone who has spent time in therapy should be aware that unconscious fear, guilt, shame, and aggression are compelling motivators in our lives. Freud spoke of making the unconscious conscious; it is recognition of the power of these unconscious feelings that has the most immediate practical benefit for us.

that allows us to modulate emotions and stress responses. While other brain centers assist in processing incoming information, it is the neocortex that allows us to formulate a plan to respond to the information, weighing both short-term and long-term consequences—a process that is usually completely unconscious, as when we are constantly analyzing and responding to incoming data while driving a car. Although other animals are also capable of complex chains of behavior—such as when stalking prey—it is "man the toolmaker" whose higher cortex allows him to learn absolutely foreign chains like driving, typing, or programming the remote (though this, for some like me, may represent the upper limit of cortical functioning).

Orbitofrontal Cortex: The Seat of the Self

The orbitofrontal cortex (OFC), the tips of the two middle fingers in Siegel's hand model of the brain, is in a unique position, only one neuron away from both thoughts and feelings, from the hormone cascade that initiates the stress response, even from brain-stem functions like heart rate, respiration, and immune response. The OFC is intimately involved with emotional responses, both their physical manifestations and what we think about them and how we experience them in consciousness—which makes sense considering how intimately the OFC is linked with the neocortex, the limbic system, the endocrine system, and the brain stem. The orbitofrontal cortex regulates the hypothalamus, which sends hormones throughout the body, and states of alertness and arousal, which are mediated by the brain stem. The OFC thus is a central regulatory structure between the three major areas of the brain, and between the brain and the body. It helps to regulate emotion and the unconscious emotional communication that goes on between people; according to Schore, it is the repository of Bowlby's internal working model (described shortly, under "The Developing Mind"), or what I call the assumptive world. The right portion of the OFC, which is enlarged, functions as an executive control system for the entire right brain. A recent journal review concludes, "The orbitofrontal cortex is involved in critical human functions, such as social adjustment and the control of mood, drive, and responsibility, traits that are crucial in defining the 'personality' of an individual." The structure and functioning of the OFC are thought to be highly dependent on the imprinting function of the mother in regulating the infant's emotional state; the OFC is not fully formed until the child is about eighteen months old, and keeps developing through childhood.

Along with other structures the OFC is deeply involved in autobiographical memory, self-awareness, and what psychologists call "theory of mind." This is the ability to use our own knowledge of our motivations to picture the world from another's point of view, which perhaps is a distinctly human ability. You can see this developing in children, ironically enough, when they try out their first lies on us at two or three—lying means they have become self-aware enough to realize that they know things we don't. Logically, then, the OFC is also implicated in the development of a sense of right and wrong. It seems to be essential to our sense of our own identity through its connections with the hippocampus and autobiographical memory.

Scientists who study the effects of childhood emotional trauma believe that one of its most devastating effects is to interfere with the connection between the right and left sides of the orbitofrontal cortex. Normally, emotional memories are retrieved by the right orbitofrontal cortex and encoded by the left. REM sleep is essential for this integration of memory. But when trauma interferes with the connection, a stable and coherent conception of the self cannot be fully developed; our story of our self is incoherent, confusing, unstable. There may be memories of childhood, but they are cut off from their emotional meanings; the adult may never be able to develop the ability to make sense of his or her emotional experience or to empathize with and understand the behavior of others. In adults with lesions in these brain areas, there is severe impairment of the ability to follow common social rules and cues. When the OFC has been stressed because of psychological trauma, it becomes weakened in its ability to divert emotional signals from the low road of automatic response to the high road of thoughtful response.

Other effects of childhood trauma are also devastating to the OFC and other structures of the brain. The OFC's responsiveness to neurotransmitters like serotonin, dopamine, and opiates may be permanently reduced, confusing the body's response to pain and pleasure, perhaps contributing to problems with chronic pain and vulnerability to addiction. The corpus callosum, the connection between the hemispheres, is damaged or impaired. The cerebellum, which provides a soothing function to the limbic system, is damaged. The hippocampus may be shrunken, impairing the ability to process explicit memory. These effects are the result not of physical, but emotional trauma, likely caused by the excess production of stress hormones such as cortisol, which can kill nerve cells.

There is evidence to suggest that it's not just trauma, but constant everyday stress, that can activate the low road more and more often. Then, under the principle that "neurons that fire together wire together," the low road of fear, irritability, lack of insight, poor judgment, or disorganized or aggressive behavior comes to feel normal. The Perpetual Stress Response programs us to behave more childishly and impulsively, making it less likely that we'll find peace, trapping us in the central vicious circle of perpetual stress.

The OFC is also implicated in overall mood. Richard Davidson has been studying the relative activity of the left and right lobes of the prefrontal cortex—an area that includes the OFC—and has found that more activity on the right is associated with unpleasant or depressed moods, while more activity on the left means happiness and enthusiasm. People who consistently have greater activity on the left typically have few troubling moods and recover rapidly when they do. In one rather famous example, Davidson tested an advanced Buddhist monk, highly skilled in meditation, and found that he had the greatest difference between left and right lobe activity of anyone yet tested.

The Brain and the Stress Response

Robert Sapolsky's wonderfully readable book *Why Zebras Don't Get Ulcers* is the best overview of how stress affects us physically. I'm summarizing here what he, and some other experts, have to say. These scientists who study the effects of stress on the body have found virtually the same pattern in all mammals, so our frightened impala, the lab rat, and the programmer working twelve-hour days have a great deal in common. One similarity we share is what scientists call the "dose effect" of stress—a little is good, too much is bad. This is due to how stress hormones affect the body.

When a stressful event occurs, or when we perceive danger, the brain immediately signals the release of hypothalamic, pituitary, and adrenal hormones. It signals the adrenal glands (just above the kidneys) to release cortisol and adrenaline, and the sympathetic nervous system to release norepinephrine all over the body. As a result, your heart beats faster, the hairs on the back of your neck stand up, you sweat, your stomach churns, and your bowels loosen. These same chemicals increase blood pressure so that oxygen and glucose can be delivered to muscles and other tissues that will need them; prompt the spleen to release more red blood cells, again helping deliver more oxygen to the muscles; prompt the liver to produce more glucose for quick energy; make the lungs take in more oxygen; release endorphins to dull pain; and constrict the blood vessels to reduce bleeding (this is what makes your hair stand on end). Sapolsky says, "in a fight-or-flight scenario, epinephrine [adrenaline] is the one handing out the guns; glucocorticoids [cortisol, etc.] are the ones drawing up blueprints for new aircraft carriers." Adrenaline acts within seconds, while cortisol and other glucocorticoids work over minutes or hours. Cortisol also impacts the immune system, sending immune cells into storage convenient to where they will be needed most. Your vision improves, your attention is focused, your memory improves, and you feel alert and powerful. This is a marvelous, complex orchestration of the body to help us deal with danger. After the danger is passed, there is another complex regulatory system that returns things to normal. This process of maintaining equilibrium is referred to as allostasis. When we feel that the danger does not go away, the mechanisms underlying allostasis get damaged, and we lose the ability to return ourselves to normal.

I've alluded to the HPA (hypothalamic-pituitary-adrenal) axis above. We have learned over the last twenty years that this response is triggered not only when we see external danger, but also by our own immune system. Cytokines, which are proteins produced by immune system cells, trigger the hypothalamus to signal the pituitary to secrete another stress hormone, ACTH. The presence of ACTH prompts the adrenals to produce more cortisol. High levels of cortisol shut off the production of cytokines—which makes sense, under normal conditions; it's the system returning to allostasis. But when cortisol levels remain high, as they do under chronic stress, cytokines are not available to perform their major function, which is to fight infection. One study found that small wounds took an average of nine days longer to heal among people taking care of a loved one with Alzheimer's, compared to a matched control group.

Bruce McEwen and his colleagues have demonstrated the effects of continuing stress on lab rats by confining them in small cages during their normal resting periods. At first, their cortisol level spiked up normally, the usual stress response. But as the rats became accustomed to restraint, their cortisol production switched off sooner each day. After twenty-one days, the rats began to show the effects of chronic stress. Their immune systems were compromised. They became anxious and aggressive. Nerve cells in the hippocampus atrophied (see Figure 9), and the production of new stem cells in the hippocampus stopped. The same effects have been shown in the human hippocampus.

So these stress hormones serve vital purposes in helping us cope with danger, but prolonged exposure is damaging to many parts of the body. Too much cortisol thins the lining of the stomach (making us vulnerable to ulcers), thins

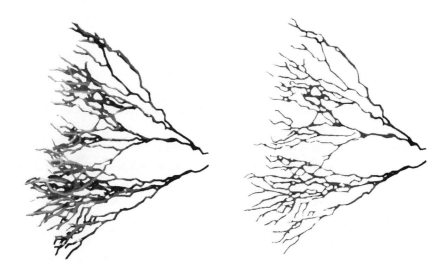

Neurons from the rat hippocampus, before and after a stress induction experiment. (After Sapolsky, 1968.) (Credit: Kerry Gavin Studio)

Figure 9

the bones, and damages the reproductive system; it suppresses the immune system, kills immune cells, and makes us vulnerable to infection. It interferes with how we store fat, sending more of it to the abdomen, which is not only unsightly but is also a greater health threat than other kinds of fat.[3] We turn to sugar and other comfort foods because they actually put a brake on the chronic stress response, but we put on weight and damage our health. Other stress hormones interfere with the production of growth hormones and insulin; without growth hormone, adults are more vulnerable to fragile bones and, without insulin, to diabetes. Monkeys under social stress are likely to die from excess cor-

---

3 Cortisol sounds like a killer, but in the form of cortisone it has saved me from many a painful itch; and with other steroids in inhalable form it saves many lives from asthma. Like everything else in the body, its damage and benefits depend on why, where, when, how much is used.

tisol secretion, which damages the hippocampus as well as the heart and stom-ach. People with PTSD are more likely to smoke, because nicotine releases dopamine, a neurotransmitter with calming effects on the brain. Men in com-bat training have lower testosterone levels; women in the same situation stop menstruating. Prolonged stress damages the memory centers of the brain, in-cluding the hippocampus, the one area that we know can produce new brain cells in the adult. Dendrites in the hippocampus become shriveled. Cortisol shuts down the immune cells' response to germs and viruses, making us more susceptible to infection.

Cortisol functions as a brake on the immune system. This means that too much of it interferes with the immune response, which is why people under chronic stress are more vulnerable to colds and other infections. Too little cor-tisol can let the immune system run away with itself, resulting in autoimmune disorders and allergies. Normally, cortisol level rises in the morning and sub-sides in the evening, allowing us to sleep naturally. People under chronic stress, however, often have higher than normal cortisol levels or lose the rhythm of the natural daily cycle. When cortisol is more or less at a constant level, our rhythms are disrupted and we have insomnia. When cortisol is con-stantly too high, the brain itself—the hippocampus—becomes damaged. Be-cause the hippocampus is essential in turning off the stress response, when it's damaged severely enough we are stuck in the Perpetual Stress Response.

When we get to Chapter 9, "Getting Along with Your Body," we'll have more time to understand the connections between the brain and other systems—the endocrine and immune system, the nervous and muscular systems—that explain why difficult circumstances in childhood or emotional trauma in adulthood can do things to us like cause ulcers, back pain, allergies, fibromyalgia, rheumatoid arthritis, depression, and anxiety. But for now let's talk about the mind, which I like to think of as the music that the brain plays. Unfortunately, trauma and stress can make our music sound more like nails on a blackboard than a Mozart concerto.

The Developing Mind

Understanding how the minds of children develop, in both near-ideal and stressful situations, can give us important clues to how we can protect ourselves from the Perpetual Stress Response and how we can heal ourselves and recover from the damage already done. Though observational studies of mothers and children, and studies of the development of abused and neglected children, or clinical studies of traumatized adults, don't have that hard-edge high-tech sterile lab glamour of brain functioning, they have become sophisticated enough and numerous enough over the last few decades that we can draw some very definite conclusions. Then drawing the connections between those conclusions and what we know about the brain empowers us to find the path to recovery.

What we experience as our "self" develops in early childhood *out of our need to control our emotions.* Think about how an infant is possessed by feeling: any upset is expressed with cries, which build into screams if unanswered; with agitation expressed by the whole body; with increased heart rate, shortness of breath, reddening of the skin—the whole stress response. Babies, at first, have virtually no ability to calm themselves down; they need soothing from the adults around them. Learning to soothe the self, to control emotions, is the primary task of infancy.

The infant's relationship with the mother[4] serves as the model of an emotion-regulating system that develops into the child's own self. Mothers who are sufficiently attuned to the child's emotional state help the child calm down when overstimulated, perk up when apathetic, regain a sense of safety when frightened, and so on. But many mothers are either unresponsive to the child's needs or inconsistent (stimulating the child when they feel like it, unresponsive at other times). Other mother-child combinations are just a "bad fit"—an energetic, demanding child paired with a mildly depressed mother; a quiet, undemanding child of an overworked, distracted mother.

Attachment research is a relatively new field in psychology and child development that has enormous implications for our purposes here. It developed from the writings of British pediatrician and psychoanalyst John Bowlby, noted for his creative work with children, especially those who had been separated from their parents for long periods, because of illness or the dislocations of wartime. Bowlby was interested in the evolutionary purposes of human behavior, and he focused on the meaning of the child's staying so close to its

---

4 I'm going to say "mother" because that is the common, natural human experience; but it would be more correct to refer to "primary caregiver" because fathers, grandparents, wet nurses, adoptive parents, anyone with the necessary dedication can provide these vital functions for the infant. There doesn't seem to be anything other than nursing that the birth mother can give the child that others can't—no genetic imprint, no sixth sense.

mother during the first few years of life. (At roughly the same time, Harry Harlow in the United States was demonstrating that infant monkeys sought something more than food from their mothers; given a choice between a "mother" made of wire mesh but providing milk and a "mother" made of cloth and a hot water bottle, baby monkeys invariably clung to the cloth mother, going to the wire mother only for brief periods to eat.) Bowlby described for the first time the intricacies of communication between infant and mother, the smiling, playing, and comforting that goes into creating what he called a "holding environment" for the child. He described children's reactions to being separated from their mother and noted that some children seemed to tolerate separations well, while others were markedly distressed, and still others became withdrawn and aloof. Bowlby speculated that something about the mother's interaction with the child determined the child's reactions to separation, and he speculated further that the child's reactions to separation would have repercussions twenty, forty, sixty years later in the adult's character, temperament, and reactions to stress. More generally, Bowlby is credited with focusing scientific attention on the relationship between infant and mother—the "attachment relationship"—as forming the basis of the child's developing socioemotional mind; the most basic postulates, rules, and structure of how we conceptualize the world, which he called an "internal working model." Now we are beginning to understand how the brain, the organ of the mind, develops the connections and structure that are the foundation for the internal working model.

Mary Ainsworth, a Canadian researcher, set out to investigate Bowlby's speculations. She developed an observational procedure known, poetically enough, as the Strange Situation: a room with toys in which mother, infant, and a stranger would interact, with the mother leaving the room twice for brief periods during the observation. The first time she would leave the baby alone with the stranger, then return; then the stranger would leave, then the mother, finally leaving the baby alone altogether (for a very brief period). It was the child's reactions to the mother's returns that were of most interest. Ainsworth and her colleagues determined that infants could be reliably classified into three groups, which they described as securely, avoidant, or ambivalently attached. Later researchers identified a fourth group, disorganized attached.

- Securely attached infants usually reacted to their mother's leaving with visible distress, accepted some comfort from the stranger but remained in

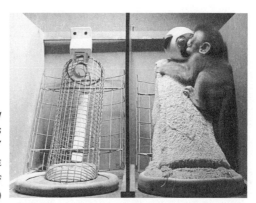

One of Harry Harlow's baby monkeys, clinging to its terrycloth surrogate "mother."
(SOURCE: HARLOW PRIMATE LABORATORY, UNIVERSITY OF WISCONSIN-MADISON.)

Figure 10

distress, and greeted the mother's return with smiling, vocalizing, or crying. They wanted to be picked up, and their distress was quickly relieved in their mother's arms.

- Avoidant infants sometimes reacted calmly to separations, sometimes with great distress. But they reacted to their mother's return as if with indifference, remaining focused on the toys in the room in solitary play. In the home sometimes these children seemed "too good."
- Ambivalent infants tended to react to separations with extreme distress, and to greet their mother's return with contradictory behavior. They wanted contact with her, but when picked up seemed angry, often kicking the mother or arching their back away from her, squirming and crying and seemingly receiving no comfort from the reunion.
- Disorganized infants reacted to separations and reunions with behavior that seemed to express intense conflict, like the ambivalent children, but did this in a highly disorganized way. There was no coherent, sequential pattern. They would approach their mother, then avoid her, then approach. When picked up they sometimes seemed angry, sometimes disinterested.

These observations have been repeated in many cultures. Securely attached infants are in the majority, with about 10 to 15 percent of children in each of the other categories. These findings would be only of passing interest, however, if it were not suspected that infant attachment has a great deal to do with adult mental health. People who were tested in infancy and found to be securely attached may be more resilient to stress as adults. They seem to be better equipped to develop satisfying relationships with other adults and to have a stable sense of self-esteem. Children who are securely attached are more curious about the world and have an expanded range of exploration. Avoidant infants when they reach their teens tend to be unpopular and avoided by their peers. Avoidant adults seem to be stuck in the left brain; they have trouble with intimacy and are not very sensitive to their own feelings or bodies. Ambivalent infants later on remain anxious and uncertain. As adults they may be preoccupied with themselves, sometimes stuck trying to make sense of leftover issues from their own pasts. Many hypochondriacs are found to be ambivalently or anxiously attached. In one high-risk sample, avoidant children tended to become victimizers as adolescents; ambivalent children tended to become victims. Disorganized infants seem to be, as adults, at highest risk for mental illness and violence; they seem to be especially vulnerable to dissociation.

A few big disclaimers are in order here. First, if children who are not securely attached in infancy remain insecure or disorganized years later, no one is suggesting that the damage was all done in the first year; in fact, follow-up studies suggest that parents remain largely consistent in how they are attuned or misattuned to their child's needs. Second, there is far from a one-to-one relationship between infant behavior in the Strange Situation and adult mental health. Life offers opportunities for children to have both healing and damaging experiences as they grow up; the result is that many ambivalent infants will have perfectly fine adult relationships, and many secure infants will have their share of trouble functioning as adults. Finally, lest mothers feel that their stresses and worries during the child's infancy are to blame for his adolescent drug abuse or difficulty finding himself as an adult, there is a recognition by researchers that what is called "goodness of fit" is the operative variable. Infants vary enormously in their temperaments, and caregivers vary in their ability to respond. So a mother who might have been overwhelmed by a difficult, temperamental child if it was born first—and thus might have played into an ambivalent attachment—may take the same child in stride if it is second or third in birth order. Or a different mother might have been spoiled by an easy firstborn, then surprised, overwhelmed, and self-blaming when dealing with a difficult second child.

Some optimistic news: Recent research has shown that, even if a relationship with one caregiver is highly disturbed, a relationship with another caregiver can provide that secure attachment that the child needs. Thus mother, father, grandmother, or others in the home can offset any problems associated with one caregiver. Researchers have also demonstrated that mothers can be rather easily helped to provide a more secure attachment through a group intervention based in the child's preschool. Depressed parents can help their children gain resilience through specific programs designed to help the child express his feelings about the parent's illness.

Perhaps the worst news about this research is that it seems that parents may transmit trauma through generations. The amount of stress a female rat is exposed to during pregnancy influences the amount of cortisol and other glucocorticoids that reach the fetus, altering the structure and function of that fetal rat's hippocampus in adulthood. Human infants who are classified as "disorganized-attached" apparently are disorganized because their caregivers are unable to provide soothing when the infant experiences fear. Because it is an instinct for the infant to approach the caregiver for safety, when the caregiver responds to the infant's needs with fearful, angry, or unpredictable responses of his or her own, the infant has nowhere to go. The baby is left alone with fear, with no source of comfort, his own instinct to turn to the parent for help betraying him. Caregivers who themselves are coping with the aftereffects of trauma or unresolved grief are most likely to be unable to provide appropriate attunement to the needs of a frightened child. And, as we've mentioned, these disorganized children seem to be at serious risk of mental health problems and violence in adulthood. Anxious parents create anxiety in their children. An analysis of videotaped interactions of parents helping children with a homework task showed that parents with anxiety disorders disagreed with their children more, ignored them more, and praised them less, than a matched control group. Further, when the children became anxious, the parents switched from withdrawal to overcontrol, apparently trying to squelch their children's anxiety.

Mother and infant who are in a securely attached relationship, when they are in a connected state, perhaps cooing or singing, are in a deeply symbiotic, primitive, instinctual state that has its echoes in cats licking their newborns and birds sitting on their nests. This is a union of two limbic systems, two brains communicating with each other without consciousness of what is being communicated. The mother is *imprinting* herself on the child's brain, "a very rapid form of learning that irreversibly stamps early experience upon the developing nervous system." Research shows that mother's and infant's heartbeats become synchronous. Their emotions, too, become synchronous, and the mother imprints emotional regulation on the child—for good or ill. This doesn't mean that the primary caregiver has to be happy or carefree or have terrific self-esteem or be intelligent or successful or available 24/7 for the infant. But he or she has to be available enough, and have the ability to merge into that deep connected state, and pay attention and respond to the child's changing needs. The most important competence on a mother's part, as Siegel has mysteriously put it, is the ability to form a "coherent autonoetic narrative"—the ability to *know herself* (autonoesis) as a consistent and predictable being anchored in relationships. Diana Fosha's language is more clear: a mother needs "an internal working model where affect and relatedness, self and other, and feeling and dealing all can operate in harmony."

The infant has the beginnings of a neural network that will embody how he will know about himself—perceiving, feeling, understanding—located in the two halves of the OFC, with projections into the limbic system and the higher cortex. Through this imprinting communication with the primary caregiver (and others) this neural network becomes built around what Siegel calls the self-as-perceived-by-the-other (*Wow, everybody loves me! I must be HOT!*).[5] As the child explores his world, there is also a growing self-as-perceived-by-the-self (*I can make that breast appear just by yelling. I can control the WORLD!*). As the child ages, of course, there are frustrations and disappointments that temper those initial grandiose feelings, though we want the child (and the adult) to retain the ability to get in touch with those feelings at appropriate times later in life. But those frustrations and disappointments become built in to the neural network that represents the self. As that happens, if the child is experiencing too much disparity between the self-as-perceived-by-the-other and the self-as-perceived-by-the-self, a structural weakness forms in that neural network. If you view the network as a tower built of steel beams, there is an area where some beams were left out, which will be permanently vulnerable to stress. Thus, if the self-as-perceived-by-the-self is just too young for trauma—still too grandiose and unprepared—something like a physical injury to the body may be permanently devastating if the self-as-perceived-by-the-other is not responsive and caring, *validating* the child's experience. We'll have more to say about validating communication later on in Chapter 10.

It's important to recognize that the caregivers do not have to protect the

---

5 Please excuse my feeble attempt to put into words what the child, of course, has no words for, what in fact are experiences so inchoate that they are beyond words.

child from trauma or milder frustrations or disappointments so much as signal that they understand how the child feels. When they can do that, the self-as-perceived-by-the-other and the self-as-perceived-by-the-self remain in harmony, and the neural network that contains the child's representation of himself continues to be built of solid material with solid connections. The child's experience of himself is coherent, and he is building that *coherent autobiographical narrative*[6] (you're going to keep hearing about this) that is his perception of himself and is physically present in the brain in that neural network in the OFC and elsewhere.

An interesting result came when scientists had the opportunity to study the effects of wealth on children's mental health. In 1996, a group of impoverished Cherokee Indians in the Great Smoky Mountains began to receive income from a casino that opened on the reservation. By 2001, each tribe member was receiving $12,000 a year, and other economic conditions had greatly improved. The researchers discovered that, compared to the years before the study, children and adolescents experienced significantly fewer emotional problems after their family income rose. After much analysis, the investigators found that only one variable accounted for the change: level of parental supervision. The wealthier parents had more time and energy to invest in their children, and it showed.

In a nutshell: if you want to be an emotionally healthy adult, your chances are better if, when you were an infant, you had a close, secure relationship with a consistent caregiver who had a stable and healthy identity. And the reason is that it takes that kind of relationship to grow a brain that works—one that allows you to express, without being overwhelmed by, your own emotions; to soothe yourself in times of distress; to understand yourself and other people; to form intimate bonds with others. So where are we today? If, as I'm arguing, today's mothers and fathers are caught up in the Perpetual Stress Response, their nervous systems fried, working too many hours, their self-confidence dissolved by anxiety, their ability to focus impaired, their ability to experience and modulate emotion damaged, what does that say for the future of the children of 2000? Can parents imprint the Perpetual Stress Response on their children in infancy, resulting in school-age children who are unable to control themselves and interact with others? And what will happen to this generation as it grows up?

---

6 I'm substituting "autobiographical" for "autonoetic" because it's less obscure; but "autonoetic" is really a more accurate term because it suggests all ways of knowing and perceiving, while "autobiographical" is exclusively a left-brain concept.

Putting Mind and Brain Together

Allan N. Schore, a highly respected neurological scientist and practicing psychoanalyst, has published an enormous and groundbreaking body of work tracing the connections between infant attachment, brain development, and adult mental health. His central thesis is that the early social environment, principally the relationship with the primary caregiver, directly influences the final wiring of the circuits in the infant brain that are responsible for the future social and emotional coping capacities of the adult. One of the reasons I am attracted to Schore's work is that he is able to account for and explain many of the observations that alert psychotherapists had discovered independently: for instance, that the majority of adults labeled "borderline" were abused as children or experienced severe disruptions in early attachment; or that many adults with addictive problems seemed to have had cold or emotionally unavailable caregivers; or that many adults with autoimmune disorders were sexually abused as children. Since these were only retrospective data, responsible therapists held back from suggesting that child abuse "caused" borderline personality or autoimmune disease, or that parental rejection was linked to substance abuse. Schore, by virtue of his encyclopedic knowledge of the literature from diverse fields—attachment research, longitudinal child development studies, brain research—has been able to provide strong support for a causative link at work. Here's the bottom line:

Negative childhood experience—not only trauma and neglect, but also simply a poor relationship between caregiver and child—results in:

- *Damage to the structure of the brain itself*, **and hence:**
- **Damage to the adult's ability to experience and control emotions**
- **Damage to the adult's ability to have a self-concept of confidence and stability**
- **Damage to the adult's ability to protect the body from psychological stress**
- **Damage to the adult's ability to develop rewarding relationships**
- **Damage to the adult's ability to focus, concentrate, and learn**
- **Damage to the adult's capacity for self-control**

Many studies support these conclusions:

- A study of four groups of women (one group with current major depression and a history of childhood abuse; one group with current major depression and no abuse history; one with a history of abuse but no current depression; and a fourth group with no history of abuse and no current depression) exposed them all to a common stressful event (delivering a ten-minute speech and performing a mental arithmetic test in front of an audience). Measures of stress-related hormone levels and heart rate were taken during the speech. It was found that abused women, both with and without current depression, experienced significantly higher stress-hormone levels and heart rate during and after the speech than did those without a history of abuse; but women with both a history of abuse and current depression had the highest levels of any group. The implication is that early abuse leads to lasting change in how the body responds to stress, leaving one more or less permanently vulnerable to development of mood or anxiety disorders and to stress-related disease.
- A study of male combat veterans with PTSD found that, compared to controls, all had elevated levels of norepinephrine in their cerebrospinal fluid; further, that the worse their symptoms were, the higher their norepinephrine level was.
- Bremner and his study group have consistently found that both the left and right hippocampus are significantly reduced in size and damaged in function among women with a history of childhood abuse and current PTSD.
- A study comparing sexually abused girls to nonabused controls found that the abused girls had altered regulatory dynamics of their neuroendocrine systems, different neuroendocrine responses to stressors, and oversecretion of corticotrophin-releasing hormone (CRH) that resulted in a reduction of CRH receptors in the anterior pituitary.
- Childhood abuse and neglect apparently interfere with the growth of GABA calming fibers from the cerebellum to the hypothalamus and limbic systems—fibers whose function appears to be helping to calm emotional irritability.
- Bruce Posner and his study group at Cornell have found reliable evidence that adults with borderline personality disorder respond to purely cognitive tasks with more anxiety and confusion than other people do, though

their success rate is about the same. The suggestion is that this is linked to child abuse experiences between the ages of two and seven, when the anterior cingulate is being fully formed. This is the brain structure that allows us to pay attention to some stimuli while ignoring others.

- Studies in rats have consistently shown that infant rats who receive more licking and grooming from their mothers are less fearful and more intelligent as adults, have better immune systems, and are more attentive mothers themselves.

Until now we've been talking about biology and psychology. For another perspective on the connections between childhood experience and adult health, let's look at public health. The Adverse Childhood Experiences (ACE) study is a project following more than seventeen thousand members of the Kaiser Permanente Health Plan in the San Diego area. The researchers have documented the incidence of seven kinds of "adverse" childhood experiences (psychological, physical, and sexual abuse; substance abuse, mental illness, domestic violence, and criminal behavior in the home) and compared them to the adult health status of the participants. The participants average fifty-seven years old, so we are talking about a *long* time for these effects to show.

The first significant finding was how common these childhood experiences are. In this middle-class sample, slightly more than half of the participants had had some form of adverse experience; one in four had two; one in sixteen had four. The researchers imply that the participants were quite willing to talk about these experiences, despite social taboos, but that no one had ever asked them before. More participants reported childhood sexual abuse (22 percent) than reported psychological (11.1 percent) or physical (10.8 percent) abuse, a surprising and troubling result. But the most common problem was substance abuse in the home (25.6 percent). The second finding was how frequently these experiences were connected: if a child had experienced physical abuse it was quite likely he or she had also been exposed to substance abuse or family violence. The surprising, if not shocking, high incidence of these experiences—again, in a middle-class sample—suggests that what we think of as "normal," in the sense of the popular conception of how things are supposed to be, is vastly different from statistical normal. Families in general, perhaps in reaction to the growing but unacknowledged impact of social stress, are a lot more troubled than we want to believe they are.

The eye-popping finding was how much impact these childhood experiences apparently had on adult *physical* health. In almost all the categories they measured, the researchers found that, quite simply, the more adverse childhood experiences a person had, the worse his adult health was. These effects were all statistically significant. So the more abuse or exposure to family malfunction you suffered as a child, the greater your risk for:

smoking	diabetes
obesity	alcoholism
no leisure physical activity	drug use
(being a couch potato)	injecting drugs
depression	promiscuous sex (fifty partners
suicide attempt	or more)
heart disease	sexually transmitted disease
stroke	broken bones
chronic lung disease	hepatitis

Some of this is no surprise. It makes sense that if you had an abusive childhood, you're at higher risk for depression or alcoholism. If you had poor role models, you might be at higher risk for being a couch potato or engaging in promiscuous sex. And we know that heart disease is linked to stress. But where do diabetes, stroke, and broken bones come into the picture? Some of the odds ratios themselves are astounding. In this study, if you had four or more adverse childhood experiences, you were 460 percent more likely to be depressed, and 1,220 percent more likely to have attempted suicide, than someone who had none.

Many readers may be objecting at this point—"This is all very well, but I picked up this book because I've got troubles, and as far as I can remember I wasn't abused or neglected." Let me say a couple of things: (1) I've talked to an amazing number of adults who recount dreadful childhood experiences without the awareness that they are talking about emotional abuse. We think of abuse as happening in only certain kinds of families. But being called names, being told you're stupid, being yelled at when you did nothing wrong, being given the cold shoulder when you displeased a parent—if these are consistent patterns, they are emotional abuse in my book. (2) Experiences of abuse or neglect are much more common than any of us feel comfortable admitting. In the general population of women, the incidence of childhood sexual abuse has been found to range from 22 to 37 percent. Again, what we think of as cultur-

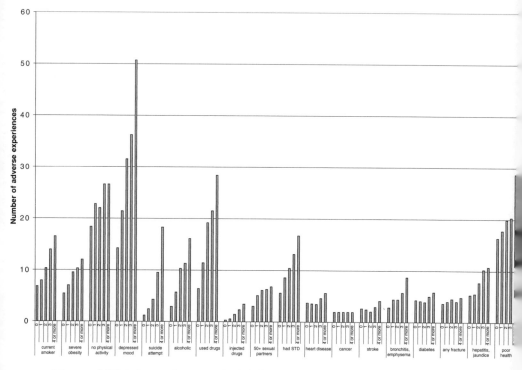

Adverse childhood experiences and adult health outcomes. Almost every adult illness except cancer is significantly related to the number of adverse experiences in childhood.
(SOURCE: FELITTI, ET AL., 1998.)

Figure 11

ally "normal" may be in fact very different from statistical normal. (3) We may be talking about very subtle effects here. A depressed or overworked mother can be emotionally neglectful though full of love and good intentions. A critical father with high standards may be fine for a resilient kid, but perceived as abusive by someone more insecure. Animal studies are relevant: Rats and other animals, separated at birth from their mothers for just a few minutes at a time, have their stress responses compromised. Well into adult life these rats will respond to stress with increased levels of stress hormones, making them more at risk for autoimmune disease. People who have a history of abuse or abandonment before age ten have the same increased stress hormone response. Babies from Romanian orphanages who were adopted before the age of four months appeared to have normal stress responses, but those who were adopted after eight months had lasting elevations in stress hormone levels.

*   *   *

Let me restate the argument: our nervous systems were not designed for twenty-first-century stress. We're full of adrenaline and anxiety, unable to relax, unable to concentrate—but strangely unaware of our condition. When it comes to raising our children, our anxiety and uncertainty impair our ability to be good parents. We can be inconsistent. We can be too angry. We can be too controlling. We can turn to substance abuse for relief, but that will impair our judgment. We may not be careful enough to protect our children as we should. Unfortunately, it's too easy for us to inflict damage on our children that will have its effects—emotional, neurological, and physical—throughout the child's life.

Psychological Trauma

One of the greatest changes in the field of psychotherapy in the past thirty years has been the growing recognition of the effects of psychological trauma on how we function. It is especially in trauma-related studies that we are beginning to see a convergence of the hard data of brain functioning with the practice wisdom of clinical psychology. There is a better understanding of just how frequent trauma *is*, and a greater interest in how it affects both the brain and the mind. There is a recognition that childhood trauma has different effects than adult trauma; that repeated or chronic trauma—which is all too often the case in childhood—is different yet from the impact of a single traumatic event. And of course, it is very hard to draw a line between trauma and stress, especially between repeated trauma and ongoing stress. In what follows I want to be careful not to assume too quickly that the conclusions of trauma-related studies apply to the effects of the Perpetual Stress Response; but at the same time we must consider that the effects of everyday stress in today's culture may be so severe that they add up to chronic trauma.

It was the aftermath of the Vietnam War that woke us up to the effects of trauma. That war seemed to result in an unusually high proportion of veterans with symptoms that were described in other wars as "shell shock" or "combat fatigue." Why so many more in Vietnam is unknown,[7] but the reasons are most

---

7 Of course, we don't really know whether Vietnam resulted in more PTSD reactions than previous wars, because we weren't looking for it in the same way. But it seems very likely that Vietnam experiences were harder on the vets than in previous wars, for the reasons cited here.

likely due to the moral conflicts the nation and many of the soldiers felt about the war; the unusually stressful combat conditions, in which it was often difficult to identify who was a threat; and the military's changed rotation system, which interfered with unit morale. Since then, however, the same syndrome has been recognized among accident and crime victims, notably battered women, survivors of sexual assault, and adult survivors of childhood sexual assault.

The formal diagnosis of post-traumatic stress disorder that was agreed on after Vietnam requires that the person have been exposed to a situation that threatened death or serious injury to self or others, and that the emotional response at the time have been intense fear, helplessness, or horror. The traumatic event then lives on as intrusive memories or symptoms. PTSD occurs even among those who *choose* to expose themselves to trauma, such as rescue workers. A study of more than two hundred individuals who had responded to a major plane crash found that, compared to other rescue workers, there were much higher rates of PTSD and depression even after thirteen months. Those who were younger and single were more vulnerable.

People with PTSD are in a chronic state of stress. The amygdala's danger-sensing system is stuck in the "on" position. The hippocampus, which normally helps us tell the difference between real danger and safety, is damaged by excess stress hormones, and is unable to switch off the amygdala. In fact, stress has opposite effects in the amygdala and hippocampus. Stress facilitates long-term potentiation in the amygdala; the neurons there sprout new branches, strengthening and generalizing the fear response. But in the hippocampus, stress interferes with long-term potentiation, damaging neurons and making it more difficult to put memories of the stressful situation away into long-term memory. Acute stress normally activates the stress hormone cortisol, which helps to turn off other somatic reactions caused by stress. But in PTSD, there is a chronically low level of cortisol and a chronic overproduction of norepinephrine; the combination of the two means a permanent state of high arousal. Thus people with PTSD are hypervigilant and always anxious; they overreact to current stimuli in ways that may appear impulsive or antisocial. Not aware that the stress is caused by old trauma, they are likely to blame current events and alienate those who care about them. Not understanding their own behavior, they feel helpless and out of control. Not able to soothe themselves, they turn to substance abuse or other pathological self-soothing mechanisms like mutilation or bingeing and purging. PTSD was probably much more common among our ancestors, who were exposed to physical danger all the time; but since no one lived long enough to suffer much in the way of long-term consequences, there was no evolutionary pressure to change the stress response. Besides, being in a hypervigilant state when danger is all around you is a good thing. Being hypervigilant when you're stuck in traffic or at home trying to play with the kids is a very bad thing.

PTSD directly affects the brain's memory centers. With PTSD, we keep *reliving* the experience, with all its sounds, smells, physical sensations, panic, fear, and confusion. Normal memories get processed, encoded, and stored by the brain as a story that captures the essence of what happened. But if you ask a PTSD survivor to tell you what happened, he can't do it very well. His memory is spotty and confused. You won't be able to understand the sequence of events and their effect on him. This is because the hippocampus was so flooded with stress hormones during and after the trauma that it was unable to perform its normal function of consolidating memory, taking the emotional memory and the historical memory and putting them into a coherent form that can be filed away in long-term memory. A recent study shows very clearly that in PTSD patients traumatic memories are stored in the right brain, the emotional, no-boundaries brain, whereas in non-PTSD patients traumatic memories are stored in the left. The PTSD experience is like the distinction between remembering and dreaming. When I remember an experience, I remain conscious that I am in the present, looking back on the past. When I dream, I'm not conscious of dreaming; whatever "I" exists is in the dream. This is the experience of reliving in PTSD.

The dissociative experiences that are so familiar with traumatic stress are partially a result of damage to the memory centers. These include feelings of depersonalization (feeling detached from current experience, or "spacing out," forgetting that one is in a particular situation and becoming absorbed in internal stimuli), derealization (feeling that current perceptions are somehow not quite real), amnesia (absence of memory of events that would normally be remembered), and problems with absorption (becoming so involved with a particular activity that time seems to stop or other activities are forgotten). Although these symptoms sound dramatic, many people are not aware of them in the moment, or dismiss them as quirks with no real meaning—part of the defensive effort to avoid experience of the trauma. Indeed, the classic dissociative symptoms include hysterical paralysis and other psychosomatic symptoms observed by Sigmund Freud and Pierre Janet—often accompanied by *"la belle indifference,"* the curious detachment with which some hysterical patients view their disability.

Yet all these symptoms do not capture the heart of the problem with PTSD, which is that the individual *does not realize he has PTSD*. He keeps reexperiencing the trauma, perhaps as nightmares, flashbacks, or physical pain; or he keeps avoiding the experience through dissociation, isolation, or phobic avoidance; but because the trauma has disrupted the memory functions of the brain *he thinks these symptoms are caused by present events.* He's reliving the past in the present.

In addition, all the dissociative symptoms are frequently associated with problems with identity or the self—pervasive feelings of being unreal, different, "weird." In child abuse studies, we find that higher rates of dissociative behaviors are correlated to more severe and longer-lasting childhood trauma, multiple perpetrators, and younger age of the victim. This makes sense if we remember that the cerebral cortex and the orbitofrontal cortex—the areas associated with healthier, more mature ways to deal with stress—are still very much under construction in childhood. Childhood sexual abuse seems to result in problems with dissociation more often than physical abuse. Conditions that interfere with the individual's ability to express negative feelings at the time of, or in subsequent reexperiencing of, the trauma seem also to be a causal factor in dissociation: threats of violence if the "secret" is told; cognitive dissonance (it's hard to believe); emotional dissonance (the perpetrator is loved by the victim); others' denial that the traumatic events really happened. Dissociation thus may be a learned response, a means of controlling the fear, rage, and shame associated with the trauma.

Freud's greatest error was his unwillingness to accept the reality of childhood trauma, especially sexual abuse. His patients were largely Viennese women from respectable, educated families. When they began telling him, in indirect ways, their family secrets (often of incest) Freud was horrified. But at first he believed his patients, and developed his treatment approach to deal as we would today with repressed trauma—that is, to bring it into consciousness in a safe and supporting setting. To his everlasting discredit, however, he later succumbed to the social pressure not to believe his patients' stories, and developed the entire Oedipal theory in response: it's not that parents are seductive or abusive to their children; rather, children have a natural sex drive that focuses on the opposite-sexed parent; and this is so shameful to them that they have to repress their desires below the level of consciousness, though they continue to experience unconscious guilt. In fact, children *do* have a sex drive, and we *do* experience unconscious guilt; but generations of women (and men) in analytic treatment were told to deny their memories of abuse and blame themselves for their own incestuous wishes.

So PTSD, which almost by definition is the reaction to a single traumatic event—or closely related events, such as serving in wartime—damages the brain's memory centers and puts us into a state of constant fight-or-flight. What is the reaction to chronic trauma—of growing up in an abusive home, of being married to an abusive partner, of living in a concentration camp? We've already talked about its effects on the brain (earlier in this chapter, under "The Brain and the Stress Response"), though you can multiply those effects depending on the severity and duration of the trauma. The effects on the mind are equally horrible—blaming the self, being unable to trust, being unable to be comforted, feeling out of control, the depression of learned helplessness, the paralysis of the will that comes from years of denying your most basic wants and needs.

We'll go on with these issues later in Chapter 7, when we take up the question of what to do about PTSD. For now, let's consider a case history that exemplifies some of the questions we've been exploring; then with that case in mind, we'll talk about how psychotherapy works.

Natalie: Putting a Life Together

Natalie contacted me a few years ago after having read Undoing Depression. *She described a difficult relationship with her teenage son and problems around the divorce from her husband, which had been going on for two years. She talked about a long history of depression, going back to childhood, and a current pattern of alcohol abuse. She had been in treatment several times and had been on many antidepressants, with little success.*

Natalie is the youngest child in her family. She grew up in the east until she was ten, at which point her mother divorced her father and moved the children to the West Coast. Natalie felt alone and terrified. The neighbor children beat her up, and her mother didn't protect her. A month after the move, Natalie attempted suicide, swallowing a poison from under the sink. She ran outside and a neighbor found her.

In Natalie's words:

Mom was interested in men. She liked dating and living with different men. I had four or five men living with us while we grew up. Two of them she married. Two of them were physically abusive to my sister. My sister was overweight and one of them made fun of her regularly and the other called her "fatso." The first one beat her. The second just hit her. Mom smoked pot and her second husband was an alcoholic and drug user. She was very interested in the physical beauty of people. She told me I should get plastic surgery to make my nose thinner, because I would be more attractive. She told me to cut my hair and wear more makeup. Her husband told me I had a fat butt. She was critical about everything I said about my career. When I told her my goals of being an artist, she told me that it was the "silliest thing she'd ever heard." I went to college and she forced me to pay rent while living in the garage. When I married, Mom disapproved of [my husband] from day one and had nasty things to say about him. She recently disowned all of her children because we wouldn't let her and her husband live with us. They are in their sixties and out of work and never did want to work to begin with.

Dad was a military guy and then went to work [as an engineer] . . . traveled a lot but kept in touch with us consistently. He called every other night for years while I was growing up. We flew to Connecticut every summer. He gave us lots of money.

What I didn't realize at first was that Natalie believed in her mother. "I was proud of my mom when I was a kid. She was an artist and I thought she was cool." Her mother seemed glamorous. When Natalie was in college, living in her mother's garage and paying her rent, it seemed like the natural order of things. She left art school to rescue her mom; she believed that she owed her mother; she believed her mother when she was critical of Natalie. "I thought I was lucky to be in the garage." It wasn't till Natalie had her own child that she realized that her mother had conned her. "I realized what kids need, starting with respect." Her father gave Natalie a sense of safety, a feeling that he'd take care of her, but he was also critical at times, and unavailable most of the time.

Natalie was always teased by her mother and family members for thinking too much and being sad all the time. She suffered from extreme social anxiety as a child. The family tells story after story about how painfully shy she was. She has largely overcome this, but instead of feeling panicky in social situations, now she feels ugly and unlovable. She did not do well in school, partly due to shyness and partly due to ADHD symptoms—trouble concentrating, paying attention, making decisions. It was differ-

ent in art, where she was a standout. She won prizes at school but her mother didn't come to the awards ceremony. She went to college but dropped out, ran away, and lived on the streets for a while. She began to abuse cocaine and other drugs. Meanwhile she also worked in a bakery. After eight years, she bought the business, which she maintained until her crisis. It was like an extended family for her; she got along well with her employees and had many regular customers who would drop in to talk.

She married her husband at age twenty, and they had their one child several years later. She said that Ken was the first person who loved her. He became a long-haul truck driver. He was loving and faithful, but needed more distance than Natalie could tolerate. He would withdraw, she would get angry and pursue, he would withdraw more. In the end, he would sit in front of the TV, high on marijuana, while she ranted and raved. She moved out, with their son, three years ago.

Son Jeff has been resentful toward Natalie since the separation. He is extremely mouthy and critical, telling Natalie she's crazy, psycho, and belongs in a mental hospital. Natalie acknowledges that there have been many times when she's been too depressed to be available to her son, but feels she's done the best she could and on the whole not too bad.

Natalie and I have been through a lot together. About two years ago, shortly after her divorce became final, she fell very hard for a man she met through the Internet. They saw each other a few times, and she decided to sell her business and move in with him, in another part of the country. I wish I'd talked her out of it. It ended very badly, and Natalie wound up back in her hometown, now broke. Since then she has struggled with employment and struggled with her son's anger for deserting him. She was hospitalized briefly when she was acutely suicidal; now she owes the hospital $5,000. She feels that leaving town was the mistake of her life. We have been trying to put the pieces back together.

When Natalie is under stress she feels isolated and strange. "The first thing I said to my [previous] therapist was that I want to connect to things. My whole life I've felt unconnected to anything—the ocean, what people are saying, what I'm saying . . . I would go to sleep [as a child] feeling that I wasn't real." She feels she can't express herself, that no one will ever understand her because she doesn't understand herself, that she is confusing, disorganized, crazy. She feels her brain going off in a million directions at once. This is an extremely scary and unpleasant feeling, full of fear, rage, sadness, and hopelessness all at the same time. It is a state psychologists call "fragmentation," a form of dissociation. When Natalie is not in this state, she still feels isolated and strange because she believes no one else ever feels this way. It contributes to a constant feeling of depression and hopelessness. She fears that she is too intense for anyone, that what she wants in a relationship is impossible. In fact she seems to lack the membrane most people have that protects them from the petty insults of the day. I tell her that she craves connection to help her with her feelings of being defective and helpless in a terrifying world. I tell her that her experience—of having a mother who presented a false self to the children, who essentially conned Natalie—is an uncommon thing, and that it has had an effect on her brain, and fragmentation is Natalie's experience of that state.

At the same time, Natalie has an active and inquiring mind. She reads whenever she can, and she is always trying to figure things out: herself, her son, the divorce, and the world. She has a terrific sense of ironic humor. She is very direct with me, wanting to know what I think on a multitude of issues. She also wants to know my feelings and my mind, what I think about her behavior and decisions, how I ended up OK despite my past. With a very few exceptions, I try to answer her directly, because I feel that she needs a mentor, a companion; she doesn't believe (and I try not to pretend) I'm perfect, but she wants to know how to get through life while depressed, how to parent, how to make decisions.

Natalie's sense of connection with me is very important. When she feels understood and contained, she functions better; when there is a disruption, she is vulnerable to depression or drinking or impulsive behavior. I try to walk a middle ground between the strong characters, like her mother and the previous therapist, who have abused and taken advantage of her, and the weak characters, like her husband, who have provoked her rage by their retreat from her. It is a case in which I feel I am trying to provide the secure attachment she has always lacked, a strong base to build on while Natalie tries to recover and grow. Therapy never can provide the reparenting that people sometimes wish for, a new relationship with a new parent that will undo all the damage that came before. But it can sometimes help a discerning adult recognize the damage, recognize that it wasn't normal, and find ways to grow and heal.

Natalie's situation is a case where I see all the effects of a distorted relationship between child and primary caregiver that I listed previously:

- *damage to the structure of the brain itself, and:*
- *damage to the adult's ability to experience and control emotions*
- *damage to the adult's ability to have a self-concept of confidence and stability*
- *damage to the adult's ability to protect the body from psychological stress*
- *damage to the adult's ability to develop rewarding relationships*
- *damage to the adult's ability to focus, concentrate, and learn*
- *damage to the adult's capacity for self-control*

The exception is that Natalie's stress does not have much direct effect on her body. Natalie enjoys being fit and enjoys regular exercise, at least when she is not too depressed to function. There are lucky people like this, who have abilities or strengths that remain unimpaired even though much of the rest of their life is full of trouble.

Natalie is an example of the difficulty of making arbitrary distinctions in diagnosis. On the surface, her childhood experiences of parental divorce and moving across the country seem hardly sufficient to qualify for PTSD; but how do you explain a child of ten who swallows poison in reaction? On top of that, her unique experience, of having a mother who was indifferent to her, exploited her, and deceived her, is clearly traumatic; and her symptom picture very much includes the dissociative problems associated with PTSD. And then how do we classify her? Does she "have" depression, a substance abuse disorder, a borderline personality disorder, a dissociative disorder, ADHD, PTSD? How can we put a complex individual into a shoebox?

This is one of those situations where therapy provides support and foundation while the patient grows and repairs herself. I try to protect Natalie from making bad decisions and reinforce her healthy decisions, and in that context we talk about how to make decisions. I try to help her learn to tolerate disturbing feelings through mindfulness and detachment, and she visualizes new neuronal connections in her brain. The list goes on. Recently Natalie has developed a new understanding of her flight away with the Internet man: it was an attempt to save herself. It was only when she returned that she truly faced the end of her marriage, with all the guilt and self-blame Natalie attaches to putting her son through what she herself went through. Now that she's recovering from the guilt and no longer feeling that she committed an unpardonable sin, she can forgive herself some and begin to move on. We don't know how things will turn out, but they are mostly going in a good direction.[8]

Psychotherapy

One of the great controversies is how psychotherapy works. Clinicians and researchers argue about it endlessly. Without denying the controversy and the

---

8 Natalie and I are very fortunate that she has an insurance policy that pays almost all the cost of her therapy without asking for too much paperwork or putting artificial constraints on her benefits. She has had to make some very real sacrifices in order to make her monthly payments. I am fortunate I haven't had to confront the issue of having a patient whom I've encouraged to depend on me who can't pay for treatment.

complications of the issue, it's vital for us to try to understand it at this point, because I'm basing my model for how you can help yourself with perpetual stress on how I understand psychotherapy.

The arguments about how therapy works usually boil down to science versus art, tangibles versus intangibles, the therapist's skill versus the therapist's personal qualities. Should we be practicing, as many argue, "empirically based treatments," standard forms of treatment that have been proved to be effective? Or is therapy more about the relationship between the therapist and patient? If the patient doesn't like or respect the therapist, can any treatment, even that backed up by the most science, ever be effective? In the best, most controlled and "scientific" research, there have always been these embarrassing findings that keep pointing back to the intangibles. A huge NIMH-funded study of psychotherapy for depression demonstrated clearly that three empirically based treatment methods were all more effective than a control group. The therapists in the study had been hand-picked—were nationally recognized as experts in their own particular treatment method—so you would think that their skill was instrumental in achieving these results. But it turned out also that the degree to which the patients experienced their therapists as empathic, caring, open, and sincere *at the end of the second session* significantly predicted outcome at termination—a pretty strong suggestion that the intangibles were important. And this has been typical of the findings in the research: you can't get those messy *feelings* out of the way and make psychotherapy a pure science.

As the twentieth century was approaching its end, leading theorists in both the psychoanalytic and cognitive camps were rethinking their aversion to considering "the relationship" as a vital element in successful therapy. Analytic leaders like Steven Mitchell and Irwin Hoffman, influenced partially by a postmodern skepticism about the infallibility of science, were talking about analysis and therapy as a shared effort, two people wrestling with some of the most difficult life questions, with little in the way of guidance and certainty. Cognitive theorists like Jeremy Safran and Zindel Segal were investigating approaches as diverse as Harry Stack Sullivan's humanistic adaptation of Freud and the mindfulness skills of Tibetan Buddhism. There seemed to be an emerging consensus that psychotherapy has two sources of strength: the relationship between the two people involved *and* the expertise of the therapist.

To me, one of the simplest and yet most helpful ways of describing how therapy works is that, over time, the patient begins to internalize the therapist's attitude toward himself. He begins to think and feel about himself in the same way he sees the therapist thinking and feeling about him: more tolerant, more curious, more forgiving; less critical, less harsh, less blinded by the assumptions of the past. More affectionate, more spontaneous, more alive. The therapeutic relationship becomes something akin to Bowlby's "holding environment," where the patient can shed some of his character armor and view himself and the world without the defenses and assumptions that have made things so distorted to him. Abuse victims, constantly in a state of hypervigilance and fear, can find comfort because the look on the therapist's face and the sound of her voice go right to the terrified reptile brain and calm the nervous system. The therapist focuses on the feelings that underlie the content of what the patient says, and thus engages the right hemisphere of the patient's brain— the right hemisphere, which is so overshadowed in today's overstimulated, problem-solving world by the left. The right brain learns to contemplate the left with compassionate curiosity. The damaged orbitofrontal cortex is gradually healed. The patient develops a more mindful attitude toward himself— tolerant, patient, curious, loving, not judging—which leads us to why I think "mindfulness" is a way out of the Perpetual Stress Response.

But the relationship is not enough. The therapist's expertise is absolutely necessary, for two different functions. The first is in creating the conditions that allow an encounter between two strangers to develop into a holding environment for the patient. Perhaps Freud's greatest discovery was that the patient will inevitably resist doing what's good for him; the same defenses that allow us to get by every day without being overwhelmed by awareness of our stress and pain will be used by the patient as resistance to the therapist's efforts to get him to address his below-the-surface feelings. The patient will expect the therapist to treat him in the same traumatic or neglectful way that the important figures in his life have, all along, and the therapist has to prove him wrong. The patient doesn't check his character armor at the therapist's door; it comes off gradually, as a relationship of trust builds. And that is what I want you to do, reading this book. There is nobody here but you and me. Give me a chance. Play with these ideas. Look at yourself honestly. There is no disgrace in being burned out by perpetual stress. Take a hard look at what it's doing to you, and give yourself the opportunity to change your life.

The second function of the therapist's skill is in guiding the patient as he gets to know a world unfiltered through his old assumptive system. The therapist will be challenging mistaken assumptions, distortions, patterns of destructive thinking and behavior, and helping the patient find fresher, less distorted, less constricting ways of functioning. The therapist tries not to impose his own values and beliefs on the patient, but can save the patient a lot of grief otherwise spent in trial-and-error learning the new world by suggesting practical shortcuts. When I helped Mary Alice Brown see that her depression was an expectable reaction to the stress she was under, when I gave her concrete advice about how to handle the children more effectively, this is what I was doing. When I listened very carefully to Natalie in her states of mental confusion and helped her see that she was making more sense than she thought, I was giving her structure and hope. That's where the rest of this book goes, after we learn about our emotions and mindfulness; we'll be addressing things like identifying destructive assumptions, distorted thought patterns, difficult relationships, and how the body reacts to stress. And we'll be giving you structure—the knowledge that there are different, healthier, more effective, more human ways to handle these things—and hope. Remember how the brain can change with experience. You can lay down new neural pathways that undo the damage that's been done, and help you better handle future stress.

As a therapist who's interested in the science behind the art, this is the most exciting period I've ever worked in. Thanks to all the new discoveries about how the brain works, we may finally be at the point in time where the language of psychoanalysis and psychotherapy—the id, the ego, the self, self-objects, object relations, defenses, drives—can begin to be translated into the structures and functions of the brain. We're beginning to understand how *mind* emerges from *brain*. There's a long way to go, but I'm thrilled about the future. I feel like Keats, "On First Looking into Chapman's Homer."

> Then felt I like some watcher of the skies
>   When a new planet swims into his ken;
> Or like stout Cortez when with eagle eyes
>   He star'd at the Pacific—and all his men
> Look'd at each other with a wild surmise—
>   Silent, upon a peak in Darien.

The fact that Keats should have named Balboa, not Cortez, just adds to the magic. What should we expect?—he was only twenty-two.

Part Two

What to Do

Repairing the Emotional Brain

The brain was not designed to benefit individuals, but their genes.
—Randolph M. Nesse and Kent C. Berridge

THE difficulty of being human is that we are animals, and at the same time we are more. It seems as if we have two brains. One is guided by senses, emotions, and experience, a highly developed tool to help us fit into the world of nature. That brain can help us be as alert as a sparrow or as fit as a thoroughbred. The other, growing on top of the animal brain like an unwieldy cabbage, is what we use to solve the problems only humans can.[1] That brain gives us memory and self-consciousness, the power and the need to impose order on the universe. Our challenge is to make sense of the world when our two brains tell us different things. In our artificial and constructed world, that happens far too often. Is it safe to drive at 75 mph—more exactly, how do we cope with stimuli flashing by us at a rate we weren't designed to apprehend? What do I do about hating my job when I need it to support my family? Am I supposed to love my father when he gets drunk and attacks me? Contemporary life may have eased our most primitive fears, but it's left us with fears that are diffuse, confusing, and perhaps insoluble.

Understanding that our nervous system, including our emotional responses, didn't evolve to keep us happy, but to keep us alive so we could pass

---

1 It's not this way, of course. As I've said, the two brains are highly intertwined, and the idea that the limbic system feels and the cortex thinks is proving to be much more complicated than that. Please permit metaphorical use here. For a more radical view that sees the brain and nervous system and endocrine and immune systems as components of a network, with the mind in the network and not in the brain, see Candace Pert's comment on page 330.

on our genetic material, explains a lot. There is a famous passage in *Catch-22* where Yossarian and Lt. Scheisskopf's wife are debating the purpose of pain. " 'Why couldn't God have used a doorbell to notify us, or one of his celestial choirs? Or a system of blue-and-red neon tubes right in the middle of each person's forehead?' " asks Yossarian. But the neon tubes wouldn't get us to remove our hand from a stove as quickly and reliably as the sensation of pain does. Our nervous systems are smarter than we are. As with pain, emotions are designed to be red flags to us.

Emotions exist to focus our attention on the thing that stimulates the emotion. They prime us for action, to respond to the stimulus. They are ancient, atavistic reactions to stimuli of danger and pleasure, the way our human brains register the same reactions that dogs, horses, and rats experience to the same stimuli. Emotions are the connecting link between mind and body, a message sent by the organism in both directions at once, a physiological change with a psychic overtone, a change in mental state that is also expressed somatically. Emotions give us a self: they tell us what we want, and they give us the problem of getting the world to give us what we want, and out of that we build ourselves. They are powerful forces felt in brain, mind, and body. Remember how a baby displays its feelings. It is *possessed* by feeling—the infant shows its emotional state all over its body, with its eyes, mouth, face, voice, arms, legs, skin, movement, posture. We adults learn to control that display, but it takes a lot of energy to do that, to be calm and cool. *The central problem for most people living in the twenty-first century is that we need to experience our emotions more deeply while still maintaining control.* Stress keeps us trying to use the left brain, the logical half, that we've been taught to rely on; but we need to attend to our feelings without being exclusively guided by or overwhelmed by our emotions.

Emotions are compelling innate responses. Paul Ekman, who has spent a lifetime studying emotions, has finally settled a long debate, showing that emotional expressions (face and body language) are the same across all human cultures. Different societies have different "display rules"—conventions about how to show emotions—which make expressions appear different to the casual observer. In Japan, for instance, there is great prohibition against showing negative emotions. If the experimenter sits with a Japanese subject while showing a horrific film about auto accidents, all the subject will show on his face is a polite smile. But if the experimenter leaves the subject alone, he will show the same expressions of horror and disgust that Westerners do. "In private, innate expressions; in public, managed expressions." We don't *learn* to grimace in pain or cry when sad or smile when we are happy; these responses are *hard-wired* into our brains. Emotions are mediated by the release of chemical messengers between cells not only in the brain, but throughout the body, most importantly between the nervous system, the endocrine system, and the immune system. Emotions provide vital information for recovery from stress-related medical conditions, and our emotional state is enormously important for our ability to recover from any disease.

Our self, the part of the mind that has consciousness, makes decisions, and registers feelings, develops first out of the infant's need to control emotions. Most of us have been around a baby who, for some reason, cannot be soothed for a while. It's a frightening experience for the adult, but for the baby it must be torture at ten thousand decibels. The first real challenge for an infant is to learn how to modulate or control feelings. Initially, adults, principally the primary caregiver, do it for the child; gradually, the child learns to do it without help; and out of this grows the mind. We spend the rest of our lives then dealing with the same issue: how to have feelings but not let them run away with us. Controlling our emotions always takes psychic energy. Too often, we stop *deciding* to control and just control mindlessly, rarely letting others in on how we feel. Worse yet, we can disguise our emotions to ourselves, not permitting our own selves to be aware of our feelings—but those hard-wired responses are still firing in our nervous systems. We're still secreting the neurotransmitters of emotion; our faces, voices, and bodies are primed to express our emotions, but we're not permitting them to do that. Think of the psychic energy involved in that degree of control; think of the stress on our systems.

As we grow from infancy to adulthood we learn to respond emotionally to stimuli much more complex than simply pleasure and pain, food and danger. We develop emotional responses to TV commercials, political figures, the subtle nuances of facial expression from our spouses and bosses. But emotions always tell us important things about our values. They are always about goals. If we don't value something, we aren't going to feel anything about it.

Much of contemporary life gives us the message that emotions are dangerous, but this is like shooting the messenger: emotions in themselves are valuable information; it's what we *do* with emotions that can get us in trouble. We think we're supposed to be cool and in control, but emotions by their nature are acknowledgments of our neediness and lack of self-sufficiency. So we desire to avoid these states; we often believe it is best to be autonomous, that neediness equals weakness. Extremes of emotions—grief, fear, anger, even joy—feel unsafe and embarrassing. Some emotions, like anger or hate, are thought to be bad by definition, and we try to avoid experiencing or acknowledging them. But this is a highly self-destructive strategy. Martha Nussbaum's *Upheavals of Thought* is a massive philosophical treatise on the role of emotions in thinking; one of her major theses, which seems counterintuitive on first blush, is that emotions should be central to ethical thinking. She points out that emotional reactions are the "values" by which our brains evaluate experience: good, bad, threatening, safe. Emotional reactions are in large part responsible for deciding which stimuli, out of the thousands affecting us at any time, are the ones we will give our attention to in the present moment. To aspire to control our emotions or make life decisions by logic alone is to set ourselves up for failure and to cut ourselves off from fully experiencing life. It also deprives us of vital information that the subtle parts of our brain pick up unconsciously about people and situations, information that we experience as intuition or gut reactions.

Science is now demonstrating that the animal, emotional brain is enormously sensitive to important information about the world that we need in order to see things clearly. The amygdala makes *instantaneous* assessments of strangers' faces: threatening or safe. Those assessments will bias our conscious sizing up of anyone new, without our awareness. When something happens to put us in danger, our body is aware of it before our consciousness is; we jump out of the way of danger before we are aware of feeling afraid. Rational thought is the uniquely human way of organizing our experience, but it's several steps removed from experience itself, and it's insufficient as a guide for living. Emotions are our immediate experience of reality and how we know what's important. Besides, trying to be perfectly rational is a futile task—the animal brain and the logical brain are interconnected in subtle, complex ways that science is just beginning to be aware of. We are by nature creatures of emotion, and while getting along in the world requires that we control our actions, to try to control our experience is futile and self-destructive.

At the same time, we're living in the age of perpetual stress, and that means our feelings are not always going to be the reliable guide they are naturally. We're full of stress hormones, ready to see danger when there is none, dissociated from a normal sensitivity to reality. We're like the PTSD sufferer who doesn't know he has PTSD; much of our fear and anger is about the past, but we believe it's about the present. We're perennially disappointed, because our efforts to lead the life we're told to live don't bring us satisfaction or happiness.

We're often angry, but there's no one to be mad at. We learn helplessness, we stop trying. Concluding that our emotions are unreliable, we try not to feel anything—a sure route to depression.

So we need to find our way back to trusting our feelings. We need to stop thinking of emotions as happening to us, beyond our control, as opposed to thoughts, which we think we control. In fact, though emotions are often disturbing, they are intimately a part of the self; and likewise our thoughts are less subject to choice than we want to believe. Fear and hope, for instance, are intertwined, two views of the same set of facts. When we fear, we think about the facts that presuppose a negative outcome. When we hope, we think about the facts that suggest a positive outcome. Often they are the same facts, just colored differently by emotion. For example, your type of cancer has a 40 percent five-year survival rate: do you focus on the 40 percent who live, or the 60 percent who die? It seems impossible to do both at the same time, so we swing between alternate states. But it's important because, according to some, an optimistic outlook can lead to a better outcome.

Emotions, Feelings, and Moods

Before we go on, let's have a short discussion about nomenclature. *Emotions* are our innate response to a novel situation; *moods*, on the other hand, reflect an assessment of our resources or motivation to handle the situation. A bad mood reflects a judgment that our resources aren't up to the situation; the self-focusing that accompanies a bad mood aids our attempt to strengthen our resources. The optimism that accompanies a good mood may induce us to stretch our resources, to take chances we wouldn't ordinarily take. The terms *emotions* and *feelings* are also often used interchangeably. There is, in fact, considerable confusion in the professional community about what these terms mean, so let me just be clear about how I use the terms here: *Feelings are the part of an emotional response that we're aware of.* The fear response is an example: usually we experience a feeling we call "afraid" as part of the fear response. We may or may not be aware of our hearts pounding, bowels churning, palms sweating, though these reactions are part of the emotional response we call "fear." We're certainly not aware of the cascade of hormones and neurotransmitters flowing from the brain and endocrine system into the body, nor of the fact that our immune cells make a strategic retreat into areas where they may be needed, though these are part of our fear response as well. Sometimes we experience the emotion "fear" without being conscious of feeling "afraid," and there are many other instances when we may experience unconscious emotions.

Daniel Goleman has a good example of how this works for fear: People who have a snake phobia will start to perspire when they are shown pictures of snakes. Galvanic skin response (GSR) meters are sensitive enough that they can register this perspiration before the person is consciously aware of feeling anything. In fact, slides of snakes can be presented so quickly, interspersed with other slides, that the person will not even be aware that he has seen a snake—but he will start to sweat. The body is responding with an emotion, fear, although the emotion never registers itself on consciousness as a feeling. Our psychological defense mechanisms (see Chapter 6) can operate the same way; defenses like dissociation, somatization, or defensive rage can operate so instantaneously that the person is never aware of the underlying emotion that caused the distress in the first place. So instead of feeling the fear associated with a threat, the trauma victim uses dissociation to "go away" mentally; instead of feeling the pain of grief, the somatizing patient will develop multiple physical symptoms that keep him immobilized and preoccupied with himself; the belligerent, anger-prone adolescent will experience anger as a cover-up for fear. Particularly troubling is the phenomenon of unconscious guilt, as we shall see.

We must recognize that emotions, conscious or not, have enormous influence over our behavior: *emotions are motivations.* And the more we are aware of our motivations, the more control we have over ourselves. We may be completely unaware of responding to unconscious emotions. LeDoux discusses a pair of experiments by social psychologist John Bargh, who had participants take what they thought was a language test. In the first experiment, some of the subjects read sentences about elderly people while others did not. Those who read about elderly people walked down the hall more slowly after the experiment was "over." In the second experiment, some read about assertiveness, while some read about politeness. When they were done, they were to walk down the hall to report to the experimenter, who (by prearrangement) was engaged in a conversation. Those who read about assertiveness were quicker to interrupt the experimenter than those who read about politeness. Knowing this, do you really think you're immune to food or drug commercials on television? Do you really think that violence in films and in music has no influence on violence in society? Given that defenses are often a healthy adaptation to stress, how can you defend yourself against stress that you're unaware of?

Distorted Views of Emotion

Regulating emotion is *the* issue for most people, the problem that leads most to grief—certainly in depression and anxiety. Addictions are external means of regulating emotions, and psychosomatic disease a defense against emotional experience—emotions expressed by the body, not the conscious self. Almost every patient who comes to see a therapist, or who asks the doctor for a psychoactive medication, is having a problem with regulating emotion—too much, too little, at the wrong time and place, out of control, or in conflict with how we think we should feel. We've already talked about the reasons why this is so difficult for so many people; disturbing early experiences combined with an adult stress load we don't acknowledge. Emotional regulation is right at the core of the self: remember that our earliest, infantile self develops out of the need to control our emotional experience and that the groundwork laid down at that time, for good and for ill, will be the structure we build the rest of our lives around.

Daniel Stern has been studying the interactions of mothers and infants for more than thirty years. He has documented in detail how the baby integrates emotions through empathic interactions with its mother. But when the mother does not respond to specific emotional states, infants may never develop the ability to integrate those emotions as part of the self. They remain vague states of tension. *"Associated experiences and behavioral systems may thus never be fully defined as part of the infants' sense of self,* and the pursuit of various important developmental goals (for example, intimacy, autonomy, and exploration) may be blocked." These patterns of attunement and lack of attunement from the mother and the rest of the social environment teach the infant what is, in Harry Stack Sullivan's[2] terms, the "good me" (emotions and behaviors that are encouraged, approved of, or rewarded), the "bad me" (behaviors that are disapproved of or punished), and the "not me" (emotions and behaviors that are ignored or elicit no emotional response). In Stern's example, a child whose mother does not respond with approval to the child's initiative or exploration

---

2 For more on Sullivan's contributions, see Chapter 6.

may get the idea that the world is unsafe and that a passive, cautious approach to life is best. In order for a child to feel that an emotion is "me," the emotion must be *validated*—responded to, recognized, mirrored—by the important people in his or her life. When feelings are *invalidated* they are likely to remain outside the child's ability to experience. Alice (see pages 117–119) is an example of this process; her parents were simply too old, too old-worldly, too *nice*, to accept the normal angry and upset feelings of an unhappy child. Alice as an adult is left with two separate modes of functioning: the competent, funny, lovable adult, who was recognized and rewarded by her parents, and the angry, hopeless, sorry-for-herself child who was split off and denied, and who remains outside Alice's everyday consciousness, yet still exists to sabotage her adult functioning.

For another example, many people have been brought up in families where expressions of negative emotions were punished. When they were angry, they were told they had no right to be. When they were afraid, they were teased. When they were sad, they were told to snap out of it. When they were ashamed or guilty, people piled on to make them feel worse. As a result, many of us are "negative emotion-phobic" (in Marsha Linehan's phrase); negative emotions are so upsetting that we deny their existence and lose consciousness of them. They become "not me." All we feel is a generalized anxiety, much like the dog who has learned helplessness (see the sidebar on pages 120–121). This is a common problem with depression, a difficult one to address in treatment precisely because we are so unaware of it. It takes actually feeling negative emotions to recognize that they are not so dangerous after all, and the patient fights that experience with every defense he has.

Some adults from abusive or neglectful environments feel almost nothing on their own, because nothing was ever validated; instead, their radar for others' feelings is always on. Judith Herman writes:

> Children in an abusive environment develop extraordinary abilities to scan for warning signs of attack. They become minutely attuned to their abusers' inner states. They learn to recognize subtle changes in facial expression, voice, and body language as signals of anger, sexual arousal, intoxication, or dissociation. This nonverbal communication becomes highly automatic and occurs for the most part outside of conscious awareness. Child victims learn to respond without being able to name or identify the danger signals that evoked their alarm.

Some of these children become caretakers or enablers as adults, always ministering to others and not aware of any needs of their own. But a little of this can be useful sometimes. I have a therapist friend from this kind of background, not an enabler at all, whose ability to read others' emotional states is so highly developed it's spooky. She has to be careful how she uses it; in fact, she uses little direct empathy but goes one step further and makes very concrete, on-target suggestions about clients' future actions based on her understanding. But most people from abusive environments are simply destabilized by emotions, seesawing between overcontrol and undercontrol. Emotions remain part of the "not me," but simply burst seemingly from out of nowhere onto the scene, create a tempest, then disappear again. We'll have a lot more to say about this problem in Chapter 6.

Alice: Self-Sabotage at Work

When I met Alice she was a bundle of soft addictions and a mass of contradictions. Outside of work, where she was quite efficient, she had always procrastinated horribly. Her apartment was always a mess, and she avoided having friends over because she was so ashamed of it. Her laundry was never done. She always weighed more than she wanted to, despite her years of on-again off-again diets. Her eating was chaotic; she rarely planned meals or cooked for herself, relying on take-out, so her nutrition was never good. Until we began making progress in therapy, she was deeply in debt, caught in the web of credit cards, which had her paying exorbitant interest rates, but she couldn't resist making new purchases whenever she had a little cash. When she got behind with my bill and began canceling sessions frequently, she realized how crazy this was and took steps to get her money issues under control. Despite all her mildly self-destructive habits, she doesn't drink, smoke, gamble, or engage in reckless sex. She's never been suicidal, though very depressed at times. She is the paradigm of the "good girl" (or boy) with a guilty secret—too good to be really self-destructive with a hard addiction, but self-destructive nonetheless and deeply ashamed of it to boot.

On the other hand she was the shining example of setting a long-range plan in motion and following through on it. Ten years ago, when she was twenty-eight, she decided she'd had enough of being the superefficient secretary for big shots and identified the career she wanted. She saved her money and borrowed some more, then went back to school, got an entry-level job, and diligently worked her way up to the point where now she is exactly where she wanted to be. And she enjoys it just as much as she antic-

ipated, but she doesn't make enough money—the one thing she'd omitted from her cal-culations.

Alice is quite quick and witty, fun to be around, and can be the life of the party, when she's up. But she's hypomanic (see Chapter 7). She can go into devastating lows when she lets everything go. At these times she has no energy, no joy, and feels utterly demoralized, helpless, and worthless. She can usually get to work during these periods, but it's a huge strain. Though there is definitely a cyclic aspect to these episodes, as if the high has just used up her energy and she needs to rest, it's also true that the lows are brought on by frustration and disappointment. Most of the time, Alice is caring and charming, and has a lot of friends, but hasn't had a serious boyfriend in years. The lows—one of her guilty secrets—are a big obstacle to a relationship. She'd like one very much, but at the same time is working on feeling that her life won't be ruined if she never marries.

Alice's schema is about rejection, defectiveness, and guilty secrets. She and her brother (not blood-related) were adopted shortly after birth by her parents, an older couple who were gentle and well-mannered. Her parents didn't tell her about the adop-tion, and she found out by accident in her mid twenties. Although she says she some-how always knew, still it came as a great shock to her. But her parents never did tell her brother. When she was about thirty, Alice tracked down her birth mother—to her ever-lasting sorrow. Her birth mother welcomed her, but Alice was appalled by the woman—five different children by four fathers, uneducated, stuck in poverty. One child, though, is a full sister of Alice's—which immediately raised the question: Why was Alice the one to be given away? What was wrong with her? She has never contacted her birth family again.

There is also a scar from her relationship with her brother. Alice was a good child, mostly, while her brother was a hellion. As they grew up he went out of his way to make Alice's life miserable, teasing and taunting her, terrifying her often with his at-tacks of rage, physically abusing her at times. The worst aspect, in Alice's view, was that her parents seemed absolutely powerless with him, in fact were abused themselves, and were not able to give her a sense of safety from him. Alice often kept to her room, hiding in her "midden"—the family's term for the mess she kept of clothes, books, and odds and ends. She left home at seventeen to get away from her brother, though she missed her parents very much. She has re-created the midden in her own apartment. It's probably a holdover from a childish need to find permanence—remember she al-ways felt she was adopted—in a collection of possessions. So the midden—which I see metaphorically in all her bad habits—represents a certain security as well as shame.

Though she loved her parents, she also was, and is, extremely angry at them, mostly for not protecting her, but also for not being there emotionally for her. As I said, she was generally a good child, but there were times when she also ran roughshod over her parents, and they just seemed helpless. They were old-worldly, "too nice" to teach her how to control herself, even too nice to survive in today's culture. Her father especially couldn't recognize or validate her anger; now she has it all dissociated into her black moods, part of the "not me" she is ashamed of. Her father also couldn't validate her ambition. We speculate that something happened to him to make him see the world as a dangerous place. He was always after Alice to stay near home, stay in the suburbs where it's safe, be satisfied with a steady job, don't set her sights too high—but Alice needed someone to validate her wish to be special. She has been caught in the bind of feeling both hatred and love for her parents, and she learned to cope by swinging from one extreme to the other.

Alice never felt that she belonged anywhere. But this is largely because she was always putting on an act. She felt that she had to dazzle and entertain. She couldn't let anyone see her midden, her adoption, her birth family, her meltdowns, her angry or jealous feelings. This was a truly vicious vicious circle, because she exhausted herself keeping her façade up, making the meltdowns more frequent, making her guilt more severe, making her doubt herself even more.

This is a case where Alice has blossomed and grown simply from the therapist's nonjudgmental attention. I've never condemned her midden or her disorganization, and she's lost the need to maintain them. I've been there to help her through her black moods, heard her guiltiest secrets, and they don't torment her so much. I've been interested in and encouraging of her ambition and determination, and she's continuing to make excellent progress in her work. The insights Alice has gained about how the old issues from the past are still here in the present have, I think, largely been helpful not because they've led to new awareness or freedom from the symptoms, but because they help her organize her experience. A storyteller at heart, Alice has been developing that coherent narrative of herself—the ability to tie together emotional memory with historical memory so that the emotions aren't floating around dissociated, ready to leap out and grab her unexpectedly, with the slightest provocation. Alice has become able to look at the "bad self"—angry, ugly, lazy, selfish—with some sympathy and objectivity, to see that it is not so horrible but only human, that it is not in her genes but in her reactions to what's happened to her. In other words, that it's a part of herself she can accept and doesn't have to keep split off.

There are also plenty of experiences in adulthood that reinforce our perception that we are not supposed to feel what we feel. On the most basic level, so-

Learned Helplessness

The observation that it is possible for humans and animals to learn help-lessness—to reach the conclusion that their behavior has no impact on their situation—has had an enormous impact on the field of psychology. It has contributed greatly to understanding depression, and its discovery drove a stake through the heart of simple-minded behaviorism, the doctrine that thoughts and feelings are irrelevant because our behavior is determined merely by what is rewarded and what is punished. Martin Seligman tells the history of the learned helplessness idea in his book *Learned Optimism*.

It started, as many scientific discoveries do, with an observation that couldn't be explained by then-current theories. In the psych lab of Dr. Richard Solomon at the University of Pennsylvania, the dogs weren't doing what they were supposed to do. Experimenters had been training them to associate a mild electric shock with a bell, so that later they would react to the bell with fear, as if it were the shock itself. Then the dogs were to be placed in a "shuttlebox"—a cage with two compartments, one with a shock, one without, separated by a small barrier—to see if they would jump into the safe compartment at the sound of the bell. But instead, these dogs didn't try to escape, they just lay down and whimpered.

Seligman, then a fresh young grad student new to the lab, and another student, Steven Maier, were the only people to be interested, rather than annoyed, at this finding. They wondered if the animals had somehow formed the concept that they were helpless against the shock—despite the fact that behaviorism preached that mental phenomena like thoughts, feelings, or "concepts" were completely irrelevant. Seligman and Maier devised an experiment to test their idea. They put three groups of dogs in the shuttlebox. The first group could escape when they were shocked, but the second could not, and the third group wasn't shocked at all. After one day's training, on the second day all three groups were tested in a situation where they could escape the shock. The first group quickly jumped over the barrier, as did the third, after some initial confusion. But six of eight dogs in the second group just lay down when they were shocked—even though escape was right in front of their noses.

Seligman and Maier published their results, introducing the concept of learned helplessness. Other researchers found the same phenomenon at work in humans. People were put into a room with an irritatingly loud noise, and a series of switches. For half the group, there was a pattern of flipping the switches that would turn the noise off; the other group couldn't turn off the noise. Later, these same people were given a shuttle-box situation: hand on one side, irritating noise; move the hand to the other side, noise stops. Amazingly and distressingly, most of the people who had been helpless in the first situation didn't even move their hand in the second!

The theory of learned helplessness was later amended to account for the dogs and people who never gave up—consistently about a third of each sample. Seligman and his colleagues introduced the concept of attributional style. Certain people who interpret their experience in a mindful, empirical, open-minded way tend to be relatively immune to the effects of learned helplessness. We'll have more to say about attributional style, and how to protect yourself from learned helplessness, when we reach Chapter 8.

Learned helplessness is devastating to people. Wives caught in a controlling, abusive marriage often internalize the husband's view of themselves—lazy, no-good, incompetent—so they don't seek help when it's readily available. Children, of course, are even more vulnerable. The same process goes on in a milder way with employees of abusive or mind-controlling bosses, who begin to believe they couldn't get a better job. The effects on self-image, initiative, and hopefulness of relationships like these is devastating and, in the case of children, often permanent. Learned helplessness leads to depression, but even worse it can lead to a depressed, victimized character style, a person with no self-esteem and no hope for ever feeling better.

cial norms appear to make the average whitebread American feel uncomfortable when we are around someone expressing strong feelings. One of my most enlightening experiences in learning to become a therapist was a summer job I had in graduate school. I had to listen very carefully to recorded tapes of my first-year classmates trying to do therapy with their clients; I was expected to code each interaction according to a scheme my instructors had worked out that had to do with their particular method of treatment. As I did this I heard, over and over again, how the fledgling therapists would change the subject or say something else nonresponsive whenever the client expressed any strong feeling. At first it was embarrassing; you would have thought we were deliberately trying to be unempathic. But as I listened more and more I could hear the discomfort and anxiety in my classmates' voices. I began to listen with new ears to everyday conversation, and I realized what a common response this is. Try it yourself: listen to friends talking together, listen to how people respond to you—you'll see that when strong feelings are expressed, people want to deflect the conversation somehow. Often they want to tell you how to solve your problem, when you're not asking for advice. They want to make an emotional conversation a logical conversation. There are exceptions; some people are naturally so supportive or compassionate that they seemingly don't have this reflex to turn away. These people, in my experience, are loved by almost anyone who knows them, because this quality is so rare and so nurturing. It's like an oasis in the desert.

Grief is one of those feelings that is consistently invalidated. Everyone else is ready for us to be over it long before we are. This is natural enough; there is no reason why others should be weighed down by our private losses. But when we consistently get the message that we should be over it already, we can begin to feel that something is wrong with the way we're handling grief, and we may try to be over it too soon. Grief denied like this comes back to haunt us later.

Fear is a feeling that we try to deny ourselves. Fear is unpleasant and destabilizing by nature, so of course we want to avoid it, but we have to recognize that it's trying to tell us important information. As my group says, "Anxiety is your friend" (see Tom's story later in this chapter). Our avoidance of fear is strengthened enormously by its social taboo. Women who feel fearful living alone, men who have anxiety on the highway—our culture's message is that these feelings are silly. We try to deny our fear, and it surfaces in other ways: a phobia, a psychosomatic disease.

The most intimate relationships develop unspoken rules about what can be expressed and what cannot. The more healthy the relationship, the more open we can be about our feelings. But more than one of my patients has expressed shock or dismay when they realize that it's only in therapy that they feel free to say what they *really* feel. Examples of taboos abound among my patients.

- Mara, who was brutally raped in her first semester in college, still has not talked with her parents about it two years later. "They can't talk about these things. I never even had the birds and bees talk. They're just embarrassed."
- When Katherine gets angry, her mom gets angrier, and quickly raises the stakes so that Katherine feels the whole relationship is in jeopardy. When she talks about feeling lonely or sad, her mother gets distracted.
- Howard spent forty-eight years with his mother as his closest companion, and they never talked about his homosexuality.
- When Natalie would try to explain to her husband that she got lonely when he was away so much, he would get defensive and angry, then withdraw, again leaving her alone.
- Joseph knows never to complain to his wife about anything she does that makes him unhappy, because she will respond with a list of what's bothering her about him, a list that somehow always trumps his.
- When Brenda was lying on a hospital bed in her living room, recovering from a broken back, she would ask her husband just to sit on the bed with her and hold her hand. He would have a thousand excuses, a million things to do. She would get so frustrated that she'd end up throwing things at him, then dissolving in tears of impotent rage.

When things like this happen, when we try to communicate with someone and get shut down, we feel the powerful emotion of shame. Shame is thought to start out as an adaptive response of the infant whose cries for its mother go unheeded. After a while, the baby will stop crying and withdraw into itself, conserving its energy—the precursor of feeling shame, and the precursor of depression. When we consciously experience shame as an adult, the feeling is extremely uncomfortable; we feel caught, exposed, naked and vulnerable. Shame dissolves self-esteem like an acid bath. The recovery literature has made "toxic shame" a catchphrase, but it might be more than mere metaphor; the brain registers rejection the same way it registers physical pain. And there is research to suggest that the experience of shame elicits a higher cortisol response to stress. Cortisol—the neurotransmitter that in excess kills brain cells. Shame is such a powerful negative experience that we will go to great lengths to avoid it, even learning not to express—or experience—our feelings. Shame, like other emotions, can also go unconscious, so that all we experience is a sense of meaninglessness and alienation at the same time as a desperate desire to please others. Our defenses also can operate on these shameful feelings, so that they become focused on some aspect of the self rather than the whole self: our weight, our skin, some illness that expresses both shame and rage at the same time. Gwen, given away by her mother at eight, always made to feel unloved and unwanted, is on the surface the antithesis of shame: she'll say whatever she's feeling to whoever is around, in direct, colorful, and obscene language. She doesn't take anyone's crap. But in my office she sometimes lets me see her cry about her weight, the visible symbol of her unlovability.

As Marsha Linehan observes, when our feelings are consistently invalidated, we can do one of three things: (1) leave the situation; (2) change ourselves so that we come closer to others' expectations; or (3) prove to others that their expectations are invalid. As I've suggested, one of the most damaging aspects of the Perpetual Stress Response is our denial of the stress, the consistent invalidation we receive. We are all expected to be happy consumers, working longer hours so we can buy more things, deprived of sustaining relationships, cut off from values like family ties and respect for others, sent to the doctor to get a pill when we begin to show signs of burnout. When our entire culture makes us feel invalidated, leaving is physically impossible and changing the culture's expectations is next to impossible. That leaves us trying to change ourselves so that we "fit in." We're forced to find ways to make our feelings go away. Though sometimes it serves a purpose to be able to do this for a while, in the long run it's a very bad idea. *Emotional experience is what gives meaning and purpose to life.* Without it, we're sterile, empty, and dead inside.

Consciousness and Unconsciousness

When we try to make our feelings go away, they never seem to really disappear, just retreat into that vague realm we call the "unconscious," ready to be retrieved whenever there's a reminder: "a stone, a leaf, an unfound door; of a stone, a leaf, a door. And of all the forgotten faces." The unconscious is the basement where we store what we don't want but can't get rid of.

Consciousness is a slippery concept. We assume that other species lack the kind of consciousness we have—that there is no awareness of an "I" that is choosing or thinking or feeling. We also assume that consciousness like this is a relatively recent development for humans—maybe, as some think, it developed around Shakespeare's time, or Christ's, or Homer's, or maybe 160,000 years ago.

Memory and consciousness are intimately intertwined. We don't know to what extent, if any, other species have explicit memory, the kind that can be called upon deliberately. My dog seems to have a memory of my son, because when he sees him every month or so he greets him excitedly, not like a stranger. But can my dog conjure up a mental image of my son, which is what we mean by explicit memory, or is it simply emotional conditioning, excitement being paired with seeing him? "To be self-aware is to retrieve from long-term memory our understanding of who we are and place it in the forefront of thought," writes Joseph LeDoux. Without memory to give us a representation of ourselves in the past, would we be able to conceive of ourselves in the present?

There's another meaning for "unconscious," which describes most of our brain's work: simply automatic, nonvolitional, requiring no input from our conscious mind. These are not repressed memories or the Freudian concept of the *Unbewüsst*, full of forbidden desires; I mean simply operations of the body that the brain attends to without bothering to inform consciousness—breathing, registering visual images, digesting, secreting hormones, initiating the fight-or-flight response—abilities that we're born with. And things that we learn consciously but don't have to attend to any longer because they've been relegated to a nonconscious part of the brain—identifying visual images, walking, typing, driving. There are also emotional habits that we learn very early in life that become unconscious with practice—not feeling certain emotions that we believe are unacceptable to important people in our lives; reacting with anger instead of hurt feelings to an insult; seeing only the weeds and not the flowers. Some of these correspond to identified defense mechanisms (of which more to come in Chapter 6), while others are so simple and basic that they have no names. But they contribute to our character. When we try to push a feeling into our unconscious, it comes at the price of distorting reality.

The entire emotional brain operates unconsciously. One of the major themes of this book will be that through *mindfulness* we can develop more awareness of our unconscious habits and use the higher cortex to control them. We respond to others' facial expressions and body language without conscious awareness, apparently through a specialized function in the amygdala. The right brain and the limbic system instantly and immediately evaluate experiences as good/bad, pleasure/displeasure, safe/dangerous. The right brain contains a dictionary of nonverbal behavior, allowing us to unconsciously respond to emotional cues from others. More than the left hemisphere, it is responsible for the autonomic nervous system, which controls our fight-or-flight responses. The orbitofrontal cortex operates on an unconscious level, generating the unconscious biases that guide our behavior before conscious knowledge does—what we pay attention to, and how we interpret it. The OFC *is* Bowlby's "internal working model" of relationships, what I call the "assumptive world."

Each of us has an assumptive world, largely unconscious, which we have constructed for ourselves (see Chapter 6)—the complex set of expectations, values, and images of the self and others that enables us to make sense of things and predict what will happen next. The assumptive world is a heuristic, a manual for how people and things work, an interconnected set of shortcuts that enables us to size up situations and make decisions quickly, without much conscious thought, based on past experience and our interpretation of that experience. I assume people will like me, you assume they won't. We're both likely to find plenty of support for these kinds of assumptions, since many are self-fulfilling prophecies. Assumptions like these are generally unconscious. They're not always inaccessible, we can identify some if we reflect or challenge ourselves, but they're automatic, like driving a car. Assumptions also affect the way we think and what we see. What the architect sees when he looks at a building site is different from what the gardener sees. If we think of the self as a fluid, adaptable to the environment, put into a container that we develop throughout life, we all have different windows in our containers, defining what we can pay attention to and what we can't.

Though we couldn't function without defense mechanisms and an interlocking set of assumptions about the world, they restrict us and can hurt us. Defenses can make us miss important cues our emotional brain is trying to tell us. Assumptions can simply be wrong; they can be vastly different from reality. Obviously, the more rigid our assumptions, the more likely they are to be wrong at least some of the time. We have greater freedom, greater ability to determine our own actions, to the extent that we are unconstrained by defenses and inaccurate assumptions. We're going to be talking next about how to live with emotions without defenses, which will help us experience reality more accurately. The bigger concept, becoming more mindful of our defenses and assumptions, will come in the next chapter.

Exercise 2. **Becoming Aware of Unconscious Emotions**

In *Undoing Depression* I discussed a simple method for how people with depression could get under the surface of their minds and become aware of how emotional reactions, which were repressed, surfaced later as brief depressive moods. I presented a tool called the Mood Journal, which is really useful for understanding *any* mood change, not just brief depressive episodes. Here it is, slightly revised.

Mood Journal

Instructions: When you detect a shift in mood, write down the change (e.g., from neutral to sad, sad to glad, happy to irritable), the external circumstances (what you were doing, where, with whom), and the internal circumstances (what you were thinking about, daydreaming, or remembering).

DATE, TIME	MOOD CHANGE	EXTERNALS (WHO, WHAT, WHERE, OTHER UNUSUAL CIRCUMSTANCES)	INTERNALS (THOUGHTS, FANTASIES, MEMORIES)

(Continued)

In that book I argued that brief depressed moods—which too often lead to *long* depressed moods—are always due to an unfelt feeling. Something happens that would have made a "normal" person have an emotional reaction; but the depressed person, trying too hard to control his emotions, doesn't allow himself to experience feelings. Instead, these feelings surface later as a mood change.

The same applies to any unexplained change in mood. Try it the next time you find yourself in a different mood for no apparent reason. This will usually happen with unpleasant moods—sad, irritable, angry, choked up, lonely—but it's possible with pleasant moods too. The key is to pay close attention to what's going on around you at the time, both the externals (what are you hearing, watching, paying attention to; what's going on in the background that could be distracting you) and the internals (what are you thinking about, remembering, fantasizing). I will bet you that if you pay close attention to the externals and internals you will realize that something happened to make you feel a certain way—though it may not have immediately seemed important or even registered on your consciousness—but you didn't experience the feeling. Instead, you experienced a mood change that seemed to come from "out of the blue."

Nothing comes from out of the blue. There's always a reason for our feelings and moods. The reason may seem silly or trivial or embarrassing to your conscious mind. You may feel it is too painful to think about. But your unconscious is trying to send you a message: "Pay attention, dummy. This is important."

As with all these exercises:

> *The more you practice, the easier it gets.*

Developing Emotional Control

As we've said, the infant learns how to control emotions through being mirrored and comforted by adults. The older child benefits from caregivers' empathy, their ability to read how the child is feeling. Adults will (hopefully) name the feeling for the child, draw the connection between the child's experience and the feeling (*you're angry because Daniel took your toy*), and teach other methods of regulation like problem solving or distraction. As adults, we continue to try to regulate our own feelings, sometimes in healthy and effective ways, sometimes in not-so-good ways. Each time we do this successfully, we are constructing ourselves, continuing to lay down and reinforce neural pathways that we can rely on in the future when we're in trouble.

Cognitive therapy has many strategies for controlling the thoughts and feelings that accompany upsetting emotions; we'll discuss this in Chapter 8. Some have suggested, though, that instead of the specific techniques, what is really effective about cognitive therapy is that all the techniques are teaching us to recognize upsetting thoughts and feelings as mental events (expressions of emotions), not as "the truth." It's just the same old mental habits that keep getting us in trouble, not moral imperatives. When we become used to the idea that upsetting thoughts and feelings are simply replays of the same old tape, we may even get bored with the tape.

I have suggested to patients, when they find themselves getting overly worked up over something, that they visualize the upsetting emotion as an old-fashioned steam locomotive. *You're standing there on the station platform, and into the station comes this huge, noisy monster, doing sixty miles per hour, with steam and lights and bells—it's an overpowering, awe-inspiring experience that gets your attention every way it can, all the senses are involved, and it is much bigger than you are; it feels like it will just suck you along with its momentum. . . . But you are standing there on the station platform, and you have* some degree of choice *about whether you get on or not.* The degree of choice is a tricky subject we'll return to later when we discuss responsibility and will power; but it's true, we all have some choice in the matter of whether our emotions will sweep us away or not. Maybe we can't be perfect, most likely sometimes we won't have enough self-control to keep from getting on the train; but we know that every time we do stay on the platform, we make it easier to stay on the platform next time. Every time we make that choice, we build up habit strength, we reinforce the neurological connections that help us stay in control, we make it a little easier to stay in control the next time. I have an exercise that will help you do this, but it requires that you be familiar with mindfulness skills. You can look ahead if you want to, though; it's Exercise 11 in Chapter 6.

Learning to live with emotions as a responsible adult requires a paradoxical strategy, as Marsha Linehan and many others have pointed out. We need first to be sure that we can experience and identify the emotions that are built into our bodies and brains; if we can't do this, we literally don't know our own selves, what is important to us, how to function in the world. But once we can do this, we must be able—when it's necessary—to pull ourselves back from the chain of disturbing thoughts, memories, and feelings that can keep feeding the emotional state and prevent us from attending fully to the changing situation. One key to resolving this paradox is to develop the skill of detachment. When we can detach ourselves, we can experience our feelings without being taken over by them. We can say, *I am feeling angry [or scared, or excited, or hurt] right now, and I need to pay attention to it. But the anger is not me, and I will probably feel differently soon.* By paying attention to the feeling, we gain important information that will help us make better decisions. And by recognizing that the feeling will not take us over, we gain a perspective that can keep a part of us in control even in the most difficult circumstances. Detachment is a vital skill and a component of mindfulness, which we will explore in much more depth in the next chapter.

I spend a great deal of my time in therapy encouraging people to "trust your feelings." It's a cliché, but it's valid. Most people have spent most of their lives learning not to trust themselves, trying to feel something different from their own experience, trying not to feel at all, or indeed *not* feeling because they have had the capacity conditioned out of them. They really do need to get in touch with their feelings, and then learn to listen to and trust themselves. But then they'll ask me something really difficult, like "How do I know which feelings to trust?" This comes from people like Natalie, who left her child behind to chase a man she barely knew, or Benjamin (in Chapter 6), who can go from feeling wildly grandiose to feeling like a complete failure in the course of an hour. The advice on regulating emotions is useful, because it can help people detach and distance themselves from the pressure to act that many feelings carry with them. But the best guideline that helps in questions like this is to know what's most important to you; have an accurate assessment of your core values (see Exercise 3). If you really feel that your family is the most important thing in your life, perhaps you won't be tempted into an affair; if you really feel that your dignity, your self-respect, is important, perhaps this will help you avoid compromising situations. If you really buy into the goal of putting your financial house in order, perhaps you won't spend money impulsively.

Above all, we do *not* want to get caught up in vicious circles of unpleasant emotions. This happens with depression all the time. When we're feeling really depressed, we're likely to *do* something depressed—eat a box of candy; get drunk and pick a fight with someone; call the person who's rejected us and really make a fool of ourselves. When we're through, we feel more depressed than ever. The same cycle occurs with anger. If you can discharge your anger in an effective way, great. But if you act in haste you'll be unprepared; you'll either

Exercise 3. **Identifying Values**

Take five minutes in a quiet place with a pencil and paper. When you are focused, write down a list of up to ten things that make living worthwhile for you. You can do this quickly and impressionistically, because you'll have the opportunity to change the list later. If you're really overwhelmed and feeling like there's nothing good in your life, think of what would make things better. Try to avoid thinking of what you "should" prioritize and stick with your own feelings. If being famous is more important to you than being charitable, that's OK. No one but you will ever see this, and if you distort the picture to try to make yourself look good, you'll only hurt yourself. Be as individualistic as you want to be; I was surprised to see that things like gardening and good food made my own top ten. If golf or keeping the house clean or watching reruns of *Seinfeld* are important activities to you, so be it.

Now put your list away in a place you'll remember it. Wait a week, and do the exercise again. Don't look at your old list. Then wait another week and do the exercise a third time. After you've done the third list, you can resurrect the first two and put them together. Don't be surprised if the lists are very different. One of the reasons we repeat the exercise is to overcome the effects of your mood on a particular day, to get around the censor that sometimes makes us forget what's really important.

Putting the lists together should result in a longer list of anywhere from a dozen to twenty items. You may be able to combine some, to see that some are just examples of a bigger concept. Now comes the hard part: try to put these items in order of their importance to you. Take another sheet of paper and write the numerals 1 to 15 (or whatever). Choose the item on your list that feels most important, and write it next to the number 1—and so on. Don't make yourself crazy over doing this; obviously there are going to be hard choices. Is good health more important than love? Is financial security more important than self-respect? There are no right or wrong answers to these questions, and we're not locking you in to the choices you make now. But you should be able to put these values into a rough order, so that you're comfortable recognizing that, say, items 1 through 4 are really more important to you than items 8 through 12.

(Continued)

If you are a real glutton for punishment, you can now do a time study on yourself. Carry around a little notebook for a week, and make regular notes on how much time you actually spend in activities that express or contribute to your highest priorities. Most people will be quite dismayed at the fact that items that aren't even on the list seem to take up the greatest proportion of their time. But you can skip this step if you want, because you probably already have a good sense that this applies to you as well.

The application of this exercise is the last step. Try to spend more time every day in activities that express your highest priorities or bring you the greatest joy. That will help you feel that you have a sense of direction and purpose in your life, that you have greater self-control, that you are able to act in accord with your highest values.

Explore what gets in the way of change with compassionate curiosity (discussed in Chapter 5). Use a therapist, if needed. Change is never easy. It's important to recognize how we convince ourselves we are too busy to do what we love and value. We box ourselves in. You only get one sweet and precious life—how will you spend it?

---

really hurt someone or act like a total jerk, or both. Then you'll feel angry *and* depressed. Jealousy feeds on itself; if you give in to every impulse, you might get charged with stalking. At least you'll be ashamed of yourself later. There is a vicious circle of fear, too, which we're going to describe next. In the grip of an unpleasant feeling, it's almost never a good idea to follow through on your first impulse. Remember that powerful emotions distort our perception of reality; we're likely to see things that aren't there, and miss things that disagree with our emotional state.

The Upside of Unpleasant Emotions

There are many unpleasant feelings we can't escape from; they're hard-wired into us. Anger and fear are what we experience in our minds while our bodies are experiencing the fight-or-flight response. Guilt and shame have to do with feeling defective, a failure, an outsider. Envy and desire are uncomfortable states, perhaps also wired into us, that frequently lead to negative consequences. Jealousy serves a strong evolutionary purpose. We want to guard our mate so that *our* genes are the ones passed down, nobody else's. But jealousy

Learning to Control Emotions

- Get the facts. Make sure you understand the situation. Don't jump to conclusions.
- Talk it out with sympathetic and objective others.
- Avoid mood-altering substances, including caffeine and alcohol.
- Make sure you're not hungry, angry, lonely, or tired (HALT—an acronym from Alcoholics Anonymous).
- Don't let ANTS (automatic negative thoughts) run away with you.
- Detach. Step back and watch yourself. Go into observer mode.
- Sit with the thought or feeling; use mindfulness to observe it. Perhaps it isn't what you thought at first. Some emotions are more than one layer; something different might be seen underneath if you observe carefully.
- Remind yourself of your core values. Don't do something that's going to make you feel guilty or ashamed later. Don't do something that's going to hurt people you love.
- Resist emotional behavior. Impulsive, emotional behavior maintains or heightens the unwanted emotion and usually leads to adverse consequences. Doing nothing is usually better than doing something stupid.
- Counter physiological arousal. (If too excited, scared, or angry, use relaxation exercises to calm down. If too lethargic, bored, or detached, do something like exercise or listen to loud music.)
- Refocus attention. Distract yourself from upsetting emotions through physical or mental activity. "Move a muscle, change a thought."
- Do something useful. Accomplish something else, something that is of value to you and is not related to the upsetting emotion.

can drive us crazy; we all know examples, some tragic, some tragicomic, of people who have been driven to extremes because of jealousy, often unfounded. Rejection is also inherently painful. We're built to seek status, to find the most attractive mate. Many men and women, after a divorce which they themselves sought—after they had concluded that their spouse was a complete louse and they'd be much better off without them—have complained to me that they feel surprisingly depressed when the divorce is final. It's that rejection gene in action. And we've mentioned the Hedonic Treadmill before, another unfortunate aspect of human nature: the pleasure of gaining something seems to be outweighed by the pain of losing it. As Jimmy Connors said, "I hate to lose more than I like to win." Losing anything meaningful to us brings pain. When we have unpleasant feelings like these we have to accept that they're part of human nature, and use our higher cortical functioning to make sure that our feelings aren't out of proportion; and if they are, to distract, rationalize, argue with ourselves to make sure we weather the storm without hurting ourselves or others.

Fear

Fear is a very useful feeling. It keeps us out of danger, in subtle ways as well as the obvious ones. It's essential in social interaction. When monkeys, which are highly social animals, have their amygdalae (fear centers) removed, their responses are complex. Earlier research showed that amygdalectomy in dominant monkeys resulted in their almost immediate reduction to the lowest position in the pecking order in the tribe. The king of the hill became the monkey picked on by everyone else. It was thought that these monkeys showed an excess of fear. But newer research is suggesting that removal of the amygdala results in an almost complete loss of the fear response. These monkeys will pick up and handle snakes (monkey fear of snakes is hard-wired into the brain) and walk right up to strange monkeys and initiate grooming or sexual behavior, very unlike normal monkeys, which take time to get to know each other. Surprisingly, as long as they're kept in pairs, normal monkeys seem to like the uninhibited behavior of the experimental monkeys. But put the fearless monkeys in a complex social group, and they'll get in trouble; they'll try to copulate with the highest-ranking females and they won't respond to the warnings of the most aggressive males; pretty soon everyone is mad at them.

The same is true in humans. Patients whose amygdalae have been removed can't differentiate between "trustworthy" and "untrustworthy" facial expressions (as rated by neutral observers). They appear to be unchanged in most respects—their intellectual and social functioning seems the same—but they always come to bad ends, because they're so gullible. Eventually they'll run into someone who will badly take advantage of them.

Men, like monkeys, depend on the fear response to keep social functioning harmonious. When men at a cocktail party or sporting event are bragging about their car or their golf score or how their son got into a prestigious college, they're not really talking about penis size, as some think. They're really

Unconscious Feelings

Some fascinating research has confirmed for me once and for all that "hunches," "gut instincts," "feelings in your bones" are real and should be attended to. Antonio Damasio and his colleagues at the University of Iowa have been studying a group of patients who've had their amygdalae removed because of uncontrollable seizures, tumors, or other pathology. As we've said, the amygdala seems to be a central processing point for fear responses, among other things. It's been known for a long time that people who've had their amygdalae removed follow a peculiar course. Though they continue to seem like themselves—their personality, memory, fund of knowledge, reasoning power all seem unchanged—they usually get in trouble in life. It turns out that they are gullible (therefore easily influenced by people who take advantage of them) and that they have a hard time organizing their futures.

It's been hard to demonstrate these phenomena in the lab, because the effects are subtle and long-term, but one of Damasio's colleagues came up with a gambling game that shows something about what's going on. The subject is essentially playing a game like blackjack with two separate decks. One deck is rigged so that in the long run the subject wins money; the other deck is rigged against the player. Subjects playing the game are asked at regular intervals if they have any hunches or explanations about what's going on. They're also hooked up to a circuit that measures their galvanic skin response (GSR; it's part of the traditional lie detector). GSR is essentially a measure of moisture on the skin, and it rises when the subject feels stressed. The experimenters found that patients who'd had amygdalectomies never "got" the game; they never caught on that one deck was good and one was bad, and so would go on playing both at random. They also showed no change in GSR as they played. But when normal subjects were tested, after a while people would begin to have hunches, and so they would start playing the good deck more, and they'd win more, and their hunches would be confirmed and would turn into explanations.

(Continued)

As expected, the GSR of normal subjects began to rise as they played from the bad deck; the fascinating finding was that GSR for these people started to rise *before they were aware* they had a hunch or any slightest idea about how the game worked. Something operating on an entirely unconscious level was telling them they were at risk. We raised the subject of unconscious feelings previously; this is a prime example of how one of these feelings—call it fear or apprehension or suspicion—can develop and influence our behavior without our awareness.

saying "I could drive you out, humiliate you, if I wanted to. I'm superior to you. You defer to me." Men with functioning amygdalae can accurately estimate each other's power, and who defers to whom gets worked out with little overt conflict. Alcohol, of course, inhibits the fear response and makes our estimates of each other less accurate, which is why there are so many fights in bars.

Fear is a very useful response to both social and physical danger. But when we're caught in the Perpetual Stress Response, our bodies are constantly full of the chemical messengers of fear, and we have trouble distinguishing real threats from imaginary ones. There is a terrible irony; now that culture has made us safe from most real threats to life—cave bears and woolly mammoths, starvation and disease—many of us are still in a more or less constant state of fear, often without being aware of it. That is the reason why everyone is so concerned about self-esteem; if you're constantly afraid, even if it's largely unconscious, you can't feel good about yourself. School programs that warn about stranger danger but don't protect kids from bullies, then have the kids repeat insipid self-affirmations in an attempt to build self-esteem, are doomed from the start. The body can't express the neurotransmitters of fear and of good feeling at the same time. Fear inevitably wins out. Men who've had the fear center—the amygdala—in their brains removed have the highest self-esteem in creation. They're convinced that they are perfectly wonderful fellows who can do no wrong, despite the fact that their lives inevitably fall apart in a heap of bad decisions and failed relationships. Breaking the vicious circle of stress will restore our fear responses to normal, and our self-esteem will inevitably recover. But learning to pay more respect to genuine fear responses will lead to better decision making, as our gut feelings and intuitions provide valuable information about people and situations in our lives.

The common understanding is that anxiety differs from fear in that fear has an obvious cause—a real threat to one's physical safety. Physiologically speaking, there is no difference. "Anxiety" covers a lot of ground, though, from the panic reaction of an arachnophobe confronted with a spider to the existential angst of Kierkegaard. In psychoanalysis, the supposed source of this nameless anxiety has changed over the years: Freud initially argued that it came from the conflict between a wish and a fear. Others have focused on the child's experience of separation anxiety as a basic fear revived whenever we feel unprotected. Heinz Kohut talked of fragmentation anxiety, the feeling that the self is literally falling apart under stress. Irwin Hoffman, an analyst who gets right to the point, believes that the basic anxiety is fear of death. Buddhists talk about fear of emptiness. I think whether we're talking about death or emptiness or fragmentation or disconnection or meaninglessness, we're talking about aspects of the same thing, something I have trouble putting into words—a loss of the self, being swallowed up by something, dissolving into nothing, going crazy, falling apart, dying. . . . These are all faces of the anxiety we feel when we wake suddenly at 3 A.M., which we try desperately to keep out of awareness.

One effect of the Perpetual Stress Response is to keep us so busy mindlessly trying to keep up with all the details of life that threaten to overwhelm us that we can lose awareness of this basic anxiety. But too many of us burn out under the strain, and anxiety catches up.

Too many of the people I meet are always running mindlessly, afraid of fear; afraid of something they can't identify, always working to keep it out of consciousness. Afraid to stop and look behind or ahead because if they stopped, they might see they're going in circles, rats in their exercise wheels. Buddhism looks at Western attempts to fill (by consuming) or cure (by finding the right pill) or explain away (with a psychological explanation) the emptiness as wasted effort. Emptiness—anxiety—is just part of life. We can't get rid of it any more than we can shed our skin. Instead, we can learn to sit with it and be still—meditate. Looking at emptiness, anxiety, death, fearlessly makes us stronger. The monster that has chased us forever looks smaller when we turn to face it. We give emptiness the fuel it needs to grow by our attempts to create a self-sufficient self—or by attempts to find the one right person, running away from our aloneness.

* * *

Most of our suffering is caused by the fear of fear. We fear the things we desire the most—the loss of the self in intimacy, in religious experience, in the joy of creativity; the audacity to try our hardest, to do our very best—and so we construct barriers to those experiences, always finding some excuse for not pursuing what we say we want. We're constantly engaged in the endless dance of intimacy, trying to get close but afraid of what will happen when we do. We chase success, but the higher we get the more vulnerable we feel. We can fear that we're not good enough, that we can't compete, that we'll get punished, that we'll be exposed, that our wants are shameful—but these dreaded outcomes rarely occur, and when they do, we get over them. Still we spend our lives avoiding risk.

Mark Epstein relates how the Buddha and Freud both understood the fear of death. One of Freud's short essays relates a beautiful mountain walk with two friends, a poet and a politician. Neither was able to appreciate the beauty of the day simply because of its transience. "The proneness to decay of all that is beautiful and perfect can, as we know, give rise to two different impulses in the mind," wrote Freud. "The one leads to the aching despondency of the young poet, while the other leads to rebellion against the fact asserted." We can either become depressed by transience, or we can try to deny it (as our present culture does). Freud understood that his friends were each trying to prevent the inevitable experience of loss, while he was trying to find a middle way for himself. Epstein says that acceptance of loss is at the heart of the Buddha's teaching. "It is possible to cultivate a mind that neither clings nor rejects, and . . . in so doing we can alter the way in which we experience both time and our selves." Notice the word "cultivate" in that last sentence. Achieving this kind of acceptance takes time and work; we'll get further direction on this in Chapter 5. Meanwhile let's just note the recent finding that Buddhist monks may be the happiest people on earth.

Tom: Reading Anxiety Differently

Tom is a single white male in his late thirties whom, at the time of this writing, I had been seeing for more than two years. He suffers from depression and panic attacks. He lives with his father in their suburban home. His mother suffers from severe Alzheimer's and lives in a nursing home. He is notably small in stature, about 5'3" and of slight build, but is an avid runner and triathlete when he is not paralyzed by depression. He has dated, more frequently when he was younger, but has never married.

The therapeutic impasse for Tom had become his difficulty getting and keeping a job. His panic attacks, obsessional thinking, and depressed thinking all get in the way. Before I knew him Tom had held two jobs for some years, one working in an office for a large corporation (which he left because he was bored), and one working in retail sales, which he left because of mounting anxiety—he was getting increasingly upset by dealing with difficult customers. Since entering therapy, he left one difficult and demanding sales job after just a few days of panic, then found a job as a laborer which he held until he was laid off. He is underemployed, with a master's degree that he pursued while he was working, a high normal intelligence, and good social skills.

Tom was bullied unmercifully in middle school, by one particular tormentor—these bitter memories come back when he's feeling anxious or depressed. High school and college were much better for him, and he made several friends with whom he has maintained relationships. After college, he entered a military officer candidate school, which led to his first panic attack. He did well and found his colleagues and instructors supportive, but he had trouble with one particular subject. Nearing his graduation, he began to obsess about the responsibilities he would have as an officer, and eventually withdrew. He remains full of shame about this incident, as well as subsequent panic attacks, which have usually been precipitated by trips away from home, job stress, or interpersonal conflict.

Tom had been prescribed many different antidepressants with little result (antidepressants have often been found to be effective with symptoms like Tom's, and are preferable to tranquilizers, which are addictive). Nevertheless, because of his manifest distress I referred him to a psychiatrist, who had pretty much the same luck. At the time of the events of interest here, he was taking an SSRI and a mood stabilizer. About a year into treatment, I invited him to join a depression support group I run, where he became an active and valued member.

After Tom was laid off from his laborer's job, we reached a real impasse that lasted for some months. In the spirit of trying to be helpful, I suggested he look into employment with the federal government, thinking that he might find a variety of jobs, many with little stress. He became fixated on one particular job, and then filled months with procrastination about applying for that. He bought study guides for government service job testing, would spend weeks studying, then decide he had the wrong guide. He would get on the government website, and his computer would break down, or he would obsess about how to answer the questions. I really can't describe all the ways Tom wrestled with getting this application done, because my mind doesn't work that way, but he was a master at procrastination. However, his delaying tactics only made him more depressed and ashamed of himself.

What seemed to start to change things for Tom came from comments from a relatively new group member. She pointed out that his panic attacks had actually served a useful function for him: that they had usually occurred in situations where he felt unsafe and was trying to force himself to do something he really didn't want to do; that perhaps he should respect his anxiety more, and learn to live with it, perhaps by finding a very low-stress job, perhaps by considering that there is no disgrace to not working when you don't have to.

The group member's line of thinking got me stimulated too: Had I fallen into Tom's trap, feeling that it was my job simply to help him beat his anxiety to death? I picked up the subject in the next individual session. Me: The anxiety has been useful, a friend; it's no disgrace to quit a bad job. *Tom:* I can't see it as a friend. But I do realize I've been feeling bullied and picked on by my own anxiety. *He went on in a depressed vein, feeling that his whole life has been full of cowardice. I expressed sympathy but disagreed strongly with his comment about cowardice, pointing out incidents I knew of when he had taken an unpopular stand or stood up to people (notably a mugger in the park when he was out cycling). I also asked him why he had not been able to tell his parents about the bullying when it was going on.*

The following week Tom was still noticeably down, saying he'd been on autopilot, trying to avoid upsetting feelings. But he'd been having trouble sleeping, fighting the urge to track down the bully from middle school. The next week he felt a little better, back to being frustrated with his job search. We talked about how his job search had now become the bully; his daily self-torture about approaching the computer and the website, trying to complete the application, had gotten to the point where he was in real turmoil every time, bad enough that he could only spend a half hour a day wrestling the computer. I suggested he give himself two weeks off from the job search. I referred to other patients who had seemed to benefit greatly from giving themselves a vacation from their struggles.

The next week Tom reported that he had had difficulty not looking at the government jobs website, and also at the Sunday want ads, and wondered if I had been using reverse psychology on him. I denied this and said that I simply thought if he took a break from the pressure he might find a new approach to the whole situation. He got back to my question from several weeks earlier about not telling his parents about the bullying, saying he realized that his mother (pre-Alzheimer's) had been extremely anxious herself, in fact highly overprotective of him; that if he'd told either of his parents what was going on, she would have just made him feel worse and been of no help at all. He remembered in his last year of college, planning a trip with some friends. Her worrying and catastrophizing had been so extreme that he finally caught it and canceled the trip. When he announced his interest in officer candidate school, it was the same thing, worrying and catastrophizing. Her tone and timbre stick in my head, like a bully hanging over my shoulder. *But then when he left OCS, she just made things worse.* You looked so good in your uniform, we were so proud of you, what will we tell the neighbors? *Her tone, he said, was either hysteria or criticism. Which, I said, was exactly what he does to himself.*

At the next session Tom reported that he hadn't been able to stay away from the federal jobs website; in fact he'd become interested in another job there and started filling out an application. When his computer froze up he called the 800 number at the website, spoke to someone who was very helpful, and went to the public library and completed (!) the application on one of its machines. He said he felt like he was having a breakthrough in psychotherapy, that somehow connecting his anxiety to his mother meant that he was able to disengage from it a little, not feel like it defined him but was only a part of him. Somehow things that had looked intimidating in previous months now seemed to look interesting. Tom followed through, had several interviews and tests, got his job, and moved to another state.

The group's collective memory retained the idea that anxiety is your friend. It's trying to tell you something that you ought to pay attention to. Tom had distorted his natural anxiety into some external bullying force, something that picked on him and made his life miserable. Once he got used to the idea that anxiety was a natural human process, it lost its hold over him.

Anxiety is your body trying to give you a message. If you don't heed it, it may up the pressure. It is a signal, and it can be a friend. Unfortunately, most of us either ignore it or try to override it or misinterpret it, and therefore miss the lesson.

Anger

Daniel Goleman (author of *Emotional Intelligence*) and the Dalai Lama and others have talked of reducing "destructive" emotions—principally anger. I have to disagree with the implication that anger is innately and inevitably destructive. In the Buddhist tradition as I understand it, destructive emotions are destructive not because they are upsetting or lead to negative outcomes, but because they distort reality. Excessive desire blinds us to the negative aspects of an object, just as excessive aversion blinds us to the positive. In this sense, all emotions, anger certainly included, have the power to be destructive. And anger can fuel secondary emotional states like envy, greed, or begrudgery, which are by their nature destructive.

But anger is perfectly useful in the right place. It's the psychological response to getting our toes stepped on, the rush of adrenaline to the muscles and body that makes us ready to attack or defend ourselves. Society needs us to control how we express the anger response; but the belief that anger itself is a problem, a destructive emotion we would be better off without, is wrong-headed. Without anger we would have no righteous indignation, have no sense of fair play and justice, and be unable to defend ourselves when attacked. Fairness seems to be innate and intimately connected with anger. Children generally don't need much cueing from parents to have a sensitive sense of justice; much of the play of even the youngest children is about "the rules"—what's fair and what's not. New research has shown that monkeys also have a sense of justice; monkeys who had learned to earn tokens for food became outraged and literally went on strike, refusing to work anymore, when they saw their neighbor monkeys getting more desirable rewards than they got.

Further, without anger we would have almost no humor. Listen carefully to any comedian's monologue; if you get beneath what makes you laugh, you hear the anger. Humor is almost always "making fun" of some person. Sometimes it's the self, but frequently it's about someone we all have some mixed feelings about—political figures, for instance. Or someone else who takes themselves a little too seriously. Of course this can go too far, and humor can be cruel and feed prejudice. But humor also can be a classic adaptive defense, taking anger that might be dangerous in its pure form and turning it into laughter, another kind of emotional release; humor makes our enemy look weak and foolish, so we don't have to kill him or fear him.

None of this is meant to deny that anger creates terrible problems for us. It gets stirred up at inappropriate times by "schema attacks" (when something has happened to make us confuse the present with the past—see Chapter 6). We can hurt the people we love most because the anger response short-circuits the thinking parts of the brain. Or we try to deny and repress all anger, but it never works, and we feel guilty and ashamed for our revenge fantasies or irritability—a direct route to depression. Some of us are "anger addicts"—either always blowing up at people, then feeling embarrassed and ashamed at our loss of control, or silently collecting grievances and nursing grudges while pretending to the world that everything is fine (these people are full of shame too, but often it's unconscious). Anger can be seductive; it can make us feel powerful and self-righteous when we're feeling demoralized by too much stress. It's often used as a defense against other feelings, such as fear or guilt or shame. Many people, mostly but by no means all of them men, have learned to get angry whenever they feel vulnerable or feel they have slipped up and are in danger of exposure. Sometimes this strategy pays off, and these people end up with some real authority over others; but of course no one can ever get close to them. Being anger-prone increases risk of both chronic heart disease and heart attack, perhaps because although the blood pressure rises, the output of the heart does not rise proportionately. The heart of an anger-prone individual must work harder to achieve the increased blood flow that the stress response commands.

When we indulge too much in anger, we inevitably feel bad afterward, and we get caught in another vicious circle of addiction: anger→shame→anger→ shame→anger. We get angry all over again, blaming the person we were first angry at for the shame we feel about our anger, instead of taking responsibility for our own behavior. We need to recognize that anger is a valuable part of human nature, and train ourselves to use it effectively when necessary but to direct it at the appropriate targets. Shame and guilt, while appropriate expressions of our conscience, can also become powerful traps that keep us stuck in self-loathing.

Psychology has wasted a lot of time arguing about what anger is. Freud had postulated that there is a destructive force within us, an innate drive he called the death instinct, which manifests itself as anger. He had to construct this argument in order to fix some gaping holes in his overall theory of how the mind works; and though few really believed in the death instinct, because Freud's authority was so great everyone has had to scramble to figure out what anger really is without disrespecting him. It took Heinz Kohut, Freud's intellectual heir and "Mr. Psychoanalysis" in the 1970s and '80s, to say there really is no death instinct. Instead, Kohut argued, real rage, the destructive anger that gets out of control and makes us hurt the ones we love, is our reaction to an assault on the structure of the self—or what we *perceive* to be an assault. Something that makes us feel in danger of coming unglued. It's usually a narcissistic injury, a blow to our self-esteem, a threat to the little world we rely on to keep us together. A put-down, real or imagined. The threat of loss of the love or respect of someone we depend on.

These things can be microscopically small. A laugh, a look in the eyes, a failure to respond in the usual way. Ask anyone who's ever tried to soothe someone who's in a drunken rage or suicidal crisis. The person's self-esteem is so *out there,* so on the line, he'll challenge you to prove you love him, prove that he's not worthless, prove that life is worth living. And any response you give that shows the least fatigue, frustration, or disinterest is a terrible narcissistic injury; you'll spend the next hour trying to convince the person that you didn't really mean it.

One does not have to be drunk or suicidal to be wounded and enraged by small things. A person can have an angry heart, perpetually hurt and defensive, carrying around old grudges and scars that threaten to burst wide open with the least provocation. If this describes you, then something is seriously wrong with your assumptive world; you're distorting your experience of reality way beyond the limits of acceptable distortion. Read Chapter 6 and try very hard to understand what's wrong with the way you're seeing things.

But in today's world, most of us have a vulnerable heart. The Perpetual Stress Response has us full of anxiety, which dissolves our self-esteem. The things we're told to value—material success, acquisitions—are easy to lose. They're subject to the Hedonic Treadmill, so that we always need more in order to keep feeling good about ourselves. And they don't repair the orbitofrontal cortex, the damage in the brain that represents our fragile psyches, in the way that meaningful relationships, living up to a set of standards, or having a rich spiritual life can do for us. The result is that *we're always vulnerable to narcissistic injury—and rage is a common response.* When we're feeling hurt, excluded, vulnerable, or damaged, rage is a powerful countermeasure. We no longer feel weak, we feel powerful, full of righteous indignation, ready to damage those who've hurt us—but too often, the hurt was unintentional, the rage is way out of proportion, and we hurt those who love us.

A great many of the problems we have with how we express anger can be prevented, if only we use the skills of assertive communication, as I outline in Chapter 10. Those skills get conflicts settled as they arise, so that we don't have to fulminate until we explode with anger we've tried to stuff. Most of the other problems caused by anger are helped by a mindful attitude; mindfulness teaches us to identify what the trouble is, to refrain from taking it out on the wrong person, to not pick a fight about taking the garbage out when the trouble is that we're feeling unloved. What's left of anger needs to be managed by developing the skills of self-control. As we will see in Chapter 6, self-control isn't one of those things you either have or don't; we all have some, and we can get more through practice.

Guilt and Shame

Though these are painful states, they serve a very important purpose in helping us function as social creatures. You can make a good case that guilt, not agriculture or the wheel, may be the foundation of civilization. As a therapist I spend so much of my time helping people who punish themselves and constrain their lives with an overdeveloped sense of guilt that it's easy to forget the other side of the coin. Guilt is our emotional experience of right and wrong. Guilt, when you've done something wrong, is good for you, provided it lasts only a reasonable amount of time and that it brings about a change in behavior.

Implicit in that thought is the idea that guilt should always be about behavior. One of the most common psychological mistakes people make is feeling guilty over thoughts or emotions. Sexual fantasies, for instance, are harmless. Angry feelings, thoughts of revenge against those who hurt us, are unavoidable. But many people think less of themselves for sexual or aggressive feelings. This is unfortunate because revenge or sexual fantasies do no harm, and may even do us some good. If anything, we're entitled to feel proud of ourselves for exercising self-control.

Unfortunately our struggles with guilt and shame are much more complex than that. Thoughts or feelings that trigger guilt are also subject to defenses that keep them out of consciousness. We may briefly entertain lustful, angry, or other unacceptable thoughts or feelings only to have our internal censor kick in to suppress conscious awareness. You might assume that if we're not conscious of the unacceptable impulse we wouldn't feel guilty about it, but you'd be wrong. It happens all the time that people feel guilty about things they're not even aware of. You don't get the pleasure of the fantasy—the imagined tryst with the object of desire, the daydreamed shootout with the bully—but you do get to feel guilty about it. It's one of God's—or evolution's—mistakes; I can't see the value in it.

This is the kind of guilt that constricts people's lives, makes them depressed and unhappy with themselves. One way that therapy works is to bring the unconscious impulses, the precursors of guilt, out into the light of day. *So you sometimes have sexual fantasies about people other than your spouse? Is this a terrible thing? Just who is hurt by this? On the contrary, perhaps you deserve to feel a little pride that you have these impulses yet choose not to act on them. You have an ethical code that you strive to live up to. Surely that is better than trying to pretend you don't have feelings.* One of the major goals of therapy is to extend the range of conscious decision making that people have in their lives, reducing the range of behaviors, thoughts, and feelings that are governed by unquestioned habits and assumptions.

So in what sense is guilt good for you? Guilt, when applied to behavior, is the little alarm system that tells us when we are not living up to our own standards. Where our standards come from, and how much ours are like others', is beside the point for now. Guilt is what we feel when we have let ourselves down. Without it, we would be in an amoral world in which everyone could act on the impulse of the moment. And how to make sure that guilt only lasts a few minutes? I believe the Catholic Church teaches that forgiveness of sins requires two things: sincere repentance and a firm intention to amend. Repentance—guilt—by itself is not enough. I've known many people whom I've felt were truly remorseful for their actions, but repeated them again at the next temptation. We can feel sorry for these people, but we can't trust them. It takes a determination to do better next time to allow us to put guilt away. Next time we may fail again, but if we truly wish to change our behavior, eventually we will succeed.

Psychologists have written reams trying to differentiate between guilt and shame, but the best way to describe the difference is to evoke our own feelings. Robert Karen gives a gut-wrenching example: A professional man, divorced, in his fifties, stands on a subway platform eyeing an attractive young woman. For a few minutes he fantasizes asking her out—his suave charm sweeps her off her feet and before you know it they are in bed. He feels powerful, manly, irresistible. Then the fantasy is broken: she notices him watching her and shoots him a look of such disgust that he is instantly deflated. He suddenly feels that she sees him as he secretly fears he really is: pathetic, vain, a lonely old man who can't form a real relationship. Though he quickly forgets (represses) the experience, he is thrown off stride for the rest of the day; he feels depressed, cranky, unable to engage in productive activities, without understanding why. This is unconscious shame.

To me this example conveys the essence of shame. It is a deep, pervasive experience of loathsomeness or disgust about who or what we are. Where guilt, hopefully, is about specific actions that may be put right or forgiven, shame is about our core identity; the experience of seeing ourselves from another, harsher perspective, in the worst possible light; or of fearing that others see the secret self we keep hidden away and only remember when we're forced to.

It's interesting to me that shame seems to be linked with seeing and being seen. Heinz Kohut, whom we talk about elsewhere in connection with narcissistic disorders, taught that children need the experience of being *mirrored* by their parents. Children need to look in their parents' eyes and see themselves reflected back with love and approval. Parents cannot do this constantly, of course; but parents who routinely show disapproval or disgust when their children are showing off, demanding attention, may be teaching the child that there is something shameful about wanting to be special. According to Kohut, such children may grow up unable to feel joy or pride and thus remain depressed and empty; or conversely they may engage in compulsive attempts to gain attention and recognition from others. These attempts are doomed to failure because the adult feels secretly there is something shameful about the need in the first place.

Sometimes it seems as if we are trying to create a society that is free of shame in the hope that it will help us all feel good about ourselves; certainly the recovery movement, by focusing so much on "toxic" shame, seems to ignore the fact that shame is useful. Shame has value in that it implies modesty, respect for others, an awareness of one's own limitations. This, I think, is the kind of shame that we learn as an inevitable part of growing up, of becoming a civilized adult instead of a wild child. On the other hand, feeling good does not necessarily lead to growth, either of the individual or of society. Our collective shaky self-esteem is, to me, more a factor of our continual unconscious fear generated by the Perpetual Stress Response. Feeling good, then, results less from banishing shame than from facing fear.

Still, there is a destructive, pathological shame which we would do well to try to eradicate. Parents need to have the capacity to experience the joy of the child's unabashed narcissism, the LOOK AT ME! that every child demands. When we have so many single-parent families, when so many people are struggling to make ends meet and coming home stressed out, when parents are not getting their own needs met in the marriage, that can be a tall order. But it can be so refreshing to shrug off adult burdens for a while and enter the shame-free existence of the child. We should all do it whenever we can.

Mindfulness, the Core Skill

I have selected *mindfulness* as the primary core skill to help us escape the Perpetual Stress Response; I hope my reasons for doing this become clear as the chapter continues. But let me explain a little now.

Perpetual stress has many effects on brains and bodies, but its most immediate and perceptible is to put us into a state of *mindlessness.* You know exactly what I mean: reacting without thought; always in a rush; always in a state of tension that action can't alleviate; irritable, preoccupied, anxious, depressed. Not being fully aware of the present, always preoccupied by the next thing on our list. Perhaps this is worsened by physical pain or a state of distress or unease in the body. Mindlessness is a vicious circle, because acting mindlessly never can resolve the distress that fuels it.

Sometimes we get a wake-up call that breaks the vicious circle. An unexpected message from an old friend; a just-miss car accident that leaves us shaken; hearing an old song on the radio that takes us back in time. Our reactions to such events are predictable: we tell ourselves we've got to change, got to appreciate life more, not always be so busy with the details that we miss the big picture. How many times has this happened to you? How many times have you changed your life as a result? Don't blame yourself; the power of that vicious circle is formidable. We obviously need something more than an occasional reminder to escape.

The stakes are higher than just learning to appreciate life a little more. If we can find ways to be more mindful, we can protect ourselves from the Perpetual Stress Response, with all its attendant damage to the mind and body. New research is showing that mindfulness practice actually does rewire our brains, by building new neural pathways that restore brain centers to their more natural state. We'll talk in later chapters about the healing power of relationships, the need for meaningful work, and other methods of helping our brains develop immunity from stress—but these ultimately work by helping us become more mindful. Practicing mindfulness has been shown to affect how the brain deals with emotions, especially in the prefrontal cortex (PFC), the area containing the orbitofrontal cortex, the seat of the self. People who've been trained in mindfulness meditation have an increase in activity in the left prefrontal area—not just while meditating, but consistently—the part of the brain that processes positive feelings and controls negative feelings. The left PFC contains a set of neurons that specifically act to modulate messages of fear and anger from the amygdala. The more we practice this effect, the easier it gets; we learn—without consciousness of learning—to control disturbing emotions.

Mindfulness, to me, just means becoming more alert, thoughtful, deliberate; not reacting automatically to emotions; more curious, more ready to look beneath the surface, more ready to withhold judgment; kinder, more patient, more tolerant. These are difficult qualities to achieve when we're always running around putting out fires; but if we can't achieve them that is our destiny, one fire after another.

In *Undoing Depression* the eleventh of the twelve principles for recovery I proposed was "Practice Detachment." I was impressed by the emphasis Alcoholics Anonymous places on developing a detached attitude toward life's problems, as described in the Serenity Prayer:

> God grant me the serenity to accept the things I cannot change,
> The courage to change the things I can,
> And the wisdom to know the difference.

Depressed people, and most of the rest of us, spend a great deal of time and effort trying to control things that can't be controlled. We get caught up in our emotions, get frustrated, get angry, get stubborn, and before you know it we've made ourselves miserable. If we could only stand back and look at the problem objectively, without the emotional heat, we might see that it's not something we can control; or that there's a better way; or that even if there is a better way, we're spending too much time and effort on something that we really don't need to be doing.

Detachment is a good word for this, because we become *attached* to our problems like Captain Ahab to Moby Dick, and we need to consciously let go before they drag us down into the deep. But since writing that first book I've become aware that mindfulness is a more basic attitude we need to cultivate. Mindfulness both makes detachment easier and prevents us from becoming overly attached in the first place.

Mindfulness is a tool to increase self-awareness; as therapist Hope Payson puts it, mindfulness teaches how

> to observe oneself without the usual judgment or criticism. Negativity has a way of shutting people down. Criticism and judgment awaken all one's defenses—denial, projection, or that foggy unfocused feeling that stops you dead in your tracks.
>
> Mindfulness is the process of simply trying to witness and observe one's thought processes, behavior, and reactions to others without judging. It is the ability to see oneself with an increased clarity; and most importantly, with compassion or lightness. A kind of, "Wow, I'm seeing a pattern in my behavior of rejecting others—it's subtle but it's there" versus "I can't believe what a jerk I am being, no wonder I have no close friends" or "People really can't be trusted, they're always pushing me away." By kindly observing ourselves we have a better chance of learning to adjust and change. It is much easier to make changes based on compassion or more positive means instead of negative—like the feedback we get from others. It's a lot easier to accept when it's presented in a loving or productive way. Doesn't it make sense that the feedback that we give ourselves needs to be provided in the same fashion?

Achieving mindfulness takes practice, because it means taking time to turn off the logical mind—the part we're most secure about. All our highly developed skills in analysis and critical thinking are useful, at times, when applied to the self; but when that's the only way we look at ourselves, it backfires. Just as we need emotional support as well as guidance from loved ones, we also need emotional support from ourselves. For most people, a willingness to accept the value of mindfulness means acknowledging that our view of ourselves has been distorted for some time. "It's a recognition that we've been trying to bake the cake with all the ingredients but sugar; mindfulness supplies the sweetness and flavor we need to add to our understanding of ourselves."

Regular, daily meditation is the best way to achieve mindfulness, and I highly recommend it. I'll provide a simple method for meditation shortly, and

---

Exercise 4. **A Taste of Mindfulness**

Extend your left forefinger, touch it with your right forefinger, and close your eyes. Now explore the surface of the left forefinger using the right. You will notice the ridges and whorls on its surface, and you will get a mental image of its location in space. You may "see" your left finger in your mind's eye.

Now stop and reverse the process. Explore your right forefinger with your left. You will notice the same things about your right forefinger, and get the same mental image of it.

Before you read on and start thinking, take a few moments to let this experience settle in.

OK, now start to think about this: Why can't you notice the ridges of the right forefinger when you are using it to explore the left? Why don't you develop the same mental image of the right that you do with the left? And then, when you reverse the roles of the fingers, why does your focus stay on the finger that is being felt, rather than the one doing the feeling?

It's a mental trick. We have "decided" that one finger is to be the active agent of feeling, the other is to be the passive object of being felt. We can reverse their roles, but we can't do both at once. Our "decision" affects what we perceive, very definitively and dramatically.

Now, explore your mind with your mind. I don't mean exploring one hemisphere with the other; your mind is a unity for this purpose. But in the same way you decided that one finger was to be the object of exploration, make your mind the subject of mental exploration. Pay attention to what it's doing. What is it thinking about? What is it aware of? How is it in connection with your body? What is its mood? How alert is it?

The heart beats, the stomach digests, the brain thinks; don't think about what it's thinking, observe its thinking.

This is the beginning of mindfulness.

I hope you will experiment with it. There are other means to cultivate mindfulness, which we'll also discuss. Some people seem to have a mindful attitude naturally; psychotherapy helps teach it; and performing psychotherapy on others certainly encourages it. Frank, intimate conversation helps you gain a better distance and perspective on yourself. A rich spiritual life certainly helps. But before we go on and talk about how to learn mindfulness, please take a few moments and let yourself experience Exercise 4.

The Relaxation Response

To introduce our discussion of meditation and mindfulness, let's start with something simple and very well documented. The relaxation response (RR) is a connected series of changes in various organs (lungs, heart, muscles, brain) in response to a specific, regular relaxation routine. It was first described by Herbert Benson in 1975 and has been thoroughly investigated since. Benson was intrigued by the fact that regular practitioners of Transcendental Meditation (TM) had lowered blood pressure and reported many other healthful effects. Benson sought to take the religious and mystical overtones out of TM and investigate whether the relaxed state that meditation seemed to bring about had healthful effects that could be documented. He has demonstrated that attaining the RR results in lowering of metabolism, blood pressure, heart rate, rate of breathing, and muscle tension, and an increase in slow brain waves—just the opposite of the stress response. And he and others have shown that regular practice in RR has any number of positive benefits:

- People with hypertension experienced lower blood pressure and less need for medication over a three-year study period.
- People with chronic pain had less pain, more activity, less anxiety and depression, and fewer doctor visits in the two years after completing the training than they had before training.
- Seventy-five percent of patients with insomnia became normal sleepers.
- Women with PMS experienced a 57 percent decrease in severity.
- Patients with anxiety or mild to moderate depression became less anxious, depressed, angry, and hostile.
- Patients with cancer and AIDS experienced decreased symptoms and less nausea and discomfort associated with treatment.

Benson is an early pioneer in mind-body science. He has been careful to do effective, unbiased research, which has brought much greater acceptance in the medical community to the effects of stress on the body and the hope

The Relaxation Response

Attaining the relaxation response is not difficult at all, but, like all these skills, it requires practice. Here is Benson's "generic" technique:

- Pick a focus word or short phrase that suggests a calm state for you.
- Sit quietly in a comfortable position, in a place where you will be free from distractions.
- Close your eyes.
- Relax your muscles.
- Breathe slowly and naturally, from your belly, not your chest. As you do, repeat your focus word, phrase, or prayer silently to yourself with each breath.
- Assume a passive attitude. Don't worry about how well you're doing. When other thoughts come to mind (as they will), just let them go and return your attention to your breathing and your focus word.
- Continue for ten to twenty minutes.
- Don't stand right away. Continue sitting for a minute or two, allowing other thoughts to return. Then open your eyes and sit for another minute before rising.
- Practice this technique once or twice a day.

There are numerous variations on the routine used to get to the RR state. Some use visualization, some use progressive muscle relaxation, some do it while walking. Many people find that use of a taped guided relaxation session is helpful. Benson's books and *The Relaxation and Stress Reduction Workbook,* by Davis, Eshelman, and McKay, are good resources for other methods to achieve RR. Benson offers guided relaxation tapes through his website at www.mbmi.org.

for nonmedical interventions to undo those effects. Symptoms like those just described, which the relaxation response is effective in treating, are all stress-related. They are the effect of living under conditions which our bodies and brains, immune and nervous systems, are not designed for. They also can be treated with medication. But meds have their side effects and may have long-term effects we don't know about yet. Most important, meds merely enable us to continue living in the same way that overstressed us in the first place.

Mindfulness Meditation

While the relaxation response is purely a physical state, mindfulness meditation leads to something more.

Daily meditation is the best way to achieve a mindful attitude, and its benefits are well documented. Jon Kabat-Zinn has been a leader in research into the benefits of regular mindfulness meditation for twenty years, and his books *Full Catastrophe Living* and *Wherever You Go, There You Are* are wonderful resources. He has described mindfulness in famously succinct terms: "paying attention in a particular way: on purpose, in the present moment, and nonjudgmentally." He and his associates developed an eight-week stress reduction and relaxation program (now generally called Mindfulness-Based Stress Reduction; MBSR) at the University of Massachusetts Medical School, and have treated thousands with the method. It's a rather rigorous program; participants meet in a weekly group for two hours of guided meditation and discussion, with one all-day session as well, and homework of daily meditation for forty-five minutes (fully described in *Full Catastrophe Living*, and Kabat-Zinn has tapes and instructional materials available through the website www.mindfulnesstapes.com). Kabat-Zinn and others have had very promising results using the program (with some special adaptations, depending on the problem) with all sorts of issues: major depression, chronic pain, anxiety and panic, bulimia, psoriasis, fibromyalgia, mixed neurosis, mood and stress symptoms in cancer patients, and stress, anxiety, and depressive symptoms in the general population. Studies new in 2003 showed that MBSR produced brain changes associated with positive moods and an improved immune response among healthy volunteers, and it decreased stress symptoms and improved immune response in cancer patients. Though some of these studies have been criticized for small sample sizes and lack of control groups, I can tell you that if a drug was showing such promising results, there would be plenty of money to conduct the studies with sufficient numbers and controls to guarantee results—and a lot of publicity once the results were in.

The application of mindfulness meditation techniques to depression is being investigated by Segal, Williams, and Teasdale, with very encouraging results. Their book, *Mindfulness-Based Cognitive Therapy for Depression,* contains a step-by-step guide to an eight-week group treatment program designed specifically for patients with chronic depression. As we will describe later, most patients with depression have many relapses; but with MBSR, after one year, patients in the treated group had half the relapses of patients in the control group. The authors are cautious to suggest that MBSR is not likely to be a generic technique that can be effectively applied to a broad range of psychological problems; rather that when these techniques are learned they are also given in a specific and clinically sound context of understanding about the problem. In other words, it seems to be necessary to have a cognitive framework for the problem, with mindfulness helping to change attitudes to fit the new framework.

These authors also note that, like the saying in Alcoholics Anonymous, just because mindfulness is simple doesn't mean it's easy. They believe that mindfulness means getting the brain to process information in a completely different and incompatible way from our normal goal-oriented way of thinking; Segal and his colleagues call it shifting from "doing" mode to "being" mode. They stress that the doing mode is our habitual pattern, and that the being mode is foreign territory for most of us. Without proper instruction, learning "mindfulness" can just become another goal we strive for in doing mode; we obsess and learn the method without the message. The beginning meditator's concern with "doing it right" is commonly understood in all meditation approaches to be wrong in itself; it's only in learning to give up such concerns that we take the first step toward nonjudgmental thinking.

The Importance of Practice

Ages ago, Plato argued that virtue is a habit; that the more one behaves in accordance with accepted values, the easier it is to continue such behavior. It won't be long now before we have pictures of the brain to confirm this. Being in a rut is more than just a metaphor. Bad habits wear grooves in our brains, those long-term potentiated circuits, electrical and chemical connections that become our brains' preferred methods of operating so that it feels comfortable and natural to take the easy way out. With continued stress, our muscles atrophy, our joints stiffen, and our brains settle into convenient but constricting, paralyzing patterns of thought and feeling. Nothing new happens in our awareness unless we work hard to make room for it.

Exercise 5. A Simple Mindfulness Meditation

There are many approaches to mindfulness meditation. Here is a simple one, which I've tried to strip to the basics.[1]

- Find a quiet place where you will not be interrupted for a half hour or more. Turn off the phone, the TV, the stereo. If you have pets, close the door. I find it helpful to turn on a fan, both for the breeze and for the quiet noise.
- Sit in a comfortable position. If you want to sit on the floor, it helps to have a thin pillow under your butt. Tuck your feet under your knees, but don't strain. Sit upright, with your back straight. Let the weight of your head fall directly on your spinal column. If you want to sit in a chair, try to put your feet flat on the floor. Again, sit upright, with your back straight.
- Close your eyes, and start to breathe slowly and deeply. Not so deeply that you strain yourself, just comfortably. As you breathe, you may find it helpful to focus on a word or phrase, timing it to your breathing. "In . . . Out." You can change this to suit your mood. When I'm fighting craving, I think "Wave . . . Rock." Other times I like "I am here . . . I am home." You will find phrases that are good for you.
- Focus on your breathing. As other thoughts or feelings come to mind, let them pass, and return your attention to your breathing. Visualize these distracting thoughts and feelings as bubbles rising to the surface of a calm pool of water. They rise, burst, and disappear. The pool remains calm. Return your attention to your breathing.
- Don't judge. Don't try to do it right, just try to do it every day. Remember that the distracting thoughts and feelings are the normal noise in your brain. It takes practice and skill to get in touch with the quietness underneath.
- When I'm preparing for meditation, and when I feel restless, I like to remember the perspective of Anh-Huong Nguyen, a Vietnamese follower of

---

1 I should warn that for some people, especially those with unresolved PTSD issues, mindfulness meditation can be just too upsetting. It can be a time when flashbacks occur. If this is you, I strongly recommend you work with a therapist to help you integrate these experiences. Meanwhile, follow my other mindfulness tips.

Thich Nhat Hanh: "If you have a fussy baby, do you shout at the baby? Do you get angry at it? Do you shake it? No—you *build a cradle* for the baby." That's what we have to deliberately allow ourselves to practice: to treat ourselves with care and concern. That's also what meditation does for our restless, anxious minds; it builds a structure we can feel safe in.

- When you are ready to stop, open your eyes. Stay seated for a few moments while you appreciate the calm state you are in.
- If you have to use an alarm, make it something quiet, not jarring. Jon Kabat-Zinn has a tape with nothing on it but temple bells at regular intervals; it's much nicer than any alarm clock.

You will find yourself frequently distracted by intrusive thoughts—sometimes nagging thoughts about what you have to get done today, sometimes memories that may be pleasant or unpleasant. You may also be distracted by emotions—primarily impatience and anxiety. *Remember that these intrusive thoughts and emotions are the effects of stress on your brain.* You will not be able to make them go away without practice, which may take months. It may help to visualize, for instance, putting these thoughts into a box or on a list that you can look at later. Just don't get upset with yourself because you do get distracted; don't tell yourself you're not doing it right; just return to the focus on your breath. Judging yourself is another habit, one you can put aside while you're meditating.

There are many other forms of meditation. Many people, especially those with anxiety or muscular tension, like the "body scan" method. There is a "mindfulness of pain" meditation, and a walking meditation. A favorite for many is the "loving-kindness" meditation, in which you first focus on the feeling you had as a child when someone deeply loved you, then focus on returning that feeling to the other person, then imagine directing that feeling to the whole world. In the Appendix you will find some interesting leads.

As with all these exercises:

The more you practice, the easier it gets.

The new neuroscience is convincingly demonstrating that practice and ex-perience make lasting changes in the electrical and physical structure of the brain. The area of the brain devoted to the "reading finger" of Braille readers is much larger than that for their other fingers, or for the corresponding fingers of controls. Though the studies haven't been done in humans yet, it is safe to assume that the exquisite sensitivity of a piano tuner or a wine taster is a result of practice expanding the complexity and even physical size of the correspon-ding areas in the brain. The coordination skills of physical movement, from skiing to typing, require corresponding changes in brain tissue.

Most human problems are examples of vicious circles in action, as the re-spected therapist Paul Wachtel and others have pointed out. In depression, your low energy and lousy mood make it very difficult to do the things that would make you feel better. In anxiety, your hypervigilant watchfulness guar-antees you'll find things to worry about; the same is true in nonspecific illness, except that your watchfulness is focused on your body. Addictions are by defi-nition vicious circles; your drug creates a craving for more. Personality disor-ders also; the ways you characteristically use to seek love or success or happiness guarantee that you will fail. I have no doubt that soon *we will find neurochemical sequences in the brain that underlie these patterns and are themselves vicious circles;* indeed, that's what we're talking about with the Perpetual Stress Response. Constant stress results in an overproduction of stress hormones that wear down the body's defenses against stress. These patterns aren't easy to break. They will require diligent practice. I suggest you make up your mind to practice mindfulness meditation for a half hour every day, six days a week. Give it a month, at least, and I'll bet you'll start noticing some benefits.

Mindfulness and Buddhism

The Buddhist doctrine of *karma* is popularly understood as a vicious circle: what goes around, comes around. When you have bad luck, it's because of your own actions at some time in the past (perhaps in a previous life). But karma is better understood as a feedback loop, because you have the power to choose how you respond to bad luck, or to good luck. The Buddhist concepts of *skillful action* and *unskillful action* describe ways to perpetuate or change your karma. "Skillful" on first reading may seem to mean ethical and compassionate: it's skillful to speak the truth, to respect the rights of others, to rise above envy and competition, to wish well for others. But calling these attitudes skills pays them proper respect—they are not easy; we have to practice; the more we practice the better we get. These *are* skills, not inborn character traits. Practice, though it may be hard in the present, makes things easier in the future.

One thing about cultivating mindfulness: *It seems too simple.* On the other hand, *few people can do it.* It seems too easy to have any real effect on what's bothering us, which seems so overwhelming and confusing by comparison. Perhaps this is one reason why few people can do it—we don't take it seriously. But another, more significant, reason is our own defense system; our minds find distractions, obstacles, and arguments against doing what is good for us. If you seriously sit down and try to do this for a few days, you will find that it's not as easy as it looks. You will want to stop. But practice is essential. You're going to be challenging years of what life has taught you about how to deal with your emotions. You'll find that there are an amazing number of obstacles that get in the way of your practice. This is *resistance*—which we'll talk about much more in the next chapter—and it's normal. Don't beat yourself up over it. Remember Plato; the more you practice being virtuous, the easier it gets.

Mindfulness is a value that we tend to associate with Buddhism. But meditation, or some form of it, is practiced in almost all religions (that's what contemplative prayer is), and the extremes of mysticism and asceticism that we now attribute to Buddhism have a long history in Christianity, Judaism, and Islam. Meditation and the ascetic life were practiced in India long before the time of Buddha (born c. 563 B.C.). Buddha himself was a rich prince who, appalled by poverty and suffering, renounced his patrimony and took up the life of a hermit in the woods. It did not bring him the understanding he sought, but a period of intensive meditation did, and after this he began teaching others. (*Siddhartha,* Hermann Hesse's fictionalized account of Buddha's early life, is good reading.) The Buddha taught that we suffer because we believe that things are permanent and can be relied on for happiness, and because we believe we have a permanent self that exists independently of others and makes us who we are. Instead, he taught, we must free ourselves from illusion and see things, and ourselves, as they are—constantly changing. Buddhism in many ways seems more like a psychology than a stereotypical Western religion because it focuses on living *this* life "skillfully"—free from desire, anger, fear, and other negative mind states. There is relatively little emphasis on the next life, or on worshiping a divine being, or on seeking spiritual ecstasy. Instead, you'll find lots of practical advice, along with the familiar Zen *ko'ans,* or paradoxes, designed to make you think mindfully.

The fundamental difference between Buddhism and the secular[2] Western view of man is succinctly described by Mark Epstein:

> In Western theories, the hope is always that emptiness can be healed, that if the character is developed or the trauma resolved that the background feelings will diminish. If we can make the ego stronger, the expectation is that emptiness will go away. In Buddhism, the approach is reversed. Focus on the emptiness, the dissatisfaction, and the feelings of imperfection, and the character will get stronger.

From a Buddhist perspective, Cartesian dualism—the belief that there is a *self* separate from our physical bodies—is itself a defense, a developmental failure, a denial of transience. We share the delusion that if we just train our left brains to be good enough, we will somehow master the world—a world that is so inherently full of suffering that we will not be able to perfect it no matter how hard we try. A standard introductory Buddhist text says: "Meditation is not a matter of trying to achieve ecstasy, spiritual bliss or tranquility, nor is it attempting to become a better person. It is simply the creation of a space in which we are able to expose and undo our neurotic games, our self-deceptions, our hidden fears and hopes."

From this point of view, Western religions can reinforce some immature defenses. The belief that there is an all-caring or all-wise god, the ultimate authority who will judge us all, reward the virtuous, and punish the wicked, is absent from Buddhism. Likewise the idea that evil is the product of some outside force. Buddhism doesn't suggest that there is any other life than this one or that there are forces more powerful than men. Instead, we are here alone and this is our one chance. Buddhism suggests a method for living in a world of fear and pain, nothing more than a method. On the other hand, it doesn't ask for us to make a leap of faith, a challenge that people find increasingly difficult in today's secular world.

Mindfulness is a tool to get underneath our defenses. When we can observe ourselves closely, experiencing our feelings but not reacting to them, we don't

---

2 We should emphasize the word "secular." Jesus' teachings (and the early Christian church's) emphasize giving up this world: "Go thy way, sell whatsoever thou hast, and give to the poor, and thou shalt have treasure in heaven: and come, take up the cross, and follow me" (Mark 10:21).

have to pretend that we don't feel. We learn to accept our emotions without being guided by them and without being afraid or ashamed of them. Mindfulness emphasizes an attitude of nonjudgmental acceptance. Things that enter our mind during mindfulness practice—thoughts, feelings, physical sensations, moods, perceptions—are to be observed carefully but not evaluated in terms of good or bad, healthy or sick, wise or silly, useful or useless. Learning to interrupt the habit of judging takes practice. So many of our problems are caused by our defenses springing into action automatically to protect us from a feeling or from reality. Negative emotions—anger, grief, guilt, shame—are a problem for everyone, but especially for those with depression, anxiety, or chronic pain conditions. Blocked or stuck negative emotions are frequently manifested as depression, anxiety, or pain. Mindfulness teaches us that no emotion, no reality, is negative; it just *is*, and it's wise to accept it. This acceptance removes the need for defenses. Besides, who would you rather have making the decisions in your life: your automatic, mindless defensive system or your full, responsible consciousness? Mindlessness is the opposite of mindfulness—being swept away in an emotional state or schema. Mindlessness is being controlled by categories ("he's only a [whatever], what does he know?"), by habitual thinking (going through the motions of reading or listening without paying attention), or by acting from a single perspective when a changed point of view might yield a new solution (thinking "outside the box").

Consider the following question to Benjamin (see Chapter 6): *What if you really look at this fear that you are somehow a fraud, destined to failure? What if you just face it?* He didn't need any more insight into the origins of these fears; they clearly came from his emotionally crippled parents, who would first encourage his great ambitions, then bitterly castigate him for acting like he was better than they were. But he needed to overcome somehow the procrastination that accompanied his fears. Facing a fear robs it of its power. We prove to ourselves that we don't have to keep running away. Confronting one's own death allows you to make realistic plans for the future.

Other Paths to Mindfulness

Daniel Goleman: Emotional Intelligence

Daniel Goleman's 1995 book *Emotional Intelligence* has become so familiar now that it's not news to most of us that "emotional intelligence"—however it's defined and measured—is much more powerful in predicting happiness and success in life than mere IQ. Old definitions of intelligence measured abstract reasoning power, factual memory, and other attributes of the higher cortex. Emotional intelligence has much more to do with getting the cortex and the limbic system, intelligence and emotions, communicating clearly with each other and working together. In Goleman's terms, emotional intelligence refers to several related abilities:

1. *Knowing one's own emotions.* The ability to recognize a feeling as it happens. As we'll discuss in Chapter 6, we have all kinds of ways—defenses—to disguise emotions from ourselves. Others of us have been so damaged by trauma or limited by a deprived childhood that the ability to register emotions on the brain has been pruned away.

2. *Managing emotions.* To Goleman, this means controlling feelings so that we can calm ourselves, so that we don't get swept away by intense feelings of the moment—anger, fear, depression.

3. *Motivating oneself.* As I've said, emotions are motivations. Goleman suggests that an important aspect of emotional intelligence is the conscious use of self-control to get what we want—for instance, the use of positive self-talk to help us get through a difficult exam.

4. *Recognizing emotions in others.* This includes empathy, the ability to feel what others are feeling, and desire and attention—the understanding that others' feelings are important.

5. *Handling relationships.* Goleman is referring to social skills, much of what I'm referring to when I talk about controlling how we display our emotions so that others understand what we mean.

Mindfulness, as I'm using the term, is closely related to the concept of emotional intelligence. It means using the whole mind to observe both the emotions and the intellect at work; feeling emotions deeply without either being overpowered by them or denying their existence. At the same time, it means using the information provided by our emotions to help us make better decisions, communicate more clearly, connect to others more intimately. Goleman's extremely useful book takes an informative and educational approach to these issues, while I advocate looking more deeply within yourself and practicing mindful thinking until it becomes automatic. Goleman, in this book and his later publications, has a great deal of extremely vivid, concrete, and practical advice for how to develop greater emotional intelligence. I emphasize the role of the Perpetual Stress Response in generating mindlessness, while Goleman is more likely to accept current cultural patterns as the givens within which we must work. We are coming at much the same subject from our own assumptive worlds, with some differences in our thinking about what the basic problem is, and with slightly different goals, but the two approaches are highly complementary to each other.

Ellen Langer: The Creative Aspect of Mindfulness

While daily meditation is the best way to achieve a mindful state, it's not the only way, and it's not a guarantee. Mindfulness is a revolution in the brain, a huge change in how we think, feel, and see the world. Ellen Langer's approach to mindfulness comes from a non-Buddhist tradition and is concerned with how our environment facilitates (or hinders) a mindful attitude. She is interested in mindfulness as the process of developing new perceptions, rather than staying stuck with habitual, mindless patterns of thought, old rules, routines, and expectations. This can lead to diverse consequences, such as becoming more sensitive to one's surroundings; becoming more open to new information; creating new distinctions and categories for structuring perception; and greater awareness of other perspectives in problem solving. For her, "the subjective 'feel' of mindfulness is that of a heightened state of involvement or being in the present."

In one famous experiment, she gave a group of nursing home residents a plant for their rooms. Half the group were told they would be totally responsible for the plant; they were also encouraged to make as many decisions regarding their own care, the setup of their rooms, and so forth as they could for themselves. The other half (the control group) were told the plant was just a decoration, and the staff would take care of it. They were encouraged to rely on the staff to make all their decisions for them. Eighteen months later, the experimental group was more active, vigorous, and social than the control group, and their physical health had actually improved, while the control group's had worsened. Most surprisingly, only 15 percent of the experimental group had died in the interval, versus 30 percent of the control group! Findings like these have led to vital changes in how nursing homes are run. Other research along this line has focused on methods of increasing mindfulness in business and education. Langer and her associates have found, for instance, that simply introducing objects in a conditional way ("may be" instead of "is") enables participants to use the objects in more creative ways.

Langer's thinking, while it also emphasizes the nonjudgmental element of mindfulness meditation, emphasizes the creative aspects of mindfulness as well. I wonder if an overlooked element in studies of MBSR might be that practice in mindfulness enables participants to be more creative in finding solutions to their own problems. They would benefit not only because MBSR training helps them cope with stress more effectively, but also because they find creative solutions that help reduce their overall stress level.

Jeffrey Schwartz: Mindful Control of Symptoms
Jeffrey Schwartz, a psychiatrist at UCLA, performed a revolutionary feat in 1996 by demonstrating that psychotherapy results in changes in the brain visible on PET scans; as far as I know, the first such demonstration. His book, *The Mind and the Brain,* contains a fascinating description of how he accomplished that. He was able to combine two key personal interests: the mind-body problem[3] and Buddhist mindfulness meditation. He decided to work with patients with severe obsessive-compulsive disorder (OCD) because they exemplify the mind-body problem so well: they *know* their symptoms are bizarre, they experience their urges as coming from outside their will, yet they cannot will themselves to resist. Schwartz and others in his group were able to demonstrate that, for people with OCD, the "alarm circuit" in the brain is stuck in the *on* position; the circuit that is supposed to let us know that a situation is new, or needs attention, doesn't turn itself off in OCD like it normally does when we've performed an action that should tell our brain we've taken care of the problem.

Schwartz began to work with that knowledge and his interest in mindfulness with his group of severe OCD patients. He began to teach them mindfulness skills, in the hope that learning to watch their thoughts objectively might help them learn to detach: *it's not me, it's my OCD.* This became the first step, Relabeling, in what eventually became a four-step process. Showing his patients their own PET scans, with the overactive alarm circuit highlighted, led to the second step, Reattributing: *it's only a brain glitch, it's not reality.* The third

---

3 A perennial problem in philosophy: how does the mind, which has no physical existence, affect the body? We've had bizarre explanations from Descartes: "all experience and action potential pre-exist in the brain"—to Skinner: "there is no mind" (see "Descartes' Error, Skinner's Fumble," on pages 499–500. Current brain research is certainly showing how the brain affects the body. The question of how we form a mind, consciousness, and will, is more complicated. Allan Schore (see the reference list) is coming closest to the answer.

Jeffrey Schwartz's Four Rs, Adapted for Depression

- *Relabeling.* Recognize that the catastrophic thoughts, the choked-up feeling, the impulse to isolate, *is* the depression. It's an old habit, a set of circuits in the brain that have become wired together as a result of depression. Practice mindfulness to differentiate between your true self, with your knowledge of what is good for you, and the self-destructive impulse, the dark cloud closing in. The despairing feeling is a false message, due to a jammed transmission in the brain. *You* are separate from the depression.

- *Reattributing.* The faulty brain circuitry will persist for some time, but recognize that it's really only static in your system. No matter how real they seem, the depressive thoughts, feelings, and impulses are due to a certain set of neurons firing together, producing a false reality in your mind. With practice, you can lay down new circuitry that will replace these faulty circuits.

- *Refocusing.* You are in control of what you pay attention to. Shift your focus from the depressive thoughts to interfering or adaptive behavior. Physical activity is very useful. So is reaching out to a friend, if you focus on talking about something other than your depressed feelings. This is the most difficult task, and will require lots of practice. It can help to start with a simple, comfortable distraction: a walk; needlework; music. Practice refocusing often enough that it becomes a habit. It can be very helpful at this point to have a success team (see Chapter 10) to encourage you.

- *Revaluing.* Keep practicing mindfulness until you reach the place known to the Buddhists as "wise attention"—the ability to see things as they really are. Not everything in your life will work out the way you want it to, but does that inevitably make you depressed? If you can rewire your brain to replace the depressed circuitry, maybe things are different than they have seemed to you. Perhaps disappointment, loss, or rejection, while sad and painful, do not have to cast a dark cloud over your whole life.

step, Refocusing, was a logical extension: *lay down new brain circuitry*. When you become aware of an OCD symptom, shift your attention to something distracting, pleasant, and good for you. Patients began to carry around diaries describing what kinds of distractions were effective, and sharing the information. Physical activity was usually helpful; something that required attention—gardening, needlework, even computer games. Schwartz asked his patients to be sure to give themselves fifteen minutes after the awareness of a symptom before they would allow themselves to act on it. During this time they found (as many others have; see the discussion of mental control in Chapter 8) that it was much easier to think of something else rather than simply *not* think about their obsessive thought. The fourth step, Revaluing, took patients back to a fundamental message of Buddhist meditation: wise, or skillful, attention. Wise attention means seeing things as they are, not being caught up in feelings about how things should be. It's Freud's reality principle, the first of Buddha's Four Noble Truths, the Rolling Stones' dictum: *You can't always get what you want*. For these patients, I think, it means something more than controlling symptoms; it means taking responsibility for life as it is.

Schwartz's work, with that of some others, has given me the support I needed to make the claim I made in the introduction to this book: that we have the power to change our own brains. The choices we make in how we live, what we value, and what we pay attention to, affect our own neural circuitry. It's important to note that Schwartz's OCD patients were able to do this largely on their own, without much in the way of "deep" psychotherapy. They put a lot of hard work, and much time, into it, but the methods were essentially didactic and experiential. It gives hope that wise self-help can have the same effects. I have been so taken with Schwartz's work that I have adapted his four-step model and am using it with some of my depressed patients. I firmly believe that depression and other psychological ills also manifest themselves in faulty brain circuitry—perhaps not so clear and consistent as OCD, but there nonetheless—and that if depressed patients can really get their minds around that concept, and if they learn mindful awareness, they can benefit greatly.

Marsha Linehan: Dialectical Behavior Therapy

Marsha Linehan's Dialectical Behavior Therapy (DBT) is a highly structured and detailed program for treating borderline personality disorder, borrowing from many sources. I believe it is an extremely useful resource for many patients, far many more than those diagnosed as borderline. Linehan is also informed by a Zen-based perspective: her use of the term "dialectics" refers to the Hegelian concept of the continuing search for "the" truth from the interaction of opposites. Each interaction generates a new truth, which in turns generates its own opposite, leading to a new interaction. She's interested in paradox: the patient is told he's perfect just as he is, but he has to change; the therapist's style vacillates between warm acceptance and blunt, irreverent confrontation. The treatment approach combines psychoeducation, individual psychotherapy, and a lot of homework. Mindfulness skills are emphasized as essential; taught in psychoeducation, reviewed and emphasized in individual therapy, and practiced over and over in the homework.

Linehan teaches three "what" mindfulness skills (observing, describing, participating) and three "how" skills (taking a nonjudgmental stance, focusing on one thing in the moment, and being effective):

- *Observe.* This means learning to pay attention to events, including emotions, without being either mindlessly swept away with them or mindlessly trying to avoid them. "Watch your thoughts coming and going, like clouds in the sky."
- *Describe.* We need to learn how to describe experiences in words. This helps teach that thoughts and feelings are different from the events that precipitated them. In practicing describing, we are forced to learn to step back from experience. "Call a thought just a thought, a feeling just a feeling."
- *Participate.* This suggests being fully aware, fully in the moment, as opposed to mindless drivenness or distraction. "A skillful dancer on the dance floor, one with the music and your partner."
- *Take a nonjudgmental stance.* We need to stop putting labels on experiences—this is good, that's bad; he's a worthwhile person, she's useless. This skill emphasizes noticing how we constantly judge, and learning to stop that process. Judging leads to categorical, rigid, mindless thinking. "When you find yourself judging, don't judge your judging."
- *Focus on one thing in the moment.* Most of us are constantly distracted by too many things at once to do any one thing effectively. We need to practice controlling our attention so that we are mindful of what we are doing. "When you are thinking, think. When you are worrying, worry. When you are planning, plan."
- *Be effective.* This refers to doing what works in a given situation, rather than doing what our emotions tell us we "should" do. It means "playing

the game." DBT reframes doing the effective thing rather than the "right" thing as a skillful response, not simply giving in. "Play by the rules. Don't 'cut off your nose to spite your face.' "

Marlatt and Gordon: Relapse Prevention Therapy

Another approach that incorporates mindfulness skills is the Relapse Prevention Therapy of Marlatt and Gordon, which was specifically designed for addiction problems but has been found helpful by individuals with other issues, including depression. Addiction is seen as an inability to accept the present moment—always being distracted by the search for the next high. Mindfulness skills are used to help the patient learn to stay in the present, learn to ride the waves of craving rather than struggling against the tide, a technique known as "urge surfing."

Living Mindfully

The goal of practicing mindfulness meditation and developing these skills is to achieve the state that Buddhists call "wise mind"—an integration of the logical mind with the emotional mind—a goal I push for throughout this book. It's what Allan Schore is describing when he suggests that, in many emotional disorders, the left and right portions of the orbitofrontal cortex aren't integrated, so that a stable and coherent self is not formed. Linehan's results with borderline patients strongly suggest that guided practice in mindfulness skills can help to heal what has been a lifetime of dysfunction and pain.

I feel it necessary to give one little caveat: Detachment can be carried too far. The advice of the Stoic philosophers—*Value only that which no one can take from you*—may sound appealing, especially to those who have been hurt a lot. If you can restrict your wants to the most basic things, if you can value only your own attainments, it seems like no one can hurt you. But what kind of a life is this? Even in Zen, which values detachment and teaches the impermanence of objects, there is an acknowledgment that loss hurts and that we can't transcend that. Acceptance of loss means acceptance of the feelings that go with it. Satori, enlightenment, doesn't mean that we're going to be blissed out with oneness from here on in; the desire to seek bliss—an invulnerability to sadness, fear, or anger—through meditation or Zen practice is another resistance at work, an effort to find a new defense.

With problems as diverse as chronic pain, anxiety, addiction, and negative emotional states, mindfulness teaches the patient to sit with, observe, and experience the symptom while resisting the urge to seek relief. This is similar to the process behaviorists call "extinction," which means breaking the connection between a response and the stimulus that formerly cued it. When a rat that has learned that a light means a shock finally stops trying to escape after a long series of trials with no shock; or when an acrophobic patient no longer experiences panic in a tall building because of gradual exposure—that is extinction. Researchers have recently learned something interesting: extinction is not forgetting. "Extinction is an active learning process, a repatterning of new memory over an old one that takes place in the smartest brain area of all, the prefrontal cortex," writes Bruce McEwen. In extinction, a new brain circuit is developed that takes the "high road" through the logical brain and overrides the "low road" connection from the amygdala directly to the stress response. Attention is the key. Focusing attention on a specific task, like paying attention to color, or movement, results in increased electrical activity and increased blood flow in the brain areas that correspond to color and movement. Focusing on experiencing the fear without responding apparently has the same effect.

We've talked about the need to control emotions at the same time as experiencing them as the central problem that brings people to therapy, and the central issue around which the infant develops a self. Mindfulness teaches us to sit with emotional states in a way that progressively helps us observe, tolerate, and explore feelings and emotion-laden thoughts. For years, therapists have called such exercises *structure building*. Perhaps at some time in the near future, we will be able to show that this is more than metaphor, that new circuits and structures are indeed constructed in the brain when we train ourselves in mindfulness skills.

One way I think this happens is that being mindful provides a kind of validating experience to the self. When we were discussing how the infant mind forms a self-concept, we talked about how the self-as-perceived-by-the-other and the self-as-perceived-by-the-self need to be congruent in order for a stable neural network representing the self to develop. The self-as-perceived-by-the-other is congruent to the self-as-perceived-by-the-self when our external experiences *validate* our internal experiences; when other people in our lives show that they "get" how we feel. And perhaps in experiences with music, or nature, or our spiritual life, there is that same validation sometimes. Achieving a state of focused mindfulness, as in mindfulness meditation, may mean that the self-as-perceived-by-the-other and the self-as-perceived-by-the-self become one and the same. We provide a "holding environment" for ourselves: we *hold our own self in our own mind's eye,* without judging, with compassion, with focus. As we have speculated about the effect of validating experiences from others, the neural network in the brain that represents our self is thereby strengthened and repaired. Both neurologically and emotionally we become coherent, together, stable. We add to the coherent autobiographical narrative, the story of our selves, that is so important for integrity, the ability to stand up to stress.

People who practice mindfulness find that they are much less moody. Developing the ability to watch the mind with a little detachment as thoughts and feelings come and go means that those thoughts and feelings lose their power to distract us. Moods are a thought-feeling state where our feelings are reinforced by our (frequently obsessive) thoughts. When we're in a bad mood, the only things we can think about are things that reinforce the mood. Mindfulness breaks the power that these thoughts have over us, and teaches us to look underneath the bad feeling with compassionate curiosity. Instead of obsessing mindlessly, we look at the bad feeling from a different perspective. It may be one of detachment, realizing that moods are self-limiting and will change soon enough by themselves. Or it may be one of creativity—*Let's see what this is all about. Let's trace the connections here.* Knowing that bad feelings never come out of the blue, they always have a reason, we can identify the reason for this one. If it's silly, we can laugh at ourselves. If it's serious and painful, we can help ourselves. We don't have to stay on the bad feeling–bad thought merry-go-round.

One interesting discovery has emerged from mindfulness research. Richard Davidson, a leading brain researcher based at the University of Wisconsin, has documented that the brain has a set point for mood. After studying hundreds of individuals, Davidson has shown that when people are feeling stressed— sad, angry, anxious—both the amygdala and the right prefrontal cortex (PFC) are very active. But when people are in positive moods, those sites are quiet and the *left* prefrontal cortex is active. Davidson tests individuals over time with fMRI techniques and develops a ratio of right/left PFC activity for each. As you might expect, there is a normal distribution: most people have a mixture of right/left activity, while there are a few at each extreme. Depressed people tend to have not enough left prefrontal activity, anxious people tend to have too much activity in the right. At a conference with the Dalai Lama, Davidson had the opportunity to use his fMRI techniques on a Tibetan monk who had been meditating all his life—who turned out to have the most extreme difference in left-right PFC activity of anyone then tested. According to this measure, the Buddhist monk was in the happiest state yet found. More promising still, Davidson and Jon Kabat-Zinn have been able to show that a mindfulness training program with healthy volunteers results in shifts in PFC activity to the left, as well as improved moods and motivation, after only eight weeks.

There is good reason to believe that mindfulness came more naturally to our ancestors. They had much more time than we do for the right brain, the contemplative, creative side, to be active. There were many times when they just had to be patient, waiting for the fish to bite, the rain to stop, the wound to heal. There were long nights together with stories and magic. They felt a part of the natural world, a kinship with the animals who lived around them. I don't believe it's an accident that Buddha came along at a historical time when the pursuit of material wealth had first become possible. He came to remind people of the old ways. We are in far more difficult times now; the push toward materialism, the emphasis on the left brain, is much stronger, and we need courage and discipline to look around and consider old ways again.

Compassionate Curiosity

"Compassionate curiosity" is the phrase a colleague of mine uses to describe how the ideal therapist should view his patient, and how we should view ourselves. It is a phrase I find loaded with meaning. It implies a kind detachment, an inquisitive affection. What a shift in attitude that would be for almost everyone I know! We don't tend to view ourselves kindly. Most of us treat ourselves like inconsistent parents treat their children. Much of the time we indulge and spoil ourselves; we let ourselves off the moral hook, we make promises to ourselves we know we won't keep. But at the same time, another part of our minds is always judging, criticizing us, finding that we don't measure up. We vacillate between spoiling ourselves and punishing ourselves. Compassion implies patience, gentleness, love, grace, mercy, concern. It suggests giving up judging but at the same time wanting the best for ourselves. It suggests empathy, a willingness to feel everything that the self feels, without fear but with confident strength.

Curiosity suggests a little distance from the self, a desire to understand objectively why we're feeling what we feel, why we're going through what we do. It's good to question ourselves. It's good to pause and reflect. We need to study ourselves somewhat; not necessarily to rake ourselves over the coals, but to

Zen and Psychoanalysis

For far too long, experiences that might be called religious, mystical, or transcendental have been either ignored or viewed with suspicion by psychotherapy. Cognitive therapy, the predominant viewpoint in American academia, has largely ignored any study of the subject. The Freudian point of view, which heavily influenced most therapists whether they're aware of it or not, has tended to treat transcendental experiences as regressive. The value system was that man's highest calling was found by renouncing "childish" feelings—including religion and spirituality—and moving grimly into adulthood, a life of duty rather than beauty. People experiencing a mystical connection with the universe or a sense of inner peace were often dismissed as regressing to a primitive feeling of loss of identity, fused with the mother—in Barry Magid's phrase, "back on the tit."

Now that attitude is changing somewhat. Two wonderful recent books by psychiatrists who are applying their own interest in Zen to their work with patients are Barry Magid's *Ordinary Mind* and Mark Epstein's *Going to Pieces Without Falling Apart*. In addition, Jeremy Safran, a highly respected cognitive-behavioral psychologist, has published *Psychoanalysis and Buddhism*, a collection from a number of authors.

Magid puts it in a nutshell: "the common goal of Zen and psychoanalysis is *putting an end to the pursuit of happiness*." In other words it is when we find ourselves believing that, in order to be happy, we need something—a new car, a new relationship, a cure for our pain, enlightenment—that we are starting a battle we can't win. Not that we should want nothing, but that happiness sneaks in the back door when we accept life as it is. Epstein has an observation that fits the theme of this book: "The traditional view of therapy as building up the ego simply does not do justice to what people's needs actually are. Most of us have developed our egos enough; what we suffer from is the accumulated tension of that development." It's the left brain striving to constantly do better, get more, escape shame and guilt, that wears us out. We need to stop and face our demons.

Psychoanalysis is quite different from regular psychotherapy. Analysis means sessions three or four times a week, on the couch. The patient is expected to use free association—to let the mind wander where it will, with nothing held back—with relatively little input from the analyst. Though it might sound insipid if you haven't been through it, the mind reaches some scary and painful places. Free association, the passive attitude toward the mind, is much like meditation. Meditation teaches us about the noise in our heads, the overwhelming volume of thoughts, and also can lead us to much of the pain we've repressed. Eventually we begin to detach, to accept feelings, and to see how much of the mind's noise is distraction. But full detachment is not a realistic goal; even after enlightenment, we remain vulnerable to the world. *After the ecstasy, the laundry,* in Jack Kornfield's phrase. Both analysis and meditation train us to face, tolerate, and learn to live with intense emotions and experiences. We develop a confidence that we will neither tear ourselves apart nor collapse into nothingness, that we can handle stress. Both teach us to identify, explore, and overcome resistance. Both teach us to explore our assumptive world, the prejudices, assumptions, attitudes, habitual thoughts, and responses that are the essence of mindlessness.

look inside with compassion and interest. Why did I snap at my wife? Why do I get bored with this patient? Curiosity suggests we look a little deeper than we usually do, not just slap ourselves on the wrist and say I'll do better next time. *Why?* What's the stress? What am I feeling? Why am I afraid to look?

You have to apply this attitude not only to the self, but the self in the situation that it's in. It's too easy for us to get distracted, to take our eyes off the ball. We're overprogrammed, overbooked, overscheduled, overworked, overstimulated, overripe, and overdone. We don't get enough guidance about what's really important in life; instead there's all this noise in our heads, thinking about what we've got to do, buy, accomplish, score, just so we can continue keeping all these balls in the air. Why do we do this to ourselves? Are we afraid of something? Compassionate curiosity suggests we take ourselves by the hand, walk off to some quiet place, and ask ourselves, gently, lovingly, why?

It may be that, in the end, the only thing we can control is what we pay attention to. Before psychology became an experimental science, William James and other giants of nineteenth-century psychology believed that to be the case.

They came to that conclusion after a lifetime of introspection, very close observation of their own minds in action, which was the only tool they had. In the present moment, all our choices boil down to what stimuli we attend to. We are not often aware that we have a choice, because we are in a mindless state where we are dominated by the urgency of our thoughts. Practicing compassionate curiosity should help us gain perspective, help us stand outside ourselves and watch our brains in action, identify that much of the noise in the head is just noise.

Psychotherapy and Mindfulness

Remember we have talked about the role of the right hemisphere of the cortex: it's the most active during the first three years; it's the seat of our "working model" of relationships; it's where the unconscious is; it's vital in emotional regulation. The infant and mother, when in synchrony, are communicating directly right brain to right brain, bypassing the mother's consciousness, and imprinting on the child's mind a feeling of being held and loved and the basics of how to express and control emotions. Though not every psychotherapist would agree, I think this is also the state most of us strive for with our patients—a deep empathic communication, a wordless union. Mind reading, in a way, although I think the ability to know viscerally what the other person is feeling actually goes both ways in the ideal therapist-patient relationship.

As I've said, therapists argue about what makes psychotherapy work. Is it the method, our overt communication with the patient, what we were taught in school? Or is it the relationship, the so-called nonspecific element in treatment, the encouragement and support the patient receives from us almost as a side effect? Even the most comprehensive research studies on how therapy works have left us with more questions than answers. Most reasonable researchers agree that both elements play a part; but then we still don't know exactly how "the relationship" helps people, and how we can make those elements even more effective.

Enter Allan Schore, with his encyclopedic knowledge of psychotherapy, the mind, and the brain. His theory is that therapy helps the patient by providing the same kind of synchrony that the child had with its mother, which then results in the same kinds of changes in the right brain that the mother-infant bond creates: a feeling of being held, a feeling of being understood, and an enhanced ability to control emotional experience. These elements have profound effects on the patient. As Jerome Frank observed long ago, most patients are, more than anything else, demoralized, ready to give up. The sense of being understood, of not being rejected but treated sympathetically, is a big step toward restoring morale. It is also a step toward looking at the self mindfully, objectively: *Everyone is telling me I'm nuts, but it all makes sense to the therapist. Maybe everyone else is wrong.* And it's a step toward believing we won't be destroyed by the emotions which seem so intense, so damaging. *He seems to think I can make it for another week. Maybe I can.* Even cognitive-behavioral therapy, which focuses on teaching patients to change their negative thinking patterns, may get some of its benefit from the inadvertent effect of teaching patients to observe their thoughts carefully. Thoughts can come to seem more like transient mental events than imperatives or absolutes. In other words, psychotherapy teaches mindfulness, both deliberately and accidentally. This awareness reinforces the "practice wisdom" that therapists have followed for a century: *Process, not content. Follow the affect. Listen to your own associations. Watch how you feel.*

I think it's quite likely that antidepressants also help the user become more mindful. Many patients have reported on what they see as a subtle change: they still have the same worries and resentments, but these things have lost some of their power. They start obsessing again about the same old things, but now the obsessing seems boring. They aren't derailed so easily by perceived slights; they're still watchful for slights, but it just doesn't seem so important anymore. People in these states have achieved a degree of detachment from their problems, which seems almost puzzling at first. They didn't expect *this* to happen, and they are confused by the growing awareness of how depression dominated their thoughts in ways they were completely unaware of. As far as I know, not much has been written about this effect of antidepressants, but many of my colleagues have observed the same thing. I don't advocate antidepressants as a shortcut to mindfulness; detachment is only one element of a mindful attitude anyway, and the drugs create too many problems to be used unless they're really necessary. But it does seem that for some people who are absolutely stuck, hopeless, and obsessed with their problems, medication might help them gain a different perspective that could be a first step toward mindfulness.

Theresa: Getting Started

Theresa is a young woman in her late twenties, self-employed as a contract writer in advertising. She lives with her boyfriend, a commercial artist. I have been seeing her for about a year. She came in initially at the behest of her boyfriend, after she had spent most of a summer sleeping, crying, paralyzed, wanting to die. She was already coming out of this when we started treatment. I referred her to a psychiatrist who prescribed an SSRI, and her functioning has been much improved, though she still is consciously fighting her blue moods. She only needs to work about six months of the year in order to be financially comfortable. When I asked her what she would like to be doing with the other time, she referred to a screenplay she has been fitfully working on for a few years, something very autobiographical.

Theresa is the youngest child and only daughter among five brothers, a chaotic Italian family from suburban New Jersey. Her father, who left the family shortly after she was born, has been a continual source of disappointment to Theresa, from not showing up for visits to not paying for college, as he'd promised. Her mother worked and was completely overwhelmed by six children. During latency and early adolescence, Theresa was repeatedly sexually abused by her oldest brother, Vincent. The house was full of drugs, violence, and parties. The sexual abuse stopped when Vincent moved out. Somehow Theresa did well in school, got herself into a prestigious college, got a prestigious internship, and has been quite successful in her career (with little effort, she feels).

After college Theresa sought treatment, which focused on the sexual abuse and was very helpful, though Theresa says that after a certain time she "decided she had to be better," moved in with her boyfriend, and dropped out of therapy. During treatment she confronted her mother with what had happened to her and established clear limits: she would never see Vincent again. But it remained a source of frustration to her that her mother seemed to forget about the issue. Neither ever discussed it with the other brothers, though Theresa has always felt they must have known that something was going on.

The incident of interest here developed over some weeks. The precipitant was that one of Theresa's other brothers announced his wedding in the summer, with Vincent as best man, and the question immediately was could Theresa go? She was not close to the brother being married and did not really care about missing the wedding, though she resented having to exclude herself from a family function because of Vincent. After several weeks of anxiety and paralysis, Theresa decided to tell her mother she would not attend, and let her mother handle the brother being married. The mother dithered for a while, then called Theresa to say she had decided to explain to the brother being married about Vincent's abuse of Theresa. Theresa immediately had an anxiety attack: the cat's out of the bag; I'm not in control of the information anymore; Vincent is going to kill me. *She made the mistake of calling her boyfriend for support, forgetting his long-standing attitude toward her family:* what do you expect, why do you bother about them, forget them, write them off *(as he had done with his family).*

Just prior to these phone calls we had had a session that focused on mindfulness: detaching from thoughts and feelings, recognizing that they're transient, they're not you, you don't have to get overwhelmed by them. The train comes roaring into the station but you don't have to get on. I told her about Schwartz's work with OCD patients, how exercising willpower under the right circumstances seems to result in changes in the brain. In the subsequent session Theresa reported that after her phone call to the boyfriend she took a nap, crying herself to sleep; but that when she woke up she decided to get to work—if the cat was out of the bag there was nothing she could do about it, and being productive might help her feel better. When her boyfriend came home she was a little cool toward him, and he tried to pick a fight (feeling guilty, she assumed), but she refused to get sucked in. After he calmed down she told him calmly and directly how unhelpful he had been when she was upset, and he apologized sincerely. Then, she reported proudly, she'd fixed her chronic oversleeping problem by taking the clock out of the bedroom. When she didn't have the clock to bargain with and argue with (by resetting it each time it went off), she got up naturally when she'd had enough sleep. She was feeling better than she had in months. "But I didn't will myself out of depression," she laughed—a comment I understood as an ironic semidenial of how easy this had seemed.

This is an example of how consciously making the effort to attend to ourselves mindfully can help us make better choices. The effect of growing mindfulness as a habit, a strength brought on by regular practice, is much more difficult to illustrate. In Theresa's case, it would be a mistake to assume that mindfulness would protect her from the painful feelings stirred up by the news of her brother's wedding. But it would have helped her with the anxiety and paralysis that followed, and would probably have made her less reliant on her boyfriend for emotional support he couldn't provide.

There is more about Theresa, more difficult problems, and her recovery, in Chapter 7.

The World We Create

The crucial thing to live for is the sense of life in what you are doing, and if that is not there, then you are living according to other
peoples' notions of how life should be lived.

—Joseph Campbell

EVERY mammal experiences the same basic emotions we do: fear, aggression, pleasure, a parental instinct, the sexual drive. Endorphins (the body's own morphine, the source of good feelings) are present in the most primitive verte-brates. Higher animals may share our most complex emotions, including love, sacrifice, shame, envy, anxiety, and depression. These feelings are mediated by the same neurotransmitters in the same nervous system in all mammals. In most species, emotional responses are inborn messages from the nervous sys-tem telling the organism something important about survival: Danger?—run away. Prey?—attack. Sexual object?—approach. Juvenile?—protect.

Animals (we think) don't have the detailed memory we do, and so these feelings are all about the present moment. But because we have memories and the desire to organize our experience, when we feel something our feelings are not only about the present situation, but they also bring up memories (in both the historical and the emotional brain) about every past situation that was like this one. When we feel threatened, we fear not only that we'll be hurt now, but that the hurt will reopen all our old wounds; that the hurt now will make us more vulnerable in the future. *Unlike animals, we have the curse of being able to imagine suffering. Unlike animals, we have the gift of prediction, of storytelling.*

We create stories that are meant to help us make sense of the world, to orga-nize our experience and help us make decisions. Our stories give us the power to predict the future and make sense of the past, help keep us out of danger and our nightmares under control. But far too often, our stories lead us in wrong directions. When we've been through a difficult childhood—as most of us have, because our parents were never taught how to parent—or when we've been through later trauma, those experiences deeply affect our beliefs about ourselves and the world. Our stories tend to become dominated by fears and coping mechanisms. The stories become rigid, inflexible, applicable to the past but not to the present. Too often, the stories themselves determine our future. Stories that tell us we're helpless, that no one will ever love us, that the world is too dangerous, that our bodies are against us, are very common and always tragic. But we can find compelling support for those beliefs in contemporary culture—we can blame our genetic endowment, brain chemistry, dysfunctional family systems, or too much stress for the fact that we're miserable. The Perpetual Stress Response floods us with anxiety and undermines our confidence in our ability to live authentically; we live with anxiety and pain and distract ourselves with stories about materialism and status.

All our stories nowadays also have to deal with the emptiness of our culture—which we keep being told is the best of all possible worlds—and the accompanying perpetual stress. We feel wretched, and our culture doesn't give us an explanation. It's only human then to look for a simple explanation, someone to blame—often ourselves, sometimes our parents, sometimes an enemy who keeps showing up in our lives as different individuals who all treat us in the same cruel way. What if it's none of these, but the way we live our lives? If that's the case, we have to abandon our favorite stories—no mean feat, because we've built our lives around these beliefs. Joseph Campbell writes, "the land of people doing what they think they ought to do or have to do is the wasteland." We're living in that wasteland, and it makes us depressed and fearful and it tears up our bodies. If we want to escape we have to be courageous, we have to be ready for adventure.

The world of psychotherapy today is very intrigued with the concept of stories, often called *schemas* or *narratives*. Leading therapists have found that helping their patients understand their narratives is a useful way of attacking entrenched problems. Some theorists have shown us some standard narratives, common themes and issues that link problems and diagnostic groups. But I think the concept of narrative, as it's usually understood, leaves some important things out. So I've revived some other older concepts, the *assumptive world*

Exercise 6. **My Biography**

Take a pad of paper, notebook, or your word-processing progam. At the top of each page write your name. Then on the first page, write "Age 5"; on the second write "Age 10"; and so on, using a new sheet of paper for each five-year increment up to your present age.

Now, for each age, write about what you were like. Get into a mindful state. Think about yourself with compassionate curiosity, with affection and respect; this attitude is very important, and it may take some work to get yourself in this frame of mind. If the exercise becomes boring or taxing, put it aside for a while until you can regain affection and respect for yourself. As you write, since you can now look back and place yourself in the context of other five-year-olds, twenty-year-olds, and the like, think about what made you different. Were you curious, energetic, serious, shy, happy, worried? Write a little about what you liked to do—ride your bike, study, hang out with friends, cook dinner for the family, close a deal. Write a little about the most important people in your life at that time—your parents, teachers, lovers, bosses—and how they made you feel.

That's the hard part of the exercise, the part you should spend the most time on, but once you've completed it I want you to go back to each age and answer some questions:

What was the trouble? Was there something that was making you unhappy or worried? What was making you think badly of yourself? Were you getting the message that you were unimportant, or that people didn't like you, or that you were incompetent? Did you think you were different because you were fat, or clumsy, or anxious? Were you feeling unsafe? (Note: Maybe nothing was the trouble in the early years. Maybe the trouble didn't start until your parents divorced, or you finished college or got dumped by a lover. If so, great; you've got less to undo.)

What would you tell yourself? What was life trying to tell you that you weren't getting? Now that you have the benefit of hindsight, how could you go back and help yourself with whatever the trouble was?

What was the fear? Fear is the heart of the matter. Too many of us secretly fear that no one loves us, that our lives have no meaning, that we're incompetent, that we're only faking it and will be found out one day. In one sense, these fears are an artifact of the stress of contemporary life, like a dog in a learned helplessness experiment, never knowing when he'll get shocked and without any means of control. Free-floating anxiety is the natural response. But in another sense, the content of these fears is very real, and we must eventually stop pretending and face our demons.

Now here's the point of the exercise. Look back at the development of fears over the course of your life. As you think about childish fears, think about their connection to what you're afraid of now. Like a figure-ground optical illusion, in which you can see either the vase or the two faces but can't see both at once, I'll bet that you can alternately dismiss your childish fears as silly or experience their continued hold over you in their current terrifying form. That's the conflict between the logical and the emotional parts of our brains. But I want you to develop a new attitude, one of tolerance for yourself. Remember that you are thinking of yourself with affection and respect. You can see how your fears developed when you were young; they weren't silly or childish, they had a real basis. You can't think of yourself with affection and dismiss that fear. Nor can you think of yourself with respect and be completely overwhelmed with fear in the present. You can learn to tolerate the fact that there are things that scare you, but that doesn't make you inadequate or bad. In so doing, you begin to heal the rift between how you think and how you feel about yourself. You begin the process of change.

---

and *character armor,* to add greater perspective and immediacy to the subject. If we think of our lives as a continuing drama, the stage is the assumptive world, the actors—clad in their character armor—are motivated by the stories or schemas they believe about themselves, and the plot is the narrative. The dramatic tension comes from the *core conflict* (which we won't discuss till Chapter 10) as we rework it over and over.

These are very useful concepts, but psychotherapists who use these ideas tend to ignore some important issues—the near universality of emotionally damaging childhoods; the physical and emotional effects of perpetual stress; and our cultural denial of these issues. Many thinkers play right in to the cultural denial, which only reinforces self-blame (*If you can't make it in this perfectly wonderful world, obviously you're defective somehow*). Therapists who hold these beliefs may be very effective, warm, and kind; they don't seem to be looking down on you but the premise is there, never stated but always in the background. And the patient gets the message. He learns how to cope better with his depression but he doesn't look at changing his world so he won't get depressed again. I want to give you a new message: *don't assume it's your fault.* We all have to compromise with reality but that doesn't mean we should assume reality is a given, or that it's "right" somehow because everyone else seems to be going along. *If you're unhappy it may be much more effective to change your world rather than yourself.*

So the stories you believe about yourself and the world have to be taken out into the sunlight and examined very thoroughly. Question every assumption, take nothing for granted. I'm going to give you a very standard list of stories (schemas, narratives) that have been compiled by very thoughtful and experienced therapists. If you read their books you will find a great deal of useful detail; but never let these ideas make you feel defective.

As you learn about these concepts, try to use mindfulness to see how certain themes keep recurring in your life. It can seem like we're always pushing the same boulder up the same hill—trying to get love, trying to get respect, trying to get success, trying to get peace of mind—but always failing in the same old way. We've just talked about how mindfulness can help us gain a different perspective; now we're going to talk about what applying mindfulness to our assumptions, schemas, and conflicts can teach us about ourselves.

Before you go on in this chapter, please start Exercise 6, your biography. *This is the most important exercise in the book.* Now that you know something about stress, the role of emotions, and mindfulness, you're ready to write your biography in a different frame of mind than you would have in the past. This is a mindful, reflective biography. Future exercises depend on it. But don't feel that you have to finish before you go on. Writing your biography in this way will take some time, probably more than one sitting. In fact, you may want to go back to it in the future, as you learn more about yourself. If you want, you might want to use a special pad you can keep for this, or a book with blank pages. I hope it will be the most memorable writing assignment you ever do.

The Stage: The Assumptive World

The assumptive world is our own unique way of viewing and interacting with ourselves and with outside reality. It's the set of attitudes, knowledge, beliefs, prejudices, and automatic mental and behavioral responses that make each of us different. Jerome Frank, a great humanist and an innovative theorist, proposed the concept of the "assumptive world" in 1961:

In order to be able to function, everyone must impose an order and regularity on the welter of experiences impinging upon him. To do this, he develops out of his personal experiences a set of more or less implicit assumptions about himself and the nature of the world in which he lives, enabling him to predict the behavior of others and the outcome of his own actions. The totality of each person's assumptions may be conveniently termed his "assumptive world."

This is a short-hand expression for a highly structured, complex, interacting set of values, expectations, and images of oneself and others, which guide and in turn are guided by a person's perceptions and behavior and which are closely related to his emotional status and his feelings of well-being.

Though the word "assumption" sounds purely cognitive, Frank explains that in his definition, assumptions have cognitive, emotional, and behavioral aspects. Cognition is how we might describe our assumptions; emotion is the fuel that drives them, and drives behavior; and behavior is how our assumptions make us interact with the world. The assumptive world is similar to the concept of explanatory (or attributional) style in cognitive-behavioral therapy, and elements of the assumptive world are similar to the cognitive distortions that have been so well documented by Aaron Beck and others (see Chapter 8). Whatever you call it, it is a mental model we construct in our heads explaining how the world works. It's the set of "default" circuits in our brains, the network of cells and their long-term potentiated connections that are the interstate highways of our thinking and feeling systems. Theoretically, it's possible for new experiences to establish new circuits or channels, but it doesn't happen often, because energy flows most easily through established pathways; neurons that fire together, wire together. The assumptive world is resistant to change, because it restricts our perception. We are more likely to see evidence confirming our assumptions than we are to see evidence that goes against our beliefs. The Perpetual Stress Response increases our anxiety level, which can make us more defensive, guarded, less open to new information that will upset the status quo, less interested in trying something new. Mindful awareness helps us look more objectively at our assumptions, helping us be more flexible and creative.

Paradigms and Perceptions

The concept of the assumptive world is quite similar to Thomas Kuhn's concept of the paradigm in science. A paradigm is a set of fundamental assumptions, or theories, that most scientists base their work on. Today our basic paradigm is the scientific method, but in former days it was divine revelation or the opinions of the ancients. The best-known example of a paradigm conflict is that between ancient astronomy, which assumed that the Earth was the center of the universe and that everything revolved around it, and Galileo's physics, which made the Earth revolve around the Sun. The old astronomers had had to construct some very intricate and noncommonsense mechanisms to explain why, among other things, the planets seen from Earth seem to stop in their orbits, reverse course, and go backwards every once in a while. Galileo's universe was simple, elegant, and obvious, to anyone with an open mind—but the power of the old paradigm was such that Galileo had to recant or face excommunication, and it took another hundred years for his ideas to take hold.

In science, paradigms and shared assumptions provide a common language, a very useful means of communicating; when we share assumptions with others, we feel safe and comfortable and we all understand each other. But paradigms and assumptions are very resistant to change and impose significant biases and limits on our ability to see things objectively. Because part of our paradigm about the nervous system was that the adult brain doesn't change with experience, millions of life-years were wasted for stroke patients. Medicine discouraged trying to teach them to use the affected limb because it was seen as pointless—until people started to realize that other areas of the brain could take over for the affected area if the patient were encouraged to use the limb. Because part of our paradigm about depression was that it was an effect of a punitive superego—and because it was assumed that the superego doesn't develop until adolescence—psychologists for decades overlooked the existence of childhood depression.

Since we rely on our assumptions to give order and predictability, comfort and safety, to the world we actually live in, when we have experiences that challenge our assumptions they are experienced as upsetting. Disconfirming experiences that represent a threat to our security may elicit the fight-or-flight response, but others may be a milder, even a pleasant, upset (the Cubs win the Series). Ideally, when we have disconfirming experiences we should change our assumptions accordingly. However, we have highly effective mental mechanisms—defenses, which we'll explain in more detail shortly—to protect our assumptions. One defense is repression. We can block our memories of events that disconfirm our assumptions. This was demonstrated to me recently when a visitor asked about an old family photograph I had hanging on my wall, and I suddenly remembered a painful association to the picture, which I had "forgotten" for the last five years.

Another defense mechanism is avoidance, simply staying away from experiences that may challenge our assumptions. Another is pseudoconfirmation, in which our own expectancies generate the evidence we expect. For example, a patient told me he could tell, without seeing his wife or hearing her voice, what kind of mood she was in, the moment he opened the front door. It had a little to do with the condition of the front room (if it was messy, she would be depressed, cranky, and overwhelmed), but he maintained even without those cues he could *feel* something that tipped him off—a tension in the atmosphere, the difference between a relaxed silence and a threatening silence. He was always right, he claimed. I suspected this was pseudoconfirmation, but didn't challenge him. However, I did ask him, next time he could just "tell" that his wife was in a bad mood, to pretend he couldn't tell; to go in and greet her in a friendly manner as if there was nothing wrong, and if she did act cranky, to try to respond as if he was interested in what was bothering her. He proudly reported that this strategy worked, and her cranky mood had seemed to disappear like magic—but I still wondered if the mood was there in the first place.

Beliefs Become Reality

To a great extent, our assumptive world determines our social world.[1] Over time, we're likely to choose intimates who approve of us the way we are; work that doesn't challenge us or make us feel inadequate; buddies who share our views of politics; recreational activities that are well within our comfort zone. We live in a fear-based culture that tells us it's wrong to be independent; we make that fear one of our major assumptions and look for ways to fit in, to get attention without seeming to ask for it, to find love without risking ourselves.

So the assumptive world is very much a self-fulfilling prophecy, a system that keeps our experience of the real world pretty much the same. As such, it can make our world very different from reality. It is as if we only have a small

---

1 There are other assumptions as well. There are assumptions about the physical world, which may or may not be true. A common error is the belief that an object being whirled in a circle on a string will continue its curved path when the string breaks. Or that a black card is "due" when three red cards are drawn in succession. There are, of course, assumptions about the spiritual world. Faith is by definition an assumption. There are assumptions about luck and fate which influence some of us enormously.

flashlight to illuminate the whole world on a dark night. Some assumptive worlds are more distorted than others; extremes are the paranoid, who is always suspicious; the obsessive, who has to have everything just so; the depressed, who sees everything as evidence of his own inadequacy. But all our worlds, even the most mentally healthy, are distorted and limited to some degree. As we grow older and live longer in perpetual stress, our assumptions take on greater power, and we can become more restricted in what we can see, think, and do. We develop "character armor" (discussed on page 216), which we have to drag around with us constantly, slowed down by its weight.

As I've said, becoming aware of our assumptive world is a difficult task, because it is so pervasive and so much in the background it is like the air that we breathe. But it's very much worth doing, because there's a great deal out there, much of it pleasurable, that we're missing. The cultural message, the assumptive world that we are programmed to buy into, is "Work too hard, go into debt, ignore your exhaustion, take drugs to help you cope, stay home and watch TV, go to the mall on weekends and buy things that will make you feel good." *But we can do things differently.*

Table 1 is my list of some characteristics of some common assumptive worlds; but please be aware that this is very superficial. Assumptive worlds are much more detailed and unique than this, as we will discover. I offer this both for illustration and to get you thinking about what your assumptive world might be. But I hope you can see from this how living in one of these assumptive worlds limits your vision.

Defenses

The stress of a difficult reality leads us to try to find ways to make it more palatable. One way is through the use of what psychotherapy calls "defense mechanisms," defenses for short. Defenses are a way of regulating feeling when direct self-regulation doesn't work. By definition, defenses protect us from an unpleasant reality by distorting it to make it seem more like what we want, or how we think things should be, or—most often—by simply keeping difficult emotions out of our awareness. Our perception of reality becomes skewed, sometimes a little, sometimes a lot. Defenses are the bricks and mortar of our assumptive worlds. Defenses are inevitable, and some are much less distorting than others, but we'll get into that in a bit. For now let's just remember that the

Exercise 7. **Your Assumptive World**

Do you see yourself in any of the assumptive worlds described in Table 1? It can be difficult to apply this kind of knowledge immediately to yourself. Instead, think about people you know well—your parents, siblings, spouse. Do any of them fit one of the "problems" listed in the left-hand column? If so, do you see the associated assumptions as part of their thinking or feeling? Do they indeed see or not see things as I predicted they might? Does the emotional style seem to fit? Think about other assumptions that may be part of their world; I've just listed a few to illustrate the concept. There are millions more assumptions that we rely on to shorten our thinking time. Think about people who don't have a formal "problem." Is their assumptive world also distorted?

While you're thinking about someone else, think about the degree of distortion in their assumptive world. How different is it from the way you see reality? Does it cause trouble for the individual? If it is substantially distorted, think about what kind of experience might change some of those destructive assumptions. In my opinion, most of us have those disconfirming experiences every day, but we don't allow ourselves to see them or grasp their implications. What might it take to open someone's eyes and have them really see things differently?

After having practiced on others, pay mindful attention to yourself with these questions in mind. Use your compassionate curiosity. You're at a great advantage for seeing yourself objectively and for recognizing distorted assumptions, because you already know something about mindfulness. Continuing practice in mindfulness will help you become more and more objective, your assumptions less and less distorted.

---

more stress we're under, the more likely we are to rely on defenses to get us through the night.

When we're under stress we're guaranteed to have emotional reactions about it. Most stresses are emotionally painful by definition. Too much to do and we feel guilty, anxious. Too little to do and we feel frustrated, bored. Rejection causes sadness. Threats result in anger or fear. Stuck in the Perpetual Stress Response, we should expect to feel anxious, angry, guilty, frustrated—the whole

Table 1. Some Assumptive Worlds

PROBLEM	ASSUMPTIONS	ALWAYS SEES . . .
Anxiety	Any stress will kill me. Anything less than perfect is not acceptable. If [blank] happens, it'll be a catastrophe.	Any sign of trouble. The phobic object or situation. "Bad thoughts" (obsessive thoughts).
Depression	I need to be liked by everyone. I can't do it. There's no hope. Good things are accidents, bad things are my fault.	Bad things Rejection. Failure.
Addiction	Any stress will kill me (without my drug). I can handle anything (with my drug). "Might as well." One more won't hurt me.	Opportunities, excuses to use. Reliable source of supply.
Stress-related illness	My nervous system is special. No one understands. It's out of my control. There's a new drug.	Any physical symptom. Medical news. Validation.
Borderline	I can't live without [person of the moment]. Nothing calms me down.	Rejection. Threat. Danger.
Narcissistic	If I ask for help, it shows I'm weak. I have to shine at everything I do.	Personal slights, rejections, signs of disrespect. Opportunities to show off.
Controlling	Anything that deviates from my standards is a catastrophe. I can't rely on anyone but myself.	Anything that deviates from my standards.
Sociopathic	Everyone's out for himself. Others are only good for what they can do for me.	Opportunities to victimize.

NEVER SEES . . .	EMOTIONAL STYLE
Opportunities to relax. Reassuring news.	Jumpy, restless, tense. Preoccupied, doesn't listen.
Good things. Love.	Flat, low energy, gloomy, withdrawn.
How use hurts others. How use hurts the self. How others become objects.	Dissociated. Numb. High, looking to get high, or withdrawing.
Opportunities for enjoyment.	Jumpy, restless. Intense or exhausted. Ready to collapse or looking for a fight.
How emotional style impacts others.	Intense. Looking for a fight.
Needs of others.	Grandiose: expansive, optimistic, cheerful. Depleted: empty, no energy, depressed.
Value of freedom, flexibility. How others resent control.	May be anxious or smug, self-righteous. More interested in appearances than people.
Own shame and rage.	May be outwardly charming, but full of rage, contempt.

PROBLEM	ASSUMPTIONS	ALWAYS SEES . . .
Passive-aggressive	I can't rely on anyone but myself. Other people always screw things up.	Incompetence of others.
Ideal	It's an interesting world. People fascinate me. I can handle most things, and know how to get help if I need it.	Things pretty much as they are.

gamut of negative feelings. But because there is pressure to ignore or deny our perpetually stressed state, and because we naturally want to protect ourselves from unpleasant feelings, we may try to keep those negative emotions out of our awareness through denial, dissociation, or other defense mechanisms. Unfortunately, one of life's toughest lessons is that these strategies don't work in the long run. Not only does the negative emotion usually surface in some other, perhaps disguised, way, but the use of defenses like these shapes our character. Instead of simply wrestling with a painful experience, we become someone who denies reality. Use of defenses to deny reality is lying to ourselves; and just as what happens when we start lying to others, we gradually build more and more elaborate lies to buttress the first one. These elaborate lies end up blinding us to more and more of our own experience, so that our assumptive world becomes more and more distorted, the blind spots become bigger and bigger, our character armor more cumbersome and restricting. Experience teaches us ways of dealing with adversity that were applicable in the past, and we keep trying to apply them to the present. Mark Epstein writes:

> The defense is what hurts. . . . In coping with the world, we come to identify only with our compensatory selves and our reactive minds. We build up our selves out of our defenses but then come to be imprisoned by them. This leaves us feeling dissatisfied, irritable, and cut off.

What's Wrong with Reality?

In order to make sense of all this, it can help to return to Freud. The "reality principle" was Freud's terse shorthand for the fact that reality pretty much doesn't give a damn whether we live or die; and when it comes to our happi-

NEVER SEES . . .	EMOTIONAL STYLE
How own hostility guarantees others will screw up.	May be controlling, contemptuous, or charming, injured, innocent.
	Open, generous, engaged.

ness, the universe is sublimely unmoved. That's hard to accept—in fact, it goes against our nature to accept it. Partly because our brains are so powerful, we create stories in which we are inevitably the main characters. Even if our stories have us as helpless victims of fate, doomed to disappointment, we still have an egocentric point of view—we see the cards stacked against us, when in fact the cards are simply drawn at random. An indifferent universe is more difficult for us to accept than one that is interested in us, even if that interest is malign.

Much of human nature is a distraction from this reality. Much of living is about creating meaning and purpose for ourselves. A formal religious belief system lends us meaning and purpose; but in the absence of religion, we must do it ourselves. We occupy ourselves with pursuits—happiness, sexual conquest, success. We want things—not only material goods but achievements and relationships—things to give us meaning, to give us status, to calm our fears, to keep us busy. At the same time, wanting things almost inevitably puts us into situations of conflict, because some things are forbidden, some are in limited supply and are pursued by others, some are in conflict with other things we want. The animal brain wants immediate sex with the pretty lady next to us on the bus, but the logical brain knows that would get us into too much trouble. Sometimes it's the opposite; the logical brain tells us it's perfectly safe to take a shortcut through the dark alley, but the hair on the back of our neck rises all the same. We want things, but we fear the consequences.

Our character is formed partially out of the conflict between wishes and fears. Freud believed that when we're aware of the conflict, we can make a rational decision and move on. But when the conflict is outside our awareness— we wish for things that are taboo, or have fears that are too shameful to acknowledge—anxiety is the result. (Anxiety, like stress, is a word that has been cheapened by overuse. This kind of anxiety is not the conscious nervous-ness we fear on boarding a plane or when speaking to an audience; it is a largely unconscious phenomenon of the mind and body, deep in the bones and gut. It is, in essence, the same thing as the chronic stress we feel when we imagine cheetahs behind the rocks.) Because the conscious experience of this kind of anxiety is so devastating, we use defense mechanisms to distract us or otherwise block our awareness. Though much of Freudian psychology has been rightly superseded by fresher thinking, the concept of defenses will likely live on, not only in popular use but in other schools of psychology, because it is an elegant and parsimonious way of understanding how we contribute to our own grief. But it's important to keep in mind that the original purpose of de-fenses is to protect us from stress.

The Origin of Character

Defenses are the sentences and paragraphs of our stories. In the psychody-namic view, ineffective defenses lead to the development of *symptoms* and *char-acter.* Symptoms are behavioral, emotional, or perceptual patterns that are experienced as bothersome and not a part of the self—the compulsion to go back and check that the door is locked; a height phobia; a sudden depressed mood; the ritualistic hand washing of obsessive-compulsive disorder; the suici-dal impulses of depression. Character is also built on stereotyped patterns, but these are more subtle and pervasive, and experienced as normal to the self—to hoard our money stingily; to avoid taking chances; to be always gloomy and pessimistic; the precision, control, and attention to detail of the obsessive-compulsive personality; the fearfulness and suspicion of the paranoid. The ear-liest manifestations of character are those childhood attachment styles: secure, avoidant, ambivalent, disorganized. Character is how we see the world, and how the world we create is shaped by the way we see it. Character is the as-sumptive world. The obsessive personality likes facts and shuns emotions; the hysteric doesn't bother too much with facts and lives emotions. All of us have our unique stress, our familiar anxiety to deal with; it shapes us and we shape it in a never-ending dance.

Wish plus fear equals anxiety. We want something forbidden to us, so we try to forget about the wish, and we experience anxiety. We feel the futility of our efforts to escape perpetual stress, and we experience anxiety again. We need a new word: *unease, dread, discomfort, disquiet, uncertainty, arousal. Terror. Fear.* There's no single word in English for the absence of confidence, the restless, driven worry that comes with perpetual stress. *Demoralized.* Whatever word we use, the fact is that life is hard, and we want it to be easy. We can try to pretend it's easy, by getting high. We can decide we're just incompetent, and get depressed. We can decide we're being treated badly, and become victims. We can use our own victimhood to justify becoming exploiters. *We want life to be easy, but it's not, and our troubles come from trying to find ways to make it easy.*

Defenses also protect us from emotions that are too powerful for us, or that we feel we are not "supposed" to have. These can range from fully conscious efforts at distracting ourselves (*don't think about the time remaining for the test, concentrate on answering the questions*), to preconscious "habits" that we might acknowledge the purpose of (automatically looking for something to eat when feeling lonely), to completely unconscious mechanisms (not allowing some feelings into consciousness at all). Children may go to the extreme of creating a complete "false self" to please an impossible parent, hiding the real self so thoroughly that they become masters at fooling people. When the real self comes out, as it may in situations of trust or intimacy, it may cause panic. The roots of the major unconscious defense mechanisms go back to the attachment phase; as the child learns what feelings are upsetting to or disapproved by the primary caregiver, he will make an effort not to feel those things. And, in the "use it or lose it" ecology of the brain, the receptors for the corresponding chemical messengers may get pruned, and the appropriate brain structures may be damaged or withered.[2]

Defenses Get You in the End

As we learn more and more about how emotions are mediated by the chemical messengers between the brain and the body, we're finding out that defense mechanisms are only partially effective. They may protect consciousness from difficult feelings but they don't protect the body from the chemistry of emotions. Just as defenses may keep guilt out of consciousness, but leave us with unconscious guilt that motivates our behavior without our awareness, our

---

2 When the structure necessary to experience an emotion is lost, I'm not sure we should be talking about a defense mechanism. Defense implies a compensatory effort not to feel something that we still have the ability to feel, not a loss of the ability altogether. However, debate about what is and what isn't a defense, the nature and purpose of defenses, and what it is that's actually being defended against takes up too much time and effort in psychoanalytic circles, so I will just note the semantic problem here.

body is left to deal with the chemistry of guilt. So we might feel that we have let a loved one down, but rationalize that we were simply too busy; unconsciously our guilt might make us avoid that person or even blame him for the uncomfortable way he makes us feel. Our body will tense up when we're around him, our stomach acid churn, our blood pressure rise.

Defenses are useful and helpful in dealing with trauma, but the body may pay the price later. Defenses are also necessary components for some adult tasks. For the surgeon to turn off his emotions in the operating room, or the pilot in the plane; for the musician to sublimate his emotions into the language of his instrument—these are highly valuable skills. These are examples of conscious choice, but defensive functioning is often completely unconscious. We perceive a threat to our happiness, we remember a painful event, we experience a forbidden wish, and the defense kicks in so quickly we don't know what happened. We aren't aware of the precipitant, or of the fact that we're in defensive mode.

Defenses are the classic example of one of those skills we have learned that was appropriate once, in an old painful or traumatic situation, but now interferes with our optimal functioning. *The walls we put up for protection have become a prison instead.* In therapy, we find the ironic effect in defenses, some unintended consequence that hurts as much or more than the defense helps; that's why the patient is in my office. But let me be clear: defenses are necessary. Our goal for healthy living should be to be as mindful as possible, deciding consciously what to do with stress instead of responding mindlessly—but we'll never achieve this, unless perhaps we want to move to a Tibetan monastery where there are fewer distractions. Mindfulness practice—meditation—will help us develop the neural circuitry to deal with stress more mindfully, but we shouldn't expect to be fully in control. Mature defenses (see Table 3) are helpful aspects of our assumptive world. We want to develop the ability to use defenses that don't backfire on us, that don't distort reality too much, that don't hurt others.

Just what *are* defenses? Table 2 is a list of some very common defenses, their definitions and their bite-you-in-the-ass effects: the ironic, unintended negative consequences. For example, almost all efforts to avoid negative feelings also lead to the loss of the ability to experience positive feelings as well. This is a *long* list; don't try to memorize it. It's here for reference so I don't have to define these terms every time I use them.

Then there are defenses that are considered more mature, in that they distort reality less and have few, if any, unintended negative consequences (Table 3).

Exercise 8: **Identifying Defenses**

Think mindfully about something you want but don't have, something that nags at you. Something you've been wanting for a while. Focus on only one thing, for now. Examples:

- I want to lose twenty pounds.
- I want to see Tuscany.
- I want to be less lonely.
- I want to feel closer to my spouse.

Now, think about what's in the way. What's the voice inside your head telling you? *I can't, I don't have the discipline. It's not worth the trouble. People just don't like me. She's not interested.* Don't judge the voice, treat it with compassionate curiosity; it's a big part of you.

That voice is one of your major defenses. It's usually an expression of fear, because it believes that change is dangerous. It protects you from that fear by telling you a different story about change. Sometimes it's an expression of anger—something you resent about others. It protects you from experiencing that anger too. It may be about other feelings—grief and desire are big ones. Whatever the feeling is, the purpose of the defense is to defuse and keep it out of our consciousness.

Sit mindfully with it for a while. See if you can identify where that unfelt feeling, that fear or anger or whatever, comes from. Has it been with you all your life? Did you learn it from a traumatic experience? A divorce, a loss? Wherever it came from, it's not going to kill you now, is it? It's not going to overwhelm you or send you off the rails. Emotions are just human, like toenails. Can you give the defense a name from Table 2?

When you hear that voice in the future, see if you can figure out what's behind it. Then make a decision about what you want that's not mindlessly controlled by fear or anger or any other unconscious emotion. Don't feel you have to go contrary to the emotion; it may be telling you something important. Just consider it as one of many factors in your decision.

As with all these exercises:

The more you practice, the easier it gets.

Table 2. **Defense Mechanisms**

DEFENSE	DEFINITION	IRONIC, UNINTENDED NEGATIVE CONSEQUENCES
Dissociation	"Going away": consciousness leaves upsetting feelings or situations temporarily; or traumatic memories are reexperienced without context or meaning.	In dangerous situations, dissociation obviously increases risk. Otherwise, it prevents us from integrating the past; can become a part of character—spacey, inattentive, disconnected.
Projection	Attributing your feelings to someone else (*I'm* not angry; *you're* the one who's angry here, Buster!).	Makes interpersonal relations difficult, if not crazy.
Passive aggression	Getting others to express our own anger; inviting anger by being controlling, negligent, lazy.	Inability to express own needs in a direct manner; loneliness and isolation.
Hypochondriasis*	Expressing anger and reproach by getting sick and rejecting all help.	The *true* cause of the pain, often a trauma, is never revealed.
Fantasy	Being satisfied with imaginary relationships and accomplishments instead of real ones.	Obviously, nothing ever really happens. Also, these people seem to elicit sadistic anger in others.
Acting out	Using violence or sexual behavior to distract from a state of internal tension.	Obviously, conflicts with the law and with society. Also, feeling of being out of control, dangerous.
Reaction formation	Unacceptable feelings or impulses are denied by going to the opposite extreme (e.g., an interest in pornography leads to a campaign against it).	The individual is driven into behavior without understanding his motives. Also, these people usually alienate others with their fervor and sanctimony.

---

*There is much semantic confusion about the terms hypochondriasis and somatization. Here I am using George Vaillant's definition of hypochondriasis, my own of somatization. See Chapter 9 for a more extended discussion.

DEFENSE	DEFINITION	IRONIC, UNINTENDED NEGATIVE CONSEQUENCES
Insolation of affect	Separation of narrative memory from emotional memory.	Emotions are likely to find their expression in other ways, which seem not to make sense, being separated from their context.
Repression	Conscious experience of a feeling is absent, but the feeling guides behavior (e.g., the "innocent" girl who dresses provocatively).	Others usually respond to the overt behavior, not the repression, so miscommunication is unavoidable.
Displacement	Taking threatening feelings out on a safe target (e.g., yelling at the dog when you're angry at your wife).	In some situations, this is the only safe strategy; but it can lead to cruelty, sadism, victimization, bigotry.
Projective identification[†]	Attributing your feelings to someone else—*and the other person acts accordingly.* Though it sounds like magic, Schore says this is right-brain to right-brain unconscious communication.	In depression, for instance, others correctly understand the subtext of the person's messages—the unconscious expectations he has that people will reject him, ignore him, treat him with contempt or sadism. This process also leads to the crazy, highly emotional arguments about nothing between intimate couples.
Rationalizing	Using specious reasoning to justify unacceptable behavior, attitudes, or beliefs (e.g., *Everyone does it. One more won't hurt.*).	Makes you dishonest with yourself, morally lazy; supports bad habits.

[†]These first eleven defenses are classical defenses as defined by the ego psychologists; the rest are my compilation, including behaviors and attitudes which stricter definitions might not consider defenses. But people use them for a defensive purpose.

DEFENSE	DEFINITION	IRONIC, UNINTENDED NEGATIVE CONSEQUENCES
Passivity, apathy, lethargy	To see the self as acted upon, not an actor (lack of agency).	Missed opportunities, of which the self is not even aware; victim identity.
Selective attention	Paying attention only to that which confirms our assumptions.	Restricts and reinforces the assumptive world; absence of creativity and initiative.
Somatization*	Use of the body as a metaphor to express a psychological state.	Results in pain, discomfort, disability, conflict with the medical system.
Intellectualization	Emotions are avoided by excessive intellectual activity.	Leads to a cold, dry life lacking intimacy and enthusiasm.
Externalization	Reflexive blaming of others.	Moral cowardice, the inability to take responsibility for one's own behavior; the Twinkie defense.
Rageaholism	Use of tantrums and intimidation to get one's way.	Drives others away, leads to loneliness and isolation.
Hopelessness	Not allowing self to feel hope as a way to protect against pain and disappointment.	Leads to passivity and helplessness.
Procrastination	Putting things off till the last minute gives you an excuse from really trying.	Leads to poor results, sense of being out of control, anger at the self.
Isolation and withdrawal	Avoiding social contacts.	Loneliness; also, restricts and reinforces the assumptive world by cutting off information.

DEFENSE	DEFINITION	IRONIC, UNINTENDED NEGATIVE CONSEQUENCES
Dependency	Relying on others to create a good feeling about the self.	Vulnerable to the whims of others; unable to identify own needs, wants, thoughts.
Counterdependency	Avoiding intimate relationships, putting on a show of independence.	What appears to be independent behavior is really determined by being oppositional (contrary); loneliness remains.
Porous boundaries	Assuming others know how we feel, and that we know how they feel; easily contaminated by moods and behavior of others.	Excessive and inappropriate guilt; social faux pas; passivity and dependency.
Self-defeating behavior	By procrastinating or other behavioral means, sabotaging one's ability to put best efforts forward.	Obviously, poor performance on a variety of social tasks.
Compulsions, obsessions	Ritualized patterns of behavior, or nagging intrusive thoughts, which distract from other, more painful, feelings.	Interferes with social relations and self-direction; may take over and dominate one's time.

The Concept of Resistance

If defenses work to keep painful feelings out of awareness, it's no wonder that they are at work in the psychotherapy situation too, because that experience aims directly at those feelings. Therapists have a special word for it—"resistance"—and it's important for us to understand exactly what that means.

The original hope of Freudian psychotherapy was that by gaining insight into the conflict between his wish and fear, the patient would be cured of his neurosis. As experience taught that this rarely happened, Freudian therapists focused on the patient's "resistance"—a recognition that the patient's own personality was getting in the way of achieving what he wanted. Wilhelm Reich, a

Table 3. **Mature Defenses**

DEFENSE	DEFINITION
Suppression	The conscious effort to put disturbing thoughts or feelings out of mind.
Altruism	Doing for others as we would like to be done by. Done mindfully, it gives the self some gratification and does not belittle the recipient.
Sublimation	The indirect or attenuated expression of wishes and feelings that cannot be expressed directly (e.g., writing a fictional story about fathers and sons rather than killing your father).
Anticipation	Spreading anxiety out over time by planning and taking preliminary measures. Hopefully you do this all the time, and never suspected it was a psychological defense.
Humor	Expressing aggression or anxiety in a socially acceptable form through jokes or wit.
Acceptance	Experiencing feelings without being overwhelmed by them; coming to terms with the limitations of our abilities, the inevitability of suffering, the shortness of life.

brilliant but doomed disciple of Freud's, began the tradition of what came to be called character analysis, aimed at understanding how aspects of the patient's personality interfere with achieving his goals. Character analysis is best exemplified today in the work of David Shapiro and Lawrence Josephs. But in a larger sense, all of contemporary Freudian psychotherapy is occupied with the problem of character, finding a way to lower the patient's defenses so that change can take place.

Much the same history has been repeated in cognitive-behavioral therapy and in psychopharmacology. At first Aaron Beck and others who pioneered cognitive-behavioral therapy were able to demonstrate that changing patients' thinking patterns resulted in permanent and dramatic change in their overall functioning. But then patients seemingly became more difficult. They correctly identified their self-destructive cognitive patterns and replaced them with more constructive ways of thinking, but continued in their problematic behavior or dropped out of therapy. It was resistance all over again. Now theorists like Jeffrey Young, with his schema-focused therapy, are investigating character from a cognitive-behavioral point of view. Others, like Jeremy Safran, are pushing cognitive-behavioral therapy to pursue intangibles such as emotions and the therapeutic relationship in an effort to help patients more effectively and address resistance.

In psychopharmacology, each new medication is hailed at first as a panacea, but then the bad news starts to trickle in. In depression, 60 percent of patients improve with medication, but 40 percent improve with just a placebo. And for many on medication, the improvement doesn't last. And there's just no telling which medication will work with which patient, or why. Researchers are reduced to considering diagnoses like "depressive character disorder" to suggest that the patient resists getting well. While the pharmaceutical companies continue to pursue the magic bullet, psychiatrists in the real world are trying to help their patients be reasonable about what medications can and can't do, and recognize that they have to change their habits if they want to be truly well. Medications without change or work don't result in lasting recovery. Medications can give some relief and open a door; if the patient doesn't step through it, depression returns.

The irony is predictable: each new method of helping people yields dramatic results at first, but then people themselves gum up the works. Any method of helping people change runs into the fact that the people interfere. That's resistance, and it's only natural. The reality principle is hard to face; we keep wanting to believe there is an easier way. Practice is difficult. Our wishes are not realistic, our fears are difficult to ease. Inevitably, we construct stories about ourselves to provide distraction and comfort. We build an assumptive world to live in, a world of beliefs, perceptions, expectations, patterns of thinking, feeling; living in that world seems as natural as can be, but it is not reality. We don't seek treatment or take medication to change our assumptive world, we just want relief from distress; in fact, all our security operations are operating to maintain our beliefs and buttress our assumptions. But we can only get relief by changing our world. Resistance is just grappling with the fact that change is much more difficult than we thought it would be. In Zen oneness, if we can ever achieve it, there are no resistances; there is simply a willingness to do whatever comes next. "We no longer have any problems. That is, we no longer divide our life into the good parts and the problematic parts; there is simply *life,* one moment after another," writes Barry Magid.

The Actors: Schemas, Characters, and Lifetraps

All of us believe a number of stories about ourselves that are only partially rooted in reality. We may believe that everyone loves us, or that everyone is out to get us; we may see ourselves as a bewildered innocent or a wise cynic; as a powerless victim or a capable hero. These beliefs are a big component of the assumptive world; they are the distorting lenses through which we process our experience, and which determine how we see the reality.

Take a few minutes and review your biography, Exercise 6. By looking back at yourself as affectionately and objectively as you can, you can see what made you unique and worthy of love, and also what was troubling you at that time. As you do this, you can see how your assumptions developed, and you can (through practice) gain greater objectivity about yourself. To help with this, I will discuss a number of common scenarios that I've seen in my practice, and character styles as understood by other theoretical points of view. James Mann, a uniquely gifted therapist, referred to these scenarios as "the present and chronically endured pain"—our old wounds that we keep hoping are healed, only to find them reopened when we face stress again.

The old injury leads to a current fear. The old injury—which we may have repressed, denied, or otherwise minimized—has created the myth that we are vulnerable and defective. The current fear—which we're usually not even aware of—is related to the old injury, perhaps just a fear of being reinjured in the same way, but also maybe of our own rage getting out, of having our vulnerabilities exposed, or dozens of other possibilities. Our bodies have adapted to our belief in our vulnerability, always in a state of tension. Besides the old injury and the current fear, and our bodily adaptations, there are the very real difficulties of contemporary life which feed them both.

Here are some of the stories I've heard repeatedly over the years:

- *The caretaker.* A parent was sick, depressed, or alcoholic; the child learned to manage her own anxiety by being reliable and tending to the needs of the parent. Too often, children like this find themselves in the same role as adults, at work or in the family. It's whistling in the dark, pretending that there is nothing to worry about. Frequently, caretakers get sick themselves, developing chronic illnesses that don't respond to treatment. Karen (see Chapter 7) is an example of a caretaker.

- *The charmer.* Again, a parent was dysfunctional, or there was a lot of conflict between parents. The child learned that by being entertaining, or beautiful, or otherwise providing a distraction, he or she could reduce the stress at home. People like this develop an acute awareness of the needs of others and are always "on stage," ready to provide a diversion whenever there's tension. But sometimes, conflicts need to be resolved. And the charmer goes through life pleasing everyone else, at his or her own expense.
- *"Poor me."* This is someone who's learned that being sick, hurt, or incompetent is the only way of getting attention. In contrast to roles we will discuss shortly in which the child has literally been the victim of abuse, this is usually a role that's fostered by a parent who has encouraged an unhealthy dependency in the child. People like this have not developed the circuitry in their brains that allows them to see their own part in the disasters that keep happening to them.
- *The hero.* In contrast to the victim, this is someone who is counterdependent, who has learned not to seek help from others because it's never as good as what he can do himself. This belief is a self-fulfilling prophecy. The hero has learned to stuff all his own fears and needs, at great cost to his physical and emotional health. Jane Jones (also in Chapter 7) has some of the hero about her.
- *Sleeping beauty.* Waiting for Prince (or Princess) Charming to come along. The problem is that so much need for love has been loaded on to the prince's shoulders that any real relationship is bound to disappoint. These people sometimes secretly believe themselves to be deeply defective, and hope for a magic solution that will undo those fears. They don't realize that it's only by getting involved in the nitty-gritty of everyday life that their belief in their defects will be cured.
- *The nerd.* Psychologists are finally beginning to take seriously the effects on children of being bullied and teased by their peers. While we see the tragic result in school shootings, the millions of children who suffer lasting damage to their self-esteem go largely ignored. These are often children who are physically awkward or small in stature, or seem to have a deficit analogous to a learning disability for social cues (Asperger's syndrome). Too often, they become contact-shunning adults stuck in dead-end jobs because their dreams and aspirations have been beaten out of them. Occasionally, they turn out to be rocket scientists or Bill Gates. Tom

from Chapter 4 fit this category not because of nerdlike qualities but because of his small stature.

- *Richard III.* The child who is stuck with jealousy or envy faces a terrible handicap through no fault of his own. It may be that other children in the family were actually favored by the parents. It may be that because of some difference (like Richard's humpback) they feel inferior and excluded. Whatever the cause, when these children grow into adults who are chronically envious, they have miserable lives, never being satisfied and always feeling cheated. They project their own self-doubts and insecurities onto others and have a hard time taking responsibility for themselves.
- *Verbally and physically abused.* These children have been betrayed by the people who were put on earth to love them; but often the child needs to believe so strongly in the parents' love that he believes it was his fault he was abused. Because he's never had appropriate models, he can't control his own rage and anger, so he abuses those who love him as an adult, confirming his sense of self-blame. Because he can't trust anyone, he remains isolated and bitter.
- *Sexually abused.* These are children who are suffering the aftereffects of trauma. They are hypervigilant and can't relax. They are subject to flashbacks. They go away mentally when they're under stress. They often have physical problems, especially autoimmune diseases. Because their rage and pain are so intense, they fear all emotions, which often means they can't feel or want anything. Theresa (in Chapters 5 and 7) is an example of this scenario in action.

Lifetraps and Character

Those are just some of the situations I've encountered often enough to notice patterns. People with bigger theories than mine have noticed similar kinds of patterns, in which you also might find yourself. We certainly like to create categories for ourselves—it goes all the way back to astrology, if not before. Categories give us a sense of control and understanding, sometimes also a cop-out. "I can't help being emotional, I'm a Scorpio." Enneagrams are another popular kind of category now, with nine different personality types and a lot of expensive workshops. The Myers-Briggs typology, which actually has some validity, is often used in organizational consulting, and is a great icebreaker. But there are really only two approaches to personality which we should pay attention to. Unfortunately, here some of our terms become confusing and overlapping, so please bear with me while I try to explain.

Harry Stack Sullivan, the influential but abstruse American psychoanalyst who developed the school of psychotherapy generally referred to as "interpersonal," used the word "personification" to describe a cognitive template or structure that controls perception. A personification is an element of what I call the assumptive world. According to Sullivan, people divide experiences into those that belong to the self, and those that don't—these instead belong to the "not me." The personification of the "me" is a set of beliefs and assumptions about the self that is acquired over time in a self-perpetuating fashion—that is, new information and experience that conflicts with an already formed personification is relegated to the "not me." Sullivan used the concept of "selective inattention" to describe how information that conflicts with established personifications is ignored, resulting in an inability to learn from experience.

Likewise, Sullivan believed that our perceptions of others are influenced by personifications based on similar experiences in the past—thus, we are likely to view others with suspicion when our past experiences have resulted in a personification of others as untrustworthy. Perhaps the most basic tenet of interpersonal psychotherapy is that of the circularity of experience: problematic behavior is likely to resist change because it is based on beliefs or attitudes that are continually confirmed by the interpersonal responses of others to the problematic behavior, and by selective inattention to results that disconfirm the belief. When we show that we are suspicious of others, they are likely to conclude we are being deceptive or dishonest, and so treat us accordingly; those who treat us kindly despite our hostility, we assume to be good at dissembling. Flexibility of personifications of both self and others implies being open to new experience, hence a greater degree of mental health.

So, for Sullivan, there are personifications of the self and personifications of others, which form much of what I call the assumptive world—the intra- and interpersonal parts. However, the term "personification" has been superseded by the term "schema"—see Jeremy Safran's *Widening the Scope of Cognitive Therapy* for an explanation. Like personifications, there are self-schemas and other-schemas. Researchers have been able to demonstrate that schemas have some demonstrable effects: for instance, that people are more likely to pay attention to and remember events that are consistent with their self-schemas than to data that is in conflict (just as Sullivan predicted). Or that we seek feedback that confirms our schemas and avoid feedback that conflicts. "Schema" has become an academically respectable term, shown to have some utility as a theoretical construct.

But "schema" gets used in different ways by different people. Jeffrey Young, an influential writer and therapist following in the cognitive-behavioral tradition of Aaron Beck, uses the term "lifetrap," which he says is the same as "schema." But a lifetrap is much more than just a set of beliefs and assumptions. It includes a person's past experience (how she got to be this way), symptoms, and repetitive patterns of behavior, especially the self-destructive patterns that have her making the same mistakes over and over again. It's pretty much the same as what common language (and the psychoanalytic tradition) refers to as *character*. Young's use of the term this way—and the popularization of his approach by Tara Bennett-Goleman in *Emotional Alchemy*—is not a problem except in terms of creating a little confusion about semantics. In fact, I think it's fascinating and wonderful that we find the cognitive-behavioral and psychoanalytic traditions—always armed camps in the past—coming together to address the problem of why we tend to keep stepping in the same hole, over and over and over again. *Because this is the thing no one can figure out.*

So *schema* (in Young's usage) is very close to *character* (in the psychoanalytic tradition). Tables 4 and 5 describe what schema and character types mean in terms of the assumptive world.

If you want to find yourself in these tables, ignore the labels in the left-hand column and focus on the assumptions in the second column. Do any sound familiar to you? If so, do you think your perception of the world might be affected in the way I've suggested? Do you think that other people might experience you as somewhat of the emotional style I've linked to the assumptions? You may find some of these categories abhorrent; please try to put these feelings aside. Believe me, people who fit what might seem like the more repulsive categories have very good reasons for being what they are. But hopefully you might find yourself in one or more of these categories; or find something to wonder about. Take that wondering and use it for Exercise 9, coming up shortly, which may help you better understand your own schemas and how they affect you.

Beware of Categories

You may be surprised to see all these categories for personality or character when I've been talking about the virtues of mindfulness, one of which is to help us abandon categorical thinking. There is a contradiction here. It's dangerous, but it's also handy, to think in terms of categories. It's dangerous because it reinforces our habits of judging, of closed-mindedness, of not seeing the uniqueness of individuals once we've placed them into categories. It leads to prejudice. But it's handy because there *are* certain personality traits that seem to go together, that seem to be a result of the same kind of experiences and, most important, lead to the same outcomes. Categories sometimes give us the power of prediction.

But remember that these categories are only brief sketches, generalities, about certain types of functioning that go together. You are more than one schema; most of us walk around the world with many tapes playing in our head at the same time. Circumstances may get you to act like one personality style at one point, a different style when circumstances change. You don't fit neatly into any category; no one does. And you have a lot of power to change how you respond, what you see, who you are. Experience and practice change the brain, and thereby can change our personalities.

I think it's best to see personality styles, character defects, lack of will power, schemas, and narratives as all examples of vicious circles in action. Whatever our theory about the origin of the problem (bad culture, bad parents, bad wiring, bad thoughts, trauma), these are all self-fulfilling prophecies, deeply ironic. We create the conditions that cause our own misery. Our defenses work both to perpetuate the vicious circle and to limit our vision so that we can't see how it operates. Insight in psychotherapy works by creating a charged emotional relationship with a great deal of trust so that eventually the patient can see—through the therapist's eyes—how the vicious circle operates. But insight isn't enough, because these patterns become hard-wired into our brains and bodies. So we have to practice, over and over, doing things just a little differently. Sometimes change in psychotherapy comes without insight. In Ericksonian hypnosis, the therapist mystifies the patient, confusing him enough so that he has to act differently. In behavioral treatment, the therapist teaches the client to modify events early in the vicious circle so that the cycle is broken. With antidepressant medication, some patients find their energy and outlook so much improved that they stop some of their depressogenic habits.

What may seem like enduring character is more constructively viewed as habit. A study of 180 borderline patients found that more than 10 percent made dramatic improvements over a period of two years—something that's not supposed to happen at all. Borderline personality disorder is usually assumed to

Table 4. Young's Lifetraps (Schemas)— Impact on the Assumptive World

LIFETRAP	ASSUMPTIONS	ALWAYS SEES . . .
Abandonment	Destined to be alone. No one can love me. You're going to leave me.	Chemistry, excitement in partners who will abandon. Rejection.
Mistrust and abuse	No one can be trusted. (Unconscious: It's my fault, I'm bad, I brought it on myself.)	Abuse, betrayal. Others' ulterior motives. Chemistry, excitement in partners.
Dependence	The world is a dangerous place. I'm not safe. I can't handle this.	Danger, threats, crime. Looks for others to depend on.
Vulnerability	The world is a dangerous place. I'm not safe.	Danger, threats, contamination. Acutely aware of bodily sensations.
Emotional deprivation	Feelings are dangerous. No one can love me enough.	Rejection, disappointment.
Social exclusion	I'm different, I'm defective/superior. No one can like me. It doesn't matter what I do.	Opportunities to fit in. Others' evaluations (always negative).
Defectiveness	I'm different, damaged, inadequate.	Envious, jealous. Need to prove something to the world. Value of success, status.
Failure	I'm a failure, stupid, incompetent. No use trying to change.	Often living in a fantasy world. Sees the real world as simply impossible.
Subjugation	Others will always control me. Life is an ordeal, and I'm a victim, a martyr.	Wants to please others, anticipates their needs.

NEVER SEES . . .	EMOTIONAL STYLE
Possibility of rewarding life alone. Possibility of happiness with less exciting partner.	Clingy, needy, possessive. Or angry, aloof, chip on shoulder.
Goodness in the world. Effects of own shame and self-blame— isolation, defensiveness.	Volatile, quick to rage; dissociated, confused, hypervigilant, anxious, depressed.
Necessity of daily survival skills. Possibility of rewards in independence. Never experiences pride regarding independence.	Reassurance-seeking, indecisive, passive. Fearful, phobic. Hypochondriacal. May rely on drugs for relief.
Possibility that life has joys or pleasures to offer. Never sees the odds of health realistically.	Fearful but cold. Incapable of enjoying self. May be miserly, may be OCD.
Value of settling for an imperfect relation- ship. Never sees effects of own coldness on others.	Can't express needs directly, but may demand attention. Always disappointed in people.
Others who feel different, insecure. Others who like or respect oneself. Need to set own course.	Passive, avoidant, schizoid. Self-conscious, anxious to please.
Dissociated from shame, unaware that it is a prime motivation. Never sees own realistic positive qualities.	Presents a false self to the world, which others may like—but since it's not the real you, it doesn't provide reassurance. Problems with intimacy—let people in, then reject them. Devalue those who love you.
Value of trying things differently. Never sees own self-sabotage, which may be extreme.	Isolated, schizoid. Anxious.
Own aggression, which is usually expressed passively, often somatically.	Anxious to please, avoids confrontations. But air of resentfulness, martyrdom.

LIFETRAP	ASSUMPTIONS	ALWAYS SEES . . .
Unrelenting standards	I must be perfect at everything I do. Weakness is a sin.	Opportunities to shine. People to reflect glory on the self.
Entitlement	I'm special, entitled to everything I want just by virtue of being me.	Opportunities to shine, show off. Opportunities to indulge self.

Table 5. **Character Styles—Impact on the Assumptive World**

CHARACTER	ASSUMPTIONS	ALWAYS SEES . . .
Obsessive-compulsive	Everything has to be perfect all the time.	Any sign of disorder. Any deviance from the rules.
Hysterical	I'm worthless; my gender is worthless. I can only get attention by being needy.	Attention from the opposite sex. Any emotional excitement.
Depressive/ masochistic	Someone must be able to take care of me. No one is capable of taking care of me.	Slights, rebuffs, rejections. Psychosomatic symptoms.
Narcissistic	I'm special, and I should take every opportunity to shine.	Opportunities to show off. How oneself is so much superior to others.
Paranoid	Everybody's out for himself. No one can be trusted.	Threats to safety, security, self-respect.
Schizoid	My own inner life is where the action is. Real people are too messy.	Incursions on own rigid boundaries.
Antisocial	Other people are just tools to be used.	Opportunities to take advantage of others.

NEVER SEES . . .	EMOTIONAL STYLE
Value of relationships. Value of relaxation.	Perfectionistic, competitive, driven. Compulsive, workaholic.
Needs of others, or effect of own self-centered behavior on others. Need for self-discipline or limits.	Self-centered, arrogant, impatient, irritable. Feels victimized when expected to take responsibility.

NEVER SEES . . .	EMOTIONAL STYLE
How need for control drives others crazy.	Flat, rigid, cold. Not in touch.
Own desires to be seduced.	Seductive/innocent. Always misunderstood. Outraged innocence.
Own responsibility for rejection.	Gloomy, self-centered, boring. Victim. Reproachful (no one can help me).
How own grandiosity causes resentment.	Pompous, arrogant, entitled. Not interested in others.
Genuine concern from others. Self-fulfilling nature of paranoid fantasies.	May be outwardly pleasant and charming, but always in control. Under pressure, may be intimidating and coercive.
Opportunities for value of real relationships.	Shy, timid, self-effacing.
Value of real relationships.	Charming, slick, seductive.

be a life sentence. But these patients, in the first six months, changed so much that they no longer qualified for the diagnosis. The researchers noted that most recovered because of relationship changes; some developed positive relationships; others extricated themselves from difficult, destructive relationships. Some conquered their drug abuse. They were able to reduce the stress in their lives, they no longer needed their self-destructive habits, and they got better.

Say Joe was raised by a cold and critical father who was never satisfied with Joe's performance, and a mother who was not sufficiently forceful to counteract the destructive impact of the father. Now clone Joe and watch as he goes in either of two obvious directions: Joe A. may go along with his father and become perfectionistic and critical of himself, with no tolerance for errors or imperfections. Joe B., on the other hand, may rebel and fight with any attempts by others to put themselves into roles where they may judge or evaluate him; in the jargon, he has "authority issues." Joe A. may become quite successful in employment but is likely to be rather cold and joyless, and prone to depression whenever things go wrong. Joe B. will probably not find success in conventional employment because he will find himself in power struggles with any boss; and he may find intimate relationships difficult because he will feel controlled by the reasonable expectations of others. Either way, from a psychoanalytic point of view Joe is likely to be considered fixated at a primitive stage of development. We might consider Joe A. to have an obsessive-compulsive character, Joe B. to have a paranoid character. Joe A. has Young's Unrelenting Standards lifetrap, Joe B. that of Entitlement.

These classifications have an unfortunate tendency to reify problems, to turn them into some condition that Joe *has* rather than something that Joe *does*. They also go into much more detail on how Joe got to be this way than on how he can change. But if we view these patterns as habits, I think we are in a position that facilitates a different way of looking at things, a focus on the present. Because Joe's problems—depression or anger—are caused by present events, not past ones. Joe A. is constantly on the alert for any way he might fall short of perfection, and he is sure to find many. Joe B. is constantly on the alert for any way others might be trying to judge him, and he is sure to find many. The solution for both Joes is to develop awareness of how their assumptions control their vision, to learn methods of emotional self-control so that they are not as reactive, and to develop greater tolerance for the emotions they are defending against, the desire for love and respect. Then to keep on practicing until these new perceptions and behaviors are stronger habits than the old ones.

Exercise 9. **Identifying Schemas and Conflicts**

In today's world, we're constantly programmed to ignore, deny, stuff our emotions. If we want to become whole again, we have to recapture the ability to experience reality completely, with our body in the form of feelings and with our mind in the form of thoughts. Here are some suggestions about how to get started:

- Monitor your associations. Learn to develop an observing eye that notices where your thoughts go when you're not paying attention. When you're driving or walking or falling asleep, for example, does your mind dwell on successes or failures? Do you keep returning to instances of shame or humiliation? Do you constantly worry about whatever is the next item on your mental list? These are good clues to what is frightening you.
- Pay attention to your dreams. Keep a pad of paper by the bedside and write down whatever you can remember when you first wake up. Look for themes. Are you lost, or trapped? Is there a childhood scene that keeps reappearing?
- Look for patterns in your life. Are you always exploited? Disappointed? Rejected? Do you keep people at arm's length?
- Listen to yourself. What is the story of your life—the one you deeply believe, the story that shows up in your emotions, behaviors, and relationships, the undertow that pulls you and compels you?
- Where does it hurt? Sometimes there is a symbolic meaning to physical symptoms. Digestive problems may mean you're trying to swallow something you shouldn't. A backache can mean you're carrying too heavy a load. Chronic fatigue can be a way of saying you're scared and overwhelmed. Breathing problems may mean someone is cutting off your air supply.
- Talk to your intimates. Are there things your best friend would tell you if you gave permission? Are there ways you keep shooting yourself in the foot, which others can see but you can't?
- Look back at your biography (Exercise 6). At what point did things start to

(Continued)

go wrong? At what point did you begin to be afraid, or feel that you were different or defective? What was going on around you at that point? Were your parents having trouble? Was there trouble in school? Were you ill? Did something harm you or scare you and you got no help for it?

As with all these exercises:

The more you practice, the easier it gets.

Schema Control

I like Tara Bennett-Goleman's notion of "schema attacks"—the emotional hi-jacking that occurs when something triggers one of our old tapes.[3] It's an emotional reaction that is very sudden and very intense, and way out of pro-portion to the event, if we could look at the situation mindfully. The problem is that a schema is in control of our brains, and we distort events to match the emotions. We've taken the emotional low road, and the amygdala is temporar-ily in charge, sending out the messages that fill our bodies with fight-or-flight hormones, restricting our vision and heightening our awareness so that we find more evidence of threat. This kind of thing can be very visible: someone says something we interpret as a challenge—at a party after a few drinks—and suddenly we're all over the poor guy, daring him to put up his dukes. It can also be very quiet and internal: someone else says something that makes us feel excluded, and we're flooded with feelings of inadequacy and loneli-ness. The precipitant can even hit us in the unconscious mind, so that we're not aware of what triggered the attack; or our defenses may work well enough to make us repress the precipitant, but not well enough to hold back the flood of emotions.

I've always resented the Pollyanna types who want us to believe that every adversity is a learning opportunity; but these schema attacks *are*. They give us a direct opening into our unconscious, the old fears and resentments that are

---

3 Of course the notion of a "tape" being played automatically in our brain in response to certain stimuli goes back to Eric Berne, the author of 1964's *Games People Play*. Berne was an original thinker and astute observer whose popularity and irreverence sabotaged his ever achieving re-spectability; but many of his ideas are still in both popular and academic use.

Getting Out of a Schema Attack

- Stop whatever you're doing and pay attention to your body.
- Control your breathing—deep inhales and exhales—so that excess carbon dioxide doesn't contribute to the panic.
- If you're in a difficult social situation, get out of it. Excuse yourself and go to the bathroom or go outside for a walk. If being alone is contributing to the problem, try to get in touch with a friend.
- Nothing comes out of the blue, and there was a trigger for this schema attack. You don't have to figure out the trigger right now, but remember that you're not crazy. There's a very good reason you're feeling this way right now.
- Remember that the feelings will pass. Your mind and body want to return to a relaxed state. Ride the feelings like a wave.
- Control your thinking. When you have thoughts that are expressions of the schema—*I hate him! No one loves me! I'm going to fall apart, right now!*—DO NOT GO THERE. Distract yourself with other thoughts—*This will pass. I'll be OK soon.* Pay attention to your breathing.
- It will help enormously if you've learned the relaxation response or a mindfulness meditation technique well enough for those behaviors to go on automatic pilot. Make a deliberate effort to engage that automatic pilot.
- Remember that this experience is giving you the opportunity to learn something about yourself, a direct window into your own unconscious. When you're calm, don't just forget the experience, but look at what set it off, what it felt like deep inside, and what old memories seem to be connected.

still loose in there, the contaminants that are still secreting toxins without our awareness. After you come out of a schema attack, try to look at the whole experience mindfully: What was the precipitant? What kind of schema did it trigger? How did it affect your vision and hearing? What other effects did it have in the body—headache, gastric upset, muscle aches, fatigue? What words would you use to describe the feeling? Does it stir up old memories? What got you out of it? If you can connect it to old experiences, bring these into mindful awareness, and allow yourself to feel the feelings associated with the experience. It's your attempt to keep those feelings out of consciousness that's giving the schema the energy it needs to keep tripping you up. If you can stop trying to not feel, your schema attacks will lose a great deal of their power.

Emotional states are naturally self-limiting; the body and the nervous system have elaborate methods for homeostasis, for returning to a relaxed state. We have to avoid the vicious circles that prevent homeostasis, by controlling the content of our thoughts, controlling our breathing, and relaxing our bodies.

Transient attacks like these are not the worst effects of schemas, in my opinion. Far worse is the gradual stifling of the self that comes with thinking in rigid patterns, seeing only what confirms our worldview, responding mindlessly and defensively to anything that might shake us up a little. Wilhelm Reich used the vivid metaphor of "character armor," which we put on gradually throughout life thinking it will protect us from the world. Character armor is our own individual set of defenses, beliefs, patterns of behavior and thinking and responding to anything that feels like a threat—and that's anything that disagrees with our assumptions. Character armor is the neural circuits that we use so often they seem like second nature. We think our armor keeps us safe. But instead, it imprisons us, makes us rigid, opinionated, dogmatic, self-justifying, afraid of the new, afraid of feeling.

There are species of crabs called "decorators"—they will attach pieces of shell, coral, and other seafloor junk to their shells to protect themselves from predators. It makes them pretty safe as long as they stay in one place. But if they start moving around on the sea bottom they look quite silly, and out of context like this their armor makes them visible and vulnerable. That's the problem with character armor; it binds us to where we are while the world changes around us. Most often these days, our armor is structurally weak because it has us ignoring or blaming ourselves for the effects of perpetual stress—the feelings of meaninglessness, anxiety, depression, and physical symptoms that we can't explain because we're culturally blinded. There was a fellow recently who built a concrete structure atop his bulldozer and went around destroying all the public buildings in his small town in Colorado. When the SWAT team finally cut through the concrete they found he'd killed himself inside. He'd had a long dispute with town officials ever since they permitted a cement plant to be built next door to his muffler shop, forcing him out of business. He's already become an Internet folk hero to those who feel constantly pushed around. It's a perfect metaphor for the tragedy of character armor, the loss of ability to see things from more than one perspective, the slow and steady progress down a self-destructive road from which you can't retreat. Everyone described him as a loner; apparently all the meaning in his life came from his job and his welding skills. We all have to be watchful that our own character armor doesn't become too much for us, weighing us down so that once we gain momentum we can't change course.

The Plotline: Coherence, Narratives, Myths, Stories

As we've said, the stories we believe about ourselves—often unconsciously—become self-fulfilling prophecies. They are the plotline of our lives.

"Narrative" is often used these days instead of "story" because it is a postmodern buzzword. It's natural for us to develop stories about ourselves to help us make sense of the world and explain our experience. Attachment researchers believe that it is the parent's ability to form a consistent narrative of their own experience that allows him or her to provide a secure base for the child, the holding environment that every child needs. One of the major tenets of postmodern thought is that "objective" reality is very, very difficult for us to grasp—if it exists at all. So people use the word "narrative" (or "text") to suggest that a story—even one that purports to be complete and objective—represents just one point of view.

But narrative also means something very concrete. If you ask a PTSD victim to describe what happened to him, very often he simply can't. His account will be vague, confused, incomplete, contradictory. He may be flooded with emotion, or he might not show any upset at all. He'll likely be frustrated that he can't be more articulate. Other than this he may be completely unimpaired. He can tell you about other highly emotional, but nontraumatic, events in a clear and understandable way. The reason is that trauma scrambles the hippocampus—the area where short-term memories are temporarily stored before being filed away in narrative fashion. The hormones of fear, when they are too extreme, interfere with the hippocampus's function of tying emotional and historical memory together. That's what the attachment researchers mean by a consistent and coherent narrative of our experience.

"Stress" is the result of conflict between the animal brain and contemporary culture—the id and the superego, the impala chained down in front of the cheetah, the conflict between our senses and our conscious beliefs. In large part our stories are an attempt to control stress. We are taught to be logical, rational, objective when things are difficult. But when we do that to the exclusion of feelings, our stories are lacking vital information. The animal brain, the id, is more correct and sensitive than we acknowledge, contemporary culture more flawed, contradictory, impossible. The logical brain attempts to resolve these conflicts by creating explanations, stories, beliefs, assumptions; but it too is not as reliable as we want to think, influenced by our emotions and constrained by the assumptive world and its neural pathways. We have to get to know both our emotions and our habits of thought (and behavior) so that they don't work on us unconsciously. When we do, we'll have reliable information about ourselves and the world, and the stories we develop to explain things will be more truthful and lead us toward the things we value.

Daniel Siegel's hypothesis in *The Developing Mind* is that we build a *coherent autobiographical narrative* of our own existence through coordinating the left and right hemispheres' picture of ourselves: the left brain's ability to explain things and link facts in a linear fashion combined with the right brain's emotional and autobiographical processing. Putting the two together results in a complete and fairly accurate set of beliefs about the self. Then when we have a bad dream we know what it's about; when someone pushes our buttons we understand why. We can make decisions unencumbered by prejudices and false assumptions. We have the experience of being both in our mind and in our heart at the same time.

The autobiographical narrative is built on the self-image that the infant forms based on its interaction with its mother or other caregivers, and it continues to incorporate our experiences with other people as we go through life. When these interactions are validating, when we feel that others understand or respect our experience, we gain coherence. We lose coherence when we feel invalidated—ignored, disrespected, attacked, thought of as weird or strange.

My dreams are full of rivers, roads, landscapes, and junctions. I'm always traveling, driving, flying, boating. In reality, in my conscious life, I'm very good at orienting myself. I have a great sense of direction. If I drive somewhere once, I can find my way there again. Instinctively, I preferred the landscape of Chicago, where all the roads run either north-south or east-west, and the lake is always east, to the road system in New England, which follows Indian and stagecoach trails. New England makes me a little nervous this way.

I seem to be drawn especially to rivers. Both my father's house in the Chicago sub-urbs and later my own first house were on riverbanks. As a child I lived just a few blocks from the Ohio River. My maternal grandfather used to walk me down there to watch the boats go by. In his youth he had followed the river down from Pennsylvania in search of employment. We saw some of the last of the old paddle-wheelers. I was very intrigued by the current, the notion that the river is always flowing downstream, that it links cities and people in some magical way. I connected with Huckleberry Finn like a brother. I was also intrigued by the fact that the river was always changing. When I learned Heraclitus's aphorism You can never step in the same river twice, *I knew immediately what it meant.*

As I discussed in Undoing Depression, *my mother killed herself shortly before my sixteenth birthday; I have nightmares of being trapped in the basement with her body. When I learned to drive soon after, I made it my business to be a* good *driver. To this day, I've never had an accident. I wanted to be able to get away, to know where I was going, and to get there quickly if I needed to. I think the appeal of rivers is that you just get in a boat, and the current takes you away. It's very comforting.*

Dreaming of rivers and roads and junctions, I think, is my way of trying to put a disturbed narrative together. In the dreams, things just flow and merge, peacefully and calmly. You can get away if you need to, but you don't have to worry about it.

Narrative can be understood to mean the "story beneath the story" that we live out on a daily basis. There is the story we tell the world about ourselves—what we have chosen for work, our lifestyle choices, and the persona we present to others. It is the clothing we wear for the world. Underneath this layer of our personality is another story, the story that drives much of our emotional life, the deeply ingrained beliefs that color how we view the world and how we re-act to it. It is this story we refer to when we use the word narrative. It's the as-sumptive world cast in the form of a story about ourselves.

The Tragic Flaw

A disrupted narrative is a recurring theme, our character rather than our con-scious self, the unconscious assumptions and distortions in how we perceive reality, the "tragic flaw." If *The Odyssey* is about exile and return, it's Odysseus's own overweening pride that banishes him in the first place. If *Hamlet* is about betrayal and revenge, it's Hamlet's own character—the combination of hesita-tion and impulsivity—that leads to tragedy. If *The Catcher in the Rye* is about an adolescent grieving for his brother, it's Holden's character—his moral outrage and deep distrust—that makes it hard for him to heal. Character is the force that drives the story. We're fascinated by narratives in literature because we have some unconscious awareness of how our own tragic flaws lead us to grief.

A disrupted narrative is an example of what James Mann called "the present and chronically endured pain." The old injury leaves scars in our brain, neural circuitry that makes us afraid in the present. We interpret this, often wrongly, to mean there's something to be afraid of now. The old injury—which we work to keep out of consciousness—still makes us feel vulnerable. The current fear, which again is usually unconscious, derives from the old injury. Maybe it's fear of being reinjured, worse, in the same way, but it can also be our fear of our own rage. We load present circumstances with the baggage of the past.

A distorted or self-destructive narrative is usually a sane reaction to an insane or difficult childhood. It is our mind and brain trying hard to adapt and survive emotionally and sometimes even physically. Often these narratives, like defenses, are a double-edged sword, helpful to us at times and damaging at others. Many people learn to become extremely self-sufficient as a result of a neglectful childhood. Self-sufficiency is a wonderful trait, but taken too far it can create a person who cannot accept the help and support of others. A person with this narrative carries into the world a story that says *I can only rely on myself.* As a result they never allow themselves to trust others completely, and they create an isolated lifestyle. Many times this is not done consciously, but a pattern emerges where the person always ends up alone. They pick the wrong partners, they leave relationships too early, they pick occupations or interests that make close relationships difficult, and so on. Rather than focusing on the environment or the "string of bad luck," narrative work looks at the patterns or behaviors that help create these situations over and over again.

It is impossible to create change in one's long-standing habits without first understanding what they are. Understanding one's narrative can be another tool to help one grow, change, and heal the emotional wounds of the past and the present. It is also a way of preventing the creation of new loss and pain.

If you've done a thorough self-examination as a result of Exercise 10, you may be feeling pretty demoralized right now. The list of ways in which old injuries and current fears affect our lives can seem overwhelming. But these are the myths you have about yourself, expressions of the way your brain has been programmed. Life experience has got you believing that you're helpless, hopeless, out of control, unlovable, too angry, too passive, too fat, too drunk, too needy, too incompetent, too you-name-it. Or that your body is fragile, dam-

Exercise 10. **Injuries and Fears**

We've discussed many schemas, assumptions, and character types. There are consistent themes in our lives—always feeling rejected; inadequate; in trouble; overworked; unappreciated. James Mann referred to these scenarios as "the present and chronically endured pain"—our old wounds that we keep hoping are healed, only to find them reopened when we face stress again.

Before you go on in this book, get yourself into a mindful state. Then take a piece of paper and write down some ideas about the old injury and the current fear. You may want to jot down just a few words or write paragraphs—either is fine. You may feel you know pretty definitely what is going on with you, or you may be clueless. Hopefully not entirely clueless, because Exercise 6, your biography, should have given you some strong hints. Regardless, this is not a test. Your answers are likely to change as you read the rest of this book, and at later points in your life, and that's fine too. We are trying to get you in touch with your own unconscious, a slippery devil who is constantly changing shape. But take the ideas you have at this point and let them loose in your mind for a while. Think about some of these questions (you may want to jot down some notes on the same sheet of paper):

- How much of my life is controlled by/in response to these vulnerabilities and fears? On a pie chart, how much area would they take up? 10 percent? 50 percent? 90 percent?
- Is it now in my DNA? Is my body expressing my fears and vulnerabilities? Or my attempts to protect myself from them? Or my protests against them? Or my anger at the people who make me feel this way?
- Are my senses affected? Do I see things from a distorted perspective? Do I take offense where none is intended? Do I not recognize danger? Do I rarely get excited? Do I not hear compliments? Do I see the weeds and not the flowers? Is there a bitter taste in my mouth when others are feeling joy?
- How about my relationships? Do I always fail at intimacy? Am I consistently disappointed, or disappointing? Am I constantly fighting the same battle, but with different people?

(Continued)

- Do I have an addiction? Do I keep resolving to cut back on alcohol? Am I using prescription drugs like painkillers or tranquilizers habitually? Is there a compulsive nature to my shopping, eating, dieting, spending, sexual habits?
- Is my thinking clear? Can I organize the information I need to make a decision? Can I concentrate and focus well, or am I always distracted? Or do I obsess about details and lose the big picture? Am I able to make decisions and stick to them? It's been proven that people with depression make characteristic logical and perceptual errors, have trouble concentrating, and are beset by repetitive negative thoughts. But anxiety, stress, and physical illness also distort thinking in much the same way.

---

aged, sick, ugly, loathsome. Or that the world is too scary, too angry, too cold, too selfish . . . you get the idea.

Resist the temptation to give up at this point. These attitudes are only myths. Their power comes from how they've gotten into your bones. You're going to learn how to overcome these myths, one step at a time, and develop new, more accurate beliefs about yourself and the world. And remember that mastering the current stress in your life will reduce the impact of these issues. What you see before you right now is a big mountain, shrouded in mist. Trying to take it all in at once makes it seem too big. Instead, concentrate on your journey for the next step, the next day, the next week.

You're pushing against the vicious circle, trying to slow it down and reverse it, beginning an *adaptive spiral* in which one good thing will lead to another. Positive events will result in positive feelings, positive moods. Positive moods lead to creative thinking, new solutions. Starting out on the adaptive spiral means setting a reciprocal process in motion, in which our new, more effective coping behavior changes our perception of ourselves and our new self-image facilitates more successful behavior. But at this point this is only fragile change, and the journey is daunting. Take it easy, one step at a time.

Benjamin: Irony Like Fine Wine

Benjamin is a bright, engaging man in his early fifties. Once a very successful author, he's been fighting writer's block for the past eight years, after his last book received some highly critical reviews and failed in the marketplace. His moods can go from sui-

cidal to grandiose in the course of a few hours, depending on how others are treating him and how his work is going. He tortures himself with obsessive thoughts about the past—what he should have done, what he should have said—and the future—how he'll respond to criticism. His deepest fear is that at bottom, he is a fraud with nothing original to say.

Benjamin had the parents from hell. Jewish refugees from the Holocaust and the war, they escaped to Israel, where Benjamin was born and spent the first few years of his life. Later they emigrated to New York. His father became a butcher; his mother worked in an office. Hardworking and frugal, they eventually bought a small apartment building in the Bronx; just two years ago they retired to Florida. From this exotic background, Benjamin blossomed in American education. He commuted to Erasmus Hall for high school, then went on to Harvard on scholarship. His parents couldn't stand it. While Benjamin acknowledges they always valued education, forced him to do his homework, and hid his baseball glove when they felt he was wasting too much time, his success seemed to threaten his father. His mother would always find the A minus among the A's. The contradictory, crazy-making message to him was always Try your best, but you'll never amount to much anyway. You'll never be as smart as your father or as hardworking as your mother. But you have to try!

After graduate school Benjamin found a teaching position and pursued his writing. His first novel was a critical success but got no attention. His second was a solid success. Benjamin met his (non-Jewish) wife, got married, and moved to England, where he continued to teach. With his earnings from teaching and some income from the second book, he and his wife had a wonderful time in England and Europe. He worked meanwhile on his third book, which turned out to be a minor blockbuster. The movie rights went for well over $1 million (though the movie was never made). Ben and his wife bought a small farm with a luxurious home a couple of hours from New York.

Ben's parents were appalled. "Sheep!? What do you want with sheep?" They tut-tuttted about the house, the mortgage, the eight different salad dressings in the fridge, the way Ben and his wife spoiled the children. It was only during this time that Benjamin realized they had a problem with his success. His father started pontificating at every opportunity, talking about how he was acknowledged as the best butcher in the Bronx, how he'd never missed a day's work, about what he'd learned watching the History Channel. Ben might be educated and successful, but he would never have the kind of instinctive intelligence that made his father so special. Ben's mother nagged at him to lose weight and made other critical comments about his appearance, his wife, and his children.

Ben and his wife had two children and lived well for a few years, until a combination of bad investments, a lot of borrowing, and the failure of Ben's next book burst their bubble. His parents could hardly contain their glee. To their credit, they largely refrained from rubbing Ben's nose in it, but he began to drive himself mad with their internalized voices. They both took the opportunity many times to lecture him on good money management. He sold his big house and moved into a much smaller one in town.

He came to see me after things had gone on this way for a while. Ben is a charming, amiable man, erudite but unpretentious; he retains a lot of his Jewish ironic humor, often used at his own expense. He has atrocious work habits: he'll stay up till three watching old movies and eating junk food, set his alarm for seven, then go to his office fortified by several cups of coffee, where he will spend the morning on the phone dealing with creditors and one or more of the hundreds of deals he has in the works. In the afternoon, when he expects himself to write, he naps, then feels horrible about himself. He's been known to bang his head on the wall in frustration when there are too many bills and he sees no way out. When he's depressed, nothing he's ever done looks good; his previous novels seem to him to be tricks he's played on the critics and the public.

We understand that Ben's parents put him in a damned-if-you-do, damned-if-you-don't situation about success—even about independence. Ben's mother has said that his youngest brother is the "best" son because he calls them every day, but in Ben's eyes he is a nebbish who has never left the nest. Thus one of the primary unconscious assumptions in Ben's world is that independence inevitably leads to disaster. He tried for many years to prove this wrong, and even was successful at it for a while, but now it's got a hold of him and won't let go. He went for about four years without being able to put a word on a page. He drives himself crazy going to cocktail parties and fundraisers at his children's expensive private school, where all the talk is about the new wing on the house, or the trip to Switzerland for the skiing, or the big party in the Hamptons. He knows that the talk is insipid, but it all makes him feel like a fraud, as if he's in this company under false pretenses.

Ben's Achilles' heel is his narcissistic vulnerability. At times, when a critic pans him, or someone he has to work with in publishing is uncooperative, he goes mildly off his rocker. He'll brood over his injury for days and weeks. His thoughts will be dominated by revenge fantasies. He's acted on some of these in ways that have ultimately proved embarrassing or self-destructive. He's never worked with the same editor on more than one book, because he burns them out; from his point of view, they never take him seriously enough. He's earned a reputation in publishing as a difficult author, and that has hurt his earning power. Much worse, though, is the fact that these obsessions dominate his thinking, making it next to impossible to work. But although he can't as yet complete another novel, Ben does work very hard on small writing projects. It never comes easy, the work is always torturous, but he keeps at it doggedly to keep the family's head above water.

I'm including Ben's story in this section not only because he's an example of the destructive effects of assumptions and schemas, but because he's a fascinating example of the problem of self-control. As an author, Ben is acutely aware of how character drives the story. He knows only too well that he gets derailed by relatively small slights, and that this is very destructive to him. But he feels he can't help himself. No matter what he does, his mind always returns to the current irritant.

We've analyzed Ben's problems six ways from Sunday. He hates his parents but still desires their love and approval, a common human predicament. Of course Ben feels very guilty about his hate; is his writer's block a way of punishing himself? Does he hurt them by hurting himself? Deprive them of the opportunity to puncture his balloon of self-esteem by puncturing the balloon first? Or is he simply displacing his rage at his parents onto people in the present who injure him in the same ways they did, albeit in much more minor ways? Does he project all his deep insecurity onto others who are only raising minor issues? Clearly, his assumptive world primes him to be on constant guard for traitors, betrayers, backstabbers; and in the deeply ironic way of projective identification, people inevitably live up to (or down to) his expectations.

What was there about his success, about spending so lavishly, marrying a goy, moving to the Waspish environs of the Hudson Valley and raising sheep? Why did it need to be so obvious a rejection of his parents' values? Did he want to show them that he didn't need them? If so, it backfired, because within a few years he was asking them for money. Was he spitting in God's eye, daring cosmic irony to come and get him?

Worst of all, Benjamin fears that at bottom he really is a fraud. His obsessions with revenge distract him from this fear, but never adequately enough. When he's criticized or let down, all his fears come spilling out, immobilizing him with terror. His rage is a defensive distraction; it's much safer to be full of indignation than to let yourself feel vulnerable. But here's the vicious circle: by distracting himself from his fears, he can never face them and prove something to himself. He knows his rage is in essence an escape from his fears, and each time it happens it dissolves some more of his self-esteem. Several times, I've gotten Benjamin to stop and face his fears. Are you really a fraud? What does that mean, a fraud? Have you just been fooling everyone? *Each time, Ben is able to answer firmly in the negative, and he's freed, for a while, from all his mindless fear-based behavior.*

Our analysis has helped a great deal. Ben is more productive now. He sees clearly what's going on, how his sensitivity works to cause trouble for him, when he used to be stuck in a big amorphous mess of confusion and hopelessness. This allows him to have a better perspective and feel more in control and hopeful. He's been able to restrain himself much better from pursuing some impulsive scenarios that would have got him into more trouble. But he can't stop his obsessions and revenge fantasies.

Ben and I have made a catalog of revenge movies, the kind where for the first two-thirds the hero allows himself to get beaten up and pushed around by the bad guys, usually because he's taken some vow to show restraint; but inevitably he reaches his breaking point. Then there's a ritual donning of his battle gear, and he goes in and cleans house (think Shane*). Ben loves these movies—there are dozens of them—and we agree that these are a good outlet for his imagined revenge fantasies. But they're not real life, because in real life there are always consequences to blowing up. If you destroy your parents, you're out of luck, because you still want them to love you.*

We've been working on mindfulness. Benjamin has become aware that when he has a good day, a bad one follows inevitably. When he allows himself to feel good, he ex-pects to get punished. He's gotten much better at isolating the irritant, the critic or the obstacle, and seeing it as a relatively small part of the overall picture. He really likes my "flytrap" exercise (Exercise 11) and is trying to use it—not to belittle or write off his enemies, but to capture and control the annoying thoughts that buzz through his head when he's trying to be productive. He's been trying to apply this, but his life and work habits are so chaotic that he can't fully work on a mindfulness routine.

This is the way I find psychotherapy works for very difficult problems. It's taken the patient a lifetime to get where he is, and it will take us a long time to undo the damage. Ben has made a lot of progress. He's much more productive now, and we're both hope-ful that a project soon will pay off for him both financially and critically. A develop-ment like this can set an adaptive spiral in motion, a cycle of success that can lead to internal healing. Until that happens, we're doing something akin to untangling a knot-ted ball of string, clearing the confusion and the mess out of the way one piece at a time so that the person can emerge from the knots and see that his problems are manageable and understandable.

Free Will and Self-Control

Our stories, narratives, and schemas are meant to help us make sense of the world, to explain our experience and help us make decisions. Because our viewpoint is narrow and our experience is limited, we tend to overpersonalize what happens to us, to believe that random events are connected to us in a per-sonal way. We are the central character in all our stories. When bad things hap-pen to us, we are too likely to assign responsibility to ourselves. My job is to understand the stories people tell me about themselves, and help them rewrite those stories to have happier endings. It's not easy because we have only limited awareness of our own stories. They are largely unconscious—assumptions, distorted perceptions, patterns of automatic behavior, habits of dealing with emotions that seem so natural that they feel like basic parts of the self. In the therapist's office, stories are told not only by what the patient says but by how he looks and what happens to him; by the presentation of the self and by repetitions of the same problem over and over, including in the relationship with the therapist.

Some of my patients, but by no means all, seem to be magically affected by what their parents or other loved ones think of them; they act as if they are cursed, doomed to live under a hex, a voodoo spell. *You'll never amount to much. Why can't you be happy, like your sister? You're to blame.* Others have other explanations for being stuck: it's their genes, or their brain chemistry, or their unconscious self-sabotage, or their history of trauma or deprivation, or their personality disorder, or their addiction. They seem to be damaged, not by what others wish on them but by accidents of birth, biology, and fate. In many cases I have helped them formulate these explanations, relying on the best of psychoneurology to help relieve some of the guilt and inadequacy they feel at repeating the same mistakes over and over; but sometimes I wonder if I have helped them find forgiveness at the expense of responsibility.

Of course it's not just the distressed few who find their way to the therapist's office who are influenced by stories like these. Developments in psychology, genetics, neurology, and medicine are vastly increasing our awareness of unseen forces that influence our behavior and personality, challenging basic premises about how we make decisions. We dismiss old beliefs in witchcraft and demons, but we have new demons now—twisted chromosomes, inadequate serotonin, neural pathways, attachment disorders, trauma, missing psychic structure.

The problem that we're trying to find a solution for is that of personal responsibility and self-control. We all do things we'd rather stop. We all have secret guilts and shames. A touch of voyeurism. Too much drinking. Little dishonesties, small cruelties. Daydreams of revenge. A pattern of destructive relationships, a depression you can't snap out of, nagging irrational fears that wake you at 3 A.M. The belief you'll never be good enough; the belief you're already better than everyone else. We'd stop if we could, so we feel out of control. But we have more control than we think, because we *do* stop, most of the time, before we go too far. We satisfy our voyeurism on the Internet instead of peeking through windows. We fantasize tearing our enemies limb from limb, and stop at fantasy. The depression drags on, robbing us of joy, but rarely making us stark raving mad. Personal responsibility, uncomfortable as the thought may be, is not an all-or-nothing quality, but a matter of degree. Is there some essential difference between us and the boy who shoots up his high school, the mother who drowns her children, the pedophile at the playground? *Do we have enough self-control to keep us legal, but not enough to make us healthy?* Yes, exactly, that is often the case: that's why we are a society of laws. Laws represent society's expectations of just how much self-control a "normal" person should have. Society, by instituting laws, seems to accept the idea that self-control is something we have a limited quantity of. Next question: Do we have a fixed quantity, or does it fluctuate? (For more discussion of these issues, see *Descartes' Error, Skinner's Fumble* in the endnotes.)

Again, we create myths and stories to help us with these complex questions. *People are born gay or straight. I can't lose weight, it's in my genes. I can't help being depressed, it's a mental illness. I didn't want to hit her, but I lost control. I'm a loser, an alien, a reject; misunderstood, victimized, helpless. I'm special, gifted, entitled to what I want.* When things are too ambiguous, when we can't explain why we don't act as we should, we rely on myths like these. Science has made real progress. There is less ambiguity than there used to be, but there's plenty left, and science has given us new excuses with which we can rationalize our weaknesses. The broad issue—to what extent are we responsible for our own choices?—is much more than an abstract philosophical question. It pervades our thinking about ourselves. Historically, eras when individual responsibility was celebrated—the Reformation, the Enlightenment, the American Revolution—have been ages of advance. By contrast, eras when individuals were thought to be mere pawns of larger forces—the Middle Ages and the Soviet era come to mind—were times of backwardness and repression. The gradual weakening of individual moral responsibility, from Freud's doctrine of the unconscious to the adoption of the Twinkie defense, pervades our culture to a much greater extent than we realize. The bottom line, which I share with Stephen Mitchell and others, is that it's a mistake to view free will as an either-or. Much of what we do, feel, think, and see is determined by forces we're not aware of; but in the present, we do have some control, some degree of choice. A worthwhile goal is to free ourselves as much as possible from these unseen forces, including our own character armor, and strengthen and broaden our capacity for self-control.

You have probably noticed by now my annoying tagline at the end of most of the exercises: *The more you practice, the easier it gets.* That, I think, may be the one way we can strengthen our self-control and expand our power to exercise choice. Though there is plenty of confusion in life, in most circumstances we know what is good for us, what is the right thing or the wrong thing to do. In the present moment, you can decide between them. The more often you do the right thing, the easier it gets to do it the next time. We know this now; we have visual proof from studying the brain: the brain makes new connections as we practice. We strengthen those connections with more practice. *The more you practice self-control, the easier it gets.*

Exercise 11. **Self-Control with Upsetting Feelings**

This is the exercise I promised in Chapter 4, when we were discussing how to avoid getting overwhelmed by negative emotions.

First, be sure you use this the right way. Don't use it to avoid thinking about something you really should be thinking about, like an upcoming deadline or a fear you should investigate or an angry situation you have to address. Don't use it to keep from going off half-cocked, catastrophizing or exploding. There's a better exercise for this situation, but it requires mental control skills, so we have to wait for Chapter 8. But *do* use this exercise when, for instance, you're really upset about a situation at work, you've talked it out six ways from Sunday, and you've made up your mind what you have to do—but here it is the weekend and there's nothing you can do till Monday. Or you're waiting for the results of your test and there's nothing to do but wait. This is for upsetting feelings—fear, anger, maybe guilt or shame or lust or envy—that you just can't do anything about right now, but can't stop obsessing over.

Are we clear? Here goes.

Get yourself into a mindful state. Be in a quiet place, no distractions, comfortable position. Get your breathing regulated. Give yourself a good ten or fifteen minutes so that you can feel deeply relaxed.

Look at what's bothering you, but don't look at it too closely. Look at it from a mindful distance. Don't get into the details. Look at yourself with compassionate curiosity. Look at how this feeling irritates you and annoys you. It

(Continued)

comes and goes like a housefly that has decided your aroma is just the most wonderful thing in the world. It buzzes around your eyes and ears, lands on your skin just heavily enough to irritate you, flies off for a few minutes, and just when you go off guard, here it comes again. You wave it away, try to smack it, but it's too fast for you.

You have a secret weapon, though.

You have a little flytrap. It's built like a little capsule, a tiny oval-shaped thing in two pieces that slide together. Flies can't resist your flytrap. You set it down, and pretty soon the fly wanders in. You put the halves together, and now you've got him. He can buzz around in your little capsule, but he can't bother you anymore. The buzzing is now tiny and distant, the voice like Mickey Mouse three rooms away. You can ignore it.

Now, think of your disturbing emotion as the fly. It's been buzzing around in your brain, scaring your amygdala, setting off the stress response, jangling the circuits in the cerebral cortex so you can't concentrate or think properly. Just put it in your little flytrap. *Encapsulate* your disturbing feeling in a little container so it's quiet and harmless and can't move.

Visualize taking this little capsule and moving it into the back storage area of the brain, the part you hardly ever use, the part that remembers your phone number from twenty years ago and is still upset at your brother for cheating at Monopoly. You can leave the capsule there as long as you like.

When you get twinges of that disturbing feeling, imagine it rattling around in its little container like the tiny worm in the Mexican jumping bean. It's happy and warm in there, and you can leave it alone.

When it's time to address the situation that led to this disturbing feeling, the feeling is there in your capsule. It hasn't gotten any bigger or more dangerous while you let it be. In fact, maybe it's gotten a little smaller because you have been able to visualize it as a little fly or a tiny worm.

As with all these exercises:

The more you practice, the easier it gets.

Common Human Miseries:
Anxiety, Depression, PTSD,
Personality Disorder, Addiction

I'VE taken Freud's cold words as the title of this chapter, but please don't get the idea I take these problems lightly. I've spent my professional life helping people with these issues, and I have my own struggle with depression, and I know that the misery they cause can be truly dreadful. But I want to make the point that they *are* common, thanks to the fact that our nervous system hasn't evolved to keep up with social change. The stress response was designed to help us escape those cheetahs—to dump everything out into an intense ten minutes of struggle. It was never designed for constant stress. The Perpetual Stress Response has us pouring neurotransmitters and hormones into our bodies that dissolve brain cells, stop new brain growth, play havoc with our digestion, damage our immune system, and wind up our muscles and bones as tight as a rubber band ready to snap. Our minds, not understanding what's going on, desperate for an explanation, create theories. The theory of depression is *It must be me*. The theory of personality disorder is *It must be you*. The theory of anxiety is *There must be something out there*. PTSD says *I'll hide from it*. The theory of addiction is *I don't care what it is, just make it go away*. Nonspecific illness says *It's my fragile body*. All those theories are false, but in the ironic way of the mind, they become true. Living based on those assumptions makes us create a life that plays them out. Our assumptive world becomes the real world. We become trapped in vicious circles and there seems to be no way out.

Then when we become aware we have a problem, the left-brain approaches we normally take just make it worse. Trying too hard to control, to feel good, to avoid feeling bad, just plays into the vicious circle. We become hypersensitive to our symptoms, and only add to our stress. Our vaunted problem-solving skills, frustrated with problems that permit no quick solutions, just make us feel more stressed and inadequate.

Conventional treatment has limited results with these problems. It's true we can make things much better for many people. Anxiety and depression can be greatly alleviated through medication and psychotherapy. People who have been literally crippled through anxiety—for instance, by agoraphobia, which makes a nightmare of every excursion outside the house, or by obsessive-compulsive disorder, which can force people to waste their lives in pointless rituals—can now expect to be able to function again. People with severe depression, who have been suicidal, unable to move, overwhelmed by shame and self-blame, can look forward to enjoying life again. PTSD sufferers can expect to have their torment greatly eased. Addictions can be beaten, but it usually takes a lifestyle change, like Alcoholics Anonymous, in addition to therapy or medication. Even personality disorders are being increasingly recognized as responses to life stresses that can be alleviated. Psychiatry and psychology have made tremendous strides in the past two decades, and can offer hope now to people who were literally hopeless before. But it's far from reliable science— the new pills and established psychotherapeutic methods are only effective with a limited number of people, and no one knows why what works for Jane doesn't work for Jill.[1]

And recovery from these conditions is never quite complete. Anyone who has ever experienced severe anxiety, depression, or PTSD knows that it's a life-changing experience. It's like an auto accident that leaves us with broken bones and internal injuries. We are shaken to the core of our being and will never again have the same kind of reliable confidence in ourselves and the way we see the world that we had before. We have to put ourselves back together after an experience like this, and we never come out exactly the same.

---

1 See Guthrie, 2000. Psychotherapy researchers have focused on efficacy—specific treatments tailored to specific conditions—as opposed to effectiveness. In the process they have restricted their applicability to a narrow range of patients who have "pure" disorders, losing relevance for the general population. In fact these patients are the ones who would be treated first with drugs if they appeared in a clinical setting, with a likelihood of good response; patients who would ordinarily be treated with psychotherapy in a clinical setting—those who decline or fail to respond to drugs— are specifically excluded from the studies.

Besides, we shouldn't want to. The old self is what got us into trouble in the first place. Our assumptions about life have been wrong, and we have to change. All these conditions are signals to us that the way we've been living doesn't work. Life has been trying to tell us something, and we haven't been paying attention; our assumptive world isn't letting new perspectives in. We may have been trying to pretend we don't care, or that we're in control, or that we're unafraid; but we can't fool ourselves for long, and our lizard brain will seize and bite us.

The first step in breaking free of these vicious circles means making sure you are doing everything you reasonably can to address your most distressing symptoms. Controlling our symptoms is necessary, but not sufficient, to regaining control of our lives. We need to get the best treatment and practice the best self-care we can, understanding that there are limitations to what science can do and that in some situations we have to accept living with some discomfort. Once you are certain that you are taking all necessary measures, even if you're still in distress, you have to move on. You can't wait for the miracle cure any longer; taking charge of yourself is the only miracle there is. So the bottom line is, get professional help if you have a problem you've tried to tackle yourself without success. Good psychotherapy and appropriate medications can help you greatly. They may give you the energy and optimism to go on and make some of the changes I advocate. See my advice on pages 281–283 about how to locate good help (and see the Appendix for helpful resources), and don't be ashamed of using it. You're just experiencing the same burnout we all are, the system overload of the Perpetual Stress Response. But be realistic about what to expect. You can get substantial relief from your symptoms, but you're likely to keep on stepping in the same hole if you don't change your assumptive world.

As we begin this discussion about categories of human misery, let's remind ourselves to be mindful of the dangers of relying on categories. Ellen Langer argues forcefully that categorical thinking is essentially mindless—it blinds us to differences between things in the category, and to similarities between things in different categories. It makes for stereotypes and prejudices. Few of us fit neatly into one of these categories. No one has depression without some anxiety. No one has a personality problem without anxiety and depression. Let's keep in mind that the diagnostic categories we're going to talk about serve a purpose for scientists in making sure everyone's talking about the same thing, but at the same time they limit creativity. They make these things illnesses that people *have*, with the implicit promise that they can be "cured" by outside intervention, instead of seeing that these are *part of you*, the results of a way of life that must be changed.

Anxiety

As we've said, the basic assumption of anxiety is *There must be something out there.* The cheetahs are hiding, just behind the rocks, waiting for you to let your guard down. With that belief, you're always vigilant for danger. If you have an anxiety disorder, you're constantly worried that something is going to push you over the brink, that you're going to lose control, and so you watch yourself like a hawk. You obsessively monitor your internal state, and of course you find more things to worry about. If you have to do something difficult, you die a thousand deaths beforehand, and you don't let yourself feel good afterward. Anxiety supplies itself with its own fuel; the more we worry, the more we have to worry about.

Jack is working his way up the mergers and acquisitions business. He works twelve-hour days and "relaxes" by playing with his own portfolio. He's already made his first million and is now shooting for ten. His wife divorced him a few years ago, after his second affair. His kids are in boarding school, and he rarely sees them, though he always wants to have more contact.

Two or three times a year Jack shows up at the emergency room with crushing chest pains, shortness of breath, ringing in the ears, sweating, and dizziness. After a full workup, the doctors tell him he's fine—nothing to worry about—it's "just anxiety." One doctor, who has seen a lot of men with this pattern, has taken Jack aside and given him some names of psychotherapists who specialize in stress reactions. But Jack, who is always deeply embarrassed by "giving in to panic," tries to forget about it as soon as possible. The problem is these attacks are becoming more frequent.

Anxiety is the classic stress reaction—the body's fight-or-flight response to fear, triggered when there is no objective danger. The question has to do with the conflict between the animal brain, which is sensing danger, and the logical brain, which keeps trying to tell us we're safe. The animal brain doesn't listen, and the body keeps pumping out stress hormones, which keep us miserable and wear out our parts, like driving with one foot on the brake.

These are major anxiety syndromes:

- *Phobias* are fears of specific situations (heights, enclosed spaces) or stimuli (spiders, snakes) that are far out of proportion to the actual danger represented.
- *Panic attacks* are periods of intense anxiety or discomfort that seem to come on for no specific reason. Sometimes they are experienced somatically; the person feels like he's suffocating, or having a heart attack. Untreated, panic attacks sometimes lead to *agoraphobia,* the fear of leaving the house, and people end up leading very restricted lives.
- *Social phobia* is the extreme fear of social situations, like parties or crowds, or an extreme form of *performance anxiety,* the fear of public speaking or otherwise being the center of attention. And here we have an example of the consequences of excessive categorization: because this is officially an illness now, you can take Zoloft (or other SSRIs) for it, and your health insurance will pay. It's nice that medications can help with these symptoms, but how many people *don't* feel some social anxiety? Where does shyness end and illness begin? Shyness is probably the personality trait that is most heavily influenced by genetics. Many shy children become anxious and depressed adults, but others do not; a supportive family environment seems to make the difference.
- *Generalized anxiety disorder* means excessive, uncontrollable worry and fear about mostly everything, not confined to a specific situation. The worry and fear are so dominant that they interfere with normal functioning. This is usually accompanied by symptoms like fatigue, difficulty sleeping, and muscle tension. When we get to some conditions like chronic fatigue syndrome in Chapter 9, it will be hard to differentiate between them and a kind of generalized anxiety disorder that focuses on the body as the subject of the excessive worry.
- *Obsessive-compulsive disorder* is classified as an anxiety disorder, though it's complicated. People with this disorder experience the symptoms more severely during times of stress, and they usually feel severe anxiety accompanying the symptoms, so it makes sense to consider it an anxiety problem. The specific form of the symptoms, though, may be, as Jeffrey Schwartz and others have suggested, due to a specific faulty circuit in the brain that doesn't turn off the anxiety response when we know, rationally, that there is no danger. Obsessions are intrusive thoughts or images that the patient knows are inappropriate and tries very hard to make go away: *There was a*

bump in the road. I must have hit someone. But I know I didn't. But maybe I did . . . and so on, endlessly torturing the mind. Compulsions are repetitive inappropriate acts, like hand washing or checking that the stove is off, that the person knows are silly but is unable to stop himself from performing.

- *Irritable bowel syndrome.* Because loose bowels are a natural component of the stress response, people with anxiety disorders frequently experience diarrhea (or the *fear* of diarrhea) as part of the syndrome. Repeated bouts of diarrhea, then holding in, then constipation often lead to irritable bowel syndrome. More of this in Chapter 9.

We've already talked about the chemistry of the stress response in the body (Chapter 3), which is essentially what's happening to you when you're in an anxious state. Let's look at how constant fear affects the brain, with the help of my flowchart (Figure 12). Under normal conditions when the amygdala gets a message from the senses signaling danger, it sends a message to the hypothalamus, which sends a message to the pituitary, which releases ACTH (a stress hormone) into the bloodstream. The adrenal glands, becoming aware of the presence of ACTH, release their hormones/neurotransmitters (adrenaline, norepinephrine, cortisol) into the bloodstream, which trigger all those somatic responses: loose bowels, engorged muscles, changes in the lymphatic and immune systems, more highly focused vision, pounding heart, high blood pressure, and so forth. Back in the brain, the hippocampus also senses these neurotransmitters, and begins to send out its countermessage—*slow down*—to all those organs in the body and to the amygdala. Again, under normal circumstances the amygdala and hippocampus develop a sensitive balancing act. Those *slow down* messages from the hippocampus enable the amygdala to look around and see if the danger is still there: if so, it keeps on pumping out distress signals; but if the danger is past, it does indeed slow down and the whole body begins to relax.

But, if the stress persists (as it does in anxiety disorders; this is when we're imagining cheetahs behind the rocks), the hippocampus can't keep up. With enough stress, dendrites in the hippocampus begin to shrivel up; with more, the nerve cells themselves begin to die. Vietnam vets and victims of child abuse have shrunken hippocampi. Continued stress interferes with the hippocampus's ability to consolidate memory, so we get confused and start to dissociate. And, of course, there is no brake left on the amygdala, nothing to stop it from constantly being in an alarmed state—which is what I think is left in generalized anxiety

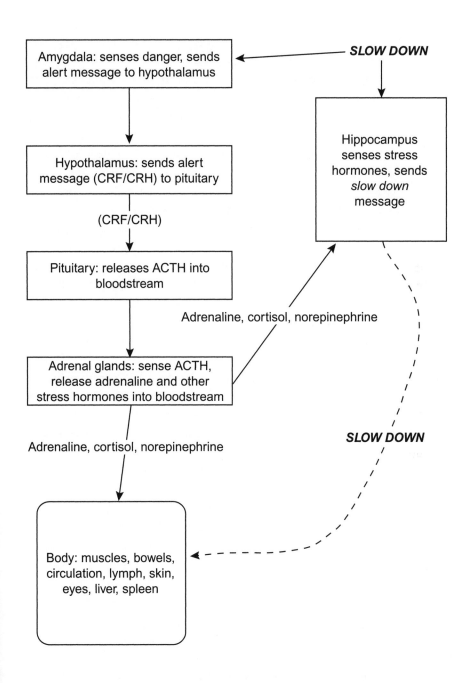

The Stress Response System

Figure 12

disorder. The hopeful news is that there's evidence that treatment—and removal from stress—can restore a damaged hippocampus.

And what, someone asks, *does this have to do with all that stuff in the last chapter about assumptive worlds, defenses, and schemas?* We're really talking about the same events, except now we're talking about what happens in the brain instead of the mind. When we're in an anxious state, the mind adds content to explain what's going on. It builds that content around our unique experiences. *I'm scared, I don't know why, this is silly. But it makes me remember the time I got so scared when I was five and Dad just laughed at me. He thought I was a wuss. I must be a wuss. I feel like I did when I used to have nightmares, and cried for help, and they ignored me. I have to get over this on my own. But I can't. Something's wrong with me. I'm different. I'm delicate.* Then these beliefs start to trigger anxiety too. *I'm not tough enough, I can't take it. Everyone can see. I made a fool of myself the other night; I felt so uncomfortable I didn't talk to anyone. I don't want to go to parties anymore.* We have another vicious circle where anxious feelings trigger anxious thoughts, which trigger more anxious feelings, and so on.

Anxiety responses are very easily conditioned (Pavlov's dog: the anxiety response is automatically triggered by any circumstances resembling the first time we got anxious) and this is very helpful for survival. When we're anxious we're highly motivated to change our circumstances (run away from the cheetah). Because we experience a great relief when we get out of the anxious situation, we're motivated to learn to anticipate danger and take precautions (build a cheetah-proof fence). Good for survival, but sometimes inconvenient: if we get dizzy and scared once in a high building, we're likely to experience anxiety next time we're in a high building; pretty soon we have acrophobia. Or if we're very nervous when giving our first speech, we may try to avoid public speaking thereafter; pretty soon we have performance anxiety. Preparedness theory suggests that our brains are evolutionarily wired to be afraid of some things (snakes, spiders, heights, perhaps being the center of attention when we're not full of serotonin) that were dangerous to our ancestors. Research has shown, for instance, that it's much easier to create a phobia of snakes or spiders than one of knives or guns, which are realistically more dangerous.

Treatment for Anxiety

Treatment for a phobia is really very simple. It boils down to getting you to experience the phobic situation in a relaxed state, then repeating this a few times until the fear response is extinguished. For the few simple phobics I've seen,

I've used drugs to produce the relaxed state. Benzodiazepines (minor tranquilizers like Xanax or Klonopin) are the drug of choice. They not only relax muscles, they also inhibit the amygdala's ability to turn on the sympathetic nervous system—the fight-or-flight response. Of course these drugs are addictive, so you have to be careful. But in my experience most phobic patients are also very fearful about the effects of medications, so they eventually just like having a pill in their pocket when they have to face the fear. The other reliable way of achieving the relaxed state is, of course, learning the relaxation response and using it as a coping mechanism as you gradually approach the phobic situation. A new high-tech way has you wearing a special headset while you watch a DVD of, say, going up in a high building; you control exactly how much height you want to expose yourself to. Whatever the method, it's just learning the "extinction" response. Remember that we said in Chapter 5 that there is proof now that extinction is not forgetting, but the actual construction of new brain circuitry that redirects fear signals from the amygdala into the "high road" of the cerebral cortex.

There's the amygdala again, the villain in the anxiety script. For, although simple phobias may be easy to treat, they are rare; the fact is that anxiety problems cause immense suffering for people who are afflicted. A significant anxiety problem will literally run your life, taking up far too much space in your head. You can waste years worrying about things that are really trivial. Trying to avoid anxiety-provoking situations means you spend your time constantly watchful. Trying to avoid fear makes you full of fear. Your self-esteem will plummet because you will beat up on yourself for not being able to get past something you think of as silly. You are likely to lose friends and alienate loved ones because they get exasperated with you. Anxiety is linked to what epidemiologists blithely call "excess mortality"—early death, primarily from cardiovascular disease and suicide. It's a major reason for substance abuse, especially alcohol and prescription drugs. One study of alcoholics found that 33 percent of them had severe, crippling agoraphobia or social phobia, and another 35 percent had milder versions of the same things. I have a theory that untreated anxiety almost inevitably leads to depression, because it is exactly the learned helplessness situation: the person learns that nothing he can do will make him feel better. Who wouldn't get depressed? There's some evidence for my theory: treatment of panic disorder seems to prevent development of major depression later on. In the National Comorbidity Study it was found that a much smaller proportion (19 percent) of people who received treatment for panic disorder developed major depression than those who did not receive treatment (45 percent).

So I urge you to get help; despite my caveats that treatment is limited in what it can do, we are good enough at treating anxiety that you have a right to expect significant reduction in your symptoms. Find a therapist who is open to working with you around medications. If you don't experience relief within a few months of starting psychotherapy, find a new therapist. See my guidelines at the end of this chapter for how to find a good one.

These are the major medication groups for anxiety disorders:

- *Benzodiazepines* (also known as minor tranquilizers: Xanax, Klonopin, Valium, Ativan, and some others) are often immediately effective in reducing the stress response and the worry that accompanies it. The only side effect is usually drowsiness and some difficulty concentrating. They wear off quickly (four to twelve hours) and symptoms return—but if you're out of a stressful situation by then, that's OK. They are addictive. For this reason, some physicians prefer to prescribe the slow-acting ones, like Klonopin, because the effect wears off more gradually; the quick return of anxiety associated with Xanax, for instance, just prompts us to take another pill. As I said, they are good for phobias, because you only need to take them when dealing with the phobic situation. They should not be used for long-term treatment unless nothing else works; there can be severe withdrawal reactions. Besides, we tend to habituate to them, needing stronger and stronger doses. They are notorious for adding to the effects of alcohol, making you get drunk much faster and often leading to blackouts. Benzodiazepines have natural receptor sites in the brain, which when stimulated release the inhibiting neurotransmitter GABA. So you're inhibiting responsiveness all over the brain, which might account for the mental fuzziness many people feel on benzodiazepines.
- *Beta-blockers* like Inderal, Corgard, and Tenormin, which are normally used to slow the heart and reduce high blood pressure, also block some of the physical symptoms of anxiety—shaking, sweating, and heart pounding. For some people, they are better treatment for phobic anxiety than benzodiazepines because they do not interfere with concentration or alertness— good for musicians and public speakers. But they don't work for everyone, and there can be dangerous physical side effects. The usual advice is to treat them like benzodiazepines—for short-term or situational use only.

- *Antidepressants* (both newer drugs like Zoloft, Paxil, and Celexa, and older tricyclics like Elavil and Tofranil) are often effective with anxiety problems. They don't work quickly, like the benzodiazepines, so they don't give instant relief. But after a few weeks, people with problems like panic attacks or generalized anxiety disorder often notice that gradually their symptoms are becoming less severe and they are spending less time preoccupied with their anxiety. They can maintain substantial relief as long as they stay on the medications, which as far as we know have no long-term ill effects. There are unpleasant side effects with all these drugs, however, ranging from diminished sexual drive or performance to dizziness, dry mouth, constipation, and low blood pressure. Another problem is that our reactions to these meds are highly idiosyncratic: what works fine for me will not work at all with you, and we have no idea why. You may have to try three or four drugs before you find the right thing, and this will take months. Some medical doctors have really educated themselves about these drugs and will have the patience to help you through these trials, but most won't, and so I highly recommend that you see a psychiatrist for any antidepressant. There is the distinct advantage to the older antidepressants that most have gone generic by now, so the treatment is much less expensive. A common treatment strategy is to give the patient in acute distress a few weeks' worth of a benzodiazepine, to help get through the crisis, at the same time as starting an antidepressant that will kick in before you're addicted to the tranquilizer.
- *BuSpar* is a drug in a unique class which often relieves anxiety in the same way as antidepressants—slowly and gradually. It's frequently prescribed for generalized anxiety disorder. Like the antidepressants, it doesn't work for everyone, and it has its side effects, though it's not addictive.
- *Antihistamines* like Benadryl and Vistaril have some calming properties and are sometimes effective enough treatment for mild anxiety conditions. They are not habit forming. I frequently suggest Benadryl for people with insomnia, and many find it helpful. All the prescription sleep aids are highly addictive and can have some unpleasant side effects.

Again, let me restate that *medications are not enough* by themselves to help with anxiety disorders. Though they supply welcome relief for many people, they are only covering up the Perpetual Stress Response. As we said in Chapter 4, anxiety is your friend. It's your body sending you an important message.

It's telling you there's something wrong in the way you're going about your life. It's telling you you've been living mindlessly, stuffing stress away down into your unconscious, where it can only express itself by triggering the fight-or-flight response. Recovery requires that we not dismiss our fears, but respect them. To respect our fears, we don't have to give in to them, but look at them carefully, mindfully. What's the animal brain trying to tell us? How is it out of sync with our world of beliefs? Maybe it's telling you to slow down, take it easy, don't take on so much.

Depression

If you're depressed, you think depressed thoughts, which lead to more depressed thoughts. You remember sad things and forget happy ones. You lose energy and concentration, so you make bad decisions and can't follow through on things. Your brain loses the ability to experience happiness. You're no fun to be around, so people avoid you. In other words, depression is not just a mood; it leads to a truly depressing life.

This is the subject I know best. I've suffered a couple of episodes of serious depression, and always struggle with feeling good, confident, and energetic. Treatment has helped me, but I have to push myself to be disciplined and do the things that I know are good for me. The story is in *Undoing Depression*. As we've said, the theory of depression is *It must be me—I feel miserable, I can't do anything right, I can't feel happy, I'm tense all the time. Something is wrong with me. I'll go to the doctor.* Unfortunately what the patient gets at the doctor's office is—far more often than not—only a drop in the bucket of the care he needs to really recover.

Depression is second only to heart disease in its health impact worldwide. The most surprising aspect about this news is that it doesn't come from any mental health advocacy group, but from the World Bank and World Health Organization, which measured the lost years of healthy life due to disease. In the United States in 1990, the cost of treatment of depression, increased mortality, and loss of productivity was estimated at $44 billion a year, higher than any disease but heart disease, greater than the effect of cancer, of AIDS, of lung disease, MS, or any other single disease entity. Nationally, there are approximately thirty thousand suicides annually, as compared to twenty thousand homicides. Every homicide is front-page news, but suicides, equally tragic and perhaps more devastating to the survivors, are hushed up because of the stigma associated with depression. One person in five will suffer an episode of major depression during his or her lifetime, and one person in five is suffering from some form of depression at any given moment. Health economists equate the disability caused by major depression with that of blindness or paraplegia. And the impact will only get worse: For each group born since 1900, the age of onset of depression has gotten younger, and the lifetime risk has increased. If current trends continue, the average age of onset for children born in the year 2000 will be twenty years old. There is good reason to say that we are in the midst of an epidemic of depression.

There are three main types of depression: major depression, dysthymia, and bipolar disorder.

Major depression is a very serious condition. If you have it, you usually know that something is really wrong, but you may not recognize it for what it is. You are likely to be very fatigued, yet you can't sleep. You have difficulty concentrating, remembering, and making decisions. Your self-esteem plummets and you feel very guilty or inadequate. You may have thoughts of death or suicide. Your appetite is disrupted. Things that normally make you happy lose their impact. You may have a lot of physical symptoms you can't explain: muscle and joint pain, digestive problems, headaches, skin problems. Women find themselves crying for no reason. Men get irritable and withdrawn, sometimes violent. The chances of developing major depression at some point in your life are estimated at about 22 percent for women, 10 percent for men.

Here's the illustration I used in *Undoing Depression:*

Nancy has major depression. Although she is able to hold down a responsible job and has raised a family successfully, most of the time she is miserable. She looks tense and sad. She is thin, shy, and worried. She's hesitant to say what's on her mind, though she is caring and intelligent. She constantly puts herself down. She believes she can't handle any stress; in fact, she copes very well, but always fears that she's messing up. She has recurrent migraines that force her to bed several times a month. She has to take a medication for these that costs eighty dollars a dose, and her antidepressant medication costs eight dollars a day. Her family is on a tight budget, and her insurance doesn't pay for medication, so she blames herself for having to spend so much money on treatment.

Nancy describes her depression as a well. When it's at its worst, she is stuck down in the mud at the bottom of the well. The mud is full of worms and rats, and it's all she can do to keep from being eaten alive. When she's feeling good, she's out of the well, able to look around at life and see opportunities and joy. Most of the time, she's part-

way down the well. Her view of life is restricted; she can see it's there, and she remembers what it's like to feel good, but she can't quite reach it.

Dysthymia is also very serious, but less dramatic. It's a depression that builds gradually, so gradually that you may not even recognize it. It means you've suffered from a depressed mood most of the time for a long period, with some of the same feelings of guilt, inadequacy, and lowered self-esteem as major depression. You also have fatigue and difficulty concentrating. You rarely feel good. You probably feel hopeless about feeling better, if you even think of feeling better. You may have some of the same physical symptoms as with major depression: pain, gastrointestinal symptoms, headache, disturbed appetite. Officially, the lifetime risk for dysthymia is 6 percent for either sex—but this is a very low estimate because to "officially" have dysthymia you have to have it for two years.

Here's an illustration from *Undoing Depression* again:

Chris fits the picture of dysthymia. A bright, intelligent woman with a forceful manner and a terrific sense of humor, she has been unhappy most of her life. Raised by an alcoholic mother and a critical father, as a child she tried to make them both happy—an impossible task. She rebelled in adolescence, getting into all kinds of trouble. Her first marriage was to a man who was alcoholic and abusive. Having found a lot of strength through Al-Anon, Chris is determined to get her life together. But she and her present husband can't communicate. Chris is very quick to anger and her husband withdraws. She struggles constantly with her sense of having a grievance against life—she knows that this, and her angry expression, drives people away, but she can't control herself.

Chris speaks of her depression as a big soft comforter. It's not really comforting, but it's safe and familiar. Sometimes she feels as if she's entitled to be depressed, to quit struggling, to snuggle down and watch old movies and feel sorry for herself.

Bipolar disorder (manic depression) yields extremes. People with bipolar disorder have episodes of major depression that are interspersed with periods of mania. A manic episode is a period of abnormally elevated mood—feeling grandiose, better than good (sometimes accompanied by irritability). During these periods you typically need less sleep (or can't sleep), have racing thoughts, take chances you wouldn't normally take, start projects you can't finish, spend money you don't have. But you also have times when you feel lower than low. Bipolar disorder typically begins in the early twenties, and the lifetime risk is about 1 percent.

One last illustration:

Walt has bipolar disorder. A big man, a truck driver, who seems pleasant and good-natured in his normal state, Walt has had trouble holding down a job for the past few years because of his erratic behavior. Sometimes he becomes sexually obsessed. He can't get sex off his mind. If an attractive woman is anywhere near, he can't concentrate on anything but his sexual fantasies. Sometimes he loses touch with reality enough to start believing that she returns his fantasies. When he's in this state, he'll spend money he doesn't have on prostitutes, on gambling junkets, on anything to impress women. He believes he's attractive, powerful, and charmed, and he feels he can do no wrong. Nothing bothers him. He can stay up for days, talking nonstop.

But at other times, Walt is severely depressed. He doesn't believe he's capable of anything. He hardly has the energy to get out of bed. He tries to go to work, but his lack of confidence makes his employers distrust him. He develops obsessive anxiety symptoms, such as going back into the house ten times to make sure the coffeepot is unplugged. He's constantly apologizing for himself.

Though officially bipolar disorder is quite rare, there are many people with major depression or dysthymia who sometimes have *hypomanic* episodes (*hypo* meaning less than), when they feel very good, have a lot of energy, may be very creative, and may be more reckless than usual. Sometimes when these people are medicated with the newer antidepressants they will experience a full-blown manic attack, a good reason to be careful about prescribing these things. I knew a man in his fifties whose daughter was in the hospital for bipolar disorder. We gave him Paxil to help with his depression. When he next had a meeting at the hospital for family members of patients, he took over the meeting, telling the psychiatrists exactly what was wrong with their program! He was very embarrassed afterward and we discontinued Paxil right away. The episode got me to realize that he often lived in a somewhat grandiose fantasy world, something that took on new meaning in light of his manic episode.

As this incident suggests, we still have a lot to learn about the chemistry of bipolar disorder. It's being diagnosed much more frequently now (because the drug companies are promoting use of their new mood stabilizers: Depakote, Lamictal, Topomax, Tegretol, Neurontin), especially in young people. There is reason to believe that bipolar is linked, or confused, with ADHD. The old drug of choice, lithium, is still often the most effective, though it has dangerous side effects. I've seen some of these drugs be very effective with some people, and have no effect on others. If you have bipolar disorder, you need to be working with a good psychiatrist who is interested in the condition and keeps up with the latest research. But since bipolar disorder probably is mediated by different neurochemical pathways than ordinary depression, pathways which we don't understand yet, I'm going to leave it here and get back to major depression and dysthymia—which are really the same animal in different disguises.

There's a lot of evidence to support this assertion. A twelve-year follow-up of 431 patients who had sought treatment for a major depressive episode found that although they remained in major depression about 15 percent of the time, still only 41 percent of their time was spent symptom-free. The rest of the time was spent in states comparable to dysthymia. This is despite the fact that patients were being treated with medication or psychotherapy in 62 percent of the weeks. Remaining in low-grade depression was a powerful predictor of relapse into major depression, suggesting that simply no longer meeting all the criteria for major depression is a very poor definition of recovery—but that's the one that's been used in all the drug trials that the manufacturers have sponsored. Most honest researchers and clinicians recognize now that dysthymia is what depressed people have when they aren't experiencing major depression, and that major depression is a stress-induced exacerbation of dysthymia.

We've talked before about how depression and anxiety are so closely interrelated; most patients have a combination of symptoms that could be considered either anxiety or depression, depending on rather small changes in emphasis. Major studies have found that anxiety and depression are likely to be found together at rates from 51 to 68 percent of the time. Medicine and psychiatry are increasingly agreeing that the two conditions are, if not the same, at least siblings. To me, it makes most sense to believe that people suffer from a general distress syndrome that causes symptoms we classify as either anxiety or depression, and that this syndrome is a result of genetic vulnerability, historical vulnerability, and current stress. It may be that anxiety is the initial response to too much stress—our panicky attempts to escape an inescapable situation—while depression represents the damage done to the nervous system, and the mind, when the stress goes on too long.

There is evidence to suggest that depression is on the increase, perhaps linked with globalization. In developing countries, young people have higher rates of depression than older folks. When we lived in small communities, each of us had the chance to be the best at something. With television, we're all exposed to people who are absolutely the best in the world. We feel envious. Perhaps envy served an evolutionary purpose, to keep us practicing and competing. But with television, we may conclude that there is no point in trying; we feel envious but hopeless, a sure recipe for depression.

It's reasonable to speculate that the reason depression exists is that it is an adaptive response, hard-wired into us because it has survival value. We've already talked about how dogs and other animals develop something that looks very much like depression in the learned helplessness situation. Human infants behave in a depressed fashion when their cries go unheeded too long. Getting depressed—which means to cease activity, become lethargic, and conserve energy—may be adaptive for the species if it gets us to retreat in the face of danger or overwhelming obstacles, or cease misguided efforts to get what we want if it's just not available, or step back from situations that just might work out if we leave them alone.

This suggests why I think depression is on the increase, especially in market economies. The Perpetual Stress Response has us full of the fight-or-flight hormones, which we experience in our minds as a vague fear or irritability that we can't shake. We do what seems to be expected of us—work hard, spend all our money on consumer goods, go into debt, leave our families and friendships behind to pursue careers, rely on alcohol and prescription drugs to make us happy, form intimate relationships that always seem to be disappointing, don't do anything to build a sense of meaning or purpose into our lives—and we still feel the same anxiety. The stress continues to burn out our nervous systems, and we feel unable to do anything that will reliably make us feel better. We conclude that we are helpless, and we stop trying so hard. But we take on a depressed identity, blaming ourselves for the situation; for many, the self-blame becomes so intense that we become suicidal. For others, it stops at losing confidence, losing initiative, losing hope.

What Depression Does to You

Depression results in damage to your body, your brain, your mind, and your world.

In the body, people with depression have elevated levels of cortisol and adrenaline, the stress hormones that wear out so many body and brain systems. In a four-year study of nursing home residents, those who were assessed as most depressed at the outset had the greatest impairment of the immune response as time went on. Depressive symptoms appear to be a significant risk factor for heart attack. Depression shortens the life span, even if the sufferer doesn't commit suicide, and increases the risk of other medical problems. Depression is significantly associated with higher death rates following heart attack, for both sexes, controlling for all other health and social variables. Depression is also associated with increased mortality for the general hospital population, across all diagnostic groups, not only cardiac cases. Patients with depression visit their MDs more frequently, are operated on more frequently, and have more nonpsychiatric emergency room visits than the general population. Depression is highly intertwined with nonspecific illness: a survey of almost twenty thousand Europeans found that 17 percent had chronic pain and 4 percent had major depression; but of those with depression, 40 percent also had chronic pain. Chronic pain, gastrointestinal problems, migraine, menstrual discomfort and dysphoria, weight control issues—all increase greatly the suffering of depression. They also compound the effects of the disease, further restricting activity, nutrition, and self-care, and reinforcing the depressive's idea of himself as out of control, bad, or weak.

In the brain, after enough depression the neurochemistry of the brain no longer repairs itself when good things happen to us. We lose the ability to produce dopamine, the chief neurotransmitter in the pleasure circuitry of the brain. The receptor sites for endorphins get "pruned." The damage to the hippocampus caused by prolonged stress probably accounts for the difficulty concentrating, learning, and remembering that is frequently seen with depression.

There is reliable evidence that long-term depression is associated with an overall decrease in size of the hippocampus by 10 to 20 percent. In laboratory animals, treatment with antidepressants has been shown to help the hippocampus regain its ability to generate new nerve cells. A recent study showed that treatment with either Paxil or cognitive-behavioral therapy results in improved blood flow to the hippocampus, perhaps leading to repair. But offsetting the good news is the suggestion that repeated episodes of depression result in shrinkage of the brain overall. There is evidence that, indeed, depression results in specific changes in brain activity that remain as a vulnerability when sad or stressful events occur to patients who have recovered.

Here's the current thinking about how depression gets into our cells (it will help if you look back at my anxiety flowchart, Figure 12): When we are stressed, the hypothalamus secretes an information substance called, confusingly enough by scientists, either CRF or CRH (for corticol-releasing factor or corticotropine-releasing hormone). CRF has the effect of stimulating the pituitary to secrete ACTH, another information substance that travels to the adrenal glands, causing them to secrete cortisol and adrenaline—the hormone of the fight-or-flight response—and steroids that help the body heal from physical injury. When the stress is temporary and the system is functioning well, there is a feedback loop in the hippocampus (that *slow down* circuit) that shuts off continued production of CRF. But with too much stress, the hippocampus is damaged, cell death occurs, and the feedback loop stops working. In depression the body keeps pumping out adrenaline, cortisol, and steroids. Autopsies of people who die from suicide almost always show a tenfold increase in the level of CRF in the bloodstream, compared to people who die from natural causes. Cortisol can be found to be elevated in the saliva of people with depression. This overproduction of CRF and other hormones eventually interferes with the ability of the body to produce and circulate the information substances that facilitate changes in behavior—so we get the impaired concentration, distorted perception, inadequate social response, flattened emotional expression, constant pessimism, inability to see alternatives, and other symptoms of depression. And we lose the ability to feel good.

One way the feedback loop gets disrupted is that, in infants and children who are under severe stress, the neuroreceptors for CRF diminish in size and number. This doesn't only happen in the brain, but throughout the body. It's the system's way of trying to adapt to too much CRF. But the hypothalamus just pumps out more CRF in an effort to compensate for the diminished response. It makes sense to believe that the same cycle develops for adults who are under constant stress. Our brains and bodies are doing what they should do in response to external danger, but since it is a danger that never seems to go away they are really only increasing the stress we feel, putting more and more adrenaline and steroids into our systems. We are like the impala chained to the ground, with the cheetah always poised to strike. This may explain why conventional treatments result in incomplete recovery from depression, why people relapse when they try to stop their medications. In order for true recovery to take place, change has to happen way down at the cellular level. That may demand removing sources of external stress and a lot of intensive practice to rewire the CRF feedback loop.

In the mind, depression causes changes in one's self-image and assumptive world that medications are powerless to overcome. The change can be so slow and gradual that the individual never notices how his life has been diminished; or so sudden and dramatic, like a nervous breakdown, that it seems to result in a permanent loss of self-confidence. Perhaps most important, we lose the capacity to feel good; depression causes endorphin receptors in the brain to shut down. With depression, we become hopeless of ever recovering, and we believe that we're helpless to do anything about it. There are well-documented changes in thinking that occur with depression: we focus on ourselves, we notice bad things more than good things. We believe that bad things are permanent, pervasive in their impact, and our own fault, while we believe that good things are temporary, limited in their impact, and just the result of chance. We try to control everything, and we feel that if any little thing goes wrong, it's a major disaster. Our minds become full of "automatic negative thoughts" which we seem powerless to control: *I can't do anything right. No one loves me. I'm worthless. What a gloomy day, I might as well stay in.* We rely on defenses like displacement and repression, so we gradually stop feeling anything at all. We're frozen, almost dead inside.

These changes also affect *your world.* People will start to avoid you. Your performance at work will suffer. Your loved ones will become frustrated and withdraw from you. If you are a parent, there's a high risk your illness will deeply affect your children. Depression will affect the course of your life: In one study, it was found that men with early-onset (before age twenty-two) major depression were only half as likely to marry and form intimate relationships as men with late-onset (or no) depression. Women with early-onset depression were only half as likely to obtain a college degree as their female counterparts, and their future annual earnings could be expected to be 12 to 18 percent lower. Children with depression have a hard time learning and may suffer real educational deficits that will have lasting effects. They also suffer socially, becoming the target for bullying, isolated from friends. Damage to their self-esteem can last a lifetime.

If you get the theme of the vicious circle again, you're absolutely right. Your depressed behavior results in changes in the real world, which just reinforce all your depressed attitudes about yourself.

Treatment for Depression

"The news that depression is a chemical or biological problem is a public relations stunt," says Andrew Solomon. He's absolutely right. The pharmaceutical industry has sold us its products with the implicit promise of a quick and easy fix. *There's nothing wrong with you but a chemical imbalance, just a little something our pill can cure. You don't have to change a thing about yourself, the pill does it for you.* It's true there is a "chemical imbalance," but that's the result of stress. Medications can help with the chemical imbalance—though no one knows exactly how they do—but if you don't do something about the stress you can't expect a real recovery.

Antidepressants have been vastly oversold, sometimes by extremely aggressive and deceptive marketing techniques. We now recognize that as many as 50 percent of drug-industry sponsored studies are never published. This means that all their efficacy claims are biased, since they don't report negative results. A recent review comparing drug industry–sponsored research to independent research has shown that industry–sponsorship creates a significant bias among the researchers—and almost all research on antidepressants is industry-sponsored. Another recent review created a firestorm of controversy within the professional community by going to the FDA armed with the Freedom of Information Act and finding out that, in all the research the drug companies had submitted to the FDA to get licensed to manufacture the new antidepressants, their drugs were only slightly more effective than placebo—but the FDA never pointed this out to the public. And the drug companies, when they published their research, did a great job of sweeping the placebo effect under the rug. The consensus now is that the newer antidepressants are no more effective than the older drugs, the tricyclics like Elavil and Tofranil, which are available generically.

The newer antidepressants—the SSRIs like Prozac, Zoloft, and Celexa and the SNRIs like Effexor and Cymbalta—are generally considered safer. They have the advantage over the older tricyclics of not being fatal if taken in overdose. Their side effects are more tolerable for most people, except for the sexual dysfunction, which can be a real problem. However, some people experience severe withdrawal reactions, including extreme anxiety, skin crawling, confusion, gastrointestinal distress, insomnia, and agitation. For some individuals (see the discussion of Jane Jones that follows) these symptoms are excruciating. The best advice is to discontinue any of these medications slowly and under a physician's care. Further, concerns have again surfaced about the safety and effectiveness of these medications with children; at this point, it's best to avoid treating children and younger adolescents with the newer antidepressants, unless strong precautions are taken to monitor suicidal and other violent behavior.

The outlook for complete recovery using the treatment methods that have been researched and demonstrated to be "effective" is bleak—because they measure recovery only at the end of the three-month treatment period—but "recovery" just means no longer meeting all the criteria for major depression, which usually means you're still pretty miserable. In the studies that follow people beyond their three-month treatment period, most patients relapse. That's why treatment has to go beyond the standard paradigm, be longer, more intensive, use medications as long as necessary, and include a strong component of education, self-help, and aftercare. In one study which followed people over five years, only half of patients with dysthymia reached full recovery, and of those half relapsed. Many developed major depression. It's now generally recognized that if you have one episode of major depression, your odds of having another are 50 percent; if you have three episodes, your odds of having more are 90 percent. But if you stay in psychotherapy, take a maintenance dose of medication, and really work on your own recovery, you can beat these odds.

Nontraditional treatments may be as good as medication. Exercise, in particular, may be highly effective. Several studies of older adults have found that brisk exercise three times a week was at least as effective as Zoloft in the short term, and that adults who continued their exercise program had a significantly greater chance of avoiding future depressive episodes. The problem, of course, is that if you're really depressed, it's very hard to overcome the inertia to start exercising. Social pressure—making a commitment to go to the gym with a friend, or joining an exercise class—may help overcome that inertia. In one study, couples therapy was more effective than medication over a two-year period, and it also reduced overall health-care costs. This study was conducted in Great Britain; unfortunately, in America, drug money funds research—and has even tainted the National Institutes of Health—so you don't see too many articles about the effects of exercise or couples therapy.

But despite all my caveats, *I urge my depressed patients to use medication.* Even though it's shamelessly oversold, there's truth in the fact that it really can help. I know people whose lives have been saved by it. A few lucky others have, within a few weeks, seen years of seemingly intractable suffering just clear up and blow away. Many find that medication gives them the energy and mindset, and a little hope, to really begin a program of recovery. Some find that their improved attitude is noticed and appreciated by those around them, and they begin an adaptive spiral (the opposite of a vicious circle) in which their improved social relations start to restore their self-esteem and ability to enjoy life.

So take your medicine. But do it with the guidance of a good psychotherapist, and a psychiatrist if your condition is in any way complex.

The ideal therapist for depression should be:

- Knowledgeable enough about cognitive-behavioral therapy to be able to use its strengths to help you, but not dogmatic about believing it's the only way to go.
- Interested and knowledgeable about the use of medication for depression. He should have a psychiatrist or two he works with and can refer to, and be willing to work with your general practitioner around medications if you choose to go that route.
- Familiar with Mindfulness-Based Cognitive Therapy for depression, and recognize mindfulness as a necessary component of full recovery.
- Able to create a spark when things get bogged down in sessions. Your therapist should make you feel that something important, something with *feelings,* is going on, even if you don't understand it right away. And he should get you thinking differently, seeing things differently.
- A person you can like, someone you experience as warm, empathic, and interested; and who gives you a sense of confidence that you're in good hands. He should be reliable, doing what he says he'll do.
- Realistic about the world. Depression is an adaptive response to living conditions that have strained us past the breaking point. Recovery is likely to involve making some significant changes in your stress load, and in how you handle it.
- Open to the idea that psychotherapy isn't the only way to get better. He should encourage you to make changes in how you deal with the outside world, for example through exercise, assertiveness, or questioning your values and assumptions.
- Available to your family to answer questions, if you wish.

Jane Jones: Coming to Terms

Jane's conflict about treatment was apparent from the first moment—she came in crying, overcome with fear and hopelessness, but at the same time angry, frustrated that she's no better than she is, here at yet another therapist's office for yet another introductory session. "I know intellectually that I'm intelligent and capable but I can't ful-

fill my potential. I've never found myself fully engaged in anything, can't think of any-thing that's turned out like I expected." Jane had been trying to make it as a freelancer in her field, had had a few successes but more rejections, and felt like she was coming to the end of her rope. She was sick of the politics of organizations, and tired of pushing herself so hard to get work, tired of starting over so many times. She was sick of her boyfriend, a ne'er-do-well who she'd been involved with for nine years despite her fit-ful efforts to break it off. She was sick of her apartment, of shelves she meant to hang one day still sitting in the corner two years later. She was even sick of her dog, an ag-gressive mutt that would attack other dogs in the crowded New York dog walks. As she described her other symptoms, I had no doubt that major depression was the correct di-agnosis. But I also had the impression of a bright, insightful, and ambitious young woman who was desperately trying to keep intact what remained of her idealism about the world, her belief that understanding leads to freedom. She had sought me out, an "expert" on depression, because she very much feared that she was sinking into a cyn-icism and powerlessness that she might never escape; at the same time she asked me plaintively for some simple guidance in making everyday decisions.

Jane made it clear that medication was a source of powerful conflict with her. She had tried psychotherapy right after college but held off on trying antidepressants until her late twenties, and reported unsatisfactory results and severe side effects with all. She was back on Zoloft now, even though it wiped out her sex drive. Just before leaving her previous therapist, she'd tried to switch from Zoloft to Wellbutrin, but reported a severe depression, wanting to die, having no energy for even the most basic tasks. She quit therapy and went back on Zoloft, reluctantly. Now she was functional again, but still in deep depression, angry at feeling she was stuck on a pill that helped her only a little, and at great cost.

For patients in as much distress as Jane, so close to the edge of not functioning at all, I advocate strongly for medication. I was glad she was taking Zoloft. As she told me of all her negative experiences with meds, I was inwardly skeptical, and I wondered about the diagnostic implications. Was Jane a hysteric, drawing attention to herself through her exaggerated symptoms? An obsessive, worried that the meds were upset-ting her delicate balance of control? A trauma victim, hypersensitive to the least intru-sion on her safety? And, I thought most likely, was I hearing in the first session the script of this therapy to come? Would I end up another disappointment for Jane, an-other in a long line of caregivers and authorities who had failed her?

That theme—falseness, unreliability, an attractive front masking inadequacy—resounded through Jane's history. Her parents had separated ten years earlier—coincident with Jane's first meltdown—when it came out that her father had been cheating for years; but they didn't divorce, maintaining a confusing façade of a commitment. Jane was furious with her mother for still being emotionally dependent on her father, for being unable to set limits with him. Her father was emotionally intrusive—insisting that both Jane's talents and her depression were legacies from him. He would provide support, sympathy, and encouragement for Jane, then abruptly turn on her, accuse her of being a weak, self-centered disappointment. Jane was raised to believe she could accomplish great things—and she often did, excellent grades and SATs, an Ivy League college—but she always felt there was too much pressure and too little support. The pressure was subtle, for the most part, and self-inflicted; Jane feared that if she failed, there was nothing to fall back on. At the same time, Jane made it worse for herself by being drawn to lost causes. The Adult Children of Alcoholics literature refers to "chemistry" to explain why women keep getting involved with abusive men, why men keep falling for abandoning women. Jane had this chemistry not only for men, but for causes. She would take up the banner for anyone who was being treated unjustly. Because of her good sense and high IQ, she was never fooled (except by men)—these were genuine social problems. But the pattern was inevitable, that Jane would lose herself in these battles only to wake up one day and find that no one cared as much as she; and that in the process she had neglected to take good care of herself. For the most part Jane did not create imaginary cheetahs; her problem was that she felt she was facing them with only the flimsy shield and fragile sword that were the best her parents—and the world so far—had to give her.

For a while therapy provided for Jane a strong, caring, and reliable other who could accept her fears and remind her to be selfish at times. We got her extricated from her boyfriend—a difficult task but one that Jane welcomed—and on the road to a new career in medicine. But after she was accepted to medical school she decided, reasonably enough, to go off her Zoloft. She had a **terrible** *withdrawal reaction, which I did not take seriously enough at first. She was beside herself with agitation, convinced she was losing her mind, unable to think; more deeply depressed than she had ever felt, absolutely hopeless. She was convinced this was a withdrawal reaction but even so the extremity of it hit her very hard. She was furious with me and with medicine, but she toughed it out over a very difficult month or so and got off the medication. It helped to validate and reassure her that I did some research and found that her withdrawal reaction was not so unusual after all. We then had a calmer few weeks and were able to part as friends before she moved away for medical school. She planned to continue her therapy in her new city.*

When I wrote to Jane to explore whether she'd be interested in having her story told, I found out things didn't end as I thought. Her first semester went well for a while, but

the schedule, new town, and loneliness got her feeling pretty desperate. After the se-
mester break, fighting a severe sinus infection, she began to have bouts of despair like
those she had had when going off Zoloft. Her new therapist convinced her to see a psy-
chiatrist, who gave her a new medication, which she took reluctantly. But things went
from bad to worse. She withdrew from med school. They tried several other medications
and combinations of meds. She found a new therapist and stabilized somewhat, but re-
mained depressed. After another doctor put her on steroids to treat an unexplained
rash, she became acutely suicidal and checked herself into a hospital.
She wrote:

The hospital was something of a turning point. It really helped me come to grips
with my depression in a way that I had not before. I understood that I needed to
focus on it and live my life in a way that respected my emotional temperament.
Things have improved steadily since then. I am now back in school, part-time.
[The school] has been fantastic about accommodating my illness . . . I am much
happier, at ease, and really stimulated by my studies and the wonderful opportunities [the city] has to offer. I worked for a great professor over the summer . . .
we hit it off and I had the chance to really prove my abilities to myself.

I'm still on [the new medication], and I battle the fatigue side effects, but not
some of the less pleasant effects of Zoloft. I plan to stay on it indefinitely . . .
certainly until med school is behind me.

Jane appears here not as a cautionary tale about Zoloft (which worked for me for a
long time with no side effects to speak of, and no withdrawal problem), but as an ex-
ample of the intricacies of the assumptive world, the mind, and the body. Jane had
never had anyone to rely on. All her idols proved false in the end. Like her father, they
promised a lot, but at the expense of intruding on her independence. Other people she
needed to rely on had always been fooled by her competent façade—"you're fine, you
can take of yourself"—or simply not interested enough to look deeper. I suspected in
the first interview that our relationship would play out the same themes. Her perpetual
abandonment filled her with rage and despair. She felt the same way about medication:
nothing was truly reliable, nothing came without sacrificing her hard-won indepen-
dence, nothing could help her without making her pay too high a price. I don't mean
that she created or imagined her withdrawal problems. They were very real. So is irri-
table bowel syndrome and the joint pain of fibromyalgia. But they are the body speak-
ing for the mind, trying to communicate something that depression alone does not say,
something to do with her anger at false gods—and her guilt about that anger—which

results in more suffering for herself. It's another example of the strange ironies of our reactions to perpetual stress. Jane's good adjustment and optimism at this time are, it seems to me, the result of her decision to let herself be helped by medication and her therapist, and at the same time to be independent and self-reliant and treat her illness responsibly.

Post-Traumatic Stress Disorder (PTSD)

Post-traumatic stress disorder is increasingly recognized as a distinct reaction to traumatic stress, and also often as the cause of the other problems we're discussing in this chapter—anxiety, depression, personality disorders, and addiction. In addition, researchers are realizing that there are important differences between the PTSD of combat experience or rape or 9/11 or other single traumatic events, and the PTSD of people who have lived for years under constantly terrorizing conditions: child abuse, spousal battering, refugee camps. So we'll discuss the two separately.

But first we need to discuss the connection between stress and trauma, perpetual stress and chronic trauma. In an effort to make sure that everyone is talking about the same thing, the scientists who classify mental disorders have set a high hurdle—for an event to be sufficiently stressful to cause PTSD, it has to threaten death or serious injury to the patient or someone he loves. But still there are degrees of stress, and it is hard to compare across individuals. Obviously, I've been arguing that the influence of the Perpetual Stress Response is so pervasive and powerful that it approaches chronic trauma; at the very least, the stress response has us so wired up and on guard—full of the hormones and chemical messengers that are generated in the fight-or-flight response—that single traumatic events are likely to have more of an impact on us than if we were relaxed and content with ourselves.

The basic assumption of the PTSD response is *I'll hide from it*. This requires a little explanation. PTSD victims develop the ability to separate themselves from the initial trauma, and that adaptation is also applied later in response to all forms of stress. Through dissociation, denial, projection, and other defenses, the PTSD sufferer keeps the impact of the stress out of consciousness; however, as we've discussed, that doesn't mean that the stress doesn't continue to work on the mind, producing other disturbing symptoms, and particularly on the body. PTSD victims, and chronic stress victims, seem to wear out their bodies more quickly than the rest of us.

Acute PTSD

We've already discussed the identification of acute PTSD and its hallmark symptom, dissociation, in Chapter 3. Other symptoms describe the individual's response to the intrusive experiences of panic and memory recurring unpredictably, and these fall into three clusters. The *avoidance* cluster includes efforts to avoid reminders of the trauma, including memories, thoughts, and feelings, as well as symptoms of emotional numbing like withdrawal from relationships, restricted range of feelings, and loss of interest in activities that used to be pleasurable. The *intrusion* cluster includes nightmares, intrusive memories of the trauma, flashbacks, and intense psychological stress at reminders of the trauma. The *arousal* cluster includes difficulty sleeping, difficulty concentrating, irritability, hypervigilance, and an exaggerated startle response. Problems with controlling anger and with unrealistic guilt or self-blame frequently accompany PTSD, and depression is very common. "The chronic hyperarousal and intrusive symptoms of post-traumatic stress disorder fuse with the vegetative symptoms of depression, producing . . . the 'survivor triad' of insomnia, nightmares, and psychosomatic complaints," writes Judith Herman. Again, though, one of the greatest difficulties with PTSD is that the sufferer doesn't recognize it for what it is. Because the emotional impact of the trauma is separated from memories of it, she keeps reexperiencing the trauma in the form of nightmares, flashbacks, or pain; but *she thinks these symptoms are caused by present events.*

Confusingly, in times of perpetual stress, present events that seem to be within the boundaries of everyday experience are often enough to trigger old trauma. All our nervous systems are already full of adrenaline and cortisol, so we're all hypervigilant, we have trouble concentrating and focusing, and our immune systems are compromised. We're full of fear already. So the individual who has actually experienced a traumatic event is stuck in a culture that doesn't allow him to slow down, take it easy, go on a psychic retreat. Pat Barker's profound and powerful trilogy about British soldiers in World War I (which features historical characters like the poets Wilfred Owen and Siegfried Sassoon and the pioneering psychologist William Rivers) recovering from "shell shock" makes it clear that the opportunity to linger in a hospital in a country retreat was in itself restorative for many. Today's PTSD survivors don't have that luxury; they're right back in our already self-destructive culture, and their alarms are always ringing.

The U.S. Veterans' Administration sponsored a huge follow-up study of men and women who had served in the Vietnam theater. They found that 31 percent of men and 27 percent of women had experienced full-blown acute PTSD reactions in later life, and that a great many others experienced partial PTSD reactions—thus, more than half of the men and almost half of the women who served in Vietnam experienced stress reactions severe enough to interfere with their functioning and their ability to enjoy postwar life. There were significant other problems associated with PTSD: almost half of all veterans suffering from PTSD had served time in jail at least once; almost 40 percent of all serving veterans developed alcohol problems; there were also high rates of depression, anxiety disorders, eating and psychophysiological disorders, and borderline personality disorders. Findings like these have led some researchers to propose a major overhaul of diagnostic thinking about mental illness and stress reactions. Bremner, notably, refers to what he calls "trauma-spectrum disorders": PTSD, dissociative disorders, borderline personality, adjustment disorder—all sharing brain abnormalities caused by trauma. Other conditions like depression, anxiety, and substance abuse are certainly linked, although the trauma may not always be apparent.

In the U.S. general population, the lifetime prevalence of PTSD is estimated at 7.8 percent—10.4 percent for women, 5 percent for men. The traumatic events most often associated with PTSD in women are rape, sexual molestation, physical attack, being threatened with a weapon, and childhood physical abuse. Those most often associated with PTSD in men are rape, combat exposure, childhood neglect, and childhood physical abuse. No event invariably produced PTSD. However, almost all women have symptoms of PTSD immediately following sexual assault. More than 30 percent will continue to have symptoms during their lifetime. (This may be a huge problem, because between 10 and 15 percent of women are estimated to have an experience of date or spousal rape.) Similar rates of PTSD are seen among children who have been sexually abused and in adult women who were sexually abused as children. PTSD is about eight times more common than cancer or schizophrenia, twice as common in women than men.

Helplessness to change the outcome may make the difference between acute PTSD and normal stress reactions. Feeling powerless to change events, people try to change their emotional reactions instead—by dissociation, by turning to alcohol or drugs, by escaping into violence. Social support is also a factor. Survivors of Hurricane Hugo in the Carolinas in 1989 and Hurricane Andrew in Florida in 1992 were studied carefully to identify the variables that were linked to subsequent psychological distress. Interestingly, injury, perceived threat to life, financial loss, and loss of personal items were less related to distress than was the performance of the individual's social support system.

Acute PTSD victims lose the ability to experience emotions as signals. As we discussed in Chapter 4, the purpose of emotions is to focus our attention on the event that causes them, usually some change in our environment: is it a threat, or an opportunity for pleasure, or something new? In PTSD, the qualitative difference between emotions seems to disappear, and everything is evaluated as a threat. Thus, the response to anything new is the fight-or-flight reaction (flight often represented by dissociation).

Many studies have documented a significant increase in norepinephrine levels throughout the body in people with acute PTSD reactions, resulting in hypervigilance, an increased startle response, and flashbacks. Heroin, alcohol, and tranquilizers like Valium are effective soothers for these people because they decrease the level of norepinephrine in the brain. Bremner and others have shown that, while an increase in norepinephrine levels in normal people improves concentration, learning, memory, and decision making, in PTSD patients just the opposite happens. Under conditions of stress, these people become more impaired.

We've talked a lot about the effects of trauma on the brain and the mind. The effects of living with a condition like acute PTSD, though, are somewhat different from the effects of the trauma itself. You experience *yourself* as being out of control, perhaps a little dangerous. You don't understand where the nightmares, blackouts, and outbursts are coming from, so you may fear you're going crazy or that something is physically wrong with your brain (it is, but it's not like a tumor or a stroke; it's microscopic, and it's reversible). You feel separated from your own past, and you're unable to develop that coherent narrative that is so important for a sense of stability and meaning. You may rely more and more on dissociation as a defense, which makes you dreamy, spacey; it's hard to concentrate or focus or learn. You also are likely to be highly suspicious of others, guarded and untrusting; and of course in a self-fulfilling prophecy you will keep finding that others fail the tests you set up for them. Your assumptive world becomes one of vigilance, mistrust, and fear.

Recovery from acute PTSD requires that patients develop the tools to reexperience the feelings associated with the trauma without feeling again that their very lives are in danger. This is a tall order, considering that most patients first have to understand the nature of PTSD, then stop trying to avoid an experience that has been absolutely terrifying to them. It requires a great deal of trust in the therapist. Reexperiencing the trauma also means that talk is not enough; insight only goes so far. The traumatic response has been highly conditioned, and there must be many extinction trials—reliving the event without feeling the panic—for a conditioned response to disappear. To relive the event without feeling the panic means that the patient must feel all his emotions and bodily states, with the confidence somehow that he and the therapist together will not let it get out of hand. Reexperiencing emotions and bodily states associated with trauma is a painful and difficult process, perhaps lasting many months. At first remembering floods the person with cortisol and adrenaline all over again; only with greater relaxation of the fear response will the hippocampus be able to consolidate emotional and historical memories, and use the higher functioning centers of the brain to consolidate the memory as a story expressed in words that captures the essence of the experience. The person can begin to remember rather than relive the experiences.

In a review of the cognitive-behavioral efficacy research, E. A. Meadows and E. B. Foa concluded that "prolonged exposure" (PE) therapy is the most efficacious treatment method for acute PTSD. Cognitive therapy techniques, relaxation training, and other methods can be used to help the patient in PE tolerate the experience. PE is, as the name implies, simply prolonged exposure to the feared stimulus, either in imagination or in reality. But many PTSD victims have developed such ingrained adaptations to their fears that this approach is not possible, and treatment consists of replacing unhealthy adaptations (such as drug abuse) with healthier ones (such as relaxation training). In other words, what helps an individual recover from a traumatic fear is simply exposure to the same situation, with the fear response inhibited through gradually increasing exposure or through cognitive restructuring techniques. It's learning the extinction response again, the same as the recommended treatment for anxiety.

This is the orthodox opinion about treating PTSD. It may be sufficient for acute PTSD, but not enough for chronic trauma syndrome. Bessel van der Kolk, one of the true leaders in the field, has alienated the orthodox by embracing unconventional therapies like EMDR[2] and various techniques that address the body more than the mind. I have to agree that talk therapy, or even PE, is often insufficient. Talking about your trauma and how helpless you feel isn't going to make you feel less helpless; the only thing that will is to do things that make you feel powerful. That includes facing your fears, but it needn't be by prolonged exposure. Good talk therapy gets the emotions going, including fear, in an atmosphere that feels safe and nonthreatening. But bodywork and EMDR often get to the feelings in a surprisingly direct and vivid way.

Much of the psychological damage of trauma comes not from the trauma itself but from the victim's efforts to avoid feelings associated with the trauma. These efforts are usually self-destructive strategies such as dissociation, withdrawal, and substance abuse. They are also doomed to fail because of the theory of ironic processes of mental control; trying not to think about a white bear dooms us to think of a white bear. And in the process we feel more out of control, ineffective, guilty, and ashamed. Acceptance of the trauma and the associated feelings is an inevitable by-product of exposure training. Acceptance means giving up efforts to control when it is evident that those efforts are doomed to fail, and a consequent willingness to accept things as they are, including one's own distressing emotions and experience.

Chronic Trauma Syndrome

So acute PTSD is pretty bad. Chronic trauma syndrome, Judith Herman's term for the effects of living for extended periods of time in conditions that create terror, is even worse, because it takes all the symptoms of acute PTSD and multiplies them. It gets so far into your bones and your brain that you are not merely scarred, but stunted and deformed in ways that seem so much a part of you that you can't be aware. And, in my experience, it's very, very common.[3]

---

2 EMDR (eye movement desensitization and reprocessing) is a controversial method developed by Francine Shapiro (Shapiro, 1989). It has the patient verbalizing traumatic memories at the same time as he watches the therapist's finger moving quickly back and forth. It seems too crazy to work, and no one has a good explanation for why it might work, but people report that it works. It may gain its effectiveness by getting the two halves of the brain—specifically, the two halves of the orbitofrontal cortex—to work together while processing emotional memories.

3 In what follows I will be talking about childhood abuse and neglect, because that's really all I've had experience with. But my reading tells me that chronic trauma syndrome also applies to, for in-

The incidence of battering by an intimate partner may range from 25 to 50 percent of women. In the ACE study of seventeen thousand largely white, middle-class people, 22 percent reported childhood sexual abuse. More than a quarter reported parental substance abuse, a problem that suggests neglect. In my experience with all my patients over the years, most have had experiences of being abused or neglected as children. It's not usually the horror stories of beatings or incest, although those are frequent enough. Much more often, it's emotional abuse: one or both parents seem to consistently undermine the child by criticizing harshly or cruelly, name-calling, emotionally battering the child when he expresses needs or wishes that are upsetting to the parents, having arbitrary rules for conduct, yelling at the child just because the parent is in a bad mood (or intoxicated, or hung over), withdrawing attention or affection because the child has displeased the parent. Or it's emotional neglect: preferring one sibling over another; not showing interest in the child's schoolwork or play; paying more attention to the television or the pursuit of a second spouse than to the child; not taking the child's normal fears and upsets seriously; being consistently unavailable when the child needs the parent.[4] Or it's not recognizing abuse when it happens: when a child has been sexually abused by an uncle or a neighbor, there are powerful forces compelling the child not to tell. But there are bound to be changes in the child's behavior, which alert parents can pick up on. One particular form of neglect is not protecting the child from abuse by the other spouse; the child feels betrayed by both. The moment that one partner abuses a child, and the other partner doesn't do anything, that child becomes an orphan. There is no one to count on.

Patterns like these are very common, and very tragic. Also very tragic is that these patterns are usually the result of parental stress, overwork, depression, anxiety problems, or substance abuse problems. No one *wants* to abuse their child.

---

stance, women who've been in abusive or exploitative relationships for long periods; runaways and prostitutes; war and disaster refugees and concentration camp survivors; and doubtless many others.

4 Parents who emotionally abuse or neglect their children all believe they love their children; and though many feel momentary remorse for egregious incidents, they also believe they are good parents. They may be better parents than their parents were, but they are not good parents. We need to raise standards for parenting in this country. We need to educate people that humiliating or scaring your child is cruel; that being emotionally unavailable is heartless.

People express sympathy for me because my mother took her own life. It's true that that was a traumatic experience, and the preceding few years had been very difficult. But people don't understand that the first ten years or so of my life were really pretty good. My parents during that time seemed, to me at least, affectionate and nurturing. There was trouble brewing, but I was blissfully unaware of it.

Many of my patients had it much worse than me, but they don't realize it. The effects of growing up with parents, or even one parent, who is neglectful, or mean-spirited and cruel, or physically or sexually abusive, or unable or unwilling or uninterested in understanding the child's emotional needs, are much more devastating than my experience. Yet because people were raised this way and had no comparison, they often aren't aware of how deviant and damaging it is.

Childhood neglect may have the most pervasive effects on adult character. Treatment can help victims of sexual or physical abuse, if they had early experiences of being cared for. Some neglected children had no such experiences; there is nothing to build on. The same may be true for victims of emotional abuse, if it was a consistent pattern—the child's very self has been undermined by the person who should be constructing it.

Abuse victims, terror victims, may internalize their tormentor's aggression and turn it against themselves. Children typically blame themselves for parental abuse; they think they did something bad, and if they can just be better, Mommy or Daddy won't do it again. One of the reasons why child protection is a burnout job comes from the strain of watching child abuse victims cry remorsefully when taken away from an abusing parent, promising to be better. And of course these beliefs penetrate the child's psyche: they continue to believe they *are* bad. Sometimes this is the motive for prostitution or other acting out. Often the belief persists well into adulthood, developing into a criminal career or deep, impenetrable shame about the self.

Rates of suicide are much higher than normal among battered women, prisoners of war, and concentration camp survivors. Judith Herman writes, "Long after their liberation, people who have been subjected to coercive control bear the psychological scars of captivity. They suffer not only from a classic post-traumatic syndrome but also from profound alterations in their relationship with God, with other people, and with themselves."

People with chronic trauma syndrome come to avoid any emotional experience, because any emotion causes an acute stress reaction. One result is the flatness and joylessness of depression. Another, more subtle but more devastating result is paralysis of the will: people lose the capacity to experience motivation, to want something, to wish for something. Theresa, whom I've talked about before (see pages 176–177), had to confront this issue as well; see the continued discussion on the next page.

Treatment for Acute and Chronic Trauma

Judith Herman, perhaps the best authority on chronic trauma syndrome, notes that recovery can only take place in the context of a relationship. The patient's relationship with the world, with everyone, has been poisoned, and only through nontoxic relationships can enough trust develop so that healing can begin. Therapy is just one of those relationships. I have known people who have been much more helped by a supportive spouse than by therapy; but such spouses are hard to find. Good therapy requires that the therapist abandon traditional neutrality and acknowledge that the patient has been wronged; "bearing witness," in Herman's phrase. It means leading the patient, who may deny or resist, into recognizing that a crime has been committed against her, and this may not be a comfortable stance for all therapists to take.

Treatment also requires extraordinary patience and sensitivity on the therapist's part. The patient will be hypervigilant for any little thing that can be interpreted as betrayal—a momentary expression of disinterest on the therapist's face; a defensive turning away from the horror of the trauma or the patient's in-the-moment pain, when the therapist is tired or just has had enough. At the same time, these micro-ruptures of the therapeutic alliance, which are inevitable, are the grist for the mill of reestablishing trust. Over time, the patient begins to learn to distinguish between merely human lapses and real trauma, and builds up a tolerance for human frailty which allows her to function in the world of relationships again. The therapist then can help the patient create a safe environment for herself, which is essential for recovery: learning to distinguish between PTSD fears and genuine fears; relearning how to trust her ability to tell the difference between dangerous people and safe people.

In the final stages of treatment the work is on reestablishing the patient's capacity for desire and initiative, qualities that have gone so far under wraps that they may feel as if they are lost forever. In a relationship in which you're terrorized, to acknowledge that you want something gives your tormentor a tremendous weapon to use against you. It will take time to feel safe enough to want something again.

Medication treatment for acute or chronic trauma reactions is much the same as treatment for anxiety, so I'll refer you to that section. There is the warning, however, that PTSD survivors are more vulnerable to the addiction problems of tranquilizers than other anxiety sufferers. The experience of calming and soothing that comes with the tranquilizer is *so* soothing and comforting to the PTSD survivor that it makes addiction understandable. The same effects come with opiate and other painkiller abuse, another particular vulnerability for PTSD survivors.

Antidepressants can be quite helpful with PTSD symptoms, but a common problem is that the person is so exquisitely sensitive to any change in his or her internal state that the side effects of antidepressants set off a trauma response. Whether to work to help the patient get through the first few weeks or give up and withdraw the medication is a delicate call, one that has to be addressed individually for each patient.

Theresa Revisited

We introduced Theresa in Chapter 5: a victim of years of childhood sexual abuse, she is a charming, talented woman who has largely recovered from the major symptoms of acute PTSD. But psychiatry distinguishes between positive symptoms (the presence of something abnormal, like hallucinations or compulsive rituals) and negative symptoms (the absence of something that should be there, like the ability to feel good in depression). It is naturally easier to recognize positive symptoms than negative. Theresa and I have only recently noticed what's missing from her life, though it's a pretty big thing: although she functions very well, she can't identify a single thing she wants. It follows then, that nothing makes her happy. *She spends three weeks in France, Christmas in Paris, touring the castles in the Loire, skiing in the French Alps—nothing. She floats through life doing her job, taking care of others, smiling at and charming everyone, and being an attractive adornment for her boyfriend. She fools everyone; it's only in therapy that she can say she feels completely empty inside. "I feel like the walking dead," she says, smiling her beautiful smile at me. "A zombie."*

In psychotherapy we talk about people's initiative; do they see themselves as controlling events in their lives, or as controlled by events? Do they feel an internal or external "locus of control"? Theresa's problem is more subtle than that. To a great extent she sees herself in charge of her life; she doesn't see herself as a passive victim of whatever life hands her. But she can't identify any desires, wants, or needs of her own, and therefore nothing touches her. This has its defensive aspects; as the Stoics taught, if you don't want anything, no one has power over you. No one can hurt you by taking away what you want. But I wonder if it's simply that Theresa has defensively repressed her own wants, or if the capacity to want has been completely expunged from her experience.

Theresa has noticed how her whole family is alexithymic—they don't talk about feelings, and they may not even feel them. At her grandmother's funeral—no tears, just awkwardness. After her mother finally told her brother Vincent that she knew he'd hurt Theresa and that he wasn't welcome in her home—when Theresa asked her mother how it felt, she said, "I should have done it a long time ago" and changed the subject. With this family background, and with fear driving out the ability to desire, Theresa has a long way to go to recapture her feelings.

Mindfulness is key. Like a chef developing her palate, Theresa will need to pay very deliberate attention to what she experiences now as perhaps only tiny perturbations in her emotional state. She needs to focus very closely on her internal experience, to watch herself like a hawk for indications of desire. I kind of like this a little; I'd like to do this again, maybe, someday; I don't like that so much. *She can practice Linehan's mindfulness skills:* observe, *pay attention without judging;* describe, *put feelings into words to help them become more real; and* participate, *be there in the moment with full attention. Eventually she'll develop normal awareness of her wishes and feelings, but even that won't be enough. She'll also need to learn to take herself seriously. She'll need to put her own desires on the same plane as others, not rationalize that it's easier to go along, that she doesn't really care anyway.*

It may seem ironic to use mindfulness to enhance desire, when most Buddhist practice (and much of this book) emphasizes freeing yourself from desire. But there are desires we need to experience: to express ourselves, to love, to create, to be fruitful. As it is now, these wishes are not part of Theresa's world.

Personality Disorders

These conditions are the bottom of the barrel of modern American psychiatry. New psychiatrists are being trained to think of personality disorders as "the patients you don't like, don't trust, don't want." Somehow there is always a moral sniff attached to these diagnoses, as if the patients *could* be better, but aren't trying. I half-joked in the introduction to this chapter that the worldview of the patient with a personality disorder is *It must be you. Whatever's going wrong in the world must be your fault, because it's certainly not mine.* This is a caricature, but there's truth in it, and that's what makes these patients so unpopular.

Nowhere else are the dangers of categorical thinking so salient as they are in considering these conditions. Any reasonable discussion of them has to consider the very real possibility that they don't exist at all, but are instead an iatrogenic myth, a series of responses generated by the way we treat these people. Another key issue is whether they are, as has often been assumed, some sort of twist in the character for which the adult sufferer is morally responsible (but not motivated to change, a particularly vicious diagnostic double whammy)—or whether they are natural and understandable outgrowths of PTSD resulting from especially traumatic experiences in childhood. And in my mind, at least, both borderline and narcissistic personalities appear to be largely responses to the changes in our social environment in the last century, the ends of continua of personality traits rather than distinct illnesses. Let's frame our discussion with these issues clearly in mind.

Personality disorders, by definition, are diagnosed as an enduring pattern of character traits that are clearly deviant from social norms. The assumption used to be—and still is, in the minds of many therapists—that personality disorders are differentiated from other emotional disorders by the observation that the individual does not feel symptoms; rather, his problems are manifested in his behavior. Except for the sociopathic personality, this is nonsense. Both borderline and narcissistic personalities are vulnerable to great pain, depression, despair, rage, and anxiety; it's an inevitable part of the condition.[5]

Let's begin our discussion on the premise that these are real conditions.

- *The borderline personality* is characterized by highly unstable interpersonal relationships, based on an extreme fear of and sensitivity to abandonment. Emotions are intense and extreme. Moods are intense and extreme. Self-image varies from extremes, depending largely on how secure one feels in a relationship. There is a lot of impulsivity, action taken with little thought for the consequences. There is a lot of self-destructive behavior: suicide attempts, substance abuse, eating disturbances.
- *The narcissistic personality* is really of two types. One is the grandiose person who acts as if everyone else is a lower form of life, who feels naturally

---

5 There are other personality disorders as well, notably the schizoid, the paranoid, the dependent, and the obsessive-compulsive. I'm not going to discuss those here because they seem to me to be extremes of continua of pathology that is both not well understood and not clearly stress-related.

entitled to special treatment, and who may descend into intense childlike rage if his wishes aren't met. The other is the extremely sensitive person who is shy, self-effacing, and depressed, but retains a fantasy world wherein his specialness is recognized, and who often seeks another person to attach himself to and idolize. Both usually lack empathy, the ability to understand others' needs and feelings. Both can treat people like objects, only good for what they can do for you.

- *The antisocial personality* (formerly sociopathic) is the guy who scares us all. These are people who do not feel much in the way of emotion whatsoever, and one effect of that is that they feel no empathy for others. They are quick to use violence, intimidation, or manipulation to get what they want. There is a reckless disregard for both the law and the truth.

Allan Schore's thinking is that both borderline and narcissistic personality disorders are manifestations of brain circuitry that failed to develop optimally during the first two years of life. The foundation of the borderline personality may be laid down at about five months, when most children "hatch"—that is, they begin to withdraw from their symbiotic bond with the primary caregiver and take greater interest in the world around them. This is a result of the maturation of the brain and central nervous system; children are learning to see, and are distracted from the mother. Mothers who are vulnerable or depressed may be hurt or confused by what they interpret as a rejection from the baby, and may in turn reject the child. When the baby is distressed, the mother is no longer able to provide the communion that enables the child to integrate self-regulation. When the baby is excited, the mother cannot provide the mirroring the child needs, the opiate receptors in the child's brain get pruned, and the child is no longer able to experience joy. Attachment researchers have found some links between adult borderline personality and ambivalent or avoidant attachment in infancy, which supports this line of thinking. Thus we have the borderline, who vacillates between uncontrollable distress and empty depression, who desperately seeks intimacy at the same time as intimacy stirs up fears of abandonment.

The narcissistic personality is more confusing, because of its two types. Both types are really all about controlling the opposite poles of shame and grandiosity, which are always threatening to flood the individual with extremely painful or dangerous feelings. In infancy and toddlerhood children are learning to deal with these feelings—children often feel, and should be allowed to feel, unique, powerful, superhuman, full of energy and life; but at the same time they also will feel vulnerable, puny, embarrassed, and ashamed. Again, in Schore's view, it is the relationship with the primary caregiver that helps the child learn to modulate such feelings so that they can be experienced but not overwhelm the self, to turn such feelings into useful and appropriate skills like creative energy or a wish to make amends when we've wronged someone. Mothers who are narcissistic themselves may provide only a contingent kind of mirroring of the child's feelings; may treat the child as a selfobject embodying their own immature wishes to be special, and hence encourage the child to continue in his grandiose status; or may turn away from the child when he's feeling grandiose, teach him that such feelings are not acceptable at all. Again, it is the orbitofrontal cortex that seems to be involved, not only in forming a stable self-concept, but in regulating intense emotional states. The mother's brain is a template for the child's brain to develop on.

The antisocial personality is perhaps the most tragic. People in an extreme state of addiction act like sociopaths, because they have reached the point where their drug means more to them than any human relationship. But the sociopath has more or less always been this way, and he usually gets there for good reason. There is mounting evidence that most violence-prone individuals have had intensely traumatic experiences as children and infants—psychological, physical, or sexual abuse—usually at the hands of trusted caregivers. The "disorganized" attachment style, in which infants seem to have no idea how to respond to the minor stress of the Strange Situation, has been found largely in two types of children. The first group are those who are currently living in situations of abuse or neglect; the second are those whose primary caregivers appear to be damaged by the effects of trauma (current or past) themselves. Children who were classified as disorganized, followed into adolescence, have been found to have high overall psychopathology, with apparent predilections for violence. It's not hard at all to understand how a child is traumatized, and the brain damaged, by abuse at the hands of trusted caregivers; when the person you look to for comfort when you're upset is also a threat, and may punish you for needing help, it's no wonder that the brain centers that are supposed to modulate fear and aggression are damaged. But these "second-generation" effects are more troubling—when the mother is herself so traumatized that she responds to the child's need for comfort with fear of her own, or with dissociative experiences like freezing or emotional withdrawal, the child is unable to use her as a template to develop mature ways of controlling fear and aggression.

PTSD and Personality Disorders

But Schore's viewpoint is incomplete. To his concerns about how the infant relates to the mother, we have to add the very real impact of later trauma on the child. Every one of my patients who could be considered borderline has a history of childhood sexual abuse, and I know that many therapists would confirm that experience. Every one of my patients who could be considered narcissistic had parents who were strange, bizarre, depressed or grandiose or intrusive. I've never treated a true antisocial personality, but the people I have treated who have committed antisocial acts were all the victims of physical and emotional cruelty at the hands of their parents. My patient who finally admitted to sexually abusing his two-year-old daughter was repeatedly forced, as a child, by his father to fight his brother, tied together at the wrists, until one of them could no longer go on. He told me this, then collapsed into frank psychosis, and has hopefully never been released from the psychiatric hospital. Where is a man like that to go for peace, if not into the reliable dullness of heavy psychiatric medications?

Clinical experience bears this out. Judith Herman reports that 81 percent of her borderline patients had histories of severe childhood trauma. Van der Kolk reports that only 13 percent of his borderline patients did *not* report childhood trauma; and of those, half had blocked out all childhood memories. If more traditional therapists missed the connection between borderline personality and sexual abuse, perhaps they didn't ask. Linehan reports a study of psychiatric inpatients with a history of sexual abuse: 44 percent had never talked to anyone about the experience before. We've just talked about the effects of trauma and terror on the mind and the brain—how much worse can it be than to come at the hands of those who should love and protect you? No wonder there is difficulty trusting, difficulty controlling feelings, unstable self-esteem.

Thus patients with borderline and antisocial personalities, and perhaps narcissistic, are also suffering from chronic trauma syndrome, with all its attendant disruption of the brain's emotional regulatory system, which in turn leads to difficulties in the body's stress response, including the immune and endocrine systems. They also can be expected to have the same kind of difficulty storing and consolidating memories because of damage to the hippocampus, and therefore to be unable to construct a coherent narrative about their experiences. Their memories will come in the form of reliving, rather than remembering.

But before we go on to talk about treatment for these conditions, let us consider carefully the possibility that they do not exist at all; or if they do exist, it is only as a result of the way our conventional mental health system treats and categorizes people. There is evidence to support this idea. Self psychologists long ago argued that if you treated borderline patients well enough, you couldn't distinguish them from narcissistic patients. And Heinz Kohut had already shown that narcissistic patients, previously thought untreatable, were in fact quite treatable if you just took their needs seriously (more on this to come). There is new research that shows that some borderlines, at least, recover naturally—something that is not supposed to happen at all—when their social environment changes, suggesting that their conditions may be much more a reaction to their living conditions than a permanent character trait. Borderlines may have come by their unsavory reputation largely because their doctors didn't *like* them (because they tend to be extraordinarily sensitive to the doctor's attitude toward them, making them demanding and difficult patients) and consequently didn't treat them well. Their reputation for manipulation, for twisting the truth, for threatening suicide, may have been a result of their frustration with getting what they needed from their doctor—respect, attention, and a real effort to help ease their distress.

There is a radical strain in psychoanalytic circles today, suggesting that there is no such thing as personality at all: that the individual doesn't exist except in a social context. It is like Heisenberg's uncertainty principle applied to humans. You can never tell exactly what or where a subatomic particle is, because the mere fact of observing it changes it. By extension, we can't presume to define a person as some sort of freestanding individual, because we always see him in a situation where he's reacting to his environment, including us. This movement has had the very healthy effect of getting therapists to pay more attention to the ways they influence, and are influenced by, their patients, and not to assume that the therapist is the unerring arbiter of truth. Even so, I can't give up the notion of personality; it's too convenient and useful a concept. These "personality disorders," it seems to me, *are* understandable reactions to the interaction of the patient with the world, and the therapist is one exemplar of the world. The patient's side of the interaction that causes the trouble is very easily understood in terms of the assumptive world the patient has constructed, and the way his brain responds to social stress and abandonment; both of which were formed in reaction to the parenting he received and the traumas he experienced as a child.

So I think it's most useful to treat these problems as "real" conditions, but I wish we could find other names for them. Abandonment-reaction disorder. Vulnerable-self disorder. Unsocialized disorder. In any case, how does one recover?

Treatment for Personality Disorders

Let me say at the outset that I don't how, or if, one recovers from full-blown antisocial personality disorder. We like to call these people psychopaths and lock them up. I do know that young people with antisocial tendencies can be helped if they are put in an environment where "normal" expectations apply: where good behavior is recognized and rewarded and bad behavior is punished in a consistent, fair, and reasonable way. That suggests to me that antisocial personality is a spectrum disorder, not an either-or disorder. In other words, you can be a little, or a lot, antisocial. So some must be treatable. James Gilligan, who has spent his professional life as a psychiatrist in the Massachusetts penal system, makes a strong case that the men he works with are at bottom deeply damaged by what's been done to them, usually the most horrific forms of cruelty to children. Their self-esteem is so fragile that they feel they have to be ready to kill if anyone shows disrespect. Their lives matter so little to them that they have no reason to hold back.

One requirement for successful treatment is that you have to *like* the patient, at least a little. Kohut understood his narcissistic patients' demands for his attention as the understandable reactions of frightened and insecure children who could trust no one, instead of as the obnoxious insistence of someone who believes he's special. They could then trust him, and he could help them. Marsha Linehan's Dialectical Behavior Therapy (DBT) for borderlines is full of her dedicated refusal to judge her patients. Instead she insists that the therapist, above all else, be prepared to *validate* the patient's experience, to see that the most bizarre behavior makes sense when viewed through the patient's eyes.

DBT often works, partly by the paradoxical strategy of radical acceptance we mentioned earlier: *You're perfect as you are, but you have to change.* All the patient's behavior, no matter how self-destructive or bizarre, is interpreted as something the patient has learned in an effort to solve problems in his life. The therapist and patient then collaborate in a behavior analysis to determine if the patient's efforts are successful in getting what he wants. The relationship is warm and supportive, but also very direct and irreverent. There is a radical nonjudgmental attitude; the emphasis is on doing what works, what is effective in achieving goals, rather than on what is right or wrong, acceptable or not acceptable. It is the Buddhists' "wise mind." Then there is an ongoing collaborative effort to help the patient learn new skills: emotion regulation, interpersonal effectiveness, distress tolerance, mindfulness, and self-management. (You will have seen Linehan's influence at work in some of the exercises in this book.) All the while there is explicit acknowledgment of the patient's real distress, and the shared goal of alleviating it as quickly as possible.

Medication for these conditions is roughly equivalent to medicating chronic trauma syndrome: tranquilizers can give some temporary relief from upset (but you have to watch their addictive powers); antidepressants are somewhat helpful with many people but you never know which, or why, so you may have to experiment a lot. Since borderline personality is so often confused with (or may be the same as, an idea we don't have the space to go into) bipolar disorder, mood stabilizers can also be helpful. Borderline is also confused with, or may be the same as, ADHD, but no one suggests stimulants for these patients; they're just too potentially upsetting to a chronically upset person.

If you think you might have a personality disorder and want to find a therapist, you really should shop around. You need someone who is experienced and knowledgeable about your condition, *and* you need someone you like and feel confidence in. If you're borderline, you probably shouldn't trust too much your first impressions, so this is doubly difficult. Please feel that you have a choice, and that you are not at the mercy of the first therapist you meet. See my advice for how to find someone at the end of this chapter.

Addiction

If you drink too much, or have any addiction from heroin to shopping to computer games, it's likely you started this activity to help with feelings of boredom, emptiness, or loneliness, but the act of indulging makes us feel ashamed and out of control. It doesn't solve but only adds to the problems that led us to our vice in the first place. If we don't know any way other than drinking—or whatever it is—to help us feel good, we're doomed.

Karen enjoyed her work as an RN for most of her career, but in the last few years she was increasingly unhappy with changes in the field—too many patients, too much paperwork, defensive medicine, never enough time for the direct patient care she loved. She started to dread going to work. When she injured herself helping a patient who fell, she took a long leave of absence. Her recovery was very difficult. Nothing seemed to help. She eventually was told she had fibromyalgia. She was unable to move without great difficulty, couldn't sleep because of the pain, and became depressed, hopeless, and angry. Her brother's death at this time made her more depressed. Periodically she would get sick of her situation and force herself to exercise in hopes of getting back on her feet, but she would always overdo it and end up in more discomfort. She became dependent on stronger and stronger medications to help her ease the pain and get some rest. She grew increasingly depressed, isolated, and eccentric; eventually her medical appointments became her only social contacts.

The conditions of our lives result in our bodies being overloaded with glucocorticoids and other substances that destroy the pleasure circuitry of the brain and put us constantly on high alert. Under those circumstances, it's not surprising that people turn to alcohol or drugs as a way of escape. These substances are attractive because they give us a reliable way to feel better quickly. Alcohol, in particular, is a very serviceable drug. With moderate use, alcohol can be counted on to loosen your inhibitions, make you feel better about yourself, and enjoy your current experience more. For a while, at least, and that's the problem; because after those initial pleasant effects wear off, alcohol will make you dull, sleepy, and irritable, and vastly impair your judgment and coordination. There's not a single drug of abuse that doesn't reach back and bite you like this in some way. Some people are able to use them carefully so that (from their perspective, at least) the benefits outweigh the damage done. But for many people, the drug's effects are so tempting, and its withdrawal so painful, that addiction is the result. The fact that, after millennia of experimentation and research, no one has ever found a drug that just makes you feel good without any ill effects is enough to make you believe in a divine plan. Because such a drug might mean the end of civilization. Who would strive if there was a pill to make you forget striving?

Let's look at hard, "physical" addictions (alcohol, drugs, and tobacco) before we go on to explore behavioral, or "soft," addictions. All addictive drugs (including alcohol and tobacco, prescription drugs like painkillers, tranquilizers, and amphetamines, and street drugs like cocaine, marijuana,[6] and Ecstasy) have a direct connection to the limbic system, causing the release of dopamine, a neurotransmitter associated with feelings of euphoria. They also have in common the fact that our brains and bodies habituate to them, so that it gradually takes more and more to get the same effect. The habituation response also means that we will go through a period of physiological withdrawal when we try to quit. In addition, regular use of any of these substances has negative consequences for the body. They are all toxins, poisons—if you ingest too much at any one time, you will die. Since they are toxic, regular use stresses the liver and other organ systems that help us filter poisons. Long-term use produces alterations in the brain that increase vulnerability to relapse and maintain craving even months or years after the last use. Nerve cells in the dopamine and opioid systems are damaged, and at this point we don't know if the damage can be reversed. Bottom line: Addiction changes the brain. The addict has a new definition of "normal," which is built around the effects of the drug.

There are complex nature/nurture questions about addictions, most of which we still can't answer. We know that there is a purely hereditary link for alcoholism among men, but we don't know much about the heritability of abuse for other drugs. Nurture certainly plays an important role. Remember Schore's conclusions from Chapter 3: difficulties in the child's relationship with the primary caregiver *in early childhood* result in lasting effects, including damage to the adult's ability to have a self-concept of confidence and stability, and damage to the adult's capacity for self-control. The ability of the brain to weave together emotional and historical memory into a coherent self is damaged, so we have an adult who never feels coherent, stable, "together." These effects result in an adult who is particularly vulnerable to drug abuse. One of the very first effects of using any intoxicant is a feeling of enhanced self-confidence. With that comes an altered perception of the self as cool, invulnerable, wise, and insightful. When you add reduced self-control to the mix, you have an individual who finds intoxicants especially pleasurable and doesn't have the internal mechanisms to resist their temptation. Alcoholics Anony-

---

6 I'm aware that some people think marijuana is not physically addictive. I don't know, so I'm going to duck the controversy. I certainly know that many people use marijuana like alcohol, infrequently enough that it seems to be a pretty harmless high. But I've known others who have been highly dependent on it, and in denial about their dependency, exactly like alcohol or any truly addictive drug.

mous is full of people who will tell you that they knew from their first drink that this was an experience they'd never felt before—because, I think, they had been operating with a damaged self that never had felt capable, stable, poised. They found a solution for the Perpetual Stress Response in the bottle.

That's the way it is with any drug of abuse. You develop a relationship with the drug. You fall in love with it, but then it becomes like a dysfunctional marriage; you love it, you hate it, it lets you down, it betrays you, but it still provides enough gratification to keep you in thrall. It soon becomes your primary relationship, and friends and family take a back seat. You may not notice this, or might not care. You develop a whole assumptive world built around the primary idea that your relationship with your drug has to be preserved at all costs. You use all the traditional defense mechanisms, especially rationalization and selective attention, plus the avoidance supplied by your drug, to not be aware of the effects your use of the drug is having on yourself and the people you care about. You alienate friends and family, but you don't care, because you're telling yourself you're fine as is. Their disagreements with you, in your eyes, are about anything other than your substance abuse. You lose your job, but that's because the boss is a jerk, not because you're so hung over your work performance is dismal.

This is why Alcoholics Anonymous (AA) works, while less radical methods don't; because it provides a completely new assumptive world. And that's what any means of recovery from any drug has to provide, because your character armor has been built on the foundation of your drug use, and you have to start from scratch. AA reparents people. It provides enough rules and structure and social life that you can "fake it till you make it": stay sober long enough just going through the motions, following the rules, until the rules—the Twelve Steps—get into your brain and become a part of you.

There is a large component of mindfulness in the Twelve Steps, and an oral tradition holds that Bill W., the movement's founder, had some exposure to Eastern philosophy. To admit you are powerless over your problem and turn it over to a higher power; to make a fearless moral inventory of yourself and make amends to those you've wronged; to continue to pray and meditate in search of a spiritual awakening. Most of all, to make a commitment to practice the steps every day for the rest of your life. Practicing these skills on a daily basis will force you to consider yourself as an object: to detach yourself somewhat; to experience your cravings as cravings that come and go, triggered by everyday experience or memories or associations, rather than imperatives that must be obeyed. The paradox of AA is that by "admitting you are powerless" over your disease, you gain power over it. It's a very Zen-like stance. You give up the delusion most of us share, that you can control all of your life that you want to, and you focus on controlling this one small part of yourself, your substance use, simply making up your mind that you're not going to drink today. In doing that, the mindless struggle to control everything drops away, and you realize that getting by one day at a time is plenty.

The AA approach has been changing with the times. I'm very glad to see that most AA chapters recognize that depression is a serious problem among alcoholics and that antidepressants are not addictive drugs, while they rightly remain very skeptical about use of tranquilizers, painkillers, muscle relaxants, sleeping pills, and other potential drugs of abuse. As the Twelve-Step program has been applied to other addictions, the doctrine of total abstinence has had to be modified accordingly. Overeaters Anonymous can't tell people to avoid food altogether, but I have one patient who's been helped enormously by OA with the idea that she is being abstinent when she is following her food plan. People with chronic pain can perhaps consider themselves in recovery if they are taking painkillers exactly as prescribed, though this requires the participation of a savvy doctor. If you're a workaholic you're not likely to stop working, but you can recognize the distinction between working normally and working addictively. The support of the sponsor, the meetings, and the method can sustain you in what is clearly going to be a lifelong struggle.

There are other addictions that are harder to explain. In an addicted state, we're so habituated to a substance or an activity that we experience a powerful craving when we're without it, and only feel good when we have it. Some substances, like alcohol and heroin, are so inherently pleasurable that almost anyone can become addicted. The feeling of euphoria, omnipotence, invulnerability is so seductive that we can recognize that it takes self-discipline to turn away and get back to reality. From that model, it can be hard to understand how things that are not inherently pleasurable, in fact sometimes painful, can be addictions. But people become addicted to all kinds of dangerous and destructive things—stressful jobs, bingeing and purging, self-mutilation. How come?

There are also "soft" addictions—so-called because the addictive potential of the drug or behavior is not immediately apparent; but at the same time the effect is not by definition unpleasant. I'm referring largely to behavior patterns like gambling, sex addiction, shopping and overspending, procrastination, television or video-game addiction, workaholism, and other forms of behavior that can take on an obsessive quality. Obviously, there are degrees of damage and risk here: gambling can be highly addictive, and the damage that it does to one's life can be terrible, whereas with television addiction it's likely that no one is hurt very much but oneself. By putting them all together this way I do not mean to imply that they are equally grave, but that there are similar mechanisms involved.

Remember that in today's world we are full of stress hormones, constantly ready for fight or flight. An addiction creates for us the cycle of tension→ release→guilt→tension→release→guilt. It gives us the sense of a little mastery over our stress. Animals in the laboratory can be trained to give themselves a mild shock if it will prevent a more unpleasant one. Eventually they start giving themselves a mild shock without any cues, almost as if it's pleasurable. The process of shocking the self has developed a functional autonomy, a life of its own; it's become an addiction. In the same way, creating a state of tension and release in ourselves through spending more money than we have, putting off projects until the last moment, even cutting ourselves with a razor, gives us the feeling of mastering stress and allows us to avoid (temporarily) the bigger stresses of relationships, achievement, and purpose.

For people who feel dead inside, stimulation like this can be very attractive. Teens and adults who cut themselves usually report that the cutting and the bleeding shows them that they are feeling *something,* and something is better than nothing. Feeling dead inside seems to be an increasingly common response to the vast emptiness of our culture, to the disempowerment that comes from being shuffled impersonally through the school system, the lack of engagement when parents are too busy or stressed or self-involved. No wonder kids turn to cutting or other self-destructive behavior; no wonder adults sedate themselves with comfort foods or pursue Internet fantasy relationships.

The feeling of guilt is also important in sustaining the cycle. We feel so bad about slipping up that our guilt becomes fuel for the growing tension that will ultimately be released by indulging in our addiction again. AA has the right philosophy: if you slip, don't waste a lot of time castigating yourself. Tomorrow you have a fresh start all over again. But people with depression or anxiety and addiction use their indulgence as another stick to beat themselves up with.

Most people with chronic pain problems drive themselves crazy with worry about becoming dependent on their painkillers. This kind of guilt and worry gets us nowhere, in fact sends us backwards. There is a difference between remorse, which is what we should feel when we've done something destructive, and the kind of neurotic guilt that just feeds the vicious circle. It takes a responsible adult to feel remorse, but anyone can feel guilty. In the twisted world of the addict, we feel truly guilty, but feeling guilty is just another stress that can only be relieved through indulging in the addictive behavior again. To my mind, this vicious circle is the only explanation why behaviors such as bingeing and purging or self-mutilation can be rewarding.

Many people are addicted to their work because of a variation on this cycle; jobs in industries with many deadlines (such as publishing or broadcasting) or that require highly focused attention under stressful conditions (such as finance) create a kind of "adrenaline addiction." The daily or weekly challenge of the job makes for a very intense "flow" experience (discussed in Chapter 10), which even if it causes ulcers is very satisfying. People suddenly deprived of this experience through illness or job loss often go through a marked withdrawal period, sometimes leading to major depression. Procrastination is based on the same cycle. The procrastinator is perpetually raising the stakes on his deadlines, pushing the task further and further off until the time is so short that pulling it off seems like a triumph. A more mindful kind of triumph would be to work hard and devote adequate time to the project so that the end results are truly substantial.

Other soft addictions have some built-in rewards, though they may be hard to spot. The rewards of gambling are obvious—the occasional payoff. Sex addictions involve sexual gratification, of course, but they are also highly dependent on the tension→release→guilt→tension cycle Compulsive eating brings with it the feeling of satiation and a temporary relief from the Perpetual Stress Response, and compulsive shopping can be a pastime in a sterile existence.

Mihalyi Csikszentmihalyi, the author of *Flow* and a leading researcher into what makes us happy, discovered inadvertently that television watching shares some special qualities with addictive drugs. People report feeling relaxed, passive, and less alert while they are watching TV. When they turn it off, the sense of relaxation ends, but the passivity and dullness continue. Viewers come to associate the sense of passivity and dullness with turning the TV off, so they leave it on. In the same way, tranquilizers that leave the body quickly, like

Xanax, are considered more addictive than those that leave the body slowly, like Klonopin. The fact that withdrawal can be perceived and feels aversive makes us more likely to want more drugs—or television.

Drug-seeking or other addictive behavior is cued by stimuli that serve as triggers, and it can be helpful in recovery to recognize and control these triggers. Of course, with drugs, the sensation of the drug leaving the body is the biggest trigger, but recovering addicts recognize that they need to be very watchful about other triggers. Family gatherings, conflict situations, stepping into bars, a poker game, a sunny Saturday afternoon—these are all triggers for drinking, and the recovering alcoholic knows he'll either have to avoid these situations or endure the pain of his thirst repeatedly until the stimulus-response connection in the brain is broken. Loneliness, boredom, and anger are big triggers for overeating and overspending. In the case of self-mutilation, a feeling of dissociation seems to be a trigger; people often report that they cut themselves in order to feel real again. With all these triggers, the two-pronged strategy is to (1) avoid the trigger as much as practical; and (2) learn other responses to the trigger. Other responses can be distractions (visiting a friend instead of eating or shopping) or simply leaving the situation (why stick around in a family conflict that really doesn't concern you?) or, in the case of emotional triggers, learning how to express feelings in a safe and constructive way. Obviously, a mindful attitude can go a long way in helping gain the ability to identify triggers.

Getting Help

We've talked about a broad range of human problems here in this chapter; let me close by offering some tips about how to get the help you need in order to overcome them.

How do you find a good therapist? There's no telling. People with crackpot theories can be effective. You're more likely to get help, though, from someone with a good professional education and a lot of experience, someone who's flexible and not dogmatic about their approach, someone who is willing to work with your doctor or a psychiatrist to include medication in your treatment plan.

If you do your research, you will find that cognitive-behavior therapy is usually recommended, especially for anxiety and depression. That's because CBT has been demonstrated to be effective in careful research trials, while other approaches generally haven't. But this is a little deceptive. In order to achieve the kind of reliability necessary to pass the tests of scientific evidence, CBT researchers have done what medication researchers have also done, which is to concentrate on efficacy rather than effectiveness. What this means is that they have carefully selected their patients to exclude those with any other complicating conditions, and they have (generally) limited their total research period to a short time, often as little as three months. These conditions greatly improve your odds of finding that whatever you're doing has some effect, but they're far removed from the real world, where most people have more than one problem and they're likely to struggle with their condition for years. This not only has the very unfortunate effect of making research clinically irrelevant, but it tilts the playing field in favor of methods like cognitive-behavioral therapy, which are highly structured and can be put into manualized form so that every therapist is doing pretty much the same. Bottom line: Every therapist should have some knowledge of CBT, but I'd much sooner recommend a psychodynamic therapist who has twenty years' experience and is warm and flexible over a cognitive-behavioral therapist who is fresh out of school and believes life is simple.

As far as the personal qualities and skills of your therapist go, review my recommendations on page 253 for finding a therapist to help with depression. You should find someone who you like, who you have confidence in, who you feel likes you, who treats you respectfully, who seems warm and open but competent and knowledgeable. You should ask what kinds of treatment approaches they practice; if they only talk about one method, go find someone else, because you need someone who is flexible and practical. You should ask if they can help you find a doctor for medication, should it be necessary, and they should have several doctors' names in their PDA or Rolodex. You should ask how treatment works, and they should be able to give you an answer you understand. I know the therapist's office is very intimidating; you feel like you're being evaluated from the moment you enter the room (as the comedian David Steinberg used to say, "Everything counts!"). But put your intimidation aside for the time being and check this person out to see if they will really *talk* to you. Judith Herman writes, "The first principle of recovery is the empowerment of the survivor. . . . Others may offer advice, support, assistance, affection, and care, but not cure. . . . No intervention that takes power away from the survivor can possibly foster her recovery, no matter how much it appears to be in her immediate best interest." Don't trust a therapist who wants to make decisions for you; likewise don't trust one who is remote or aloof from your pain. Trust one who seems to be genuinely interested in helping you make your own decisions.

About how to find someone: ask for recommendations from friends, from your doctor, from your clergyman. If you find yourself shunted to a psychiatrist who only does medications, that's a good place to start: ask the psychiatrist who he or she thinks might be a good talk therapist for you. Ask your insurance company who's on their "panel" in your area; at least you get someone who's licensed and has the proper professional background. Look for self-help groups on your problem, and ask the members who they recommend. If you're in a metropolitan area, see if there's someone who's written a book on your subject, or on therapy in general, and don't be afraid to call them. These people always have junior colleagues, usually very competent, whom they will refer you to. Be prepared to shop around, to see three or four or more different people until you find the one who feels right.

Medication treatment for these conditions can be horribly expensive, especially if you have no insurance. Most of the pharmaceutical companies have a way for your doctor to get free or low-cost medications for you, but the doctor will have to do some paperwork. It may be simpler to get your medications from Canada, at least until we have real health-care reform. There is also a website called Needymeds.com that seems to give good advice and promises to keep up to date with all the current ways of getting low-cost medication.

AA and other Twelve-Step programs are the best approaches to self-help for addictions. For anxiety and depression, we've never been able to develop a comparable network of support. However, major cities usually have some self-help groups, like the Mood Disorders Support Group in New York, and you can locate these via the Web. There are a lot of Internet-based self-help sites, too many for me to give any specific recommendations. Healthyplace.com is a good place to start. I'm not aware of any self-help resources for people with personality disorders, unfortunately.

Karen: Addiction and PTSD

I described above how it was that Karen became involved with painkillers, but her story is really not that simple at all. Like many nurses, Karen went into her career because taking care of others was in her blood—"It's a symptom, not a profession," she says.

It's the caretaker family role I described in Chapter 6: the child's own emotional needs are ignored at home, but she gets some mastery and gratification from taking care of a dysfunctional parent. It leads to Young's "abandonment" lifetrap and the psychodynamic depressive/masochistic character. In Karen's case, the dysfunctional parent was her mother, and alcoholism was the problem.

Karen's father left the family very shortly after she was born. (He never expressed any interest in her until he was dying, and then he wanted her to take care of him! These patterns are incredibly deep-rooted.) Karen grew up with her mother, who began her slow descent into alcohol, and her older brother. Things always seemed chaotic; Karen remembers escaping, going out for walks by herself at a young age, hiding in the woods and fields, to get away from the yelling at home. She remembers her mother, in an adjoining room, crying to herself at night, drunk, Karen torn between wanting to go in and comfort her, and anger that her mother put her in this position. When Karen was ten, they moved in with her maternal grandparents. Karen loved her grandmother, who made a good home for them. Horses became an important part of her life, reliable friends who could help her calm down. Then her grandmother died when Karen was thirteen. Her mother's alcoholism grew steadily worse.

When Karen was about fifteen her mother set herself on fire—badly. Drinking and smoking, she fell asleep late at night and set the chair on fire. Karen remembers waking up to hear her mother sobbing in the tub, where she had gone to put the fire out. Karen and her brother took their mother to the hospital, but the brother then decamped, leaving Karen alone in the house for six months while her mother recuperated in the hospital. It took her weeks to get the nerve to clean out the tub, and to this day she is haunted by the scent of burning flesh. When her mother came home there was no one but Karen to take care of her, to change the dressings and put new salve on her wounds. Her mother was to go back to the hospital after a week but she refused, just relying on Karen to care for her. Karen knows that all this happened, but she remembers nothing from these weeks, except the medicinal smell.

This is a traumatic memory, and Karen has it dissociated. She can't remember the sequence of events, but her feelings—horror, tears, fear, rage—come back whenever she talks about it. She keeps reliving the experience in her nightmares and in her pain, but she doesn't connect them to the experience. She has the survivor triad of PTSD— insomnia, nightmares, and psychosomatic complaints. She's lost the ability to experience emotions as signals; she's only confused and upset by feelings now. She feels strange to herself, a little dangerous and out of control, and that's contributed to her social isolation. She is hypervigilant, always on the alert, always ready for fight or flight—and this has worn out her muscles and tendons so much that she is always in pain.

Symptoms can mean more than one thing. I also think Karen's somatic pain in the present is her mother's pain from the past. Karen's pain is generalized, all over her body, joints, muscles, back, legs, headaches. There is no doubt in my mind that it's real; she's not imagining it; it's not all in her head, it's all over her body. She has internalized her mother's pain, partly as a way of memorializing her mother, as we often do with incomplete mourning: we find ourselves acting like the person we've lost. She also has her mother's pain as a way of punishing herself. She will say very directly, I felt it was my job to make her happy, and she died before I could. I felt guilty for moving away from her, I knew she'd die, but I had to protect my children from her. *Nothing helps Karen's pain except drugs to the point of intoxication, just as nothing helped her mother but drinking. She makes her doctors feel helpless, just as she felt.*

But in the past year, Karen has improved a great deal. Her primary physician—who has gone to heroic lengths to coordinate care for her—and I, and especially Karen, have got her taking a regular manageable dose of painkillers, an antidepressant, and a few other meds that she needs for allergies and asthma, and no more. She's stopped her doctor-shopping and medication-seeking. She has more days of feeling good. She is beginning to work on the "push-crash" syndrome that is always exacerbating her pain. She's let me into her world much more than ever before. She understands that most of her symptoms have to do with PTSD, and having an explanation for all the strange, scary, seemingly unconnected things that were happening to her body and mind has helped a great deal.

Good Thoughts, Bad Thoughts, No Thoughts

THE twin themes of this book are (1) that stress is getting into our brains, causing severe yet unrecognized damage; but (2) by deliberately controlling our experience, we can undo the effects of stress and return to a natural healthy mind-body functioning state. The fly in the ointment is, of course, that if stress affects our brains in subtle and unseen ways, how do we trust ourselves to know what's good for us? If our brains have been infiltrated by little covert operatives of stress, spreading disinformation in an effort to disrupt our executive functioning, how do we regain confidence that we are seeing reality clearly and making wise decisions? This is a hugely complex question—I think that ultimately we need to rely on universal human values like the Golden Rule— but this book is not the place to investigate those issues. We do need to have a firm grounding in our individual values, as we explored in Exercise 3. On a more mundane and practical level, we are fortunate that psychologists have identified many common errors in thinking and perception that we are likely to resort to under stress. Other scientists and philosophers have taught us the processes involved in making good decisions. We can use this knowledge to make a habit of a continual mindful review of our thought processes, identifying how we're going wrong before we get ourselves in too much trouble. As we do this we develop greater confidence in our perspectives and mental mechanisms. We can go further yet and make long-term plans that will help us achieve our most important goals and give us the opportunity to live creative and fulfilling lives.

I've referred many times to cognitive-behavioral, or simply cognitive, psychotherapy. It's the approach developed in the 1970s that rescued American clinical psychology from the dead end of behaviorism. Cognitive therapy simply started with the commonsense hypothesis that the conscious content of our minds—our thoughts—might be responsible for emotional problems and irrational behavior. We might be unaware of this since we rarely do a systematic review of our own thought processes. Cognitive therapy focuses on the patient's problematic functioning area and provides exactly this systematic review. It was the first method of psychotherapy that demonstrated it could be more effective than no treatment, an embarrassing state of affairs that had undermined support for psychodynamic psychotherapy. Cognitive therapy proved to be an effective treatment for most patients with depression and anxiety disorders (the bulk of patients in psychotherapy). It's been adapted for work with borderline patients, with couples, and with severely disturbed patients.

In the way that we seem to have of stretching new theories beyond the bounds of reason, some cognitive theorists unfortunately pushed the idea that distorted thought processes were *the* cause of problem behaviors, rather than being content just to demonstrate empirically that correcting distorted thoughts resulted in change in the problem behavior. I'd rather view thought distortions as one more element in the system of the stress response: that the Perpetual Stress Response affects both our physical self—the brain, nervous system, and body—and our minds—our feelings and thoughts. Identifying and remedying dysfunctional thoughts is another way of addressing the Perpetual Stress Response, just as is learning mindfulness or taking better care of our bodies. These dysfunctional thoughts are the conscious manifestations of the default circuitry in our brains, those long-term potentiated connections between neurons that have fired so often together that they have become wired together. These thought patterns become completely automatic and unconscious; by dragging them out into consciousness we expose their fallacious reasoning, give ourselves the opportunity to break those hard-wired connections and replace them with new, less automatic, more deliberate ways of thinking.

Alcoholics Anonymous tells us we can't think our way into right acting; we have to act our way into right thinking. To me, this is another reminder of the need to practice. Walk the walk and talk the talk, even if you don't believe it altogether. Use your mindfulness practice now on how you think. But don't stop at observing; don't give up when you recognize how unreliable your thoughts are. Get used to thinking about your thinking, paying attention to your thought processes, opening them up to new information and new perspectives.

Cognitive Distortions

Over the years the cognitive therapists have identified a number of ways that we can make ourselves miserable, contributing to depression, anxiety, and other emotional/behavioral problems. These are generally referred to as "cognitive distortions" rather than "dumb ideas," to avoid alienating the patient. The truth is that the smartest of us are capable of some really dumb ideas, embarrassingly false beliefs or blatant contradictions, but we're rarely made aware of them because we have our intricate defensive system that protects us from seeing reality correctly. You may laugh at some of the cognitive distortions we'll be discussing, but I promise you that you, and I, engage in these constantly. Don't sneer, and be open-minded about finding yourself here.

Two days ago a bad digestive experience left me choking, unable to catch my breath for a few minutes. I started to experience a panic attack—naturally enough: deprivation of oxygen triggers the fight-or-flight response. But because I had had panic episodes in the past, which developed into a height phobia that made it very difficult for me to go up in tall buildings or cross bridges, I immediately began to catastrophize: Oh, no, it's going to start again, after all the work I did, I'm going to be having panic attacks regularly, I'll be miserable all the time! How will I get to see the kids in Brooklyn if I can't drive over the Whitestone Bridge?

In about three seconds I had gone from indigestion to never seeing my children again. Fortunately for me the episode passed quickly and I'm not worried about more panic attacks. But it was only because I was thinking about this chapter and the power of distorted thinking that I made a mental note of how quickly crazy my thoughts became. If I hadn't been trying to be aware I promise you my defenses would have distorted the episode. I would remember the panic attack but forget how my catastrophic thinking ran away with me. We all do this kind of thing, all the time. *And if I'd continued to have panicky episodes, then next time I'd have to drive over the Whitestone Bridge I would work myself into a lather beforehand and really have a genuine panic attack while driving.* Such is the power of thought.

There are several different kinds of cognitive distortion that get us into trouble. The first we'll talk about are false assumptions.

False Assumptions

These are unconscious beliefs, components of the assumptive world. Though they operate unconsciously, most people will admit ruefully that they recognize themselves in some categories.

- *If [blank] happens, it'll be a catastrophe.* My problem, straight out of the box. *Catastrophizing* like this means that you're assuming that the consequences of an undesired event will mean the end of the world, or something close to it. Of course there are real catastrophes, but the stress response often expresses itself as mindless catastrophizing, getting so caught up in the fear that you're unable to see that this particular issue might be rather trivial in the grand scheme of things. Or that there are steps you could take to prepare for the worst possible outcome.
- *Everything has to be perfect, or else . . .* This statement may end any number of ways: *people won't like me, I'll be a failure, I'll be rejected, I'll be worthless, I'll be humiliated.* These assumptions of perfectionism are particularly devastating. In research on depression, those patients who are most perfectionistic tend to have the worst outcomes. Setting impossible goals means never achieving anything worthy of your own self-respect, a sure route to misery. Perfectionism also means focusing on the details, not the meaning; the appearance, not the substance. It leads to isolation because you're certain to be picky and irritable when people mess up your plans, and because people will grow tired of your obsession with appearances over substance.
- *It's essential that everyone like me.* In adolescence we all experienced the powerful wish to fit in and be accepted; and most of us also experienced some of the pain of being rejected. Adolescence is also the time when we begin to learn that sometimes fitting in requires compromising on values and principles that may be important to us. But some adults who suffer from especially uncertain self-esteem seem to behave as if they still believe that being liked by everyone will help them feel better about themselves. It may, temporarily; but what happens when two people you care about want contradictory things from you? This kind of popularity is a thin substitute for the kind of self-respect that comes from trusting your own values, making up your own mind, and speaking up on difficult subjects even when it might alienate some people who can't tolerate disagreement.

- *Feelings are dangerous.* This is a very common assumption in depression and in some other conditions. Often the individual has been disappointed, repeatedly or traumatically, and has concluded that it's best not to wish or hope for things to be different. Sometimes people have been raised in situations where it really was dangerous to let anyone know how you feel, because that information could be used to hurt you. Regardless of its origins, this is a severely dysfunctional belief. Feelings provide us with essential information about our wants and needs; without the ability to experience feelings we lead a dismal and empty existence. It's not always wise to express our feelings unguardedly, but that's a different matter from suppressing their experience.
- *I can't live without you.* Not only does the threatened end of a relationship mean the normal experience of rejection and loss, it seems to mean the end of existence itself. By giving another human being this power over ourselves, we seem to be saying there's nothing we wouldn't do to preserve the relationship. Do we really mean this? Would we steal, lie, commit murder? Hopefully not—and if not then I *can* live without you. People who take this position are being controlled by a mindless fear that won't let them look at what life might be like without the other person.
- *I'll quit tomorrow.* This, of course, is the common belief of the addict, the dieter, the procrastinator, the gambler, anyone who has a self-destructive habit but isn't quitting. Remember I told you not to sneer: these people actually believe they mean it when they say it to themselves. They feel a little pride in the self-control they will be showing the world tomorrow or the next day. They support the belief with all these little side rationalizations that explain why tomorrow's a better day than today anyhow. This belief is what allows them to indulge today without feeling overly guilty. It's a comforting belief, especially compared to facing the hard truth: *I'm an addict, and I've lost control.*
- *My nervous system is special; there's nothing I can do about it.* This is the assumption shared by many who are suffering from nonspecific illnesses, who feel they have a purely physical ailment that Western science doesn't understand yet. They see themselves as misunderstood victims, both of their disease and of a medical establishment that wants to blame them by telling them they have a psychosomatic condition. I have also encountered this with some patients with depression, who feel their state is purely biological. It's likely that we'll never know if some of these condi-

tions are "purely" biological, but the point is that it's not a useful hypothesis. It gives you nowhere to start, nothing to work with. It's completely disempowering; the only thing the patient can do is wait for the right pill to come along. It's much more useful to be open-minded, to consider that *maybe if I try this . . .*

- *I'm defective/damaged/inadequate.* This is different from the previous assumption because it carries none of the righteous indignation of the person who feels victimized by society. In this case, the individual simply believes himself to be different from normal in some way that accounts for his troubles. It's frequently a manifestation of depression, but many people who feel this way have never had a major depressive episode. Some have been told this all their lives by parents and other family members, and it is so much a part of their reality that it never gets questioned.
- *No one can love me.* This is a variation on the "defective" assumption, restricted to the realm of intimacy. Sometimes it's a manifestation of hidden guilt or shame. More often it's the result of being raised by cold or withdrawn parents who have made you feel that your natural needs for affection and support are ugly or unnatural.
- *It doesn't matter what I do, nothing will ever change.* This is perhaps a deeper, more unconscious assumption than some others; few people will own up to this belief. But it is not that unusual. It's the cognitive expression of learned helplessness. These are typically people who have just gotten burned out on trying to change their circumstances, and have internalized the belief that they are powerless to change. Though this may start out affecting only a circumscribed area of an individual's functioning (like a dysfunctional or abusive marriage) it often generalizes, so that you end up feeling that wishes, aspirations, or goals are pointless. Of course this assumption is highly associated with depression, but many people who share this belief simply lead depressed lives without the intense negative affect, guilt, and physical symptoms of depression.
- *No one can be trusted.* This is, of course, the basic assumption of paranoia, but there are millions of people who feel this way without blossoming into full-blown mental illness. Some are people who have been hurt so badly that they've decided to withdraw from relationships. Others have taken the defectiveness assumption and projected it onto the world: *It's not that I'm defective, it's the world that always lets me down.*
- *Everyone does it.* Here is another rationalizing assumption that permits the

individual to behave in ways he knows are wrong. It shifts the blame from the individual to society: *If everyone else does it, I'd be a fool not to.* Unfortunately, it adds a big heavy chunk to character armor, because you have to keep on justifying why you're doing something that you know to be wrong. It can make you defensive and crabby, or it can just make you weak and wishy-washy.

There are many other assumptions like these: *I have to do everything myself. One more won't hurt. I can't handle this. I have to shine at everything I do. Life is an ordeal, and I'm a victim.* I hope that it's obvious to the reader by now how such beliefs naturally set up vicious circles, creating the very conditions that seem to be the foundations for the belief. If you treat people as if you don't trust them, they aren't going to trust you, and you will interpret their suspiciousness as proof that you can't trust them. If you believe no one can love you, you're naturally not going to put yourself out there in the social world as an attractive and interesting individual; you'll adopt a character style of shyness and self-effacement, and no one will be interested in you, let alone love you. If you believe feelings are dangerous, you'll do everything you can to deny them, bottle them up, distract yourself from them. Then the only feelings that break through your characterological defenses will be those that are inherently powerful and overwhelming. You'll experience them as coming like a thunderstorm out of the blue, and you'll have confirmation for your belief that feelings are dangerous. Cognitive therapy is good at identifying beliefs like these and dragging them out into the harsh light of day where their bases can be questioned and their effects identified. A disciplined, mindful contemplation of the self can provide much the same thing. But remember that these beliefs represent the hard-wired default circuitry of our brains, and that it will take a lot of practice to establish new patterns. Developing awareness of these things, while it feels good and gives us a momentary *Aha!* experience, is just a baby step on the road to learning new thought patterns.

Inaccurate Perspectives

As we reviewed assumptive worlds, schemas, and character styles in Chapter 6, we noted how these positions affect our perception: how we will always see some things and never see others. The classic example is the depressive position. In depression, we are much more likely to pay attention to negative events than positive ones, to interpret ambiguous situations as indications of rejection or failure, to ignore evidence that people love us or respect us. The cognitive therapists working with depression introduced the concept of *at-tributional style*. They have produced a large body of research showing that people with depression make common assumptions, which can be summed up as:

> *Good things are temporary, limited in scope, and sheer luck.*
> *Bad things are permanent, pervasive in impact, and my fault.*

There are three general dimensions of attributional style: we can tend to be-lieve that explanations and events are *stable* (if it happened once, it'll happen again) or *unstable* (today was a bad day, but tomorrow may be better); *global* (if it applies here, it applies everywhere) or *specific* (if it applies here, it may or may not apply everywhere); and *internal* (I was the cause of that event) or *ex-ternal* (there were many causes of that event). Obviously a bias toward either of the extremes of these dimensions can create problems for us, making it diffi-cult to interpret reality objectively. For instance, if we consistently lean toward an unstable interpretation of things, we may fail to predict future events accu-rately, leading to disaster (*It's rained for three days straight, and the water is at the door; but don't worry, it's bound to be dry tomorrow*). If we are overly specific, we can miss important probabilities or trends (*So what if Johnny and all his friends were busted for selling dope? My son is a good boy. He is the innocent victim of evil companions*). If we favor external explanations, we can avoid taking responsi-bility when we need to (*I know I'm not supposed to hit her, but she should know bet-ter than to get in my face when I'm drinking*).

People with depression tend toward global, stable, and internal explana-tions of events:

> *Everything sucks, everything will always suck,*
> *and it's my fault that everything will always suck.*

Helping depressed people identify and challenge beliefs like these is an ef-fective tool in shaking up the grip of depression. But it's not only depressed people who have skewed perspectives or make attributional mistakes. Unfor-tunately, there's not a lot of research yet systematized about the cognitive dis-tortions associated with other maladies (except for Linehan's work with borderline personalities), but I can give you some impressions.

- HYPERSENSITIVITY is at the heart of many distorted perspectives. We can be hypersensitive to *phobic cues,* making the phobic situation stand out from its background like a DayGlo sign in a peaceful forest; to *"bad" thoughts,* contributing to our low self-esteem or nagging shame; to *narcissistic injuries,* blows to our self-esteem, making us feel unstable and dependent on others for positive feelings; to *somatic cues,* little burps in the heart rhythm, for example, setting off our alarm circuits and making us feel fragile and unsafe; to *failures, betrayals, rejections, behavior that falls short of our own standards,* and many other patterns of everyday events. Hypersensitivity just means we are especially good at noticing these things. These are acquired skills, just like an accomplished birdwatcher has learned to identify species via vague shapes and bird songs. We don't realize that we are paying undue attention to these things, because our hypersensitivity has grown on us so gradually that it seems normal. We don't realize that our perspective is skewed, but it is; we're focusing on the very things that make us miserable, giving them undue weight and importance, at the same time as we're not paying attention to alternative facts that could help us feel and function better.

- BLINDNESS, the opposite of hypersensitivity, is of course equally distorting. I mean metaphorical blindness, as in: blindness to the effects of our drug use on ourselves or on our relationships; blindness to opportunities for happiness, relaxation, or joy; blindness to the needs of others; or blindness to our own needs. We have available many different defense mechanisms that can make such blindnesses possible, but they can become so integrated into our daily functioning that defenses are unnecessary. We can develop "mindless blindness," the automatic closing down of sensory and feeling inputs that keeps us stuck in the same routines day after day, hurting ourselves and others without awareness, missing out on many of the pleasures life has to offer just because we have trained ourselves not to see.

- BEING TRAPPED IN THE GRIND—never thinking of fulfillment, never planning for joy, always mindlessly following the day's routine—the "living dead" that I referred to in Chapter 1. For some of us, life is very hard, and it seems like all we can do just to meet our obligations; but we have an obligation to ourselves to sometimes lift our heads from the mud and look around: to make an effort to enrich our lives, change our routines, challenge our assumptions.

- NEVER BEING PRESENT. I mean always being preoccupied with judging, planning, juggling, to the exclusion of awareness of your moment-to-moment experiencing. Living life as if it's a tennis game, demanding such intense concentration that we can't step back and observe ourselves mindfully. The danger is that you're not making conscious decisions about where you're going because you're too busy reacting to what life hands you.

- HYPERVIGILANCE. Just a little different from hypersensitivity; I mean having one's radar too finely tuned to threats, signs of danger, signs of "contamination"—from germs, sex on television, threats to our culture, society, you name it. God knows we all have reason to be vigilant, and I can't make a simple rule to tell us when we carry it too far, but some people do just that. My patient who can't go to sleep at night until everyone else is in bed and he's made a tour of the house, double-checking the lights, alarms, and locks, knows he's going a little too far, but feels he can't help himself. We devote so much space in our brains to threats and dangers that there's not enough room left for relaxation or pleasure. We're too quick to classify things as threats when they might be benign or pleasurable, and we miss out on too many opportunities. This perspective gets into our bodies too; we go through the day stiff, tense, and guarded, and before too long our muscles and joints start to wear out.

- KEEPING SCORE is a pastime for many people who lack internal criteria that provide validation. We keep score by comparing ourselves to others in terms of financial success, possessions, lovers, academic degrees, physical fitness—all kinds of ways. Doing this kind of thing distorts our perspective on the world by making us pay too much attention to whatever it is we keep score by. We miss out on other, perhaps more meaningful, forms of gratification. We tend to see others as either competitors or losers, a mindless and hurtful classification system that blinds us to much of what people have to offer.

- THE CARETAKER'S PERSPECTIVE is an adaptation some people arrive at after a lifetime of subjugating their own needs to those of others. The self is undervalued, and meaning is found through taking care of other people. It's a malnourished self, unable to take in validation or support directly, living parasitically by caring for others. There is a big blind spot as far as one's own wants and needs are concerned.

- EXTERNAL LOCUS OF CONTROL. "Locus of control" is psychological jargon that has to do with whether you feel that you are largely responsible for your life, or whether you feel that you are controlled by forces external to yourself. People who feel that their lives are somehow out of their own control tend to be passive, to let others make decisions, to not have strong feelings or strong opinions. They are highly likely to find evidence to support their beliefs since, feeling as they do, they do not present themselves assertively or authoritatively; thus others tend to take them for granted and ignore their needs.

• THE PROJECTING SELF. There is a certain personality built around the defense of projection. Any objectionable quality perceived in the self is denied, split off, and projected outward to another individual or group. People who are excessively contemptuous of others are frequently taking their own (deeply unconscious) shame about themselves and projecting it outwards. People who are in denial about their own rage frequently spend a great deal of time and energy protecting themselves against anticipated attacks from others. Overreliance on this defense results in a highly distorted perspective on the world, where the individual is never seen as responsible for his own feelings or actions.

• EXCESSIVE SELF-CONSCIOUSNESS. There are people who are petrified in any social situation because they literally feel that all eyes are on them. They expect that they will commit social blunders and that other people will judge them quite harshly. People with depression believe that they are socially awkward even when objective observers can't distinguish them from people who believe they have high social skills. Their naturally high anxiety virtually guarantees that they will be stiff and ill-at-ease, and so *will* be likely to commit minor social blunders; and also that they will have a miserable time and have all their worst expectations confirmed.

There are many other ways our perspectives on reality can be skewed. People who tend to dissociate learn to literally not see the subjects that cause them pain or distress including their own feelings. People who prefer fantasy to reality tend to focus on only the risks and dangers of living in the real world, and minimize the benefits of having real relationships, while they exaggerate the virtues of their fantasy life. Others, like my patient Theresa (see page 266), have lost the ability to experience their own desires or feelings, and experience a very monotonous world without color or energy. Many of us are masters at selective attention as a defense, only seeing that which agrees with our assumptions, literally blinding ourselves to evidence to the contrary.

A friend recently had to judge the Cub Scouts' Pinewood Derby, an event in which the scouts (and their fathers) build small race cars and compete for prizes. As a judge, his eyes lined up with the finish line, he had to call a race against his own son; the son, positioned elsewhere, was certain that he'd won the race and that his own father was arbitrarily against him. Perspective is everything. From one point of view, we can see everything, but we're too far away to appreciate the detail; from another, we're close enough for a lot of detail but we miss some aspects of the picture altogether. Some perspectives are clouded by distortion, others have huge blind spots. As we grow older and we become more like ourselves, the danger is that whatever distortions exist in how we view reality will only become more rigid and more pervasive with the passage of time. It behooves us to develop better awareness of our prejudices and perspectives, and to learn to stretch them, challenge them, and correct for them.

Logical Errors

The cognitive therapists studying depression identified a number of logical errors that they found to be quite common among their patients. Later research—and a little introspection—demonstrated that these logical errors are by no means unique to depression; anyone can, and frequently does, make them every day in trying to solve problems and make decisions. The press of anxiety, the effect of the Perpetual Stress Response, means that we usually feel hurried and worried at the same time as we're trying to think clearly and logically—certainly not the ideal circumstances for rational thought. Though I think that excessive rationality is overrated, and that we do have to learn to pay more attention to our feelings, still if we are trying to be rational we should be as rational as we can be. If we want to believe that we've reached our decision logically, we should be sure that we've followed logical rules.

Here are some of the standard errors in logic characteristic of depressed (and nondepressed) thinking:[1]

---

[1] The flat tires and other disasters that accompany our hero are from *Active Treatment of Depression* (O'Connor, 2001).

- OVERGENERALIZING. This means assuming that if something is true under these circumstances, it's likely to be true in all circumstances. *My boss hates me. I'll never get along with management.* Or: *I had a flat on the way to the theater. All the tires must be going bad. I can't do anything right.*
- SELECTIVE ATTENTION (DISQUALIFYING THE POSITIVE). This is the process of only paying attention to information that fits our preconceptions. In depression, with its negative preconceptions, good news is selectively ignored. *Everyone said they liked my speech but there was someone in the fifth row who looked bored. It must have been a boring speech. The others are just covering up to make me feel better.* Or: *I had a flat on the way to the theater, and we missed the opening credits. It ruined the whole evening.*
- EXCESSIVE RESPONSIBILITY. This means taking responsibility for bad events but not for good events. Good things are pure luck, bad things are my fault. *I had a flat on the way to the theater, and we were late. I should have checked the tires more often.*
- ASSUMING TEMPORAL CAUSALITY. This is the formal logic error of *post hoc ergo propter hoc* (after that, therefore because of that). It's superstitious reasoning; just because one event follows another doesn't mean the first event caused the second. It also suggests that just because something has been true in the past we assume it will always be true. Overgeneralization then spreads this out so that we reach crazy conclusions: *I woke up this morning feeling depressed. I'm always going to feel depressed.* Or: *I had a flat on the way to the theater, and we were late. My date acted like it didn't matter, but she was cold to me later. It's all my fault.*
- EXCESSIVE SELF-REFERENCE. This is the belief that everyone is watching you all the time, especially when you make a mistake; and the belief that whenever things go wrong, it's because of something you did. *No one is going to listen to what I say because I'll be so anxious they'll only pay attention to my nervousness.*
- CATASTROPHIZING. If any one little thing starts to go wrong, the whole system will come unglued and fall apart. *I had a flat on the way to the theater. I must need new tires. They'll all go bad and I can't drive to work. I'll have to quit my job. I'll never find another job. I'll starve.*
- DICHOTOMOUS THINKING. This is the process of dividing experience up into categories of good or bad, right or wrong, without any shades of gray. *I got a B on my paper. The teacher must hate me.* Or: *I had a flat on the way to the theater. What a lousy car! I should never have bought it.*

- EMOTIONAL REASONING is simply taking your current feelings about any situation as the absolute truth about the situation. However I'm feeling right now is the only way to feel. Never mind that an hour from now I might feel completely differently; that will be absolutely true then. *I had a flat on the way to the theater. It put me in a lousy mood. My date said she had a good time, but she was only trying to make me feel better.*
- "SHOULD" STATEMENTS (PERFECTIONISM). This is the belief that there is one and only one correct way for things to be, and if they're not that way, that's awful. It means being made disproportionately unhappy by life's little calamities. *I had a flat on the way to the theater. I should have known it would happen. I should take better care of the car. I should have a better job so I could have a better car. I should have gone to med school instead of being an English major.*
- MAGNIFICATION AND MINIMIZATION. This means exaggerating the importance and impact of bad events, and not paying attention to, or not being aware of, good events. *I had a flat on the way to the theater. After the movie my date said she really had a good time. Too bad about the flat, it ruined the whole evening.*

It should be clear that these logical errors are quite common in anxiety disorders, as well as in depression, and that they are frequent in personality disorders, addictions, and the mental processes associated with nonspecific illness as well. These little reasoning slips are, to a great extent, what makes it possible for us to maintain our distorted assumptive worlds—because if we really applied hard logic to our assumptions and perspectives, they wouldn't hold up very long. These errors are still further examples of crossed wires in the brain, circuits that have built up through use and convenience to save us temporarily from fear and stress, that reinforce their own existence because they keep having us come to the same conclusions, but circuits that are inherently self-deluding and self-destructive.

Automatic Negative Thoughts

Aaron Beck first described what he called "automatic thinking"—our natural tendency to react to events with little evaluations, barely conscious—and noticed how in depression so many of the automatic thoughts were negative. In cognitive therapy, much attention is given to helping the patient develop awareness of these patterns of thought, rather like mindfulness helps us become aware of our continual judging. The cognitive therapist helps the patient challenge and counter automatic negative thoughts through examination of their premises and logical disputation. But many patients are helped merely by their developing awareness of these mental habits; they learn to see *there I go again* and don't especially need to challenge the negative thought. They can see that it's simply a bad mental habit. Many patients like the acronym ANTS and see how automatic negative thoughts behave like ants at a picnic, showing up out of nowhere to spoil the party. In my depression support group, members began to mime rubbing out ants with the foot when they caught themselves slipping into old thinking habits.

Automatic negative thoughts, in my experience, fall into the following five categories:

- SELF-CRITICISM. In depression, by far the most common type of automatic thought. *I sure screwed that up. I'll never get it right. He must hate me. I'm just useless. I should have [done something different].* Depressed patients in cognitive therapy are taught to become aware of the "shoulds," and to notice how they *"should* all over themselves."
- HOPELESSNESS. Often, the next logical step after years of self-criticism. *I'm no good at this* turns to *I'm no good at anything. Why bother trying? It won't make any difference.* Again, the voice of learned helplessness at work.
- VICTIMIZATION. Here is a variation on self-criticism and hopelessness. *I can't do anything right . . . but it's not my fault! It's because [my mother didn't love me, I was abused, I have a learning disability, I have ADHD, I have depression, I have a bad back, etc., etc.].* All the hopelessness is still there, but the patient has found a way out of guilt by finding something other than the self to blame. I hope that no one comes away from this book feeling that the Perpetual Stress Response is a new legitimate target for this kind of blaming.
- FEAR-BASED THINKING. This is the interior monologue of people with anxiety disorders, as opposed to depression. *I have to give a speech. . . . oh, God, I can't! I'll faint, I'll burst into tears, I'll have a heart attack. Everyone will be looking at me and I'll make a complete fool of myself.* Or: *I'd really like to ask her out on a date. . . . oh, God, I CAN'T! I'll stutter, I'll blush. I don't have the right clothes. I don't know where to take her. She'll be staring at me and I'll make a complete fool of myself.*
- DISSOCIATION. It's hard to put this process into words, since it's nonverbal.

The patient encounters something that stirs up a trauma-based association, and then just "goes away." The brain makes an unconscious decision to dissociate, just as in depression we make an unconscious decision to go into self-critical thinking, or in anxiety fear-based thinking takes over. A patient talking with a young man who appeared to be interested in her reported that her memory of the conversation was full of holes. She assumed, I think correctly, that during those blank spaces they had continued to talk, but she probably made less sense and was less emotionally connected.

A common cognitive therapy technique has the patient keep a daily log in which he or she is expected to write down all the automatic negative thoughts that occur during the specified time interval, and answer each with a rational argument. Another method has the patient use a wrist counter to simply count the number of ANTS each day. As David Burns notes, often the mere act of counting a habit like this will result in a reduction in its frequency. But these methods also are teaching the patient to be more *mindful* of his thought processes in action, to pay more attention and not take the automatic thoughts as gospel. It's the reframing method that is common to many approaches to psychotherapy: these thoughts are phenomena of your brain at work, manifestations of your illness, not necessarily true at all.

Schema Magnetism

We all know this phenomenon, though no one can explain it—except for Daniel Wegner, whom we'll meet shortly. It's when we keep stepping into the same hole over and over, despite our best attempts to avoid it. It's when you're learning to ride your bike, and you notice a telephone pole fifty feet away from you, and you could go in any direction you want but you're *drawn* to that telephone pole like a magnet. The more you try to steer away from it, the more you find yourself steering toward it. You knew the moment you saw it that you were going to hit it, and you do. In more adult terms, it's the woman who successively marries three abusive husbands, despite her basic good sense. It's when you open your mouth to discipline your son, and your father's voice comes out of your throat, despite your vows never to repeat his mistakes. It's when you've been feeling excluded or unloved, and you have the same lump in your throat that you had in fifth grade, and you find yourself making the same dumb responses that just made things worse then—getting desperate, jealous, petty. I'm using this term *schema magnetism* to mean what some describe as chemistry, the repetition compulsion, the present and chronically endured pain, a character flaw—the idea that we are somehow destined to keep fighting the same battle over and over again throughout our life, with new characters each time but the same old plot. It's another vicious circle but it's the unique one that each of us seems to have as our special curse.

This magnetism is a peculiar kind of cognitive distortion. There is no magnetism, but there is a *fascination* with the issue. We know a lot about how this works with depression. Depressed people forget about positive feedback, while nondepressed people forget about negative feedback. Depressed people underestimate their own competence, while nondepressed people overestimate theirs. People with depression are more pessimistic about their future than nondepressed people. Nondepressed people have a positive bias about themselves, predicting their own future success and the likelihood of happy events to be better than average, whereas people with depression expect more sad events to occur to them. As people recover from depression, they begin to overestimate themselves again. To the depressive, others are always more competent, more successful, more attractive, more happy. This is the Same Old Song of depression, looking from the outside on a cold snowy night into a brightly lit interior where people are laughing and singing and warm. But the point is that it's not just a state of mind; it's actually true. Depressed people *are* less healthy, less successful, less loved, and less respected than their nondepressed brethren. But it's largely because their negative expectations are self-fulfilling prophecies that have negative consequences in the real world.

I have no doubt that the same type of circular mechanism operates when other schemas exert their magnetic pull: when a woman is finding herself fascinated with a man she knows to be a cad; when we feel our present relationship is dull because it lacks the "chemistry" of the old explosive, violent, relationship; when we find ourselves procrastinating over the most important assignments of our lives, risking everything to play another hand of computer solitaire; when we find ourselves excluded again, just because we know all the answers. These are all situations where our cognitive skills don't seem to be enough to overcome the magnetism of that telephone pole.

In Chapter 6, I gave some pretty direct advice for how to pull yourself out of a schema attack. But when they keep happening, we need to go deeper into our own psyche. The telephone pole, the cad lover, the dangerous procrastination—these all have to do with a part of ourselves that we've been trying to deny. A wish to make things more interesting, perhaps; that dead feeling inside that we can escape from with a little danger. We need to take a hard look at ourselves: *What more do I want?* When we can answer that, then we have a choice: go for it, even though it may endanger what we've got; or let it go, even though we won't stop wanting it. A hard choice, but better to be mindful than to play with fire.

Mindless Categorization

Cognitive therapists generally refer to "all-or-nothing thinking" as another logical error, but I've separated it here because I think it is a bigger phenomenon. It refers to our habit of instantly judging our experience, filing it away in neat dichotomous categories of good/bad, happy/sad, dangerous/safe. It contributes to depression because we rarely achieve perfection, and if we're thinking in terms of black and white, anything short of perfection is failure. Clearly, we can fall far short of perfection and still get a lot accomplished, in fact do a very good job, but this kind of categorical thinking robs us of credit and discounts real progress.

This is a problem for all of us, not just those with depression. Mindless categorization—judging—is a manifestation of the hypervigilance we develop as part of the Perpetual Stress Response. We want to take each new input and file it away quickly so that we can be ready for the next one, always on the alert for danger or threats of danger. In doing this, we gloss over the details of our experience. We all know that God is in the details, or perhaps it is better to say that *life* is in the details, in learning to pay attention to our own unique experience—sensory, emotional, intellectual. And in exercising our curiosity. Curiosity is an innate attribute of children, and one we do well to maintain in ourselves, but judging shuts it right down. Judging plays right into closed-mindedness and prejudice. It's essentially saying that I'm the arbiter of the world and I get to decide what's good and bad. Of course, each of us is ultimately responsible for making those decisions individually, but we want to do that only after thought and reflection. Mindless, knee-jerk judging shuts down our input from the world. We start dismissing anything that doesn't agree with our prejudices, and only remembering things that agree with us. We build a closed system inside our character armor, where nothing new can penetrate. It leads to an empty life.

Inability to Prioritize

Another common cognitive distortion is our inability to prioritize, so that we are always putting out fires and never have time for the things we want time for.

There is a simple paradigm that can be used for organizing work so that more time is available for goal setting and planning. We can classify all tasks and activities on two dimensions: importance and urgency. When people do this, they generally find that they are spending most of their time in cells 1 and 2, activities that seem urgent but may or may not be important. It is especially dismaying to recognize how little time is spent in cell 4, on activities that may be very important but carry little urgency. Most people realize that, if they were able to address the important but nonurgent items, many of the urgent but unimportant things would take care of themselves. Cell 4 is preventive maintenance: getting the chimney cleaned in the summer, getting the car in for oil changes, having our teeth cleaned, setting up an automatic deduction to pay the mortgage so you don't have to scramble at the end of the month to get the payment in on time.

Table 6. **A Paradigm For Prioritizing**

1. URGENT BUT UNIMPORTANT	2. URGENT AND IMPORTANT
3. NOT URGENT AND UNIMPORTANT	4. NOT URGENT BUT IMPORTANT

Thinking about Thinking

With all these sources of error in our thought processes, the question naturally arises, can we trust our left brains at all? Can our logical skills, the powers of reasoning, actually make a difference in our lives when so much of our perception is biased? Is it possible that we might make *all* our decisions based on hunches, prejudices, and other programmed unconscious responses of the right brain, and that all our glorious logic and ratiocination is a belated cleanup effort by the left brain to justify doing exactly what we wanted to all along?

This has been the opinion of much of psychology (though we don't talk about it much in public, probably feeling it's best to let the naïve thinker imagine he's actually making decisions). In the traditional analytic view, consciousness and will were largely treated as irrelevant; that is, as epiphenomena of unconscious processes. Ironically, the same position was taken by behaviorists such as Skinner, who tended to see man's decisions as under the control of external stimuli. Cognitive behaviorism tended to put us back in control of ourselves: stimuli may control us, but we can control our stimuli. If you want to stop a problematic behavior, avoid the situations that precede the behavior. If you want to do more of another behavior, increase the amount of time you spend in the situations that precede it.

Now brain researchers are giving new ammunition for the case against self-control. Indeed, much of our decision making seems to consist of snap judgments, decisions we make on the basis of instinct or emotion. The right brain steps in a few milliseconds later to create rationalizations for our decisions.

I'm sure some clever psychologist is out there trying to design an experiment to answer the question: Do our thoughts determine our actions, or vice versa? But I think this is going to be one of those messy questions that the experimental method wasn't designed to answer. I'll stick with common sense: Thinking is both an emotional and intellectual process, the left brain and right brain combined. Our thoughts *can* determine our actions, but they do so in fact much less than we'd like to believe. Many of our actions are based on mindless snap judgments, cognitive errors, and emotional reasoning. The process of growing up is one of developing greater conscious control of all aspects of our lives, including our decision-making processes.

It should not come as a surprise to the reader at this point that I suggest we need to understand our thought processes from a different perspective than the one we take for granted. A more mindful approach to thinking is called for. When we observe ourselves mindfully, over the course of time, we see how our thoughts are constantly changing. What seemed like a huge issue yesterday has somehow gone away today; the terrible importance that we attached to addressing this problem has become detached, and the problem assumes its proper proportions. Observing ourselves mindfully, we become used to the idea of *thoughts as mental events*, things that are happening inside our brains. We stop thinking of our thoughts as the absolute truth or as moral imperatives that we must act on immediately. We see how our thoughts are influenced by feelings, the stress of the day, the weather, the background music, how much coffee we've had, how much Zoloft is in our systems, and we trust them less. That doesn't mean that we dismiss our own thoughts, or become so laid back and detached that we don't care about anything, or that we can never make up our minds because we can always see all sides of an issue. We may trust our thoughts less, but they are still vital information to us.

We can go on and practice thinking mindfully. We can consider the evidence of our thoughts and feelings together, and make our decisions accordingly. We can recognize the impact of stress in the pressure to make quick decisions, and we can practice patience, waiting until we're as certain as we want to be. Then we can observe carefully the impact of our decisions.

Mind Control

To what extent can we control our own thoughts? Tolstoy's older brother once told the young boy that he would be given access to certain great mysteries if only he could not think of a white bear. The point is, of course, that it is almost impossible to control our minds enough *not* to think of something. This is a harmless enough phenomenon when it comes to meaningless challenges, but most of us are tormented by intrusive thoughts we desperately want to control—at 3 A.M., tomorrow's presentation that we fear; when we're dieting, the thought of potato chips or chocolate ice cream; any time, the single negative element of an evaluation that seems to outweigh all the positives.

Daniel Wegner has developed a theory of "ironic processes" of mental control, which suggests that it is largely stress that guarantees we will sabotage ourselves at the worst possible time. According to this theory, our minds work through two mechanisms: a conscious mental operating process that works to get what we want (happiness, for instance), and a largely unconscious monitoring process that searches for evidence that we are not getting what we want. Under normal circumstances the two processes work well together. The monitoring process scans our experience for problems, and the operating process works to address those problems. Thus, in our quest for happiness, the monitoring process may scan and report something like "I'm pretty happy right now but I'm worried about the article I have to write." The operating process is signaled to get to work on the article, and I feel happier again. But the important implication of this theory is that the monitoring process continually oper-

ates to make us aware of events that fail to meet our goals. Thus efforts at negative self-control—to stop worrying, to not think about a certain subject, to fall
asleep, to ignore pain—are ironically handicapped from the outset because we
have a built-in process to make us aware of disturbing events. And, under
stress—say my child was sick and up all night; I'm tired and concerned about
her health—the operating process may not be able to work effectively on the
article. The monitoring process may thus become more alarmed; "I'm not
happy at all, and there's too much to do." The alarm circuits in the brain fire
continuously, and panicky, catastrophic thinking may kick in. We may become
so full of adrenaline that we can neither concentrate nor relax. The monitoring
process becomes conscious; we become focused on spotting indicators of unhappiness, and of course we can find many. So by trying too hard to be happy
in adverse circumstances, we guarantee our own unhappiness.

Wegner argues that keeping the monitoring process unconscious is a good
way of maintaining control; consider the skilled batter versus the rookie who
"chokes" under pressure. The rookie has too many things to think about, while
the experienced hitter can concentrate on the ball. I'd rather argue that we can
adopt a mindful attitude toward that self-monitoring process, to picture it as a
little radar antenna that is always on the alert for bad news, and to be grateful
for the early warning it provides—but to see it as one more part of the mental
apparatus, one that is especially sensitive to overload, one that we have to monitor carefully lest it send us mistakenly down the low road of panic.

Positive self-control, however, appears more attainable. If we cannot not
think of white bears, we can think of brown dogs instead. Distraction is a relatively effective strategy for dealing with intrusive thoughts and magnetic
schemas. We might be able to avoid that telephone pole if we were able to focus
on thinking about some other object—the finish line, for example. We can control our inputs, reducing our exposure to needless stress. Women who are exposed to repeated images of other women who are unusually attractive—as
they do when they read a lot of women's magazines—feel less attractive themselves, and their self-esteem is diminished. The same is true for men who read
descriptions of dominant and influential men. Some time ago, a researcher
studied the effects of television access in three small Canadian communities
that were just receiving cable for the first time. She found that, after the introduction of television, both adults and children became less creative at problem
solving, less able to stick to tasks, and less tolerant of unstructured time. We

can simply turn off the television and save ourselves from much of the toxic information and attitude that the medium purveys. We can learn to be mindfully skeptical about the information that creeps in regardless.

We know that we have some ability to control what we remember. When we deliberately try to suppress memories of a recent event, we make it less likely that the event will be stored in long-term memory. The prefrontal cortex is activated in suppression, while the hippocampus is deactivated, just the reverse of the remembering process.

The feeling of being in control is important to our well-being. One of the most disturbing aspects of depression is the sense that we can't stop our intrusive thoughts; we feel we've lost control of our minds, and that feels crazy. In her subversive little book *Positive Illusions,* Shelley Taylor reviews the evidence and concludes that it's the *feeling* of being in control, more than the actual degree of control we have, that comforts us and insulates us from stress. But this is not bad news. Many things can help us feel more in control. Doctors know that for the patient facing cancer treatment, the more information he has about what will happen, the better off he'll feel. We don't like surprises. Feeling that things are predictable, if not controllable, is vastly comforting in itself.

This, I think, is something like the comfort a mindful attitude brings to our contemplation of our own thinking patterns. We see that efforts to control our thoughts are largely ineffective, but we also see that our thought processes make sense, judged as an effort to understand how we experience the world through our two seemingly different brains. We need to keep in mind that our brains and nervous systems were designed for a much duller existence than we have today. In the past, our focus was largely *Do I get to eat today?* Now we not only have that question largely answered, we have a million choices about what to eat. We have, I think literally, too much information to process, and it shouldn't be surprising if our brains sometimes become overloaded. Under those circumstances, our thought processes can be forgiven for taking shortcuts, for falling into cognitive distortions, prejudices, mindless judging. Mindful understanding suggests that we simply keep working at thinking as clearly as we can, and be patient with ourselves.

Mindful Decision Making

Here's my suggested process for making the best decisions we can. This is not based on any particular model that I'm aware of, but is something that I've come to gradually over the years of reading, trying to help patients with their problems, and trying to do the best with my own:

1. *Attend.* Pay attention. Look carefully at what's going on, from as many sides as you can. Look at things mindfully, objectively, curiously. Don't get hung up on details, but don't push any awareness aside. Apply your compassionate curiosity to the situation, both the external, real situation, and what it's doing to your mind. Define the boundaries of this problem, and try not to be distracted by what seems irrelevant. If you do keep being distracted by what you think is an irrelevant detail, it's probably not that the detail is irrelevant but that you've defined the problem in such a way that it excludes an important aspect. This may be a manifestation of a gut-level hunch, the amygdala's danger-sensing system operating, and you should pay attention.

Check your perceptions. We've talked at length about the assumptive world and how it limits your vision. Do what you can to correct for that process. Talk to other people and get their viewpoints.

A great deal of the success of problem-solving strategies is determined in the first step, by how the problem is defined. Do you want to make John love you more, or do you want to be less dependent on John's opinion, or both? Is this problem specific to John, or to all your romantic relationships? Or to all relationships? The process of mindfully answering these questions will not only help you solve this particular problem, but also learn from the experience.

2. *Notice.* Play mentally with this problem as you've defined it. Let it bounce around in your mind for a while, and see what reactions get set off. Are you glad to be addressing it, or do you fear adverse consequences? Does it make you angry? Is this a conflict in values? Do you have to choose between two bad alternatives? If so, do you have a bigger problem that you've been putting off?

(Continued)

Do you feel pressure to make a decision quickly? If the pressure is coming from other people, your first decision should be whether or not to ask for more time. Often, you may have the impression that someone else wants your answer quickly when they really might not care. If they really are pressuring you, learn techniques to buy time for yourself to think. There is nothing wrong with saying *I'm going to sleep on it* or *I want to talk it over with my spouse* or even *I want to talk it over with my friend the lawyer, and he's out of town till next Wednesday.* If you're getting that much pressure, you should be suspicious.

If the pressure is coming from within you, can you silence it? Much of our suffering comes from the consequences of hasty decisions made under the press of a desire to relieve a painful situation. Can you get some metaphorical pain relief so that you have more time and a clearer head to make a thoughtful decision?

Look at the evidence. As much as possible, separate facts and feelings from conclusions, guesses, inferences. Put the conclusions, guesses, and inferences in a holding pen for now; it's too soon for them. But both facts and feelings are important data. *Be sure you know what you want.* If you go into a process unsure, you may find yourself disappointed at the outcome without having realized it was important to you.

3. *Adjust for biases.* Social psychologists have been seriously investigating the process of decision making over the past thirty years, and their conclusions should make us all humble: we're much more subject to influence, bias, or prejudice than we want to believe. Are you focusing on this issue because of something someone recently told you or that you read about or saw on television? Be aware that we can be horribly biased by this kind of personal experience. *Joe just won big on the lottery with a ticket he got from the same convenience store I go to. I'll have to buy some tickets there!*

4. *Think.* Follow each possible solution to its logical outcome. Try to consider how it will affect you and those close to you in the future. Consider both the externals and the internals. *You've been offered a job in another city. It would mean leaving behind your parents and your spouse's parents. But it's a great new job, a lot of money, a lot of job satisfaction if you do it right.* Part of the problem with a situation like this is that there is so

much that can't be known. You can do all the research in the world on the new city, but that won't tell you how you (and your spouse, and your respective parents) will feel next year and ten years from now. You have to look objectively within yourself, look at your feelings in any comparable situation, and make the best decision you can.

One useful strategy is to favor the option that leaves you the greatest freedom of choice in the future (go to college instead of nursing school), but even this isn't the best choice all the time (get a Ph.D. in philosophy instead of an MD) or for every single person (some will be happier to start a career in nursing than to spend four years on a BA).

5. *Decide.* Once you've reviewed all the possible outcomes, you need to choose the one that is best for you and for all the parties involved. Since each scenario will have its own degree of uncertainty, the best choice is the one that has the greatest value and the greatest certainty. Unfortunately, life doesn't seem to like giving us those choices. You can earn a high rate on your investments if you can tolerate risk, but you can't have a safe investment and a high return at the same time. You have to decide how much risk you can tolerate. If there's a great deal at stake, you'd do better to choose a scenario with only moderate risk and only moderate benefit over one in which you may lose everything on the chance of great rewards.

It's important to do a values check on any decision; try to make only choices that you're proud of, that you could tell your mother about. Hemingway famously said "What is moral is what you feel good after, and what is immoral is what you feel bad after," and I think he was largely right—if you are mindfully aware of your feelings and not engaged in self-delusion. If you're in a position where you find yourself repeatedly having to do things you're not proud of, you need to get out of that position.

6. *Evaluate and review.* Once you've made your decision, the process isn't over. Watch what happens. Be prepared to change your thinking as new information comes in. One of the great values of taking action is that it reveals much of what was hidden before. Don't be surprised if things seem very different from what you expected. Don't let your ego get in the way of changing your mind.

Setting Goals

We have marvelous minds, and we don't have to use all their capacity to counteract the effects of the Perpetual Stress Response. We can also use them to build some happiness and creativity into our existence. But it helps to know what makes us happy. There is a vast body of psychological research and life experience to prove one thing: money isn't it. Once we've risen above the poverty level, having more money has almost no effect on our overall happiness. This, it seems to me, is a huge social problem, since we've all been conditioned to believe in the power of wealth. *If wealth doesn't make us happy, why are we working so hard?*

I happen to think that is a damn good question. Here's an important insight from David G. Myers in *The Pursuit of Happiness*:

> What matters more than absolute wealth is perceived wealth. Money is two steps removed from happiness: Actual income doesn't much influence happiness; how satisfied we are with our income does. If we're content with our income, regardless of how much it is, we're likely to say we're happy. Strangely, however, there is only a slight tendency for people who make lots of money to be more satisfied with what they make. . . . This implies two ways to be rich; one is to have great wealth. The other is to have few wants.

If one of the sources of our unhappiness is the disparity between what we want and what we can get, sometimes instead of trying to get more we might try to want less. This may seem like a subversive concept, almost un-American. But consider how quickly the novelty wears off most acquisitions; after a short time they fade into the background of our lives, something else to be taken for granted. We're in danger of becoming addicted to the new, always needing a new toy to make us feel good. Spending money in this way can be a real addiction: we overspend because it gives us a temporary thrill, then get depressed because we're in debt, then overspend again because we're so depressed we need that thrill again. It's just like gambling; we need the adrenaline rush to make us feel alive. We're buying ourselves *consolation prizes,* just stuff we get to console ourselves because our lives aren't bringing us real satisfaction. We'd do better to save our money and use it to buy ourselves freedom when we need it: freedom to walk off the job when the boss crosses the line; freedom to take the time to learn the banjo or oil painting or French.

There is a feeling of empowerment and satisfaction that comes with going shopping and deciding that we don't need to buy anything. It's not tantalizing the self with things we want but deny ourselves; it's realizing that we already have most of what's important to us. Spending money is always a matter of choice, of one thing or another, and saving it now may come in very handy later. We can reinforce the awareness that the cost of the item doesn't really justify the fleeting joy that possessing it will bring us.

But to have few wants in America is definitely swimming upstream. Having money, and spending it, is not just about buying things. In America, wealth is a competitive sport, money is how we keep score. We seek money not to provide for ourselves but to prove to ourselves, our rivals, our fathers and mothers, both that we're special somehow and at the same time that we belong. That we uniquely deserve the accoutrements of wealth, and also that we're a member of the club.

These desires betray a deep insecurity, one that is not going to be fixed by more money or more success. Let's see what we can learn about this insecurity by looking at depression.

People with depression are rarely satisfied with their own performance or achievement, at least partly due to our tendency to overestimate the happiness or power of others. When people are told that the "correct" button-pressing pattern will turn on a light, but the light actually goes on at random intervals, depressed people soon realize that the button and the light are not connected. They're likely to turn to the experimenter and say that something is wrong with the wiring. Nondepressed people, however, develop the "illusion of control" and go on happily pressing the button in the pattern that they think works. "Depressive realism" is the phenomenon that, compared to others, depressed people in many ways have a more accurate perspective on reality. But that's not completely true. When they are asked to judge *another* person's ability to influence random events, depressed people overestimate the other's control, while nondepressed people are more accurate observers. The same pattern is found when you ask people to estimate how socially accepted they are. Nondepressed people think that others like them, even if they don't; depressed people think that others don't like them, even if they do. Nondepressed people seem to have these comforting illusions about their own efficacy, which depressed people lack; but depressed people tend to overestimate the efficacy of others.

As I described in *Active Treatment of Depression*, when we overestimate the abilities of others, we set impossible goals for ourselves. Aaron Beck described these as false assumptions: *In order for me to be happy, I must be liked by everyone. If someone disagrees with me, it means they hate me.* Some have to do with our consumer culture: *How can I be happy when I don't have that [car, house in the suburbs, trip to the Bahamas]?* Some fuel competition in the workplace: *I'm a failure if I [haven't made a million by the time I'm thirty, lose that case, don't get that promotion].* Some goals have to do with others in our lives: *If Johnny doesn't make the soccer team, he won't get into the right prep school, and that means he won't go to Yale. My husband has put on so much weight that it's an embarrassment to be seen with him.* All these aspirations have two things against them: (1) They are largely outside our individual control; all we can do is do our best, and recognize that the ultimate outcome is highly subject to luck and the influence of others. (2) They are all examples of catastrophizing, assuming that if the desired outcome doesn't come to pass, it will be the end of the world. In fact, it is possible to be quite happy if some people don't like us, if our son doesn't make the soccer team, and if our husband doesn't lose weight.

At the same time as we go about setting these impossible goals, we "know" with another part of our mind that we'll never be able to attain them. There is a preconscious knowledge lurking in the back of our awareness that we're setting ourselves up for disaster. We have our overly pessimistic view of ourselves and all our previous experience with disappointment (screened by selective attention) to tell us we'll never make it. But we try frantically to quiet that voice, redoubling our efforts to achieve. *This time will be different, this time I'll do it, and then I'll be happy.* It's the same tension→release→guilt→tension cycle that we saw in addictions. The state of tension is so familiar that it's become normal to us; we would feel ill at ease if we were to relax, rather like Csikszentmihalyi's unhappy workers at leisure (see Chapter 10, page 404). So we keep the tension up for ourselves by setting ourselves up for failure.

The pursuit of wealth gives us the illusion of control. The game of success is where we chase our impossible goals. It's an addictive process, fueled by mass media and the groupthink that doesn't challenge these meaningless values, chasing the adrenaline high and denying the hangover of futility the next day. We'd do better to stop and look for what we can do that can truly make us unique and enable us to contribute something of value to the world.

Creativity

Anne Lamott's advice in *Bird by Bird* to writers facing writer's block is to concentrate on short assignments; as we all should when faced with an insurmountable task, break it down, start small, start with something manageable. Along the way she gives us a fine description of the brain meltdown that occurs when we finally sit down to attack the task we've been dreading:

> What I do at this point, as the panic mounts and the jungle drums begin beating and I realize that the well has run dry and that my future is behind me and I'm going to have to get a job only I'm completely unemployable, is to stop. First I try to breathe, because I'm either sitting there panting like a lapdog or I'm unintentionally making slow asthmatic death rattles. So I just sit there for a minute, breathing slowly, quietly. I let my mind wander. After a moment I may notice that I'm trying to decide whether or not I am too old for orthodontia and whether right now would be a good time to make a few calls, and then I start to think about learning to use makeup and how maybe I could find some boyfriend who is not a total and complete fixer-upper and then my life would be totally great and I'd be happy all the time, and I think about all the people I should have called back before I sat down to work, and how I should probably at least check in with my agent and tell him this great idea I have and see if he thinks it's a good idea, and see if *he* thinks I need orthodontia—if that is what he's actually thinking whenever we have lunch together. Then I think about someone I'm really annoyed with, or some financial problem that is driving me crazy, and decide that I must resolve this before I get down to today's work. So I become a dog with a chew toy, worrying it for a while, wrestling it to the ground, flinging it over my shoulder, chasing it, licking it, chewing it, flinging it back over my shoulder. I stop just short of actually barking. But all of this only takes somewhere between one and two minutes, so I haven't actually wasted that much time. Still, it leaves me winded. I go back to trying to breathe, slowly and calmly, and I finally notice the one-inch picture frame that I put on my desk to remind me of short assignments.

This, it seems to me, is a wonderful account of creativity at work. Many people lament their lack of creativity, as if it's like blue eyes or the ability to roll your tongue, a genetic gift they missed out on. On the contrary; creativity is hard work coupled with mindfulness.

Most of us have had the experience of worrying a problem to death, doing all the research, gathering our notes, finding more information, regrouping, then finding *more* information, finally becoming overwhelmed. Then sometimes the next day when we wake up, or are taking our shower, or driving to work, the pieces fall into place and we see the obvious solution that totally evaded us yesterday. What's happened is that we've given our unconscious mind time to work. We've overwhelmed the left brain with too much information, while the right brain has stood back, processing the picture impressionistically, putting it together in a whole new way. It needed for us to shut down the left brain in order to do its job.

That's what mindfulness does for creativity. Creativity is essentially getting the hemispheres to work together to create a new whole out of separate parts. Mindfulness allows us to shut down the left brain, slow down, and listen to ourselves. Creativity is not just for people who work in the arts, it's for everyone, and it's one of the true joys in life. Practice mindfulness and you'll see.

Working at Joy

Silvan Tomkins, the most widely respected theorist of emotions, only identified three basic positive emotions: surprise, interest/excitement, and joy/enjoyment (the others are distress/anguish, contempt/disgust, anger/rage, fear/terror, and shame/humiliation). Even surprise is not necessarily a positive emotion, but a kind of priming response that can go either way. That leaves only two of eight basic emotions as positive. In general, science pays much less attention to the positive emotions than the negative. You don't find joy in Damasio or LeDoux's indices, but there is a lot of fear there. Martin Seligman, Mihalyi Csikszentmihalyi, Daniel Kahneman, and others have been trying to lead us to understand more about positive feelings, but they have a long way to go. Although most of us might add things like pride or love or humor to Tomkins's list, we also tend not to pay too much attention to positive feelings. They tend not to stay in our memories the way that bad experiences or negative feelings do. Sitting in the sun with your dog might be one of your top ten good things, but somehow an experience like that seems trivial when compared to all the horrible things you can think of—deaths, diseases, accidents, heartbreaks.

Maybe it shouldn't.

Most of psychology focuses on helping us overcome problems and difficulties, as well it should. But we need also to focus on positive experiences, to understand how we feel good, to deliberately bring more positive experiences into our lives. As we'll discuss later, there is good reason to believe that the normal resting state of the human mind is one of mild anxiety. On top of that, we have the effects of perpetual stress, increasing our anxiety and our helplessness to do anything about it. Given all that, it only makes sense to learn and practice the skills of joy, humor, creativity, warmth, generosity. Research tells us that these are indeed skills we can cultivate like any other skill; they get easier and better with practice. Experiencing joy is a habit. A healthy sense of humor is a strength that can be developed like a muscle. And creativity is something to practice, not a mysterious electricity possessed only by a lucky few. The Perpetual Stress Response has us full of anxiety hormones, which interfere with any positive emotion—so we have to work deliberately at feeling good.

Many people, not only those with depression, have as a major component of their assumptive world the belief that all feelings are dangerous. They've been disappointed or hurt often enough that they don't take chances anymore. They don't let anyone see their needs. They get so good at hiding their feelings that they forget where they hid them. Unfortunately, it seems to be impossible to stop feeling only bad feelings; the good ones disappear too. Then there are those who are unfortunate enough to be spending a lot of time and energy coping with psychological or physiological symptoms. They are at a real handicap here, because they are left with fewer resources to build on. They have a lot of hard work and discipline ahead if they want to genuinely reexperience life. Yet joy, humor, and creativity have to be built in to the hard work from the start, or there's no point in trying.

For example, a strange thing seems to have happened with public consciousness about endorphins, the "endogenous opiates" that are manufactured by our bodies to transmit feelings of pleasure and vitality. After an initial burst of interest, it seems that endorphins have been relegated to the role of an interesting artifact—something that happens when you exercise hard, but not very meaningful in everyday life. Talk about missing the point! Endorphins not only make us feel good after exercise, they are the transmitters for all our good feelings, from play to intimacy to awe. They insulate us from pain. They play an important but as yet not understood role in the functioning of the immune system. An abundance of endorphin receptors in the system makes us less sensitive to the negative emotions of anger, shame, and fear. Endorphin receptors are right in the limbic system, the emotional brain. We know that when infants are socially isolated, deprived of the attachment connection with their mother, they experience a permanent reduction in the number of endorphin receptors. But we as adults have a great deal of power in determining how much endorphin is in our system. Exercise helps a lot, but so do activities like music and dance, sex, good food, intimacy, self-expression, mutual aid. Church socials and softball games are great endorphin-makers. Breathing releases endorphins, as do running and laughter. Breathing helps with labor pains by flooding us with endorphins, which kill pain as well as making us feel happy. Making a deliberate effort to get out and socialize, not sit around and be prisoners of our stress, is one of the most important things we can do to adapt to twenty-first-century life.

I think it's useful to make a distinction between two major classes of positive feelings, *joy* and *fulfillment*. Joys are right now, in the moment, pure experiences of pleasure, happiness, gratification. We want to smile, laugh, dance, celebrate. Fulfillment is a more quiet state of satisfaction. It comes (sometimes) when we get something we've wanted, something we've worked hard for or sacrificed for. Something that achieves a goal, something that expresses our aspirations. We feel a sense of accomplishment, of arrival, of progress. There is pride mixed with joy in fulfillment. But since (I believe) we can feel fulfilled by reading a good book or listening to a powerful sermon or seeing our daughter graduate from law school, fulfillment can be somewhat vicarious; we can be moved by another's accomplishments as well as our own. Perhaps fulfillment engages both halves of the brain more than joy does, because there is an element of thoughtful reflection in fulfillment.

Martin Seligman, who has been doing a great deal to push the field of psychology into learning more about positive states, has a distinction between *pleasures,* which are roughly equivalent to my joys, and *gratifications,* which are activities that engage us fully in a state of flow (the state of rapt attention we feel when fully engaged in something—see Chapter 10). Like my use of the term fulfillment, gratifications engage the intellect and perhaps the body besides the pure pleasure system. But to me, gratification is too limited a concept to express the range and depth of positive feelings suggested by the word fulfillment.

Perhaps I have given the impression somehow that fulfillment is somehow better than, more mature than, joy. I don't mean that to be the case at all. We need plenty of both experiences in our lives. Fulfillment is great, but there's not enough of it, and sometimes fate will interfere in our ability to achieve the things we want the most. We need also to be able to appreciate the joys of everyday life.

A mindful attitude can help with this. Mindfulness makes us aware of transience, of how quickly things can change, how what we take for granted can

sometimes suddenly be lost forever. Mindfulness helps us accept that awareness without being terrified by it, but it also can make us more sensitive to the
little pleasures of the day. We become better able to appreciate the sensations of
the sun on our skin, the winter light in the kitchen, the smell of a good stew,
the touch of a loved one. But there are other ways as well to bring more joy and
fulfillment into our lives:

We need to remember to play.

This is one reason why pets and small children are good for us, because
they're often nudging us to get out of the chair and play with them. Play is nurturing to the self. It's a present we should give to ourselves more often. It gets
the left and right brains acting together in an integrating experience. Play can
change our moods. When we're really down, irritable, and feeling sorry for
ourselves, one of the major reasons we don't want to play is that our sour mood
will look pretty shallow or foolish if we're able to get out of it after only a few
minutes of Boggle or tickling our child. Well, guess what—that sour mood *is*
often trivial or foolish. We've talked ourselves into worrying too much or feeling sorry for ourselves or being angry about something we can't change, and
we should do anything we can to snap out of it.

Play is mindful, in a way. It takes us out of our usual roles and puts us in incongruous, less dignified, situations. It teaches us flexibility, the capacity to roll
with the punches and be ready for the unexpected. It makes us be spontaneous
and in the moment. It often gets us interacting with others in ways we're not
used to, where we don't feel as controlled as we usually do. Many forms of
play get the body involved, the large muscle groups practicing balance and coordination; activities we often neglect as adults but which are really very integrating for the two halves of the brain.

There are other ways than play to experience joy. Sensual pleasures fill us
with endorphins. Humor is not only fun, but a highly creative and mindfulness-
making experience, because it depends so much on changing our perspectives.
And then there is also the necessity of learning to appreciate small things more.
How often have you sat through a concert or a movie preoccupied with worries and aggravations? Suppose you could stop doing that, and more: begin
to appreciate and value your everyday experience, the fact that the world is
full of miracles and mysteries and things to feel good about. *We only have to
practice.*

Fulfillment is more complicated than joy. Fulfillment usually means that
mindful, deliberate activity has been involved. When we feel fulfilled, we have

been thinking creatively, challenging ourselves, taking chances, or opening up our world to new perspectives and experiences. Mindful activity is inherently pleasurable. We are curious by nature, and we possess the drive to be in control, to master our experience, to produce something useful. Mindful activity satisfies all those needs, and fulfillment is how our minds register the resulting emotions.

Fulfilling activities can absorb us completely: reading a good book, having a thoughtful conversation, figuring out why the engine isn't running right and knowing how to fix it. They can also be long-term, in the background: raising our children the way we think is right; finishing your thesis; working out a difficult problem at work; getting the promotion you've been wanting. They are often both left- and right-brained, getting us to pay attention to our feelings and hunches as well as our knowledge base and logical skills. They give us a sense of pride or mastery. They help us feel coherent—all of one piece, not scattered and distracted and unfocused.

You may notice that I haven't mentioned acquisition as either a joy or a fulfillment. One reason that getting new things isn't especially rewarding is that old Hedonic Treadmill again—we quickly adapt to the new, and want more. We're born, I think, with a nameless hunger that's always telling us *I want, I want, I want.* You can't satisfy that hunger through buying it things, because it always wants more. So another reason why getting new things isn't rewarding is that we have an awareness that it's not going to solve the problem, but we give in to our impulse anyway. We feel guilty and ineffectual as a result. Unfortunately, too many people don't know any other way to feel good, and they may be stuck on the treadmill forever.

The Coherent Narrative

All along I've been talking about the importance of building a coherent autobiographical (or autonoetic) narrative for ourselves—the ability to see ourselves over time, from childhood through now on into old age, and experience ourselves as the same person in different situations. To understand ourselves and forgive ourselves; to see our motivations and struggles with compassion and humor. The brain researchers are telling us this is an essential ability to be a good parent, and to go forward into aging without despair, with a sense of generativity and continuity. I remain semiapologetic about this concept, because it seems so abstruse and hard to pin down. In apology I submit this exercise, which I think can give us the experience of what the concept means.

Exercise 12. **Developing a Coherent Narrative**

Return to your biography. Write about yourself now. Observe yourself with compassionate curiosity, without judging. Write a brief sketch of yourself, your interests, your passions, your habits. Is there trouble now? What does it seem to be? Is there more fear than you want? Are you doing things you're not proud of? If so, you're like everyone else. I have yet to meet a perfect person.

Look at the present trouble in the context of its development over your lifetime. Perhaps this is an old wound that has never fully healed. Perhaps it is simply the effect of the Perpetual Stress Response eroding your confidence and skill. Consider this trouble as perhaps a fear that you should face. Maybe it has you running mindlessly, and you will be better off to stop and put your guard down. Whatever it is, the fear won't kill you.

On the other hand, maybe it will be your burden to struggle with this issue the rest of your life. Can you think about accepting that? Can you think about loving yourself and enjoying life anyway?

Think about yourself five years from now. Knowing what you now know about how much of the world you can control, what would you like to be different in five years? Can you make a plan that will ensure that will happen? If so, you should put your plan into action. If you can't make a plan, perhaps you should wish for something else, because what you want doesn't seem within your power to control.

Carry these ideas into your everyday functioning:

- Learn to observe, describe, and participate with awareness, without judging.
- Attend to emotions and events, even if they are distressing; feelings are what they are—they won't kill you.
- Describe events and responses in words meaningful to you. Avoid labels. This is essential both for communication and for self-control.
- Learn to discriminate between emotional states and their precipitating events. The emotion doesn't inevitably have to be associated with the event.
- Focus the mind on *current* activity; on what *works*.

Whether we have depression or anxiety, an addiction or a psychophysiological problem, we can be sure that our thoughts—and our methods of thinking—have become part of the problem. The Perpetual Stress Response reaches deep within us, deep within cell tissue to our DNA itself, and in the process it has its effects on our brain cells and circuits as well. In our minds, life teaches us certain lessons, and we draw certain conclusions—we can't help this—but they're not all accurate. They're distorted by a fear and stress which we have trouble acknowledging, and they try to explain our experience at the same time as pretending that our fears are baseless—oh, and by the way, we're perfectly innocent as well. Given these biases, you couldn't expect our thought processes to be dead-on-target all the time. Still, we retain the *capacity* for objective thought, and we have to use mindful attention to apply that capacity to our own thought processes. In doing so, we free ourselves from the most vicious circles that take root right in our own brains and keep us miserable, hopeless, and confused.

Getting Along with Your Body

Most of us will live long enough and well enough to get seriously ill with a stress-related disease.
—Robert Sapolsky

WE'VE been talking a lot about the connections between the mind, the brain, and the body. Now we're going to go into detail on how the body is affected by stress. If you are lucky enough to enjoy good physical health, no significant aches or pains, no recurring mysterious illnesses, you don't need this chapter, except for the last section on preventive maintenance. But chances are that if you're over thirty, living in a culture that produces the Perpetual Stress Response, you have some stress-related health problems. It may be one of the new "nonspecific" diseases—fibromyalgia and many others; it may be a stress reaction in your digestive system; it may be an autoimmune disorder like Crohn's disease or multiple sclerosis; it may be a chronic pain condition that doesn't respond to treatment. Even weight control and eating disorders are highly influenced by stress. Or it may be that you have a major illness like cancer or heart disease, and how you deal with stress may have some impact on the course of your illness. Whatever it is, understanding how stress—especially the stress you're not aware of—impacts your condition can be very helpful. And learning how to unstress yourself, to the extent possible, can make your life better, longer, and richer.

Try to imagine how quickly things are changing now in mind-body medicine. As recently as 1980, science assumed that the immune system was completely autonomous, closed to any influence from life experience or thoughts or feelings. Now we know that's not the case at all—*the immune system is shaped by our earliest emotional experiences as infants learning to cope with stress*—and it continues to respond and adapt to our emotions and feelings throughout our lives. As recently as ten years ago, we didn't know the adult brain grows new nerve cells. Last month (as I write this in early 2004) we learned that the adult brain changes in size and shape in response to new learning. Developments like these mean that many, many of our old ideas about illness and stress have to be reevaluated, and the process has not gotten very far yet. Unfortunately, the average MD, psychotherapist, or alternative medicine practitioner is not going to be able to use this new perspective very well, because current practices interfere with its application and it's very hard to tie it all together and discover the practical implications. It's up to the individual to digest this information and use it to prevent and recover from the Perpetual Stress Response.

We've talked about the power of assumptions and beliefs to distort how we view the world and create self-fulfilling prophecies that trap us in destructive cycles. These assumptions, beliefs, and stories are also part of our bodies. The beliefs we hold about ourselves and the world are manifested in changes in our brains and in our nervous, endocrine, and musculoskeletal systems. Science is just on the verge of being able to trace the connections between thoughts and their physiological pathways, but it won't be long. We know now that depression is tied to changes in brain structure and to hormone levels detectable in the bloodstream. Pain can be controlled by our minds, even clearly "physical" pain like surgery. People who believe in positive myths about themselves live longer, have fewer heart attacks, and require less anesthesia during surgery. Optimists' wounds heal more quickly than those of pessimists.

Social status is also an important factor in health. Monkeys who are far down in the pecking order have more atherosclerosis and are less fertile. Women who view their social status as higher than average sleep better, have lower resting cortisol levels, more efficient hearts, and less abdominal fat. Interestingly, what we *believe* our social status to be is more strongly linked to health than objective measures of status.

Pessimistic, anxious, and depressed people, besides enjoying life less, have poorer health. They have higher blood pressure, their immune systems are less effective, and they recover more slowly and less completely from surgery. They have that pathetic euphemism of statisticians, "excess mortality." One study of over twenty thousand individuals suggested that the net effect on physical health of chronic anxiety or depression was the equivalent of feeling twelve years older than your age. On the other hand, people who are hopeful have better health after heart transplants, recover more quickly from bypass surgery, have less anginal pain, do better and live longer with HIV treatment, and have generally better-functioning immune systems.

We need to address several slightly different subjects in this section, all connected by the interaction of the Perpetual Stress Response with our bodies, brains, and minds. The first is our struggle with weight and eating. Next is stress- and trauma-related disease, including what I've called nonspecific illness: chronic fatigue syndrome and fibromyalgia, mysterious conditions seemingly epidemic now, and some other illnesses that may be related. We will need to understand the immune system especially well to understand these conditions. There are other nonspecific illnesses that are generally understood to be stress-related, though the immune system doesn't seem so highly involved: irritable bowel syndrome and other digestive disorders, allergies, headache. Then there are conditions that have been thought to be exclusively "physical" in nature, like diabetes, lupus, Crohn's disease, multiple sclerosis, and some others, that are increasingly thought of as responses to stress and trauma. Finally, there is the interaction of the stress response with catastrophic illness like cancer and heart disease, where the patient's ability to cope with stress successfully can influence his prognosis.

The third major subject is how we can adapt to conditions that cannot be relieved. We'll look primarily at chronic pain conditions, which is another area where new research is shaking up old assumptions. This means we have to understand the body's pain system. We'll also look, though, at the pleasure system, for what it can tell us about making adaptation easier.

Weight Control and Stress

Our struggles with weight control, and the development of eating-related mental disorders like anorexia and bulimia, are intimately tied in with cultural change. First of all, our bodies were not designed to live with abundant food. Animals that are allowed to eat as much as they want tend to die early; study after study shows that restricting intake to 30 to 70 percent less than free eating results in improvements in longevity, immune response, physical endurance, learning ability, and delays in onset of cancer, diabetes, and autoimmune disease. Our digestive systems are designed to make very efficient use of sparse food, with the rare attack of gluttony when the harvest was in or a big animal was killed. We're designed to graze, an eating style that leaves us healthier and makes much more efficient use of food, rather than sit down to three big meals a day, which dull us and slow us down and make us vulnerable to cheetahs.

Second, eating habits are highly sensitive to conditioning—after all, Pavlov's first experiments were to make his dogs drool. We too drool at television ads, beautiful supermarket displays, high-fat and high-calorie snacks at the convenience store. Advertising (and portion growth) is largely responsible for the American epidemic of obesity that has resulted in twice as many adults and three times as many adolescents overweight now as in 1980. Obesity is a great example of blaming the victim—when society provides constant drool-inducing stimuli, we still look down on those who don't have the "self-discipline" to be thin.

Third, eating is a very emotional process. Weight problems are associated with eating for emotional reasons rather than eating when you're hungry. When we're stuck in a society that tells us it's our duty to be happy at the same time as it continually reinforces how inadequate we are, we can't win; we might as well stay in and finish the ice cream. Much of our eating is to distract us from depression or anxiety or loneliness; we eat to give ourselves a little present. "Comfort food" is not a joke; we do get comforted by a carbohydrate rush—but there is always a crash to follow. Most dieters break their diets in anger, sending a big middle finger to the world that is judging them harshly for being obese. Rationalization comes to the aid of those who want to continue overeating. Alice, whom you met in Chapter 4, observed that the three worst words for dieters are "Might as well."

It's deeply ironic to me that in our society obesity is associated with being poor. Throughout history and in the third world today, obesity has always meant wealth, because only the wealthy could afford to overeat. But in the West today, mass marketing of prepared foods and fast foods, high in carbs, fats, and sugar, lures in people who feel overwhelmed and demoralized and are looking for a quick way to feel better. The well-to-do, meanwhile, have more time to shop and prepare foods carefully or more money to eat out; and besides are preoccupied with their appearance. In my area of Connecticut, you can see the differences just by driving from town to town: in the working-class towns, the men have beer bellies and the women have big hips; in the upper-class towns, everyone looks slim and fit. In the expensive private schools, *all* the kids are slim and gleaming, if not anorexic. Obesity has important negative social consequences. Overweight people are less likely to be hired, and they earn less money than thin people. It also has important health consequences.

Low-fiber, high-fat, and high-sodium diets increase risk for heart disease, colon cancer, and high blood pressure. Obesity increases risk of degenerative joint disease.

Perpetual stress makes things worse. An overload of stress hormones interferes with our ability to store fat, sending more of it directly to the abdomen (as does alcohol: if you want to lose a beer belly, stop drinking). Abdominal fat is a greater health risk than other kinds of fats; pear-shaped people are better off than apple people. Many people report that carbs numb them out; sugar and other comfort foods are known to interfere with the Perpetual Stress Response, but of course they add to our weight and damage our health.

Scientists know that diets don't work. In the best studies, fewer than 25 percent of dieters can maintain their weight loss over a period of years. But no one can accept that fact. Each of us seems to have a "natural" weight that our bodies inevitably return to, even when we restrict intake and stay active; and for many of us, that "natural" weight is well above what society considers attractive. Yet how many people are desperately unhappy with themselves—and looked down on by others—because they carry a few extra pounds? To lose weight requires a permanent change in eating habits and activity level. The weight won't melt away, but gradually you will feel and look better. A basic knowledge of nutrition really helps. It shocked me very much to learn that the meat course in your main meal should be about the size of a pack of cards—and of course it should be *lean* meat, fish, or poultry. Our consumption of fats has doubled since our grandparents' generation, and fat makes you fat.

So give up dieting, unless you are really ready to make a permanent change in eating habits and activity level. While there are health consequences to obesity, the health consequences of yo-yo dieting may be worse. If you're over forty, and for most of your life you've been 10 to 30 percent over what the statistical tables say you should weigh, get used to it. Eat healthily and work to get yourself in shape, but don't beat yourself up for lacking willpower. Use your willpower to keep your eating moderate, and allow yourself to be proud of that.

You *can*, however, expect to be successful if you want to control emotional eating. Remember all we've said about conditioning: our nervous systems are primed and waiting to link emotions with events, like eating. If you've done it a lot, you can expect that, when you're depressed (anxious, angry, lonely, cranky, bored . . .) you'll experience the desire to eat. Work on extinguishing this connection. The first thing to do is to address the emotion, if possible. Call a friend and talk it out. Plan for how you'll deal with the person who's made you angry. If this isn't successful, you can break the connection between the feeling and the desire to eat by introducing any healthy intervening behavior. Go for a walk, clean the kitchen, call a friend. I've been moderately successful by drinking a glass of water and making a deal with myself that I won't let myself eat for a half hour. By then the desire is past, or I'm in control enough to eat something healthy.

Eating disorders are the extreme of our complex relationship with food. I believe that these conditions are metaphorical protests against stress and lack of love. To starve yourself when food is plentiful (as in anorexia) or to binge till you're blue then throw it all up again (bulimia)—these are rejections of what the world has to offer. They're also often the only thing the patient can reliably control. Yes, it's true that eating disorders are also a result of society's obsession with thinness, fashion magazines holding up frankly grotesque-looking young women as models of beauty, that makes readers excessively self-conscious of every pound. And it's also true that these conditions are *extremely* vicious circles, very tough habits to break despite our sincere efforts to overcome them. But too many of my eating-disordered patients have been victims

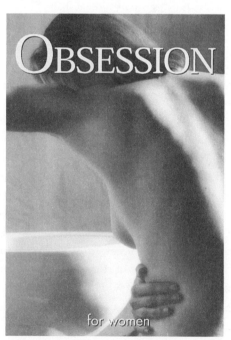

(SOURCE: ADBUSTERS MEDIA FOUNDATION)

of PTSD, usually rape or sexual abuse, for me to believe that the conditions aren't ultimately stress-related protests. My bulimic patients tell me that purging is precipitated by a growing feeling of panic, and they are rewarded for it because the body reliably feels calm afterward—often the only experience of calm in the patient's life. It's like alcohol, for some people the only reliable friend. In eating disorders, the focus on exactly what is consumed, the planning that goes into purging—these are safe distractions, something the patient can control when the whole world feels dangerous and intrusive and the fight-or-flight response is stuck in the "on" position.

Perpetual Stress and the Immune System

I first became interested in this topic when Nancy (described in Chapter 7), a member of my self-help group, began to talk about her physical symptoms and her experiences with medical treatment. There was no question that Nancy had major depression. She also had a significant trauma history, both as a child and as an adult. Physically, she suffered from debilitating migraines and a great deal of fatigue. Her MD had referred her to a rheumatologist, who told her she had fibromyalgia and chronic fatigue syndrome, and perhaps chronic Lyme disease. Nancy was intelligent but unsophisticated. She assumed that these were physical illnesses not connected to her depression. I thought it only made sense: that if I walked around for thirty years as tense as Nancy, always afraid, always hypervigilant, unable to relax, my joints and muscles would ache too, and I would always be on the edge of exhaustion. I watched over the next few years as Nancy became a guinea pig for medication: stimulants, relaxants, antibiotics, hormones, painkillers, steroids.[1] She went through hot flashes, cold sweats, deep depression, hypomanic highs, disfiguring skin eruptions, insomnia, nightmares, sleeping too much, impaired concentration, crippling anxiety, the fear of losing her mind, a psychiatric hospitalization, and I kept trying to suggest this was largely due to the medication. She'd agree, but then she'd go back to the doctor, and he'd talk her into trying something else.

I began to be aware of how many other patients of mine and in our clinic

---

1 Since I was a member of this experimental leaderless self-help group, I did not confront Nancy as vigorously as I would have if she'd been my patient. She was in treatment with another therapist at the clinic, with whom I shared my concerns about what Nancy was putting herself through. As I look back on it now I wish I had been much more direct with her.

were being treated for the same conditions. They were all being treated by us for depression and anxiety disorders. Some had better results than Nancy, but none seemed to get much real relief from their physical symptoms. I decided to try to educate myself. I learned that patients with depression visit their MDs more frequently, are operated on more frequently, and have more nonpsychiatric emergency room visits than the general population. I learned that depression is not the only emotional disorder involved with the body. Anxiety causes early death, too, and PTSD has far too many somatic repercussions. Anxiety and depression somehow result in wounds healing more slowly. In all, 50 to 70 percent of visits to primary care physicians are for psychologically related complaints. I began to wonder what people like Candace Pert, not a New Age mystic but a tough-minded research scientist, meant when they said things like "the body is the unconscious mind." Here's where I've come out:

There is a more radical view of the mind-body connection than I have pursued in this book. I've not pursued it because I don't feel confident enough of my biological skills to understand it totally, and also I think it's easier for the reader to think in the old familiar terms. But I see this view as ultimately truthful and helpful. Candace Pert puts it this way: the brain and nervous system, the endocrine glands, and the immune system are in fact not the separate organs we see, but a network of communication, linked by information substances (including hormones, neurotransmitters, and other molecules). The emphasis is on the *network,* not the constituent parts. Let's go on in her words:

> I like to speculate that what the mind is is the flow of information as it moves among the cells, organs, and systems of the body. . . . The mind as we experience it is immaterial, yet it has a physical substrate, which is both the body and the brain. It may also be said to have a nonmaterial, nonphysical substrate that has to do with the flow of that information. *The mind, then, is that which holds the network together, often acting below our consciousness, linking and coordinating the major systems and their organs and cells in an intelligently orchestrated symphony of life.* Thus, we might refer to the whole system as a psychosomatic information network, linking *psyche,* which comprises all that is of an ostensibly nonmaterial nature, such as mind, emotion, and soul, to *soma,* which is the material world of molecules, cells and organs. Mind and body, psyche and soma.

The body is not a machine to carry around the brain; rather the brain is just one organ among many that makes up our self, our consciousness. Our self is not located up in the brain pan, it's distributed all over us. Memory is not only in the brain, but in the guts, the immune system, the neuromuscular network all over our body. When we feel an emotion, it's not just a passing experience in the mind; each emotional experience changes the brain and the body a little. Each emotion is a signal that there is an important chemical reaction happening everywhere within us. How we choose to live with that experience—to stuff it, pretend it's not happening, take it out on someone else, or accept it, listen to it, and move on—has important consequences for our health.

As we've said, emotions are the link between mind and body. Emotions are mediated by the release of chemical messengers—hormones and neurotransmitters—between cells not only in the brain but throughout the body, most importantly between the nervous system, the endocrine system, and the immune system. Perhaps soon we will be able to identify exactly how these messengers work to signal the different emotions; but for now it's clear that we are a unified organism. *And it's emotions that give us a self.* "The biochemicals of emotion," writes Pert, "are . . . the messengers carrying information to link the major systems of the body into one unit that we can call the bodymind."

The body often speaks for the mind. The concept of *somatization* may seem mysterious, but we all know it. It's the child who gets sick or gets a headache, even a slight fever, before a tough day at school. It's me feeling my back tense up when I'm somewhere I feel ill at ease, like a cocktail party. Somatization refers to the experience of emotional distress as physical symptoms. It's another defense mechanism, and it serves a defensive purpose by distracting you from the real cause of your distress. It can range from the person who experiences more headaches or an exacerbation of chronic back pain during times of stress—who knows that his body is complaining about the stress he's under and that he'd better do something about it—to the person who is completely disabled by painful or crippling conditions that do not respond to medical treatment—who is completely unaware that there is any link to emotional distress. The medical profession recognizes the phenomenon of somatization, though current practice interferes with its effective treatment. Medical specialization, the practice of defensive medicine, and the erosion of the health insurance system (leading to use of the emergency room for primary health care) have contributed to the trend of patients with recurrent complaints being passed along to specialists who end up treating them with expensive palliative care. Neither the primary care physician nor the specialist wants to tell the patient directly what everyone thinks: that the symptoms are the result of stress, more emotional than physical in origin. But the further the patient goes in this process, the more time, effort, money, pain, and hope he has invested in his medical care, the less likely he is to welcome this news.

Remember what we know about the developing mind: the mother teaches the baby what emotions are, by responding to some emotions and ignoring others. She teaches the baby what's acceptable and what's not: what's "me" and what's "not me." When few or no emotions are permitted into the "me," children grow into *alexithymic* adults—who have few or no words for feelings, who indeed experience almost no feelings. Yet the chemistry of emotions still flows through their body in response to every emotional stimulus; thus they may be forced to use the body to express emotions, and they will vigorously resist the idea that a physical symptom could have an emotional basis. They may be able to describe their condition in vivid, calm detail, without any reference to stress or emotional reaction, greatly impressing doctors who believe this to be one of the most lucid and rational patients they've ever met; therefore the condition must be real. So, by virtue of the fact that the patient doesn't experience emotions, or by virtue of the way contemporary medicine treats refractory complaints, the patient's somatization becomes very real and very concrete.

In talking about somatizing I've been tap-dancing around the dirty word: *psychosomatic*. John Sarno, a respected back pain specialist, and others have commented on the irony of our aversion to the term. Our aversion comes from misunderstanding the word: it simply means mind and body are both involved. It doesn't mean the problem is all in your head. *Everyone is psychosomatic. Psychosomatic is normal.* You wouldn't want your mind not to be affecting your body, because in addition to causing problems it also gives great benefits. But psychosomatic patients do give doctors fits, because their problems don't respond neatly to conventional treatments. I think their frustration with psychosomatic patients has been translated into common speech in the disparaging, dismissive tone we associate with the term.

Here's a mindful question: are warts psychosomatic? They're not imaginary, they're very real. They're localized viral infections on the skin, quite common; most of us have had some. They can be treated with acid or freezing if they're persistent, but most warts seem to go away by themselves after a couple of years. Warts are also highly subject to mental control, because hypnosis is often an effective treatment. In one study, subjects were given the hypnotic suggestion to rid themselves of warts only on one side of their bodies. Nine of four-

Exercise 13. **Body Scan**

This is a comfortable exercise—in reality, a form of self-hypnosis—that can help relieve localized pain and also help you gain a much better awareness of your body and its mechanics: what's connected to what. It's great for relieving aching muscles and joints.

1. Lie down on your back on a pad or comfortable rug. Keep the room and your mind free from distractions for the next half hour.
2. Focus on your breathing, as in a mindfulness meditation.
3. Once you feel centered, turn your attention to the soles of your feet. Pay attention to any sensation you are aware of there. Pay attention mindfully, without judging, without explaining, without associating. Just be present with the sensation for a few minutes. Then, let yourself imagine that your breath is flowing through your body down to the soles of your feet. As you continue to breathe, you might experience a feeling like a release of tension, as if the muscles and tendons in your soles are opening up or softening.
4. Turn your attention to the rest of your feet. Again, pay attention mindfully to any sensation you are aware of there. Allow yourself to be present with the situation, without judging, without explaining, without associating. Then imagine that your breath is flowing from your lungs down to your feet. Allow yourself to feel whatever you feel—there may be a release of tension, a relaxing.
5. Proceed up your legs in the same manner—your lower legs, knees, thighs, pelvis, hips, and buttocks. Be mindful and take your time with each body part. You don't have to hurry. Pay attention to all the sensations present, without trying to make them different, without thinking or judging. Finish by breathing into the body part and notice what you feel.
6. Go to your fingers, and do the same thing. Pay attention to all the sensations you are aware of there. After you have attended mindfully, let your breath now reach your fingers. Then do the same for the palms of your hands, your wrists, forearms, upper arms. Finish by breathing into and through each part and notice what you feel.

(Continued)

7. Return to your belly. Apply this mindful attention and breathing through to your abdomen, your belly, your flanks, your lower back, your upper back, your chest, your shoulders.

8. Now visualize the organs you can sense inside your body—your guts, your stomach and esophagus; your heart; your lungs and windpipe; your liver and kidneys; your ovaries and uterus, or your prostate. Attend to each of these in turn, mindfully. Try to get in touch with any sensation you feel there—perhaps some pain or discomfort, but also perhaps a constriction, a swelling, a burning. Allow yourself to be present with these sensations without judging, without explaining, without associating. Now imagine that you can direct your breath to that organ. As the breath touches the organ and then recedes, perhaps some of the sensation goes with it.

9. Now go to your neck. Pay attention to how it feels, without judging or thinking. Allow your neck to breathe. Do the same for your throat—is anything caught in there? Let the breath reach it and let it go. Go on to your facial muscles and your scalp. You will probably find some areas of tightness. Let them breathe and relax.

10. Think about any place in your body that still has tension or pain. Pay attention mindfully to those sensations. Breathe and let the breath come down to those areas, opening up any areas of tightness or pain and creating a sense of warmth, of calm, of space. Imagine the tension flowing out as you exhale.

11. Imagine that you have a breath hole at the top of your head, like a whale. Breathe in from the top of your head. Let the breath go down all the way to the soles of your feet, the tips of your fingers, any last areas of tension. Repeat this breath a few times, allowing it to take away any tension or pain.

This exercise is not only about relieving tension, it's also about helping us get in touch with our bodies. Too many of us are living in a left-brain world, always jumping from one crisis to the next. We take our bodies for granted, and they have to do something pretty dramatic sometimes to get our attention. I think if we can practice this kind of exercise with some regularity, our muscles, joints, and organs won't have to go into severe pain or break down in order to get us to attend to them.

teen were able to do just that. How is this possible? How is it that hypnosis works, but simply telling people to wish their warts away doesn't? We just don't have answers to these questions. But clearly warts fall under the dreaded "psychosomatic" label.

The Immune System and the Mind

With that semantic discussion out of the way, let's look at how the mind affects one very important part of the body, the immune system.

The immune system is very much like radar, always scanning the body for signs of microscopic foreign invaders. Like radar, it needs to be calibrated accurately. If radar is set too high, it picks up too much "noise"—from every tree, house, tower—so the invader can't be distinguished from what belongs in the area. If the immune system is set too high, it also picks up noise, and will react by generating an immune response to things that are not really a threat. This may be part of what's happening in allergies, asthma, chronic fatigue syndrome, and fibromyalgia. But the immune system can be set too low as well. When radar is set too low, it misses important things—it doesn't "see" planes accurately. When the immune system is set too low, it also misses things, and we become more vulnerable to attack. This is why we are more prone to colds when we're under stress, and why people with AIDS, with damaged immune systems, are vulnerable to opportunistic infections.

The immune system is a complex collection of organs, tissues, cells, and transmitters that is still not very well understood. Unlike the digestive or circulatory systems, it is not made up of organs that are structurally connected and serve a single function. The immune system consists of organs like the thymus, spleen, bone marrow, and lymph nodes, which anatomists had not found much function for until relatively recently (now we understand that part of their function is to generate and store immune cells) and which communicate indirectly, through the blood, lymphatic circulation, and nervous system. Immune cells, specially designed to attack foreign bodies, flow through the blood to reach every part of the body. There are also cells that serve an immune function distributed in every organ, especially the skin; and immune system messages are also carried by the nervous system and bloodstream. Lymph cells in the bloodstream are able to respond quickly to any foreign invader—bacteria, virus, cancer cell—in the body. There are several types of cells, which serve important roles in the immune response; among the most important are:

- *Macrophages* (white blood cells, leukocytes) are scavenger cells that swallow and digest invaders, cleaning up debris from infections. They also send signals attracting T cells when they encounter an invader.
- *T cells* destroy or weaken cells with foreign antigens. They are formed from the stem cells in bone marrow, and migrate to the thymus gland, where they mature and specialize. Some T cells become messengers, others kill invaders, others kill cancer cells, and still others suppress the immune response once an infection has been eliminated. It is T cells that are damaged by the AIDS virus; without T cells any little infection we get can develop into a serious illness.
- *B cells* produce proteins called antibodies that are specifically designed to attack each unique invader. They are also generated in the bone marrow, and are found in the lymph nodes and spleen.
- *Memory cells* specialize in recognizing a new attack from an invader that has attacked before. They coordinate a rapid response from the B and T cells.
- In addition to these cell structures, the immune system also relies on proteins and antibodies such as the interleukims and interferon.

The immune system's response to acute stress has proven to be more complicated than originally thought. It had long been known that stress interferes with immune functioning; in fact, stress lowers the white blood cell count. But this didn't make sense to some researchers; from an evolutionary standpoint, why should we do without the immune response when we might need it most, to combat infection from a wound? Careful research has shown that the initial immune response to stress is to direct those white blood cells to where they will be needed most, organs like the skin and lymph nodes. Scientists who had been looking for them in the bloodstream mistakenly concluded that they had somehow disappeared instead of realizing they were hiding in storage. This phenomenon is one part of the system that allows the immune response to "learn" invaders—repeated invasion by the same germs is met more quickly and more vigorously by the immune system each time. We develop immunity to germs in this way; viruses, because of their ability to mutate quickly, are much more difficult for the immune system to learn.

The body and the immune system, if they are healthy, recover quickly from acute stress. We have lots of little thermostat-type mechanisms built in whose function is to maintain *homeostasis*, bring us back to normal from any major change. But the effects of prolonged stress, stress since childhood, are another affair altogether. A major review of the literature on stress and the immune system published in 2004 bears that out. The researchers found that experiences of acute stress may actually be good for the immune system, as if keeping it in shape. In all twenty-three studies of prolonged stress, however, stress had "negative effects on almost all functional measures of the immune system." Unfortunately, there were only nine studies of the effects of what the researchers called "distant stressors" (childhood or wartime trauma), too few to draw any conclusions.

Prolonged stress, as we've said, means too much of the stress hormones, including cortisol, floating around the body. Too much cortisol (and other glucocorticoids) has all kinds of nasty effects we've mentioned, but we haven't looked at what it does to the immune system. It causes shrinkage of the thymus gland, where new T cells and B cells are formed. It makes the T and B cells already in the system less responsive to messages from other cells about foreign invaders. And, most impressive, *too much cortisol kills immune cells.*

Consider how lifelong stress appears to be related to some aspects of health. People who had an anxious or ambivalent attachment relationship with their mother turn out, as adults, to be more likely to report symptoms and seek medical attention than securely attached or dismissing people. Remember our discussion of attachment research previously. We focused on the mother-child relationship and its impact on the child's emotional system, but there is also an impact on the child's immune system. It starts with nursing, when breast milk provides lymphocytes and other cells that serve an immunizing function, beginning by killing intestinal bugs that can cause discomfort and colic in the infant. When we cuddle, play with, or hug the child, his antibody response is strengthened—don't ask me how, but it happens. Remember that infant rats who get licked and groomed more by their mothers are smarter and less fearful as adults, have stronger immune systems, and are more attentive mothers themselves. In the same way, a child who is not "handled" very much has lower levels of immune cells in the bloodstream. This leads to increased activity by the infant's pituitary and adrenal systems, resulting in increasing levels of stress hormones (ACTH and cortisol) in the bloodstream. It's during the attachment phase of infancy, when the neurons in the child's brain are developing their specialized functions, that the nerve networks between the brain and the immune organs (thymus, spleen, bone marrow, and lymph nodes) are developing also. Although we're never aware of it, it's from our brains that these organs receive their orders and coordination. Allan Schore feels enough confidence to state definitively: *"The infant's attachment relationship with the mother permanently influences the development of the individual's future immune capacities."* The child whose caregivers aren't responsive to his needs goes into the stress response, which can flood the body and brain with stress hormones, and which can result in brain cell death, damage to the ability to control emotions and behavior, and tissue damage in the body, among other things. When the mother responds to the child's distress with soothing and comfort, stress hormones return to normal. The mother is *imprinting* on the child the ability to modulate the stress response. When the child is left under stress, stress hormones kill, among other things, the cells that produce T cells, and T cell disturbances are seen in autoimmune diseases like rheumatoid arthritis, MS, and lupus. Continuing stress in adult life means overproduction of cortisol and adrenaline, which interfere with the ability of T and B cells to reproduce.

This explains my clinical experience. The three lupus sufferers I've known were all victims of childhood sexual abuse. Almost all the patients I've known whose bodies have extreme or bizarre reactions to medications (like Jane Jones in Chapter 7) have had narcissistic or exploitative parents—it's as if their bodies can't trust and have to protest against the intrusion of meds into what has become a very important boundary. Most of the patients I've known with chronic fatigue syndrome or fibromyalgia have been depressed since childhood, though usually in an unrecognized way—they've been the caretakers in their families (see Chapter 6), the children who take care of a nonfunctioning parent while their own needs are stuffed away, denied, and ignored. When language is not yet available, the body speaks for you: it's possible that the baby who was invasively traumatized goes on to develop rashes, allergies, or diarrhea as a way of communicating "stay away from me," while the baby who was neglected develops pain, weakness, or another debility as a way of saying "take care of me."

There may be other effects of childhood stress on the body. There is a link between narcissistic personality and the "type A" personality prone to coronary disease. Narcissistic rage, and the inability to modulate it, can kill you. The vulnerability may come from the fact that disturbances in attachment result in nerve cells never fully developing in that same orbitofrontal cortex that is thought to be so important in developing a healthy self-concept. This same area controls ACTH and corticosteroid (stress hormones again) levels in the brain. The same area has been implicated in gastric ulcer, bulimia, and hypertension.

PTSD also damages the immune system. It is now generally accepted that people with PTSD as a result of childhood trauma have disturbances in the body's two main stress-response systems: the hypothalamic-pituitary-adrenal (HPA) axis and the sympathoadrenomedullary system. As a result, the individual with PTSD suffers from difficulty regulating the immune system. One difficulty is an out-of-proportion inflammatory response. Under ideal circumstances, the stress response is self-limiting. Cortisol plays an important role in this, acting like a thermostat, shutting down its own production when the stress is removed. It also checks the immune response. But too little cortisol allows the immune system to run off with itself, resulting in immune responses to rather innocuous substances, as what happens in allergies and asthma.

Acute stress has its own effects on the immune system. People who are unemployed or socially isolated are more likely to develop colds than other people. Marital strife and bereavement can weaken the immune system. Patients who report greater stress levels before surgery have slower wound healing and impaired immune responses in the wound. People who have more interactions with others, surprisingly, have a lower incidence of colds than people who are isolated. This is a counterintuitive finding because we assume that the more social contacts, the more germs, hence the more colds. But having a social network strengthens the immune system, apparently by a factor more than enough to offset the increased risk of infection. People with cancer who form strong bonds with each other through group treatment will generally live longer than those who keep to the periphery.

Damage to the immune system is not necessarily permanent. Nursing home residents trained in several different stress reduction programs, including the relaxation response, had a significantly improved immune response after a month. Caregivers of Alzheimer's patients improved their immune response after a simple eight-week stress management program that taught them how to use cognitive-behavioral methods to recognize and reframe their stresses. Patients with cancer who learn relaxation and cognitive therapy also have an improved immune response.

Damaged immune systems can be repaired because the immune system *learns*. The brain has receptors for the immune system–signaling molecule, interleukin. We've known since the 1970s that the immune system can learn, although the research was greeted very skeptically at first. Robert Ader and Nick Cohen at the University of Rochester gave mice saccharine at the same time as an anticancer drug that suppresses the immune system. Before long, when the mice were given saccharine alone, their immune-cell counts went down. This was a breakthrough finding; until then the immune system was thought to be completely autonomous and automatic. (Later, Ader and his colleagues were able to show that the immune system can also be strengthened by learning.) Now we know that the human immune system is responsive not only to learning, but to meaning; spouses of patients who died from breast cancer were found to have reduced lymph cell production. It reached its lowest ebb about two months after the patient's death and returned to normal gradually over the next year. Our own belief in our ability to control the stresses that we experience (not our actual ability, our *belief* in our ability) dramatically affects our neuroendocrine functioning in ways that can have an important impact on immune functioning.

But at this point we should be cautious in our optimism that we can heal a damaged immune system. The awareness that we *can* hasn't been around long enough for us to know reliably *how.* Robert Ader and other researchers are concerned that their discoveries in psychoneuroimmunology have been adopted and bastardized by people who claim to teach us to control our immune systems through various New Age techniques—fads in nutrition, in psychotherapy, in hypnosis, even in meditation—without any documentation at all that their methods are effective. As Ader says, these people often represent an "anti-scientific, anti-intellectual, and anti-establishment" viewpoint. My belief in and advocacy of mindfulness and other methods for healing the damage of the Perpetual Stress Response represents a hope and a clinical guess, backed up with some evidence and experience, that we can learn to control some of the disease processes that seem to be stress-related, but I must acknowledge that we still have a great deal to learn.

Autoimmune Diseases

In this varied group of conditions, the body's own immune system is turning on itself; the immune cells that usually work against foreign invaders somehow identify our own individual organs or tissues as foreign, and begin to destroy them. These diseases include multiple sclerosis, in which the myelin sheaths that wrap nerve cell axons are attacked; rheumatoid arthritis, in which

Body Mindfulness

Remember our trick (Exercise 4, "A Taste of Mindfulness") of having one finger feel the other, then mentally switching, so that you alternate which finger is feeler and which is felt? You can use the same method to have your mind—your mental finger—explore other parts of your body. When I was a kid, this is how I taught myself to raise one eyebrow, but you can do it for much more important purposes.

As part of your mindfulness meditation, take your mental finger and explore your body for the places where there is pain or tension. You probably know very well where many of these places are, but there are likely to be others you're not aware of—your shoulders or scalp, for instance. It may not be in your muscles or joints, but in your viscera—your stomach, your guts, your heart. Locate the afflicted organ or muscle group with your mental finger and explore it. Create a mental picture with the input from your finger (it may help to look at an anatomy book). When you have a good visualization of the area, let it feel warm. Let it feel relaxed. Let your endorphins bathe it. Comfort it and reassure it. It doesn't have to be so much on guard. Your mind is able to handle things; this poor organ or muscle can stand down.

Repeat this for a week. After a few days, this gets easier and easier to do. You'll be more sensitive to the afflicted area even if you're not in a mindful state. Eventually you'll be able to relax it on command. After a while, it can be much less painful or uncomfortable.

the lining tissue of the joints is attacked; and lupus, thyroiditis, Crohn's disease, scleroderma, psoriasis, and others. Some think that chronic fatigue syndrome and fibromyalgia are also autoimmune diseases. So far, no one has had much luck crafting an effective treatment for any of these conditions, though symptomatic treatments have made many patients' lives easier.

Finding ways to cope better with stress may be helpful, at least in preventing flare-ups (which characterize most of these conditions). Eighty-five percent of exacerbations of multiple sclerosis are caused by psychological stress, though there is such a long latency period—an average of two weeks—that most patients probably do not feel the connection. If a long time period be-tween stress and flare-up characterizes all of these conditions, then that ex-plains why no one has observed this before. Since we can't avoid psychological stress, it follows that we need to learn to cope—as the rest of this chapter sug-gests. I don't want to kindle false hopes here, however; these are all difficult conditions. Change, if any, is going to come slowly, as we make mindfulness, exercise, and other coping mechanisms a part of our everyday life.

Nonspecific Illness

These are the conditions that are often most troubling to patients and most dif-ficult for medicine to treat. They make the sufferer feel blamed and the doctor feel inadequate. Many have only come to our attention within the recent past, which suggests to some that they are a result of increasing stress (like chronic fatigue syndrome) or a result of new environmental conditions (sick building syndrome). But that also raises the possibility that some people have devel-oped their symptoms through the power of suggestion. Still others of these conditions, like bad backs and irritable bowel, have been around for centuries.

If you have a troubling and unexplained physical condition, of course you're likely to be anxious and depressed about it, which of course adds to the stress your body is protesting against. Worse yet, many of these illnesses—fibromyalgia, chronic fatigue syndrome, chronic pain conditions—make it more difficult to do the things we need to do to recover: to exercise, stretch, relax, play, and treat ourselves well. Nonspecific illness feeds on itself like a nuclear reactor; we become victims of a chain reaction of stress→pain→disability→ more stress→more pain→more disability, relentlessly destroying our bodies.

Two recent review articles discuss many of the conditions I have been call-ing nonspecific illnesses, under different names: functional somatic syndromes and symptom-based conditions. They're referring to:

Multiple chemical sensitivity (idiopathic environmental intolerance)
Sick building syndrome
Silicone-associated rheumatic disease (side effects of breast implants)
Gulf War syndrome
Irritable bowel syndrome
Chronic fatigue syndrome
Fibromyalgia

Chronic whiplash syndrome[2]
Chronic Lyme disease
Certain food allergies
Mitral valve prolapse
Hypoglycemia

And I might add:

Temporomandibular jaw syndrome
Chronic candidiasis
Certain chronic pain conditions

The authors note that these conditions are all characterized more by their symptoms, and the accompanying suffering and disability, than by any evident tissue change or damage. In addition:

- The symptoms do not respond to standard treatments.
- There is no known cause.
- There is no known mechanism for how the disease causes its symptoms.
- The conditions are almost entirely diagnosed by self-report; there are few objective indicators.
- It's common for an individual to have two or more of these at the same time.
- It's common for the person to have anxiety, depression, or PTSD as well.
- There is often distrust of the medical system, a sense of being victimized or maltreated.
- There is often a sense of "embattled advocacy"—the patient takes on the mission of educating others about the disease.
- There are often financial or other incentives for demonstrating the "reality" of the illness—disability payments, pain and suffering damages, and so forth.
- There is often sensationalized media attention about the condition.
- Medical clinics and specialties develop a vested interest in perpetuating

---

2 Items from here on down are only referenced in the Barsky and Borus (1999) article.

concern about the illness (but pharmaceutical companies don't, because by definition the condition will not respond to medication).

In addition, these conditions often respond to placebo. People with these illnesses often react defensively to that news, because they feel they are being told it's all in their heads. On the contrary: this is a very important clue to the real nature of these problems. Patients' conditions improve because their systems are responding to the nonspecific effects of placebo treatment: the relief that comes with a relationship with a medical professional, a diagnosis of a specific medical condition, a treatment plan, the positive expectation of getting better. These factors are interrupting the Perpetual Stress Response. The patients' endocrine systems stop producing fight-or-flight hormones, because their brains are telling the endocrine systems that the danger is past. If only we could find more such benign, inexpensive, and time-saving ways to interrupt the Perpetual Stress Response.

Now that the consumer and victims' rights movements have been so widely accepted—even formalized in the Americans with Disabilities Act—it's likely that some people are going to get very angry at me for suggesting that there are psychological factors at work in conditions like fibromyalgia and chronic fatigue syndrome. I hope they don't misunderstand. As we've said, mind and body are one; the body is the unconscious mind. Their illnesses are real, and suggesting that they have an emotional connection does not make them less real. There are psychological factors at work in all aspects of our health, including heart disease and cancer. I have no doubt that in another twenty years research will have described exactly the mechanisms by which stress affects tissue, resulting in the pain of fibromyalgia and the multiple symptoms of chronic fatigue syndrome. Hopefully it will also explain why wounds heal more slowly under stress, how depression shortens the life span, and how trauma impacts the immune system.

Consumer groups are right to distrust the medical establishment, because there has been a long tradition of dismissing patients as crazy or hysterical when their symptoms weren't easily explained. They've been badly served by Western medicine, largely because their conditions don't respond to simple treatments, the single-factor scientific model we discussed in Chapter 2. They are frequently labeled *noncompliant*—meaning they don't follow treatment recommendations to the letter. "Noncompliant" is actually a much dirtier word than "psychosomatic." What it really means is there is a breakdown in communication between doctor and patient; but the way medicine uses the word, it's all the patient's fault. David Mechanic's comment:

> Doctors, of course, typically feel the need to direct, interrupt, or cut off the patient's presentation to arrive at a diagnosis within the time realistically available.[3] The task as they are trained to see it is to maximize the needed information within the allotted time, avoiding digressions and irrelevancies. What is irrelevant or a digression, however, is often not obvious, and physicians often end encounters diagnosing and prescribing discernible conditions, but not necessarily those that motivated the patient to seek care.

In reality, the patient would be more cooperative with treatment if he really had hope, if he believed that the treatment made sense, if he had all his questions answered, if he felt that the doctor cared, and so on. But consumer groups are wrong to reject consideration of stress as a factor in disease, and the mind as the mediator of stress.

Treatment with antidepressants alone has been shown to be at least partially effective for six of the most difficult-to-treat nonspecific illnesses: fibromyalgia, chronic fatigue syndrome, migraine, irritable bowel syndrome, atypical facial pain, and premenstrual syndrome. Most patients with fibromyalgia also suffer from depression, and treatment with antidepressants and/or cognitive psychotherapy has been demonstrated to be effective in relieving the physical symptoms. Though we might think that's natural, that anyone with a painful disease like that would be depressed, research shows that something more is going on here. People with rheumatoid arthritis—another painful, chronic condition with an unpredictable course—are no more likely to suffer depression than the general population, while those with fibromyalgia almost all have depression. The co-occurrence of chronic fatigue syndrome, back pain, irritable bowel syndrome, allergies, and other stress-related diseases with anxiety and depression is also suspiciously high.

While most symptomatic treatment for these conditions is good for the body, mind, and soul, many conventional medical treatments have a real adverse impact. Exercise, relaxation, massage, good nutrition, removal of stres-

---

3 A 1999 *JAMA* study found that, on average, doctors interrupt their patients' initial presentation after 23.1 seconds (Marvel et al., 1999), suggesting that either MDs are incredibly intuitive or that they are something else.

sors—these all make common sense. But many depressed patients with fibromyalgia are being given high doses of painkillers or steroids, which have severe psychological and physical side effects. People with chronic fatigue syndrome are being told that complete bed rest is the answer, when it just prolongs their inability to function. People with bad backs are undergoing painful and sometimes crippling surgical procedures of very doubtful benefit.

Let's look at some of these conditions in more depth:

Chronic fatigue syndrome (CFS) is characterized by fatigue bad enough to interfere with the activities of daily living, which is not relieved by bed rest and has no obvious other cause. To meet the formal diagnostic criteria, the person must have the condition for at least six months. Secondary symptoms often reported include sore throat, tender lymph nodes, weakness, muscle or joint pain, impaired memory or concentration, insomnia, and severe fatigue after exertion. Since reliable diagnosis is difficult, we don't have much data on who gets it, though it seems to strike both men and women and all races. The Centers for Disease Control estimates that less than 0.1 percent of the population fits the formal diagnosis.

Fibromyalgia is assumed to be a rheumatic disease characterized by widespread pain in the muscles and joints. It is diagnosed on the basis of "tender points" at specific locations throughout the body. Fibromyalgia also is characterized by many of the same symptoms as chronic fatigue syndrome—fatigue, headaches, sleep problems. A problem with diagnosis is that healthy individuals often experience pain when a doctor presses on the same "tender points."

Many studies have documented that a great many patients with fibromyalgia also meet the criteria for chronic fatigue syndrome, and also meet the criteria for multiple chemical sensitivity and other functional conditions. It's quite likely, to me at least, that many if not all these conditions are simply different names for the same thing, some underlying condition that has not been formally named but is the body's reaction to the Perpetual Stress Response.

There is not much known about any specific physical cause for any of these conditions. Initial reports suggested that CFS was a reaction to a viral infection, but that hypothesis has been discounted. Current investigations center on stress and the immune system, particularly the overproduction of cortisol and abnormalities in the HPA axis and serotonin pathways. In both conditions, it turns out that the hormonal stress responses are out of balance (CRF-ACTH-adrenaline-steroids). The most encouraging results come from applications of cognitive-behavioral therapy and graded exercise programs.

Chronic fatigue syndrome and fibromyalgia sufferers tend to view the medical establishment with suspicion, and see themselves as victims of prejudice, for the very good reasons which we've explained. But vested interests play on those feelings. An ad for one popular book on the condition claimed "This book reveals that a devastating infectious disease is reaching epidemic proportions while government researchers ignore the evidence and the shocking statistics."

Most CFS sufferers also fit the diagnosis of major depression, or they report all the symptoms of depression except the guilt and low self-esteem. A study of twins with chronic fatigue syndrome found that there was little genetic linkage; instead, the twin with CFS was likely to be depressed or be suffering other psychological distress. Treatment with antidepressant medications, both SSRIs and the older tricyclics, is just about as effective for chronic fatigue syndrome as it is for major depression. Cognitive-behavioral therapy, added to medical care, results in satisfactory outcomes for a much higher proportion of patients.

If we had good childhood histories on people with these conditions, we might understand better what's going on. A study compared child and adult abuse and victimization patterns among three groups: those with chronic fatigue syndrome or fibromyalgia (CFS/FM); those with rheumatoid arthritis or multiple sclerosis; and a matched group of healthy controls. The CFS/FM group was found to have a much higher incidence than the other groups for emotional neglect, emotional abuse, and physical abuse, with almost 40 percent of the group having a lifelong pattern of victimization. Another study comparing fibromyalgia with rheumatoid arthritis patients found that the fibromyalgia patients had much higher rates of both childhood and adult victimization, particularly adult physical assault.

Some people are diagnosed with *idiopathic environmental intolerance* (IEI), formerly known as multiple chemical sensitivity, but this may simply be panic disorder under another name. These are people who seem to have allergic reactions to many common household furnishings and products, including plywood, carpeting, and fabrics, as well as perfumes, cleaning agents, insecticides, and the like. One study compared reactions to inhaling increasing concentrations of carbon dioxide (which can induce panic reactions) among patients with IEI, patients with panic disorder, and healthy controls. While only 5 percent of the healthy controls reported panic symptoms, the overwhelming majority of IEI and panic disorder patients did; meanwhile there were no differences between groups in heart rate, breathing rate, and other physical measures. In my experience with people who have this problem, they face a very uphill battle because they are, in essence, trying to change the world. They have developed the unconscious assumption that they are allergic to the world and need to protect themselves from it, instead of believing that they can strengthen themselves and their tolerance for stress.

I don't think I need to go on beating this drum. There is overwhelming evidence to support the idea that chronic fatigue syndrome and fibromyalgia (and many of the other nonspecific illnesses) are manifestations of the Perpetual Stress Response. Many sufferers start out with a difficult, if not frankly traumatic, childhood, which has created both a vulnerability in the immune system and a tendency to express feelings somatically. They reach a stage in life when they begin to feel *demoralized*. Jerome Frank writes:

> They are conscious of having failed to meet their own expectations or those of others, or of being unable to cope with some pressing problem. They feel powerless to change the situation or themselves. In severe cases they fear that they cannot even control their own feelings, giving rise to the fear of going crazy. . . . To various degrees the demoralized person feels isolated, hopeless, and helpless, and is preoccupied with merely trying to survive.

They don't have enough immune cells in their bodies, because they're in a state of perpetual stress. They do experience too much pain, too much fatigue, too many other weird somatic states. When you're in this state you have to get help. In America, you go to your doctor. Unfortunately, the treatment you get there is likely just to make things worse, by providing no real relief but giving you the feeling that somehow it's your own fault you're not getting better.

In order to really feel better, you need to do a few things:

- *Be patient.* Recovery will be slow. This is a serious problem you have.
- *Learn mindfulness skills* and the other ways of coping with perpetual stress that are throughout this book. Especially learn, and practice, the body scan exercise earlier in this chapter.
- *Challenge your assumptions about your body.* It's not trying to betray you or

punish you or make you miserable. It's trying to get your attention, telling you that the way you've been living is not good for you.

- *Use mindfulness to detach from your illness.* Focus on learning that it's not you, and it doesn't have to dominate your life.
- *Use mindfulness to bring more enjoyment into your life.* Try to laugh and play every day. See my recommendations for how to accomplish this in Chapter 8.
- *Take minimal medication.* Don't use steroids, which have a very spotty track record. Don't use muscle relaxants or Neurontin, a drug still trying to find its market. Don't use stimulants. But be open to using an antidepressant, which can be highly effective with few side effects.
- Use heavy-duty painkillers only if nothing else will work and be very careful about addiction. But use aspirin or Tylenol or ibuprofen as much as your health will permit.
- *Exercise daily.* Stretch the part that hurts. Build up muscle tone. Flabby muscles hurt more than fit muscles. Get yourself fit. There's no other way to beat fatigue. Do a cardio workout and get your endorphins flowing.
- *Eat nutritiously.* If you are satisfied with your weight, follow the American Heart Association's guidelines (available on their website). If you want to lose weight, follow the South Beach diet (a very healthy program). Try to fix appetizing meals that you will enjoy.
- *Sleep well.* Go to bed and get up at a regular time. Don't eat or drink too much before bedtime. Use your relaxation skills if you have difficulty sleeping.
- *Try psychotherapy.* Be sure you find someone who is interested in stress-related illness.
- *Practice, practice, practice.*

In addition to chronic fatigue syndrome and other nonspecific illnesses that affect the whole body, some are expressed only in specific organs. The gut is a popular place, because the digestive system is highly responsive to stress and emotion. *Ulcers* are a great example of the revolving door of stress-related disease. Ulcer used to be the poster boy of stress. In the 1950s, it was the white-collar disease, the mark of the poor overworked executive who had to swallow all his own resentment about working too hard, which created excess stomach acid, which led to ulcers. Then in 1983, two Australian researchers reported that they consistently found a bacterium, *Helicobacter pylori*, in the autopsied stomachs of people with ulcers. They speculated that the bacterium actually caused the ulcers, and were nearly laughed out of scientific meetings. "Dirty test tubes!" was the conclusion—the suggestion that the researchers had carelessly contaminated their work with some outside agent. But some researchers set out to prove them wrong, and couldn't. Now we recognize that *Helicobacter* is very common in adult stomachs, and is implicated in most cases of ulcer. And we have effective new drugs targeted at *Helicobacter*, which have dramatically reduced the incidence of ulcer. However, that's not the end of the story, because only about 10 percent of the people infected with *Helicobacter* develop ulcers, and about 15 percent of ulcer patients don't have the bacteria. Clearly, some other factor, like stress or vulnerability, must be playing a role. For example, the more symptoms of generalized anxiety disorder you have, the more likely you are to have an ulcer. But the revolving door has swung around on ulcer—the accepted wisdom is now that it's just an infectious disease—so there's been a substantial decline in research into the stress component.

Irritable bowel syndrome (IBS) is my favorite name for an illness. We all know our digestive systems have personalities—here is one that got up on the wrong side of the bed today, and remains overly sensitive and just plain contrary. IBS occurs in 20 percent of the adult population and accounts for half of all consultations with gastroenterologists. The symptoms are vague. The primary symptom is abdominal pain; then you can have constipation or diarrhea or both. Half of patients with IBS also suffer anxiety or depression, and those patients have a poorer prognosis than those without psychological distress. First episodes are often precipitated by a stressful event, and the patient typically experiences worse episodes in subsequent stressful periods. Treatment with antidepressants is often effective in relieving the symptoms of IBS, even when the patient isn't aware of anxiety or depression. It seems highly likely that patients with IBS have developed a specific neural pathway between the brain and the gut that makes the brain highly sensitive to any abdominal discomfort, and the gut ready to respond to any stress with the chemicals that produce diarrhea and other IBS symptoms. As with other nonspecific illnesses, there is often a history of physical or sexual abuse.

Asthma is another physical illness closely related to emotional illness, but this time to anxiety rather than depression. A recent review article concluded that, while the incidence of panic disorder is between 1 and 3 percent in the general adult population, it ranges from 7 to 24 percent among asthmatics. And conversely, among asthmatics, 70 percent reported panic attacks. This high association is not surprising, since panic attacks frequently include hyperventilation, leading to feelings of shortness of breath, which just contributes to increasing fear. The shortness of breath associated with asthma must frequently lead to feelings of suffocation, a trigger for panic.

Back in the 1950s Franz Alexander, a respected psychoanalyst, wrote of the psychosomatic component of diseases such as irritable bowel, ulcer, arthritis, and asthma, but his work was dismissed by the medical establishment. Everyone thought that the immune system operated on its own without any input from the brain, so it was thought that emotion could play no role in such conditions. And we didn't have the tools we have now to see the connections between the body and the mind. Current techniques allow us to visualize much more clearly what's going on within and between cells. We now know that nerve cells from the brain have long extensions that reach deep into the body, into the guts and the heart. And it's clear, for example, that the same parts of the brain that control the stress response play an important role in inflammatory diseases such as arthritis and are implicated in depression as well. For instance, it's been shown that treating rats that are susceptible to arthritis with low doses of CRF—the hypothalamic stress hormone we discussed in Chapter 7—reduces their vulnerability to the disease, as if they gradually build up an immunity. We've validated Alexander's guess, that traumatic events in childhood may play a role in susceptibility to both disease and depression. Unfortunately Alexander and the analysts of his time didn't have the tools to bring reliable relief to their patients. Today we have better methods of getting the mind and body reprogrammed to work together.

These conditions, like anxiety and depression, are manifestations of the Perpetual Stress Response. Too many stress hormones, over too long a period, damage the immune system, damage the hippocampus's ability to modulate emotion and stress, and damage our ability to create a coherent story of what's happening to us. People in this state feel frightened and demoralized. They seek explanations for their suffering. They respond to "prototypes," as I put it in an earlier book:

> Modern society—through the media, the glamorization of medicine, the sensationalism and fear-mongering of disease—gives them new prototypes. Sometimes the prototype—as in fibromyalgia—is not really an explanation at all, but

carries with it the weight of scientific authority. Sometimes the prototype comes from a widely shared and ambiguously frightening experience—as in Gulf War syndrome or silicone rheumatic disease—that suggests a cause even though none can be pinpointed. Sometimes a highly improbable explanation emerges only when the patient becomes thoroughly conditioned by charismatic healers and the media—as in satanic ritual abuse and multiple personality disorder. Too often, these prototypes become the patient's identity, and a life becomes organized around a disease and its treatment.

Let me be clear and emphatic: fibromyalgia, chronic fatigue syndrome, idiopathic environmental intolerance, irritable bowel—*THESE ARE NOT MEDICAL DISEASES.* They are painful and debilitating conditions, your body's reaction to too much stress, and if you suffer from one, my heart goes out to you. *But GIVE UP YOUR SEARCH FOR A MEDICAL CURE.* There are destructive processes going on within your body that contribute to your pain and discomfort, but you have to take your recovery slowly. Accept that your condition is telling you you have to live your life differently. There may be medications that can reduce your distress, and you should use them. But don't fall for the hoax that the government, or the pharmaceutical industry, or some vast conspiracy, is withholding a cure from you. There's no pill you can take that will make your symptoms go away; you have to change your life.

Mindfulness can help us resist the desire to fall for these categorical explanations. Mindfulness can help us control our anxiety, so that our fear doesn't guide our thinking. It can help us understand that this "disease" is really part of us; not some foreign invader but just our body's response to being asked to do too much. Realizing that, we can understand that our distress is a wake-up call, and we can reorganize our lives accordingly.

Catastrophic Illness

There is plenty of evidence that our ability to cope with stress has a significant effect on our ability to recover from heart disease, cancer, and stroke. There is also some evidence that the stress response may have some impact on our susceptibility to these conditions. In this discussion, however, I want to be very cautious about building false hopes or assigning blame. Some patients have been told that, for instance, if they just work hard enough at yoga or meditation or God-knows-what their cancer can be cured. When they're not cured they may blame themselves. They die feeling it's their own fault, a tragic victim of good intentions. Some patients pursue false hopes mindlessly, when they and their families would be better off preparing for death. Each situation is different. While I'm sure that learning mindfulness and other methods of dealing with the Perpetual Stress Response is bound to help anyone cope with a catastrophic illness, and may have a role in preventing such illnesses, we have to be careful about how much help we promise.

Depression is clearly linked to both cancer and heart disease. Depressed patients with cancer have higher than normal immune system abnormalities. Depression appears to be linked to higher risk for pancreatic cancer; but this seems to be a unique association among all the types of cancer, one for which no one has any explanation. However, depression does seem to slightly increase the risk for all cancers, probably because it affects the immune system, resulting in a reduction of T cells and other lymphocytes that attack tumors and other invaders. Psychotherapy for depression among cancer patients has been shown to result in longer survival time for patients with breast cancer, lymphoma, and malignant melanoma.

Some research on cancer patients reinforces the idea that psychotherapy and meaningful supportive relationships can influence brain functioning. Spiegel and his colleagues reported a controlled study in which sufferers from metastatic breast cancer were randomly assigned to group psychotherapy or a control group. Those in group psychotherapy lived an average of eighteen months longer than the controls. In a study of patients with malignant melanoma the researchers divided them into either a support group or a control group. They found the death rate was lower, and remissions were longer, among members of the support group than in the control group. This impact was highly significant even though the support group lasted a mere six weeks.

These groups helped because the members formed a deep emotional connection with each other. They were helped to face, and express, their fears in a way they could nowhere else; they didn't get false reassurance or frustration or a desire to change the subject, they got others who were in the same boat willing to look at the truth with them. They learned to control the stress response, by not giving in mindlessly to the urge to run away from it. It seems likely that with better control, there was a reduction in stress hormones in their systems, the stress hormones that kill immune cells.

*   *   *

In heart disease, some of the greatest risk factors are psychosocial: stress, lack of social support, and "coronary-prone behavior pattern." The role of stress is clear: the fight-or-flight response releases adrenaline and norepinephrine, which can increase blood pressure, increase cholesterol, and cause more rapid blood clotting. Adrenaline can constrict and block the heart's own arteries, and cause arrhythmias, which, if prolonged, can stop the heart. Too much adrenaline also means surges of high blood pressure, which scar the blood vessels. The scars are the places where the sticky plaques of atherosclerosis build up. However, learning to cope with stress can ameliorate these effects. One study of 192 high-risk patients found that after four years, those who had been taught about the relaxation response and stress management techniques had significantly lower rates of cardiac disease.

People with depression are twice as likely as others to develop coronary artery disease. Depressive symptoms are also a risk factor for heart attack, almost as great a risk factor as smoking. Depression after a heart attack increases risk of death—from 6 percent to 20 percent, eighteen months after the attack. These effects are apparent after all other comorbid features have been ruled out—smoking, alcohol use, and so on—suggesting that it is the strain that depression puts on the immune and cardiovascular system that is to blame.

"Coronary-prone behavior pattern" is a refinement of the old concept of the type A personality—ambitious, hard driving, bossy. Further research has suggested that the real factor that makes type A's vulnerable to heart disease is overt hostility. It's been found that cynical beliefs, frequent angry feelings, and acting out those angry feelings are highly related to heart disease. One study of college students found that those who tested highest for hostility at age nineteen were most likely to have heart disease at forty-two. These people seem to be prone to misinterpret any disagreement as a threat, and to react with a full-blown stress response.

We don't know for sure why lack of social support is associated with increased risk of heart disease, but there are hundreds of studies that document this effect. People who have a more limited social network, who see fewer people on a daily basis, who have recently lost a loved one, who have recently retired (and lost their social network), who have distant marriages—are all at greater risk of heart disease. So far no one has demonstrated a mechanism to explain why this is so. It seems likely to me that a social network is a good way of dissipating stress. With less stress, there is better immune system functioning, less stress hormones to raise blood pressure and increase cholesterol.

Pain and Illness

Understanding that we're not biologically engineered to live much past child-bearing age helps me understand why chronic pain is such a problem for us. Our bodies wear out. Cartilage gets used up, nerves and bones get permanently damaged, muscles get flabby or go into constant spasm. But add to this the effects of all the stress hormones percolating through our bodies in response to our social conditions, and maybe those of us who are over fifty and relatively pain-free ought to offer a daily prayer of gratitude. Currently, 14 percent of Americans suffer limitation of activity due to chronic pain, with 9 percent suffering major limitations. And 60 percent of pain sufferers are reluctant to take analgesics, partly because analgesics are only effective in about 50 percent of cases.

The word "pain" derives from the Latin *poena*, punishment, in line with the theory that pain was a punishment from the gods; and many people with pain still feel guilty, as if they've done something to deserve their pain. In my experience moral culpability and pain are independent variables, so I don't go along with the Romans. But we still don't understand how pain works. There is no generally accepted pain mechanism theory. The subjective experience of pain seems to vary greatly from one person to another, for no reason that can be presently understood. Many scientists believe that fibromyalgia and some chronic pain conditions are the result of a low pain threshold—some people are just more sensitive to pain than others.

The relationship between pain and emotion is quite complex, and science really is just beginning to understand it. Pain responses seem to be highly intertwined with the emotional brain. The intensity of pain registered by the brain is reduced by neuron systems descending from the brain to the spinal cord, systems that rely on serotonin and norepinephrine to function well. These are the neurotransmitters that appeared to be especially weakened by depression, and this may account for the high incidence of pain-related conditions among depressed patients. Brain-derived neurotrophic factor (BDNF) appears to help protect the brain from stress, slowing the rate of neuronal atrophy. BDNF levels in the hippocampus are reduced in depressed patients, and antidepressants may help restore BDNF.

We all know that in the heat of emotion (such as on the battlefield) people can be impervious to pain. We also know that when we're depressed or anxious, minor aches and somatic upsets (indigestion, a cough, a rash) can be especially irritating. Many people feel their pain diminish greatly when they are simply treated with sugar pills; one study of over a thousand patients with angina found that 85 percent reported their pain relieved by medications that were later proven to be ineffective. Another study of ten years' worth of patients recovering from gallbladder surgery at a particular hospital found that the patients who could see trees from their windows requested significantly less pain medication, got along better with the nurses, and had shorter hospital stays than those whose windows faced an airshaft. We know that the same neurotransmitters, serotonin and norepinephrine, that seem to be implicated in depression also play a critical role in pain modulation. One study of psychological complaints shared by chronic pain patients found that the patients scored significantly higher than normal on all the symptoms, but that a special cluster of symptoms—feeling that everything is an effort, disturbed sleep, worry, and low energy—were especially highly evident in the depressed patients. To me, this may be evidence that the somatization defense works—that patients who somatize are somewhat protected from the guilt, self-blame, hopelessness, and loneliness of depression, but are not protected from the physical manifestations of somatization such as lack of energy and disturbed sleep. So the perception of pain and one's emotional state are clearly related. When it comes to chronic pain, the relationship is still there, just more complicated, because chronic pain is itself a major form of stress, leading to the Perpetual Stress Response, and often leading to serious depression. For many people, learning how to live with stress has relieved conditions like chronic backache, colitis, and fibromyalgia.

Most patients with chronic pain are dealing with all the same problems as patients with nonspecific illness—they have been to so many doctors who have thrown up their hands that they feel they are to blame somehow for the pain. They get the message that it's all in their heads, "merely" a psychosomatic problem. They feel defensive and misunderstood. Since their pain isn't visible to others, they are often thought to be malingering, milking their condition. If they are dependent on prescription painkillers, they are often made to feel like drug abusers by their doctors, pharmacists, and insurance companies. With chronic back pain, orthopedists love to find a cracked vertebra or a bulging disk, something visible on X ray that confirms to them that the pain is real. But cracks and bulges are so common that if you take a dozen X rays of healthy backs and a dozen of painful backs and shuffle them together, many orthopedists wouldn't tell which is which. Seventy percent of back pain patients have no apparent injury. As many as 90 percent of back pain patients don't have a definitive diagnosis; there is a poor correlation between symptoms and objective findings. Surgery on the back is performed eight times more frequently in the United States than in Great Britain, which should make us question the value of surgery. The general wisdom is that if there is no definitive physical finding—tumor, fracture, nerve damage—aspirin and ibuprofen are as effective as anything else for pain relief.

How Opiates and Endorphins Work

We have specialized cells for pain perception all over our bodies, on the surface of the skin and deep in the muscles and other tissue. When these cells are activated, they send messages to the spinal cord via two kinds of fibers, slow and fast. The fast signals get responded to reflexively by the spinal cord without the brain's involvement at all, which allows us to withdraw our hand very quickly from a hot stove. There are also slow fibers that mediate messages of, say, muscle aches or gradually increasing heat from the same stove. When a fast fiber message comes into the spinal cord, it also triggers a local neuron in the cord, an interneuron, that shuts off the fast pain signal. The signal goes up to the brain but the interneuron stops it from continually transmitting. But when messages come in from the slow fibers, they inhibit the interneuron from firing, and pain signals are continuously sent up to the brain. This is relevant because, when we scratch an itch, we're getting the fast fibers to fire, and the interneurons shut off, turning off the brain's perception of the burning of the itch for a while. The same goes for the effect of a vigorous massage on aching muscles. Scientists have been able to help some chronic pain conditions by implanting electrodes into the fast fiber and giving the patient a little machine to activate the electrodes.

There are also descending pathways, long neurons directly from the brain, that affect the perception of pain. This is the mechanism by which

(Continued)

our emotional state affects our perception of pain. When soldiers in battle are wounded, or middle-aged men in the heat of a softball game pull a muscle, there is often little immediate awareness of the pain. When we begin a difficult workout, all our muscles hurt and we really would rather do anything else; but after a while, we start to feel really good—not only are we not hurting anymore but we feel powerful, competent, energized. We're experiencing the runner's high, the surge of *endorphins* that both blocks pain and results in a natural euphoric state. Forced heavy breathing generates endorphins too, which is one reason why Lamaze works for mothers in labor. Acupuncture also gets its analgesic effect from release of endorphins, though the mechanism is not quite clear.

In the 1970s, researchers hard at work to understand the neurochemistry of drug abuse knew that the active ingredients in all opium-based drugs (heroin, morphine, opium) were molecules called opiates. It was a major breakthrough to find that these drugs had specific receptor sites in the brain, which were located primarily in the areas that process feelings of pain. In fact, once opiates were recognized, it was not a big step to show that they block pain by activating those neurons with the long descending fibers that block the transmission of pain signals to the brain. Then, the obvious question: why should the brain have receptor sites for molecules coming from poppies? And the obvious answer: there must be similar compounds naturally occurring in the body. Robert Sapolsky says neurochemists went wild with the challenge of finding the body's endogenous morphinelike substances. It didn't take them long, either. They found three different classes of substances: enkephalins, dynorphins, and endorphins, all of which are considered *opioids* (opiates come from outside the body, opioids from within).

There is one huge difference between opiates and opioids. We get acclimated to the effects of morphine or other opiate painkillers (such as Percocet, Darvon, and Oxycontin). We gradually need more and more, both to get pain relief and to get the euphoric state drug abusers seek. But opioids have the opposite effect: the more we generate endorphins and other opioids, the more sensitive we get to them. People who exercise regularly seem to enjoy the little things in life more: relationships, tastes, other sensory pleasures. It may also be that people who have a lot of opioids in their systems, because of regular exercise, have some immunity from pain because the opioids are there to activate the nerve cells with the long fibers that block the perception of pain.

Andrew Solomon has pointed out that, in depression, there is no such thing as a placebo. If you have cancer and take a sugar pill and feel better, your cancer is probably still advancing at the same rate. But if you are seriously depressed and take a sugar pill and feel better, you *are* better—that's the only goal we're shooting for. The same is true for pain. Since we don't understand the mechanisms involved in either condition, it would be absurd for us to say *You may feel better, but our tests show that your serotonin is still out of balance, so you're still* really *depressed.* Or, for pain: *You still have too much of substance P, so you're still really in pain. You only* think *you feel better.* This points out the phony distinction between physical pain and "psychogenic" pain, supposedly caused by our minds or our imaginations. The fact that a pain responds to a placebo does not mean it was psychogenic; there are plenty of very genuine pains— with visible, sometimes horrible, tissue damage—that respond perfectly well to placebo, or to purely mental interventions like hypnosis or relaxation training. There is a physical mechanism at work in any experience of pain, whether it's from damaged tissue or a change in neurotransmitter levels or any other cause, but the mind can sometimes control the brain's response. We need to have a lot more research going into how this works than goes into research for new medications, but of course there's no one to fund it.

Not surprisingly, chronic pain is associated with depression. This is due not only to the fact that pain is a constant stressor, but also that both pain and depression reinforce negative self-focusing, which may magnify symptoms of both. Surprisingly, the intensity of pain does not seem to be a predictor of depression, but interference with activities and diffusion of pain does. This finding suggests that the effect of pain on depression is indirect—that pain causes disability and worry which themselves are depressing. It's logical then that treatment that reinforces distraction, imparts coping skills, and offers a graduated program of physical therapy *and* cognitive-behavioral therapy will be most effective.

Unfortunately, chronic pain can carry with it a lot of "secondary gain." This is the term for the hidden rewards that can accompany an illness. Pain can get you out of doing things that you really would rather not do. It tends to be an argument-stopper: *Sorry, honey, I just can't go to the PTA meeting, I'm hurting too much.* Pain can be a justification for taking painkillers, which have a subtle high, and also insulate you from stress. Some think that the body can manufacture pain in order to justify more painkillers. Pain can be a way of controlling others, getting them to do things for you and feel guilty when they're not thoughtful. These payoffs for having pain can grow on you naturally and gradually; pain becomes part of your character armor. You may not notice the change in yourself, but you can reach the point where having pain seems natural and comfortable, while changing—by setting out on a rehab program—seems scary. But you should consider how your life has changed. If you are benefiting from secondary gain, it's likely to have damaged your relationships with other people, especially those closest to you. If you keep getting out of things because of pain, with time people may start avoiding you—or resenting you. You end up more isolated.

If you have a problem with persistent, unexplained pain, you should ask your doctor for a referral to a physiatrist (an MD specializing in rehab), physical therapist, or occupational therapist (ask for one who has experience with chronic pain). These experts can customize a recovery program that fits your needs and your current state, and your health insurance will pay for it. Make it clear that you want a program that focuses on coping and recovery, not one that will just give you massage and hot packs for a little temporary pain relief.

And despite my warnings about secondary gain, strong medication is likely to be part of any pain management program. Opioid drugs are the most powerful pain relievers in use. These include heroin, morphine, codeine, and their synthetic derivatives like methadone, Percocet (Percodan), Darvocet (Darvon), Oxycontin, Dilaudid, and Demerol, among others. They all are narcotics, which is a much scarier word than it should be. "Narcotic" simply means causing sleep. In popular, pejorative use, the use of "narcotic" to include cocaine or speed (both stimulants) or any drug of abuse is a complete misunderstanding.

Many drugs can be abused, to provide a high or an alteration in mood or sensorium that is not their intended effect. Opioids are popularly viewed as particularly dangerous drugs of abuse because they are physiologically addictive. But so are alcohol, sedative-hypnotics (Placidyl, Equanil, Quaalude), benzodiazepines (Valium, Xanax, Klonopin, Librium, Ativan), and the sleeping pills Dalmane, Halcyon, Ambien, and Restoril, among others. Though we generally recognize that alcohol and these other drugs can be abused and have some addictive potential, we tend to think of opioids as in a specially dangerous class of their own, perhaps due to their derivation from opium, a particularly stigmatized drug in American culture. In fact, use of opioids for pain relief is much more medically specific and appropriate than use of benzodiazepines for nonacute anxiety. One respected pain specialist, Barry Stimmel, puts it this way:

> The prescription of a dependency-producing drug to relieve pain and allow adequate function is not only appropriate but extremely beneficial. Such a person should not be considered to be addicted any more than a diabetic would be considered addicted to insulin.

It is more often the behavior of the physician, rather than the person in pain, that causes persistent suffering. Physicians consistently prescribe inadequate doses of narcotic analgesics at too infrequent intervals, regardless of the actual cause of the pain.

So use medications if necessary, but use them wisely. Don't use them to allow you to destroy your body. Most patients I see with chronic pain of the musculoskeletal variety have it, at least in part, because of their own bad habits. They resent their pain and try to fight it. Whenever they feel good, they overwork themselves, and as a consequence feel lousy the next day. They then feel damaged and fragile, and stay immobilized for a few days, while their bodies stiffen up again and become weaker, until they have a burst of energy or another light pain day, when they will push themselves too hard again. They have their own frustration and hopelessness reinforced. It sounds so simple and obvious when I lay it out like this—they even have a name for it, the "push-crash syndrome"—and you don't have to be an expert to guess the solution, a regular exercise program.

For relief from muscle and joint pain, most experts recommend daily stretching for the whole body with some special attention to the afflicted area, combined with an aerobic workout three times per week, with a strength-building program on the alternate days. This need not take more than thirty minutes per day. It can be as simple as a half hour's brisk walk alternating with some work with dumbbells or an elastic band and stomach crunches (make sure you do these the right way). Combined with your meditation program,

I'm asking you to make room for no more than an hour a day. You must start off gradually and be persistent. Within six weeks you should start noticing some benefits like sleeping better, more endurance, and more pain tolerance. An excellent resource is Margaret Caudill's *Managing Pain Before It Manages You.*

Living with Disability

Understandably, we are all reluctant to accept the idea of constant pain and the diminished capacity that goes with it. We want to get back to our "old self." We dream about our youthful athletic abilities. We joke about the aches and pains of old age but we are whistling past the graveyard. We know, at least in the logical brain, that pain and disability are an inevitable part of aging; but when it begins to happen to us our attitude is *Wait! There must be some mistake. I'm not that old!* And of course when the pain happens when we are young, due to accident or illness, the unfairness is even more fierce.

Yet the same research that gave us the Hedonic Treadmill also demonstrated that people are remarkably resilient, once they accept their fate. Accident victims and people who have become disabled through illness generally return to their former levels of happiness once they have accepted their condition. It's a rare thing for a disability to create a bitter person from a formerly happy one, though unfortunately people who are already depressed are likely to find themselves feeling worse. The key is acceptance. It's easier for us to accept the pain and limitation caused by a condition we can understand than it is when the diagnosis is mushy—a bulging disk, muscle spasms, tension headaches. It's easier to adapt when we know bad news for certain: a sudden, permanent loss rather than gradual deterioration. Unfortunately, this is not the way we normally learn bad medical news, so perhaps we need to practice facing the worst in our minds; mindfully contemplating what the extent of the loss can be, what we can do about it, how we can adapt.

Sometimes we gain strength by facing the worst. When a painful, disfiguring, or disabling condition can't be completely healed, we have to learn the skills of acceptance, even though it feels unfair, even though it might feel tempting to linger in rage or self-pity. We have to learn how to detach ourselves from pain and adversity, how to respect them without letting them rule our lives. We have to accept that we can no longer do some things that used to bring us pleasure or pride. We have to be open to finding new activities that still challenge us, that make us work or stretch or sweat without damaging us. These skills are, after all, going to be necessary for all of us as we grow older. We have some positive role models: we can think of leaders like Franklin D. Roosevelt and his uncle Theodore, or John F. Kennedy, as men whose struggles with disability seemed to enrich their lives.

Summary: Perpetual Stress and the Body

It should come as no surprise that, since the Perpetual Stress Response has us perpetually pouring stress hormones into our bodies, with time our bodies will protest or break down. We've reviewed the effects of the stress hormones, and we've talked about some of the recognized effects on our bodies—weight problems, autoimmune disease, nonspecific illness, chronic pain. The stress hormones have powerful effects—they were designed to get our attention, to make us ready to run or defend ourselves, to prepare our organs to heal, to shut down digestion if necessary—many effects, which when they go on continuously wear our bodies down. If you're suffering from fibromyalgia it may make no sense to you that I suggest you look inside yourself for the trouble: to the sources of conflict in your life; your job, your spouse, your children—and to the sources of meaning and happiness; your friends, your church, your goals. But if you want to get off the vicious circle of perpetual stress that is exactly the kind of thing you should be prepared to do. Instead of running off to a new doctor, try meditating; try thinking mindfully about the particular stresses you have, and what you might do about them; try finding ways to put more joy and adventure into your life. Don't let "fibromyalgia" hold you back. Go to Venice or Ceylon or the Pyramids—or change your job, or visit your neighbors more—and your fibromyalgia might disappear.

Relationships under Stress

PSYCHOLOGICAL distress and stress-related illness can seem to be intensely private events, but in reality it's our relationships with other people that cause us the greatest pain. Relationships are the central issue in our lives, where healing and hurting both can happen. They are the arena where our greatest needs and our greatest fears struggle:

- The wish to be loved . . . the fear of not mattering
- The wish to be admired . . . the fear of being humiliated
- The wish to fit in . . . the fear of being rejected
- The wish to be in control . . . the wish to lean on another

Our ability to create and maintain successful relationships is the key to our happiness. But the odds—never good to begin with, so much in relationships is beyond our control—are made far worse by the culture of perpetual stress. Just go back to Figure 1 in Chapter 2, showing how "happiness" seems to decline with gross domestic product. It's because we're being taught to value things more than relationships, or to see things as ways to maintain relationships, or to see the time it takes to maintain relationships as somehow subtracting from our main purpose in life (to be successful). Given all this, we lose relationship skills; we don't value the lessons that relationships teach us, and we become clumsy, inept, inarticulate, selfish around others.

Under normal conditions we are usually able to put brain and guts together, to use both our rational thought processes and our intuitive feelings and impressions to develop a quick and coherent impression of others. Trusting our perceptions, we can act accordingly: give the hitchhiker a lift; know when our thirteen-year-old is lying; understand when our elderly loved one is confused but pretending not to be. But the Perpetual Stress Response makes us hyper-vigilant and anxious, quick to misinterpret; too insecure, too desperate to trust our feelings. Our confidence is eroded by constant fear. The ability to put emotional impressions and rational thinking together is damaged by stress hormones in the limbic system and the orbitofrontal cortex—so we're in a state of confusion, which just adds more to our anxiety. Anxiety, depression, and illness can leave us feeling self-absorbed, bitter, irritable, or just lethargic and boring. People begin to avoid us, and our relationships with those who can't avoid us become full of conflict.

Having grown up in a culture that emphasizes outward appearances, we're less likely to value more durable (and valuable) attributes: honesty, strength of character, tolerance. Having grown up in an environment that leaves us emotionally scarred, we come into any new relationship with all our defenses and character armor fully engaged. We've learned how to distort reality to maintain a shaky hold on ourselves, but it means we can't see others accurately. We expect others to play a role in a script we've been playing all our lives, and when they don't it's as if we're talking different languages.

Given all this, it's surprising that relationships do survive, sometimes even flourish. Our need for others is so great that it often can make us rise above ourselves, shed our fears, and take a chance. When it works, it's wonderful, because good relationships have the power to heal us at the deepest level. We can recover from our old wounds and abandon our fear-based schemas. Intimacy—connectedness—is even good for our physical health; loneliness is as great a risk factor for early death as is cigarette smoking.

In what follows I hope to lay out some guidelines for how to create and maintain relationships that can meet our needs and help us recover. But be prepared for some work: contrary to popular belief, trust and intimacy aren't automatic by-products of love and affection. There is a skill set to human relationships, and the more we learn and practice these skills, the better off we will be. We need to use our brains, minds, and bodies to help us learn whom we can trust, under what circumstances. We need to develop firm boundaries between what is our responsibility and what belongs to others. We need to practice love, kindness, and generosity without exposing ourselves to manipulation. We need to be able to identify our wants and needs in relationships and to ask for those things clearly and directly, without shame or guilt.

Signaling What We Mean

Our understanding of human communication has been increasing at an exponential rate, with basic contributions from sociology (Erving Goffman, Talcott Parsons), linguistics (Deborah Tannen), anthropology (Gregory Bateson), neuropsychiatry (Antonio Damasio), and even primatology (Robert Sapolsky; works by all of them are cited in the list of references). We're realizing that much of our communication is ritualized and stereotypic, guided by the emotional part of our brain without our conscious awareness, like dogs greeting or baboons grooming each other. We convey messages on a completely unconscious level, messages directly from one emotional brain to the other. These are messages about how we feel about the other person—about status, attraction, attention, respect, caring, need. They get expressed in the facial musculature, in posture, gesture, tone of voice. This is part of the music of communication, while the content of what we say is the lyrics. When we're fully engaged in communication, it's more likely that the music and lyrics will be congruent, carrying the same message.

When music and lyrics are incongruent, people have trouble understanding what we really mean; we're sending "mixed messages." We can ask someone out on a date or ask the boss for a raise at the same time we're sending messages of fear and negation. Even though our words may be clever and well rehearsed, the other person is likely to respond with the emotional part of their brain, giving us the rejection we seem to be asking for. When we're caught in the stress cycle, we have a very difficult time making our messages congruent, because—whatever else we *want* to communicate—we can't help also communicating that we're overwhelmed, scared, frustrated, in despair. Getting off the stress cycle helps us be centered enough to convey that we mean what we say, and to hear what others really mean. In Goleman and Ekman's research with the Dalai Lama, they discovered incidentally that monks who are adept at mindfulness meditation are extremely good at reading other people's emotional messages—despite the fact that they lead what we would consider very sheltered lives, largely unexposed to aggression, manipulation, or innuendo.

All human communication takes place on these two levels, words and music, text and subtext, content and process. There is the communication itself—the content of the message, what the sender consciously wants the receiver to understand. Then there is the metacommunication, equally if not more important. Metacommunication provides a *frame* for the message. The frame tells us how to interpret the content. Saying *I hate you* in a loud angry voice is very different from saying it with a big smile and a mock punch on the shoulder (after you make a bad joke) or with the invisible quotation marks that say "Don't take this seriously" (after you've won a hand at cards). Metacommunication is also about the relationship between sender and receiver. Metacommunication says things like *I care about you, I'm better than you, I defer to you, I have the right to order you.* To a great extent, metacommunication is in the "music" of speech, the tone, the facial expression, the posture. But speech also conveys relationship messages directly. Consider:

- *Waiter!*
- *Do you want to go out looking like that?*
- *Can I get you anything?*
- *I missed you.*

So metacommunication is conveyed in both words and music, text and subtext.

Or consider my favorite example, from *The Great Gatsby.* It's a hot day in the Roaring Twenties, before "cool" became a term for "hip":

"Who wants to go to town?" demanded Daisy insistently. Gatsby's eyes floated toward her. "Ah," she cried, "you look so cool."

Their eyes met, and they stared together at each other, alone in space. With an effort she glanced down at the table.

"You always look so cool," she repeated.

She had just told him that she loved him, and Tom Buchanan [Daisy's husband] saw. He was astounded.

Communicating a message with words alone is hard enough. Metacommunication brings in much more room for error. Deborah Tannen, whom I consider simply the greatest authority at analyzing communication, has this vignette in her book *I Only Say This Because I Love You:*

"When my mother says, 'I only say this because I love you,' I know she's going to tell me I'm fat." The message is just an observation about Esther's weight. But both Esther and her mother are concerned with metamessages: what her mother's comment says about their relationship. Her mother focuses on one metamessage: I want to help you improve because I care about you. Esther focuses on another: You're criticizing me. And she ends up feeling, I can't get approval from the person whose approval means the most.

This mother is trying to frame her message as one of caring, but it doesn't work. Criticism rarely does, unless the message is framed very carefully. As the example shows, history is a major component of metacommunication. Esther hears her mother's message framed by the history of their relationship, one in which she apparently never got enough approval. Our schemas and core issues skew our interpretation of metacommunication, too; Esther is sensitive about her weight, probably because she fights it, doesn't win, and feels ashamed.

Metacommunication is also about control and power; who is top dog and who is underdog in this relationship. In Esther's case, her mother is asserting her position as top dog: she has the right to give advice. If Esther were now to blow up at her mom, she might assert her equal status with a message like *Mom, don't talk to me that way*. Or she might go for pity, which would get her mom to shut up: *I know, I've tried everything, nothing works* (on the verge of tears). If Esther did blow up, a mother who starts with the attempted frame *I only say this because I love you* will probably respond with a one-down, guilt-inducing reply: *I'm sorry, it's only because I want you to be happy*. This will make Esther stop attacking, make her feel guilty, and subtly recapture Mom's one-up status. The take-home message is never yell at your parents, you only feel guilty afterwards.

Eric Berne (author of *Games People Play*, the book that started pop psychology publishing) was a master at describing these kinds of dysfunctional communication patterns in intimate relationships; his books are enlightening and may help you become more mindful about some of your interaction patterns. As I write about Esther, I find myself unconsciously adopting his playful but condescending tone. But that's a mistake, because these patterns can cause great suffering, and can become so ingrained that communication becomes almost a meaningless ritual.

Communication of content goes to the left, dominant side of the brain, the hemisphere that uses logic and likes facts. Metacommunication—both verbal and nonverbal—goes principally to the right side, the feeling side. When communication and metacommunication convey messages that support or amplify each other, we have congruent communication, and we "get" the message with both mind and heart. But when the content of the message says one thing and the metacommunication says something else, we're likely to be confused, and anxious or irritated—our fight-or-flight response system is being placed on alert, if not swinging into full action mode.

However, the fail-safe in metacommunication mix-ups is that we can *talk* about them. We can use our language skills and higher reasoning processes to sort out what caused the mix-up. Indeed, this is the greatest thing about relationships, the factor that gives them the power to heal old wounds, support us through adversity, and promote growth in wisdom and maturity. A loved one can help us see ourselves with new eyes; if our trust is sufficient, we can shed some of the character armor and be truly ourselves, a rare thing in today's world. With some continuing work on clearing up our communication patterns, we can develop the level of congruent, validating communication that allows us to resolve some of our troubling schemas and shed some of our character armor.

The Drama: Core Conflicts

Judith Herman has this to say about recovering from trauma:

> The core experiences of psychological trauma are disempowerment and disconnection from others. Recovery, therefore, is based on the empowerment of the survivor and the creation of new connections. Recovery can take place only within the context of relationships; it cannot occur in isolation. In her renewed connections with other people, the survivor re-creates the psychological faculties that were damaged or deformed by the traumatic experience. These faculties include the basic capacities for trust, autonomy, initiative, competence, identity, and intimacy. Just as these capacities are originally formed in relationships with other people, they must be re-formed in such relationships.

"Recovery can take place only within the context of relationship"—I don't want to minimize the effect of trauma, but I do think this observation applies to most of us, traumatized or not. In our culture, given the strains of parenting and the lack of support parents experience, given the state of perpetual stress most adults operate under, it's increasingly rare for a person to emerge from childhood without some pretty big scars. Somehow falling in love kindles the hope that we can be healed, that our most basic doubts about ourselves can be resolved—as indeed they can be, in a very good relationship. But starting out with that kind of pressure is a handicap to begin with; then add to it the baggage we bring in: the character armor, the defenses, the schemas we're going to ask our partner to play along with. Odds are our love won't live up to its potential unless we're very mindful about the process.

Relationships are so full of joy and pain because they stir up our "core conflicts," the wishes and fears that we bring with us, the old wounds we seek healing for. Falling in love with the same rejecting personality type, over and over again; screaming at our children exactly like our parents screamed at us, which we swore we'd never do; never quite getting the job done perfectly and on time, always feeling guilty and afraid of the boss; taking a drink after twenty years of sobriety, and waking up a week later broke, sick, and alone. Core conflicts always have us looking for a magic solution to our unhappiness. Under stress, we're highly vulnerable to the appeals of magic. Identifying our core conflicts means getting underneath our defenses, stepping back from our customary assumptive world, to see ourselves objectively and compassionately. The most basic core conflicts are the wish to be loved, and the fear of not mattering to the person whom we wish to love us; the wish to be in control, and the opposing wish, to trust another enough to cede control; the wish to show off, to feel special and admired, and the fear of failing, being humiliated, exposed as a faker and a fraud; the wish to fit in, to be part of the clan, and the fear of being rejected, driven away and isolated.

There is a hypothesis about people that most psychodynamic therapists find useful: Whatever brought the patient in the door now (the presenting problem) is just the latest example of a long-standing painful issue (the core conflict) in his life. Moreover, that same problem will be played out somehow in the relationship with the therapist (the transference problem). Say Frank comes to therapy because his wife has rejected him for another man (the presenting problem), and he's overwhelmed with anxiety and depression. As the therapist takes Frank's history, it becomes clear that Frank has always feared rejection (the core conflict), dating back to his relationship with his mother, who seemed to favor Frank's little brother. Frank tried to cope with this by becoming an overachiever, a well-educated and highly successful man. But it didn't pay off with his mother, who just seemed to conclude that the poor little brother needed her more than Frank did. Frank's coping style backfired with his wife, too, who ended up feeling that Frank was shallow and self-centered, too busy with his career to care about her. In the therapeutic relationship, the therapist might expect any number of transference problems to be created by Frank's coping style: Frank might try to impress the therapist with his erudition or wealth, and be hurt when the therapist remains neutral. Or Frank might find it too humiliating to keep on exploring his rejection fears or his devastation about his wife's desertion, and drop out of treatment. Or Frank might become desperate and demanding of special treatment from the therapist, expecting him to be available at all hours and instantly responsive to Frank's needs.

This triangle gets played out in treatment often enough that most therapists accept the paradigm. Many theorists and researchers have organized their approach to treatment with this as one of the main assumptions. The reason why the central issue is often referred to as a conflict is that we assume there is always a wish and a contrary fear operating here: the wish to be special, the fear of being nothing; the wish to conquer, the fear of being defeated—and so on. Each core conflict has these three elements: a wish or need; a fear, usually regarding a reaction that we expect from others to that wish or need; and our response to that anticipated reaction, usually a defense. In other words, an emotional habit. We long for love, but because of painful early experiences, we expect rejection. Consequently, we're always finding reasons to feel rejected, or misinterpreting others' behavior, and we can be very difficult to live with. The core conflict is a self-fulfilling prophecy, a vicious circle in action.

Gwen is an example of how core conflicts get played out. Her father died when she was eight, and her mother sent Gwen to live with an older sister. She felt unloved and rejected. She deeply wished to find parental love again, but she feared rejection once more. She defended against the conflict by (1) rebelling against her sister, the authorities in school, in fact just about anyone who was in a position to take care of her; and (2) becoming a compulsive overeater, which gave her temporary comfort from needy feelings, and at the same time made her obese, and less likely to attract love from anyone who could give it to her.

Remember that we talked about defenses as the result of an unresolvable conflict between a wish and a fear, and symptoms as the behavioral manifestation of failing defenses. Here's the same conflict again, the basic human conflict, now brought into relationships. Whatever has happened in our past life, it has brought us into the present with doubts about ourselves. We wish for a magical response from others to make those doubts disappear forever, but at the same time we fear that others will just confirm they are true. Conflicted like this, we are handicapped going into relationships. We can't state our needs forthrightly, because we are ashamed of them. We can't be honest and sincere, because we are full of doubts. It's not only when we're in trouble and seek therapy that we're troubled by core conflicts; they enter all our relationships, and the more we need from the other person, the more they are in play. *If our task in life is to construct a coherent story of ourselves, the core conflict is the tragic flaw.*

There is good reason to believe that psychotherapy derives a great deal of its effectiveness from the synchrony of communication between patient and therapist. We've already talked about good therapy creating a kind of "holding environment," where the patient feels safe enough to let down his defenses and face his fears. Daniel Siegel talks about the attunement between two brains that facilitates the natural healing, integrating force of the one; the therapist providing emotional regulation, empathy, compassionate curiosity, joy; the patient learning these abilities through the same nonverbal channels that the infant uses to learn from the parent. It is direct right-brain-to-right-brain communication. With the emotional, right brain calmed in therapy, the patient's two hemispheres can begin to work together, the emotional brain and the logical brain together developing a coherent response to intense emotion.

What the therapist provides, however, is not magic; it's simply what we all long for in intimate relationships—a validating response, a signal that the other person deeply understands how you feel, and accepts you as you are. This has much deeper effects than the simple cognitive effect of agreement. When we send out a signal to the world, our brains are looking for responses to that signal, and those responses get embedded in the network of neurons that makes up our core self. We create a neural representation of the self-as-perceived-by-the-other in our brains that is a key element in our sense of our own identity. *When the response from the therapist or the parent or the intimate partner is validating, the neuron networks that make up the self-as-perceived-by-the-self and the self-as-perceived-by-the-other are in agreement; they are* coherent. I visualize this as the twin strands of the DNA molecule knitting themselves together to form something that is greater than the sum of the parts. Our flexible and vulnerable neural networks that contain how we understand and feel about ourselves likewise combine and create something newer, stronger, and more durable when we understand that others view us as we view ourselves. Two halves of a bridge join and make a solid, lasting structure out of what were just pieces of steel. When we are getting enough of this from the world, especially our significant others, we are able to feel coherent and vital. Under these circumstances, the hippocampus and the orbitofrontal cortex, the left brain and the right brain, can work together to process emotion and memory, giving us a sense of being connected and in charge. We are piecing together that coherent autobiographical narrative. We can feel insulated from the Perpetual Stress Response.

When my son got a hit in baseball, his eye catching the delight in my face as I watched from the sidelines validated his experience of himself: Pretty good!

When a patient tells me the latest story about her jealous, competitive sister, the fact that I can guess the ending before the patient tells me is intensely validating. She feels that I, perhaps only I, deeply understand how her sister has made her life miserable.

I believe that achieving a state of mindfulness also provides us with the same validating response. In mindfulness, we're observing the left brain with the right. We're seeing all the anxiety, drivenness, obsessiveness of the left brain overwhelmed with too much information, and we're *holding* it with the right. Observing ourselves mindfully, we step back from our busy-ness and accept ourselves as we are.

Being Loved and Being Unloved: Intimate Relationships

Being in love is probably the most joyous state available to humans. Our bodies are full of happy hormones, and we feel blessed, on top of the world. We idealize our partner, we see all their virtues and none of their flaws, and this happy state spills over so that we feel pretty good about ourselves, too. Of course, with all that investment in another, we also open ourselves up to the possibility of loss. When such high emotional stakes are on the line, intimate relationships are by their very nature regressive—we can find ourselves acting, and feeling, quite childish. We become very self-centered; everything that happens is about us somehow. When there's trouble, our core conflicts are brought right back in our faces, full frontal: our doubts and insecurities about ourselves, our secret feelings that we're just not good enough somehow, that we're going to be rejected in the end. So it's very easy for us to misinterpret our partner's communication. She's feeling tired and doesn't want to go out, but we take it personally, feeling rejected again. He's preoccupied with work and doesn't want to listen right now, but we take it personally, feeling rejected again. I don't need to go on; you know what I mean.

But, if we're smart, we can *talk* about what's going on. We can prevent little things from blowing up into big things by taking the time to frame our communication carefully—*This is upsetting me and I don't think it should. Can we talk about this?* We can listen to each other mindfully, with full attention, without judging or categorizing. We can work out big problems by setting aside the time to approach the problem mindfully, trying to stay calm and not let our emotional brains run away with us. Although I talk a lot about trusting your feelings, when you're in a huge swivet with your loved one it's only too likely that your feelings will be so strong that you'll say or do something you'll regret later. So *mindful attention* to the problem is the key.

A problem that's going to arise in any intimate relationship is a conflict about power. We have the wish to be in control of things, but we also have the opposing wish, to trust someone else enough to let them take care of it all. We want two contradictory things at the same time, a seemingly unfair but perfectly human state of affairs. So who's in charge is always going to be an issue. In close relationships, we're always sliding back and forth on what Deborah Tannen calls the connection continuum—trying to be close enough that we feel some protection but not so close that we feel dominated. Much of metacommunication contains subtle (or blatant) messages of power and control. The husband's *Let me do the dishes for you, dear* makes it clear that he gets to decide when he's going to step in and help with what he considers her job. The wife's *Please wait to do your workout, I won't be ready for half an hour* may be a connection message to her, but he might hear it as a control message.

Tannen is perhaps best known for her observation that men and women speak different languages—or at least use the same language very differently. She argues that men live in a world of hierarchy and competition, and that much of male communication is about establishing one's status in the hierarchy, and gaining dominance if possible. But women are more likely to see the world as a network of connections, in which closeness is the goal, and communication is about trying to deepen connection, building confirmation, support, and consensus. Brain researchers are documenting that there are consistent differences between male and female brains, as you might expect since they are continually bathed in different chemicals—hormones. But one difference not explained by hormones is that women seem to have the left and right hemispheres better integrated. This may account for why women seem to be more sensitive to incongruent verbal and nonverbal messages than men. These differences in perspective and data processing lead to a great many misunderstandings between the sexes, because each is hearing the same communication *and* metacommunication from a vastly different assumptive world. Tannen goes right back to the stereotypical childhood play of children. Boys' play is often a contest: who's stronger, who's better, who's got more; boys win social points by athletic prowess. There's usually a single leader, but some jockeying for leadership. There are often elaborate rules, which themselves are the subject of much contention. Girls' games tend to emphasize cooperation rather than competition; jump rope, hopscotch, "playing house" all require taking turns and have no clear winners. Girls tend to punish too much initiative by complaining of "bossiness." The focus is on who's in the group, and who's out; the hurt feelings of the girl who's left out are just as bad as the boy who can't compete, but the values and methods of the groups are different.[1]

In relationships between the sexes, the differential use of language leads to a lot of problems. Women use "troubles talk" as a way of connecting, of showing support:

Woman to woman: *I'm really worried about my exam tomorrow.*
Woman's response: *I know, I'd be scared too. What's this doctor like?*
Woman to man: *I'm really worried about my exam tomorrow.*
Man's response: *Try not to think about it.*

In the first situation, the woman feels supported by and connected to her friend. They can go on talking about their health concerns for some time, and they will both feel better in the end. But in the second situation, the woman just feels shut down. She's likely to be hurt and angry. But the man is doing what he thinks she wants, giving advice so she can feel better. In the man's world, when one man reveals troubles to another, they both realize he's placing himself in a subservient position. They both know this is pretty uncomfortable, so the problem must be pretty serious. The askee does the asker a favor by getting

---

1 I know that the reader is going to say I'm using outdated stereotypes. I agree I am, to make a point. All boys and girls are different. Cooperation is evident in boys' games, competition in girls'. And the stereotypes are changing fast as girls are freer to choose how they want to interact. But let's go with the stereotypes for now, because there is still a lot of truth in them.

right to the point and moving on so their relationship can be mutual again. Women find troubles talk perfectly natural and helpful, but it makes men uncomfortable. Men don't like talking about problems they can't fix. It brings up feelings of inadequacy. Men are supposed to be in control all the time. Their response is usually something along the lines of *We don't have enough data. We don't know all the variables. So what's the use of talking about it?* The use, of course, is to feel supported and connected—but men are tuned into the power implications of having problems.

They're not as clued in as they might be, however, because the advice-giving response so common to men also registers as a put-down: *You have the problems, I have the solutions. You have the questions, I have the answers.* The woman quickly gets sick of this. She wants to use communication to make her feel close and secure, but his response has just the opposite effect; she feels distanced and somehow put in an inferior position. She'll get angry, and he won't understand why. But just let him once ask for support and get advice instead, and he'll feel as injured as if someone just stole his new Game Boy. My wife and I many years ago decided we had to make it clear at the outset what we wanted: Are we feeling vulnerable, and want someone to listen to us and share our problem and help us feel better? Or are we feeling confused, and want someone to help us sort out the problem and arrive at a solution? It's saved us a lot of heartache and aggravation.

I think there is more to this particular problem than communication and socialization, though, because I've seen men do incredibly stupid things when their mate needs emotional support. I mentioned earlier my patient Brenda, lying in her hospital bed in her living room with a broken back, begging her husband just to sit with her and hold her. He simply couldn't do it—this was repeated many times, and she ended up throwing the bedpan at him. I hear variations on this theme all the time. The woman makes it perfectly clear what she wants (which is simple enough, a few minutes of undistracted attention), and the man does everything under the sun to avoid it. It is as if men are really panicked at the idea of holding, comforting, listening. As a man, I feel a little of the same myself. I really make an effort to control it when my wife needs me, but I know she'd like more of this kind of attention all the time. Some sort of very basic fear response is being triggered in me, probably a sense of being pinned down and controlled. Or maybe this acute discomfort men feel is just a conditioned response. If these conversations have never worked out well for you, as they probably haven't, if the urge to turn away is so strong, most likely they've always ended by disappointing and upsetting the woman—then you're likely to expect the worst and get your fight-or-flight response going very early in the process. The wife's tone of voice: *Honey, could you come here a minute?* The four words that strike terror into the hearts of men everywhere: *We have to talk.*

Mindfulness is the key to any successful relationship. We've talked about mindfulness as a state of heightened awareness of the present moment, a focusing of attention from both the emotional and the logical brain on what's going on right now. It's also a neutral witnessing attitude that suspends judgments, categories, prejudices, and assumptions; we drop our defenses and are open-minded. It's that compassionate curiosity, the desire to understand tempered with love, that we now take and apply not only to ourselves, but to our partner and to the way we interact. If we mindfully pay attention to our communication, we can hear more clearly what's being communicated, and we won't need to respond in our usual fear-based, defensive, knee-jerk way. This not only prevents misunderstandings and hurt feelings, it allows both people to feel deeply connected. They give each other the validation that we all desire. There is some of that direct right-brain-to-right-brain communication that allows us to feel deeply held and allows our brains to heal from the Perpetual Stress Response.

Here are some communication skills to practice and integrate:

- Practice mindful listening. Listen and attend with an open mind, without preconceptions or defenses—no judging, no fears, no defenses. Let yourself be empathic—be here fully in the present. Listen very closely and attend to what the other is *feeling*. Let yourself feel it too. Put yourself in their shoes.
- Validate feelings and perceptions. We all want validation, the recognition that how we feel is important to the important people in our lives. Notice that you don't have to agree to provide validation: *I understand that this is upsetting for you. I see that this is really scary for you.* Validation doesn't mean that we agree with how the other person is seeing things, it means we understand how they got there. If we don't agree, and it needs to be straightened out, the acknowledgment of validation provides a solid basis for negotiation. Sometimes when people are talking about something really awful, all we can provide is validation, the "witnessing" that Judith

Herman talks about for trauma victims. We may feel this is inadequate, just a drop in the bucket—but the other person may be shaken to the core, and the simple human message of *I understand how you would feel that way* is reassuring. It means they're not crazy.

- *Validation is essential for mental health.* As I explained above, it's not simply that it feels good and reassuring to be understood. Validating responses nourish the brain. They help build a coherent neural network of self-image. When the neural representations of the self-as-perceived-by-the-self and the self-as-perceived-by-the-other are in agreement, we feel good and reassured, but most important is that our brain is knitting itself together, building that good old coherent autobiographical narrative.

- Work on congruent communication. Be mindful of your nonverbal language, and try to be sure it's in agreement with what you're saying. If you feel that your partner is giving you mixed messages, point it out, in a kind way, and ask what the contradiction means. If you have it pointed out to you, look inside yourself. Be aware, though, that some incongruity is OK—if you're using an affectionate tone to deliver a criticism, that just makes it go down easier. But if you're overtly saying something positive in a harsh or critical tone, we're all likely to conclude you're insincere.

- Give up on clairvoyance. Sometimes we think *If you loved me enough, you'd understand.* Or: *I want a relationship where we just click, we just magically understand each other and we don't have to work so hard on communicating.* Well, get over it. Sometimes we *do* meet people where there seems to be some chemistry that allows easy understanding. But wait a few months, a few years. You'll both have changed and the magic will be gone. Relationships take work. We have to pay close attention to how we communicate, both words and music, so that we are giving congruent, clear messages. Don't blame your partner for not understanding you, it's your job to make yourself clear.

- Frame your message from the start: Clearly state what you want. If you're having a deliberate conversation, state your agenda right away. *I want your help figuring out a problem. I'm worried about something and I need your support. I've been feeling that you're angry at me for some reason.* You're allowed to change your agenda, because conversations have a way of wandering and changing purposes, but be as clear as you can.

- Increase your self-knowledge. You should have this goal in any interchange. Mindful, open communication with a loved one can help us see things very differently than we have. Our partner might call our attention to something, or we might just notice it ourselves. Mindfulness is always creative, never interested in the same old answers, always looking for new ways to put the puzzle together.

- Practice active listening. It's a cliché, but it works. Reflect back what you think you heard, and let your partner have the opportunity to clarify. It's a good way to prevent the kinds of little misunderstandings that can lead to big misunderstandings. It's another way of validating.

- Don't interrupt to tell your own story. If your partner is opening up and reflecting on something especially meaningful, be very careful about sharing something of your own. Wait till you're sure the other person is really finished. You may think it's interesting that you've had a similar experience, but that doesn't mean your partner will, at least right now.

- If there is conflict, use your assertiveness skills (see sidebar on pages 395–397). Assertiveness is not aggressiveness, it's not a means of getting your own way; it's a method of communication that focuses very directly on achieving understanding and consensus.

Of course, we can't be in a perfectly mindful state all the time, and misunderstandings will occur. They can be resolved much more quickly, however, by a little mindfulness. Mindlessness in relationships is usually the reason people end up in my office.

There is a particular way that couples get into vicious circles of oppositional behavior that is referred to as, of all things, *complementary schismogenesis*. It is simply a vicious circle in which one person's insistence on having things a certain way makes the other person all the more determined not to do it that way. The different ways men and women have of thinking about power in relationships often play into this. We saw a little of it with the Browns in Chapter 2, where Mary Alice's insistence that James stop drinking made it more difficult for him to stop drinking, because it would have been "giving in" to her. It's what often causes men (or teenagers) to complain that their wives (or mothers) "nag." Typically the man will start a project in a burst of enthusiasm, but run into some difficulties and put the project aside for a while. If the project is in the middle of the living room, the wife will get concerned, and ask him when he's going to get back to it. This is experienced as nagging by the man, who will be damned if he'll let her boss him around. The project changes from something he wanted to do into something he's expected to do, and it loses all its joy for him.

For most people, the way to break this vicious circle is to reframe the communication. If the wife can understand that the husband or the teen feels he's being nagged, perhaps she can stop reminding. Or she can change the rules, find another inducement to get the project done; bribes work sometimes. Or she can sit down with her husband, take his hand, ask him to look her in the eyes, and *plead* with him to get the project done before she goes crazy. She knows he doesn't enjoy it anymore, she knows it will be a miserable chore, but can he please do this for her? That way, he's doing his wife a great favor and he's not being controlled by her nagging.

Another common set of problems in relationships derives from the fact that many people are loath to ever admit responsibility or accept blame, and it can drive their partners crazy. People (including some high-profile politicians) usually take this position because they assume that admitting fault somehow conveys weakness. On the contrary, admitting responsibility gives you the moral high ground. You are strong enough to admit you're not perfect. You don't have to beg for forgiveness, but be evolved enough to admit the occasional mistake. Taking responsibility for your behavior, and expecting the same from others, may be the only way there is to develop self-respect.

There is a dark side to how we decide whom we want to marry or choose as a life partner that is very helpful to know about, because it often explains the crises that develop later. Essentially, part of the reason we fall for the particular person we do is that they appear to us to be capable of helping us with our deepest doubts about ourselves (core conflicts again). Unconsciously we think *I have this problem about myself: I lack self-confidence, and this person seems to have all the self-confidence in the world.* Or: *I don't think I can take care of myself in the adult world, and this person looks like someone who can take care of me.* Or: *Nobody's ever paid attention to me, and this person pays a lot of attention to me.* The catch is that the other person really has the same problem, just a different defense. We know it's a defense because it's such a blatant, obvious element of their character: they're overcompensating. I put it this way in *Undoing Depression:* "As in a distorting mirror, we see our spouse's defensive system as the ideal solution to our problem; but the spouse, inside that suit of armor, is only too aware of its chinks and weaknesses, and is looking at our armor as what he needs."

> ### Exercises 14 through 16. **Communication Skills for Intimate Relationships**

Three exercises are grouped together here: one to practice regularly, another for when one person needs support, and a third for when there is a conflict.

TO BE PRACTICED REGULARLY, JUST BECAUSE IT'S GOOD FOR YOU

This is an exercise in providing validation. It's something we all need more of. Needing it is merely human. It's not weakness, it's not dependency, it's not childish. If you're so autonomous that you think you don't need this, you're kidding yourself.

1. Arrange a time and place where you both can get into a mindful state, free of distractions. It's also nice if this occurs spontaneously, but to avoid hurt feelings you should be sure early in the process that you're both committed to seeing it through.
2. Take turns. Divide your time in half, or alternate who's going to be the focus of sessions.
3. Whoever's turn it is—just talk. Talk about an emotional experience, something that happened recently to make you feel good, bad, hurt, angry, proud, whatever. Or something that happened that made you confused about your emotional reaction: getting angrier than you think you should have, feeling sad for no apparent reason. Look your partner in the eye and speak directly and mindfully. The only thing that's off limits is a complaint about your partner. For that, follow the instructions below, "When There Is a Conflict."
4. The listener has to listen, mindfully. Try to imagine how your partner would have felt in the circumstances he or she is talking about. *Don't assume, don't diagnose, don't jump to conclusions just because you know your partner.* The only responses you're allowed to give are (a) those that seek clarification and (b) those that provide validation or affirmation.
5. Both of you: Pay attention to your partner's nonverbal messages, and seek clarification if there is an incongruence. If the talker feels that the listener looks bored, or if the listener feels that the talker is beating around the

(Continued)

bush or having trouble focusing—draw it to your partner's attention in a respectful way. Don't leap to conclusions and don't take offense.

6. Suspend all judging for the duration of the session. Suspend all defenses. Speak truthfully, but respectfully.

7. The session is over when the time's up, or when the talker feels satisfied.

WHEN YOU NEED SUPPORT

This is for when one of you is having a tough time with something and would like the other's help. It's not, however, for when one of you is having a tough time with the other. That's a conflict situation, which we'll get to shortly.

1. Try to make it clear what kind of help you want. Do you want problem-solving help, ideas or advice about how to handle something difficult? Or do you want emotional support—just to be listened to or held or reassured? If you want both, that's OK, but the conversation will be more complicated.

2. Problem-solving help:

   a. *For the speaker:* Give your listener the respect of having gathered your thoughts somewhat beforehand. State the problem as clearly as possible. Be clear about what's bothering you: is it an ethical problem, a practical problem, a relationship problem, a scheduling problem? State what you see as your alternatives, and why you can't make up your mind. Remember that the problem is yours, and that you're only asking for advice, not to be taken off the hook. Very often the mere act of putting the problem into words that another can understand helps you stand back, objectify the problem, and come up with the solution yourself.

   b. *For the listener:* Give your undivided and mindful attention. Ask for plenty of clarification; this is what can help the speaker think of the problem from different perspectives. Don't be afraid to offer suggestions; you can detach from the problem and think creatively about it in a way that the speaker can't. However, you also have to understand what the stakes (feelings) are so that you don't make impractical or flippant suggestions. Be alert that the problem may not be exactly what the speaker says it is. Nonverbal communication can be a tip-off: if the speaker is more upset than the subject seems to warrant, maybe it's about being afraid or feeling a lack of emotional support. Remember that the problem belongs to the speaker, and that you're only there to give advice.

3. Support-seeking help:

a. *For the speaker:* State what you want as clearly as possible, and then explain why you're bothered by this problem. (You don't have to have a great rationale; it's fine just to want some support.) Let your feelings come to the surface, and let your nonverbal cues communicate your feelings as well. In this exercise, physical contact with your listener is just fine (if you want it) and it may help a lot. Remember that there is no judging here, of yourself or by your partner of you. Stop when you feel better, and respect the fact that though *you're* feeling nice and cozy and want to snuggle now, your partner may not feel in the same place.

b. *For the listener:* DON'T GIVE ADVICE. This is not the time for solutions, it's the time for empathy and validation. Attend very closely to your partner's feelings, use active listening (echo back: *So you're feeling . . .*), and provide validation (*OK, I understand what's bothering you*). This is a situation where you can use your knowledge of your partner to help you go a little deeper into feelings, if you think you're getting something that your partner is blind to (*You often feel hurt when you feel left out . . . is that what's going on here?*). But frame these comments as tentative suggestions and let them go quickly if your partner doesn't agree. Keep your comments to helping your partner express feelings, as much as possible. Don't rush in to provide reassurance just because you're bored already; people know when you're doing this, and it's a very invalidating response. But do provide reassurance when you mean it, and when you can be sure your partner is ready for it.

WHEN THERE IS A CONFLICT

One or both of you has a grievance.

1. Agree to take turns; don't interrupt except to ask for clarification. Give your partner your attention, and be as mindful and attentive as possible.

(Continued)

When you've heard your partner's case, make yours, assuming that you will get the same mindful attention you gave.

2. Follow the rules for fighting fairly (see the sidebar on pages 386–388). You each get one violation. If you make more than one, your partner should break off the discussion until you can stick by the rules. If you start arguing about what's a violation and what's not, just give up and try this later.

3. Follow the rules for assertive communication (see the sidebar on pages 395–397). State clearly what's bothering you, stick to " 'I' statements." Don't judge, accuse, diagnose, or make personal attacks. State clearly what you want. Make clear what will happen if you don't get what you want. But this can be as simple as *I will continue to feel awful;* I don't mean to suggest you have to have a retaliatory strategy. Remember that you have to keep taking turns, so you'll have your partner's consequences to deal with too.

4. Keep a mindful approach to the whole problem. Try to stay a little detached and maintain an objective perspective about the meaning of this conflict in terms of your entire relationship. At the same time, allow yourself to feel your feelings and express them. Don't try to deny or disguise or rationalize them—except that you have to control anger through the fair fighting rules.

5. Look for ways to *reframe* the conflict. It may be that your teenage daughter is feeling that you don't respect her judgment when you feel you're only trying to protect her from a lifetime of degradation and debasement. Maybe you should look at it from her point of view. Or perhaps you're feeling bossed around by your wife because she's been barking orders at you—but maybe she's only barking because she's under so much stress she's been in a mindless state about how she communicates. Maybe it's not about your dignity, but about her stress.

6. Most conflicts in close relationships are really caused by incongruent or mindless communication, as the above examples suggest. Try very hard to identify if there has been, or is, some disconnect between what your partner is saying in words and what she's saying in tone; or a disconnect between what she's trying to communicate and how you're receiving it. This is what people mean when they agree with relief *It was only a communication problem.* This is a good solution both because it is true, and it's also a reframing of the situation so that no one is to blame.

7. The model for resolving the *content* of the conflict is the *dialectic,* as revived by Linehan. You have one perspective on the truth (the thesis). Your

partner has a different perspective (the antithesis). Neither is *the* truth. Your task is to put the two perspectives together to form a new truth, the synthesis. The synthesis is what you both can live with. That's what you're aiming for. You're not aiming for proving you're right, or making your partner pay, or anything like that. Grow up.

8. Equally important, the model for resolving the *process* of the conflict is to preserve and perhaps strengthen the relationship. This is accomplished by providing mutual validation. You need to acknowledge that you understand, that your partner has a point. The conversation has failed, in my opinion, if you both can't reach that. If you can't, one of you is going to walk away feeling one-down, hurt, and misunderstood, and the conflict is going to resurface again, like Germany after Versailles. There may be too much anger in the room to expect to kiss and make up, but look for mutual validation.

This happy little folie à deux could go on for years, if not for stress. But it's inevitable that one of us will have a personal crisis, our defenses will melt away, and we'll be exposed. Then the other spouse will feel cheated, lied to: *You were just pretending to be strong. You're just as weak as I am.* Or the defense can go too far, as when the woman wakes up to realize that all the attention she's been getting from her spouse is really a form of control, and she has no freedom left at all. The marriage is turned on its head: What once were virtues now are defects; strengths, weaknesses.

I think all couples have to work through some version of this disappointment crisis. What *can* happen, in the best circumstances, is that each member will look at what's happening and conclude something like: *This is disappointing, but it's my own fault. I was looking outside myself for something I should find inside myself. Meanwhile I do kind of like this guy. Maybe we can work something out.* When that happens, the couple can actually be quite helpful to each other; with a problem in common, they can support each other, share strategies and tactics, make allowances for each other, and continue to provide affirmation. But too often the spouses won't look inward, the blaming process will go on, and things will end in a divorce or a stable unhappy marriage. If they divorce and haven't learned from experience, the new marriage is likely to be a recapitulation of the first. And there are, unfortunately, a great many of those stable un-

How to Fight Fairly in Love

"I don't have any idea why he walked out—we *never* fought." The fact that they couldn't fight is why he walked out. Without a way to resolve conflict, the only way to differentiate yourself is to leave. Any marriage counselor will tell you that a relationship where there are no disagreements is sunk. These people are putting on some kind of a mask, probably because they're highly conflicted about feelings of anger. Disagreements are inevitable in relationships; people are bound to want different things. After you live together for a while, you'll have had some experiences of being hurt by your partner. The combination of disagreements and old hurts is volatile, sometimes leading to the explosive fights over trivialities that leave you both shaken and scared.

   In an effort to help keep disagreements from causing permanent damage, I drew up a set of rules for my patients who were having relationship problems. Some of these appeared in *Undoing Depression,* but I've added a few more over the years.

- No "kitchen sink" arguments, in which one grievance leads to another and you find yourselves dredging up all the dreck from years of unresolved arguments. Stick to the subject at hand. If you find yourself thinking about old grievances, bring them up when you have set aside some time to work on your relationship.
- Use "I statements." "I think" or "I feel" rather than "you should" or "you shouldn't." Don't try to control your partner's behavior; rather, make your reactions part of the shared agenda the two of you must address.
- Never say "never" (or "always"). As in "You never think about me," or "You always put yourself first." Avoid generalizations. They are inherently unfair and can't be answered; they only put your partner on the defensive. If something is bothering you, be specific and concrete.
- Listen, no matter how painful it is. Try repeating what your partner said, just to make sure you heard it right. Try never to lose sight of the fact that this is someone who might tell you an important truth about yourself.
- Be assertive, not aggressive. Be very specific about what you want,

what's bothering you, how you'd like things to change. Be prepared to say what you'll do if things don't change (but don't go out on a limb in the heat of the moment). Do not threaten, nag, or intimidate. Do not call names or make judgmental statements. Cruelty is never acceptable and almost unforgivable.

- Watch your metacommunication. Sometimes you can say something that might sound innocuous enough by itself, but in context and in tone it is quite cruel. You can then disavow any cruel intent, because it's not in the text. This is a dirty trick.

- Respect personal disclosure. Over the course of a long relationship, you're going to learn a *lot* of information about each other, some of it deeply private. Some of it is going to be about your partner's secret fears and shames, things they've disclosed to you in a moment of intimacy and trust. *Never use this against your partner.* This is the dirtiest of dirty fighting, and it's almost unforgivable. You may be tempted; you may be so angry and hurt by what your partner is doing to you that you feel it's justified to hurt them just as much. But if you do, it may be the end of the relationship. It certainly is a betrayal that means you may never be trusted again.

- Never get physical. If you don't think you can control yourself, or if you think your partner might lose control, get out. Go for a walk, not a drive.

- Don't fight when drunk. Better yet, don't get drunk. But even one glass of wine can impair your judgment enough that you might say something you'll regret.

- Before you open your mouth, be sure that what's bothering you is really something your spouse is responsible for. Most fights have to do with feeling diminished in self-esteem, wounded somehow and sorry for oneself. Sometimes we don't even realize this until we find ourselves angry at our partner over some little thing. But think about whether this little thing is really responsible for the way you're feeling.

- For the children's sake—don't fight in front of them. Save it for when

(Continued)

you're alone together. If you feel that it can't wait, take this as a sign that you're too angry and need to cool down some anyway.

- Always have a way out. Have an agreement in advance that anyone can call time-out, anytime, and the partner will respect it. Sometimes when you fear you're losing control, or you can sense your partner is going to say something unforgivable, a time-out is the only saving option.

- Don't look for allies. Don't talk to the neighbors, the kids, your parents, in-laws, friends, or anyone else about the dispute until it's over. The exception is someone you *really trust* to be honest and objective. You can't trust what most people say anyway, because they are likely to feel pressured to support you, even though they may not mean it. And when you find support, you just harden your position and have more trouble listening. Your partner will justifiably feel betrayed, too, if you use friends or relatives in this way.

- Know how to apologize. The judge in the Microsoft antitrust case said, "If they don't admit they did wrong before, how do we know they won't keep doing it?" The half-hearted *I'm sorry I hurt your feelings* without admitting that you were at fault just doesn't make it. So take your share of the blame, and have a firm intention to do better in the future. And make sure that words and body language are congruent: *look* sorry as well as be sorry.

- Know how to accept an apology. Your partner is in distress, doing something difficult; allow him or her to save face. Don't drag it out, don't make it a ritual of degradation. If you're not ready yet to kiss and make up, because you haven't gotten over your anger, that's all right. Just express appreciation for the apology and let things drop for a while.

happy marriages, because each partner has a handy scapegoat in the other, an ideal target for projection of all their own issues because it's true that the spouse does have a problem. *I'm just fine:* you're *the one with the issues. If it wasn't for you, I could be happy.* But they don't break up because the mutual blaming gets each of them off the hook for being responsible for their own lives. These are the families that may look OK on the outside but generate really unhappy and clueless children.

A variation on the stable unhappy marriage happens when one of the partners breaks down under stress and steps over the threshold into the sick role. If one partner in a couple, or one member of a family for that matter, officially has a "problem," that perception can create permanent barriers in communication. I mean a problem like depression or anxiety or a nonspecific illness, openly acknowledged and out on the table. Of course it should be out in the open. But sometimes loved ones can find it easy to blame "the problem" for everything that goes wrong. The implication is *Hey, I didn't do anything wrong; you're too sensitive.* The person who already has a problem now becomes a scapegoat (or, has always been scapegoated, and the problem is the result of years of scapegoating). In any case, it makes matters worse for the patient, who has all his feelings of guilt and inadequacy just reinforced.

Although there are a great many stable (some might as well be carved from granite) unhappy relationships, I still feel that the best reaction to the disappointment crisis is to try to make the relationship work. *Love the one you're with.* Long-term relationships take work. Of course we have the wish for true love that will be so idyllic there are never any problems, but there is no such thing. Relationships call on our best communication skills. But they also give us the opportunity to practice being the best person we can be: to be patient, kind, tolerant, forgiving, unselfish, remorseful, affectionate; to seek forgiveness, to live up to our promises. Let me reiterate that these are skills. They require mindful attention, and they require practice. Few other relationships in our lives give us the opportunity to learn to be our best selves.

Living Alone

Social isolation kills. People who are less socially connected tend to die earlier than people who have wide social networks. This is true both for people in general good health and for people already at risk due to conditions like heart disease. As I mentioned before, the effect on mortality is roughly the same as that of smoking. Yet many people are alone, in the sense that they are without a life partner. We're getting near the point where more people in the United States live alone than live in families, yet we still think of solitary life as "abnormal." One very valid criticism of *Undoing Depression* is that I did not address the experience of an increasing number of people who have not found, or not wanted to find, a mate. These people are reminded every time they turn on the television that being alone is somehow abnormal; women who face the end of their childbearing years are especially vulnerable.

Yet I know people who lead a rich, full, healthy life alone, and I'm sure there are millions more of them out there. I won't pretend to be an expert on how to do this, but here are some ideas I've heard from my patients and from my reading:

As I said, the experience of being validated is essential to mental health. If that's not coming from a life partner, it's got to come from elsewhere. Some can come from within you, but that's not enough for most of us. Many single people have close relationships with siblings, cousins, or other kin that they rely on for regular, if not daily, communication. Others have a relationship with an institution that provides an experience like validation—a church, a school, a career, a cause. Validation simply means that we get an echo of our feelings from other people and the world; we feel cared about or understood or respected or at least that we made a connection. Not that the other has to agree with everything we say as much as be interested in and sympathetic to how we got to feel the way we do. Being part of a couple doesn't guarantee validation; in fact some couples have stable relationships based on hate where they do everything they can to *in*validate each other. But having a life partner does create opportunities for validating experiences that single people lack. So single people need to put more effort into finding validating experiences. That means deliberately building a social network.

A friend of mine, who always was made to feel like the oddball in her family, built a new family for herself. She invited a carefully selected group of friends—most, but not all, single—to her home one night for dinner and proposed that they form a something-with-no-name, something like a support group without the problem focus, something like a family without the kinship bonds. In other words, a network of people making a commitment to be a part of each others' lives. Not everyone invited joined, and there have been additions and dropouts over the years, but the concept has held. They gather for dinner in someone's home about once a month, and they have lots of contact with each other in pairs and subgroups between meetings. It sounds very successful, and I don't know why more people don't do something like this, particularly in New York and other big cities where there are thousands of people who share the same interests and values and problems with being alone, but have no opportunity to meet each other.

Barbara Sher, a pop psychology writer with some really good and creative ideas, has been on *Oprah* with a similar concept. Sher developed the concept of the *success team,* simply a group of people who have made a commitment to help each other achieve their goals—by brainstorming, cheering, nagging, supplying information, making introductions, whatever it takes. A success team is a small group, about six people, who usually meet weekly until everyone's achieved their goals. Though it's not an ongoing social network, obviously relationships will develop out of a success team. Members have the opportunity to share their wishes and fears in a nonjudgmental, in fact purposefully supportive, atmosphere. They'll receive some validation, as well as real assistance in achieving something important to them—something that they've been stuck on, that they probably never would have done without support. I know that in college none of my friends would have ever called a woman for a date if we didn't have each other there encouraging, nagging, daring, shaming—we were a success team and never knew it. There are lots of other informal success teams out there: artists who share studio space, writers who take turns reading their works aloud, book clubs, musical groups, and on and on.

Some success teams and support networks exist only on the Internet. The Web has created wonderful opportunities for people of like interests to connect, and for people to discover new interests themselves. Web-based introduction services for singles like Match.com are a wonderful development and serve a real need. But the Web is a mixed blessing. Some research has suggested that it contributes to isolation. One study found that greater Internet use was associated with less communication with other household members, a reduction in size of the social network, and an increase in depression and loneliness. Like most good things, I suppose, the Internet can be abused and turned into an addiction. Chat rooms and the like often provide the illusion of intimacy without the reality: no one there is necessarily being honest, no one is accountable for what they say. There's no nonverbal communication, which is really more important for loneliness and validation than overt communication. The bottom line is, don't rely on the Internet to help with loneliness, don't use it as a substitute for face-to-face interaction.

There are of course millions of other ways to build a social network—churches, interest groups, workplace relationships—but all take effort and patience. Meanwhile, the individual must maintain a sense of confidence, an immunity from depression, a barrier against the feelings that lack of connection brings—self-blame, feeling that the self is weird or strange or doesn't fit in. There are some who are relatively immune from these feelings. Some people prefer a solitary lifestyle. Some who have been intruded on too much since childhood may feel oversensitive to and resentful of the demands of others, and conclude that intimate relationships are too much work and that solitude feels peaceful, restful, and healthy. Others, who have always felt on the outside, may have too many painful memories of being made to feel they didn't belong and may find it too hard to trust, and they prefer to build rewarding lives without an intimate partner. And I don't mean to suggest that all who choose to be solitary do it for some pathological reason; I'm sure there are many who through some combination of circumstances have wound up alone and like it just fine.

One great factor at work in this is the perception of choice. If you have deliberately chosen to live a solitary life, you're at a great advantage over someone who has always wanted to be part of a couple but has not attained that goal. There is a poem by Adrienne Rich with the lines:

> Only she who says
> She did not choose, is the loser in the end.

If this is the case, the individual must work on acceptance and make the conscious decision to own the situation and make the best of it—by building a social network, by maintaining existing relationships, and by learning to enjoy what the single life has to offer. There is a wonderful book by Anneli Rufus, *Party of One: The Loners' Manifesto,* proudly celebrating the preference for being unattached. I hope she gets a movement going, a support network for loners, if that's not an oxymoron.

If validation is important to mental health, and it's more difficult to get if you're alone, it may be more necessary for singles to learn how to protect themselves from invalidation. I have a lot to say about recognizing and protecting yourself from difficult, invalidating people in a little while, but there are many other sources of invalidation, work being primary. If you're going to be single, it will help a lot if you love your work and you get recognition for it. If it's not your work, it should come from your avocation. If you're single and hate your job and don't have any real outside interests, I strongly suggest you find a good therapist, because you're just too vulnerable.

And that brings up a delicate subject, the use of an ongoing psychotherapy relationship largely for validation when there is not much validation coming in from elsewhere. It's delicate because it brings up the rent-a-friend aspect of therapy, and opens therapists to the charge of fostering dependency in their patients. Although there are dangers, I believe it's perfectly respectable to use therapy to provide validation. My relationships with most of my patients feel perfectly real to me; there is the unguardedness and give-and-take that we expect of friendship, although in respect of the patients' paying me I don't burden them with my problems. If I feel that a patient is somehow holding back from investing in or trying to find other relationships because it's too gratifying with me, or is depending on therapy to support an unhealthy, schizoid lifestyle, those are real therapeutic problems, which I am obligated to address. Many of my patients are using me like Sher's success team, focused on the difficulties of interpersonal relationships, and I am cheerleader and nag to get them out there and functioning in the world. And when all that is set aside, and the patient remains lonely and needs me primarily as someone to witness, understand, and respect his feelings and experience, I feel fine about providing that function.

Finally, I think that regular mindfulness practice provides a kind of self-validation that can be very important to people living alone. Mindfulness practice helps control disturbing emotions, so we feel more in control and respect ourselves more. It generally raises our levels of happiness and satisfaction. But most important, I think, is the experience of being held in one's own mind's eye that I referred to in Chapter 5. When we can sit quietly and observe ourselves with compassionate curiosity, detached from all our striving and worrying, we are providing ourselves with the kind of holding environment we needed as children and which we continue to need from others. We feel cared about, nurtured, and respected by ourselves.

Getting Your Needs Met

Let's return to the topic of getting along with others, focusing now away from deepening intimacy to the issue of conflict. As I said, intimate relationships are by their nature regressive; they stir up our deepest wishes and fears, and we feel like children again. It's hard to control ourselves mindfully in relationships; sometimes it seems as if the closer we get to someone, the less control we have and the more childish our arguments become. People who conduct themselves with aplomb in the business world can act like two-year-olds when their spouse treats them carelessly. Spewing our rage at the nearest target is another manifestation of the stress-fueled vicious circle. The ability to resolve disagreements, while it relies on assertive and direct communication, goes beyond communication skills to consideration of the meaning of the relationship. It may feel great temporarily to devastate your partner with the icy brilliance of your logic, but that feeling is cold comfort if you drive someone you love away. There are ways to resolve disagreements that allow both parties to feel that they have won a little and lost a little, which are often the best solutions to maintaining loving relationships. These same skills can also be easily applied in the world of work. Learning how to negotiate win-win solutions can provide a tremendous relief from the amount of stress we bring on ourselves.

The Perpetual Stress Response has us stuck in fight-or-flight mode. In situations of conflict, then, our bodies and minds are already primed to either kill the other person or run away and hide. Finding a middle course is difficult. It requires focused attention and practiced skills. Fortunately there are now plenty of resources to help you learn assertive communication. Assertive communication really is a skill that can be learned, and like most skills we get better the more we do it. It's not only for high-stakes conflict, asking for a raise, or dealing with difficult people. It involves listening carefully and attentively, and considering the other person's wants and needs. It strengthens self-esteem and builds relationships. If we treat ourselves as if we are worthy of respect, others are more likely to treat us the same way, and we feel better about ourselves not only because we have made a good case but because we have behaved well.

Being assertive suggests a clear understanding of your rights, and the skills to articulate your wants clearly and coherently. It does not mean aggressive communication—being pushy, demanding, controlling, or selfish. It does not mean submissive communication—begging for something you have a right to, whining, pleading. Being assertive does mean identifying what you want and asking for it in clear language that maintains respect for others.

Assertive Communication

There's a conflict. You want something that someone else doesn't want to give you; or you *don't* want something that someone else does.

1. Objectively evaluate your rights. What's wrong with this situation? Are you being treated respectfully but not getting your way? Or is there disrespect as well as conflict? You certainly have a right to expect respectful treatment, and that may be more important than the subject of the conflict itself. We all have basic rights we tend to forget about, including the rights to change our minds, to say "I don't know," to be treated with dignity and respect, and to experience our feelings without being invalidated.

2. Arrange a time when you want to deal with the situation. For a conflict with a loved one, a coworker, or someone you are in regular contact with, establish a mutually convenient time when you can discuss the problem. But some situations need to be dealt with on the spot, before greater damage is done, and you need to be prepared.

3. State the problem in terms of how it affects you. Make it clear exactly how you are hurt or inconvenienced by the other person's behavior. *When you leave without telling me good-bye, I feel hurt. When you eat the last of the lettuce, I don't have anything for lunch the next day. When you make dirty jokes in the office, I feel offended and uncomfortable.* This may be all you need to do. Sometimes people are just not aware of their impact on you. Use calm, objective language that avoids personal attacks. Don't volunteer speculation about the other's motives. Don't apologize for your feelings. Don't talk about the weather. The AA acronym KISS applies here (Keep It Simple, Stupid).

4. State your feelings, using congruent verbal and nonverbal language (this takes practice). This is also where "I statements" come in. *When your stereo is loud, I can't get my work done* (step 3); *I get worried that I can't meet my deadline* (step 4). *When you make dirty jokes in the office, I feel offended and uncomfortable. I shouldn't have to feel this way at the*

(Continued)

place where I work every day. (Not: *Maybe I'm silly . . . maybe I'm old-fashioned . . . I know you don't mean to offend.* Don't apologize for your feelings, don't try to mind-read. Stick to the subject.) The other person is not responsible for the way you feel, but has a right to know about it. If you don't state your feelings, you're assuming that the other person can read your mind.

5. If you need to, rehearse assertive nonverbal communication until it comes naturally to you. In any conversation, maintain eye contact. Keep your body erect. Speak in a firm tone.

6. Tell the other person what you want. Use simple, direct language. Keep it specific: *I want you to help with the dishes* (not: *I want you to show more consideration for me*). *I want you to stop the dirty jokes* (not: *I'd like you to show more respect*). Address the other person's behavior, not his personality or character, to avoid putting him on the defensive.

7. Nevertheless, listen for a defensive response. *You don't understand . . . Those aren't really dirty jokes . . . You've got a nerve.* This means your message is not getting through. If you're not getting through, just repeat. Don't get distracted. Be mindful of what your goals are, and ignore diversions like attempts to change the subject or shift the blame, or personal attacks. Stick to the issue. You may have to repeat steps 3 and 4 several times before the other person sees that defenses aren't going to work.

8. You also should describe the consequences. Clearly spell out what will happen if the other person does or doesn't cooperate. This should not be a threat, but a natural consequence. *If I can get my work done, we can go out later.* When you're dealing with someone you know to be uncooperative, you may point out the natural consequences of his refusal: *If you don't let me get my work done, we won't have enough money to buy the things you want.* Or: *If you don't stop the dirty jokes, I'll have to speak to the manager, or call Human Resources.*

9. Be ready to negotiate. Ask the other person if they have alternative solutions to the problem. Be ready to give something up in order to get what you want. Often the other person needs a way out that doesn't feel like complete defeat, and you should consider ideas.

10. If you're not getting anywhere, leave the problem in the other person's lap. *I can't change my position. Take some time to think about this,*

and get back to me. He may be so surprised or defensive in the moment that he can't think clearly, but will come up with a solution if you let him simmer for a while.

11. If you do get through to the other person, as you usually will, be gracious. Express appreciation simply and directly. And it's very important to allow the other person to save face. If he's agreed to change, *then* you can listen to defensive explanations. Don't allow yourself to get drawn into a long-winded discussion that may undo some of the good you've done, but allow him an explanation, even if you both know it's really a distortion.

Dealing with Difficult People

The world of Perpetual Stress has created a great many unhappy people. Most of them are anxious or depressed or sick, their own worst enemies. Some of them, however, have made it their business to make others unhappy too—they may be *your* worst enemy.

As a therapist, this is a subject I run into a great deal—but never hear much talk about. My patients—depressed, anxious, unassertive—seem to attract people who enjoy making them more unhappy. Bullying in the schoolyard has been taken seriously for a while, and now bullying in the workplace is attracting some attention. Just as in the schoolyard, where there can't be an abuser without a victim, some people in adult life are victims as well. They bring out the sadist in others. Of course, the sadist has a story to tell, and if we took the time to understand we could be sympathetic. But that's not my purpose here. It's rather to teach you how to minimize your stress response by protecting yourself from people who will hurt you.

You are going to run into people who won't let you win. You're going to run into nasty people who don't like you and will make it their business to hurt you, and you have to protect yourself from them. These people have a few things in common: They like power and control much more than intimacy and sharing. They're conscience-impaired. Often, they're envious of you, and it's their envy (unconscious) that makes them want to hurt you. Often, they lead miserable, joyless lives, and they want everyone to feel the same way. These are just plain nasty people (to borrow Jay Carter's term).

A mistake many of us make in dealing with people we don't know well is that we look for validation too quickly, before we know they're trustworthy. To the people we're talking about here, that is a sign of weakness, and they will use your need for validation to abuse, exploit, or destroy you. Your need for validation is something they can seduce you with; they can promise, and suck you in, and before you know it you're in way too deep. Far from seeking validation from these people, the best we can seek to do is limit how much invalidation we receive.

There are several varieties of nasty people who would like to make you miserable:

Manipulators: I've been looking for a good definition of manipulation, and can't find one. My psychiatric dictionary just says it's "behavior designed to control or exploit others to gain special consideration or advantage." But then it goes on to give the examples that capture the heart of what we mean: weeping, throwing a tantrum, threatening suicide, lying. It's emotional blackmail: the threat that if you don't do what's demanded, the manipulator will embarrass you in public, make a scene, hurt themselves, or continue to make your life miserable forever. Manipulation is controlling or exploitative behavior, yet the manipulator somehow gets to pretend he or she isn't controlling or exploiting. That's why we're so frustrated and flummoxed by manipulation; it's not a naked display of power or aggression, so we often don't recognize it right away.

Abusers: These are the people who get their way through overt violence or intimidation or psychological abuse. Living with them puts you in a constant state of fear. They work their methods gradually on you (who would consciously enter into a relationship with an abuser?), undermining your will, isolating you from family and other external supports, destroying your confidence so that you believe that trying to get help would be useless. Or worse, that you deserve the abuse, because you just can't measure up to the abuser's standards, which you've adopted as your own. It's brainwashing, learned helplessness.

Controllers: These are abusers, but their methods are more subtle. Instead of abuse they use shame and guilt. *I* know *you could do better, if you just tried a little harder. I* know *you don't mean to hurt my feelings, you're so busy. You looked so good in that picture* [fifteen pounds lighter]. *I'm only doing this for your own good.* In a bureaucracy, these are the people who constantly send your work back to you for petty corrections, all the while telling you it's for your own good. They hold out the promise of validation, but they never give it. You are very likely to want to avoid these people as much as possible, but the shame and guilt have got their hooks in you, so you feel bad about avoiding them. They are sad little people who feel so badly about themselves they want to make everyone else feel the same way.

Passive-aggressive obstructionists: These are the people who get ensconced in middle management in bureaucracies and institutions, and devote their lives to following the rules rather than selling products or whatever the mission of the organization is. *Do not get on their bad side,* for they can make your life miserable. They know more than you can ever hope to know about how the organization works, both on paper and informally. They can sabotage you in a million little ways so that your productions always look inferior to upper management. They can say little things about you that seem at first glance to be innocent, but leave you feeling completely impotent and awful.

Dependent whiners: These are people who attach themselves to you, then gradually stop functioning as a person and expect you to do the work. They often have an illness or a condition that justifies this switch, at least in their eyes. A lot of illness behavior is metacommunication, a frame the patient wants to place around communication that says *I'm sorry, it's not my fault, but I just can't [take care of the kids, mow the lawn, go to the movies, have sex, balance the checkbook] . . . you'll just have to do it. You don't think I want to feel this way, do you?*

No-shows: The alcoholic is the classic example. Lots of promise, no follow-through. *We'll go to a game this weekend. Of course I'm coming to your graduation. Sorry, I just forgot to go shopping.* Unless these people have great charm, they can't con anyone other than their own children for long, but the children suffer a lot before they wise up. And some of these people are so charming, and can be so dazzling when they're present, that we tend to forgive their absences. It's OK, unless you take it personally.

The smiler with the knife:[2] This is the person who will be your best buddy for years, will charm the pants off you, will get you to tell your deepest secrets, then use them against you when you're both up for the same promotion. These people are completely amoral, and simply feel no guilt. They don't understand your outrage at their betrayal—*That's just the way things work,* they say. Fortunately, there aren't too many of these people. Unfortunately, they're very hard to spot, except that they tend to leave a trail of bodies in their wake. So, if you

---

2 The title of an old espionage novel by Nicholas Blake, the poet laureate C. Day Lewis in disguise.

begin to hear whispers about your new buddy's track record, maybe you should look into it.

It's interesting to me that these people thrive in contemporary society. Not that they haven't always been with us. Villains are known through the ages, and I'm sure that many clan leaders were abusers and many witch doctors were manipulators. So they have a long heritage. But in creating bureaucracies and other large interlocking networks of people, we've given the difficult people lots of opportunities and lots of ways to hide themselves. Living as part of a kinship network is known to reduce the incidence of domestic violence, and it probably has the same effect on child abuse and incest. Living in small villages meant we knew everyone's history, and if someone was not to be trusted everyone knew it. But now we live in anonymous cities. And we may be creating more difficult people, because I think the overall quality of parenting is declining due to technological and social change.

There isn't much you can do except try to protect yourself from nasty people. Don't trust them, don't open up to them, and avoid them to every extent you can. But how do you recognize them?

- Watch for evasion and diversion. You can't get a simple answer. You can't get a complete answer.
- Watch for seduction, promising you too much, trying to flatter you, make you feel special. If it feels too good to be true it probably is.
- If you feel hurt but there's always an excuse: Trust your feelings, not the excuses.
- Watch for guilt-tripping and other manipulations.
- Watch for shaming—*What's the matter, are you scared?*
- Watch for isolating you, getting you to distrust or cut yourself off from others so that the nasty person is your only source of information and support.
- Watch for playing the victim—*I have to cut corners to get ahead.*

What can you do?

- Set limits, and stick to them. *I need a simple and complete answer, now.*
- Judge outcomes, not intentions. Don't allow yourself to be fooled by deceit and manipulation: Look at the end result.

- Accept no excuses.
- Use assertive communication.
- When you get cut down or attacked: *Could you repeat that, please? . . . That's what I thought you said.* Often the nasty person will back off or shade a little bit what they first said. With your action of drawing attention to the comment, you're serving notice that you're aware of what's going on. The next strategy does the same.
- A cold stare and absolute silence may also have an effect.

The old army adage is "Never volunteer for anything." Not only does it increase your chances of getting killed, it makes the higher-ups think that you're looking for something—a need for recognition, validation, promotion, to stand out from the crowd. As we've discussed, to some people your need for validation is a weakness that they can exploit. They have access to means of validation—say, promotion or light duty—and they can get you to do what they want with the promise of a validating response.

The army is the quintessential bureaucracy, and the same situation applies in every similar institution: corporations, schools, hospitals, government. Not that you should never volunteer for anything but you should be careful how others may use your need for validation. Full of fight-or-flight hormones, we feel insecure and we want to fit in, but we have a hard time being "cool" and want to make an impression. In many school settings, unfortunately, there is the unwritten rule that you can't volunteer too many answers or ask too many questions without being seen as a brownnoser. In workplace situations, where there is conflict between management and the employees, the employee who cooperates too readily with management will be made to feel the wrath of the group. Sometimes this process gets so strong and so twisted that employees are expected to cover up for each other when crimes are committed or lives are at risk, and even then the individual who speaks out often has to be protected by special "whistle-blower" status.

Many of my patients have simply made the mistake of wearing their hearts on their sleeves. They make it too obvious they want to shine, they want to be loved, they want everyone to like them. But trying to have everyone like you is a self-defeating strategy, for several reasons:

- It will never work. People want different things from you, and you'll split yourself in a million different directions trying to please them all.

- It waves a red flag at all the nasty people you encounter, who will see immediately that you're a potential victim, and set out to do you dirt.
- Ultimately, it compromises your own integrity. You're more worried about pleasing others than doing the right thing.

The last point is worth expanding on, because many people who really are desperate to please just don't understand. But, in a way, they invite the wrath of difficult people, and they turn off normal people, because they're constantly doing the right thing for the wrong reason. There is the suspicion that they act as if they like you not because they like you, but because they are so desperate to be liked in return. They will give you the shirt off their backs, not because they are generous, but because they are desperate. They have the right answer in class, not to advance the discussion or to share information, but to show off or show others up or get validation from the teacher. Pleasers are generally unconscious of their desire to show off, and will always deny the desire to show others up, but they just don't get what's wrong with seeking validation. What's wrong with it, in a setting like the classroom, is that it's a distraction from the agenda of the group, which is to have a *mutual* learning experience. In a sense, to be part of the group, each member is expected to check his individual narcissistic needs at the door, and the pleaser just doesn't see that. In a setting of mutuality, validation is expected to come from within, or from the gratification of group participation. The same applies in any bureaucracy in which a number of people are engaged in the same or similar tasks, and there is one authority, the source of validation, which must be shared by all. So the pleaser sticks out like a sore thumb; he just doesn't get the unwritten rules. And unless he can stop being so needy of validation, he's doomed to a life of isolation.

The above sounds harsh. Some of my patients are inveterate pleasers, and I think I know them well enough to know that they *are* kind, generous, cooperative, and caring, but they are *also* anxious to please. Unfortunately that often seems to be all that others see, so their motives are never taken at face value. I have to talk to them about the value of "cool."

"Cool" means not needing—or not appearing to need—validation from outside. Self-assured, self controlled. Understated, not straining to be heard. Not excited by very much. There's often an acerbic wit that goes with being cool, usually having to do with puncturing pomposity (it's not cool to make jokes just for laughs). Steve McQueen was cool. John and George were cool, Paul and Ringo were not. Keith Richard is cooler than Mick Jagger. James Dean was fascinating because he looked cool and tried hard to be cool, but you knew there was vulnerability underneath. Elmore Leonard knows all about cool. Owen Wilson puts cool on. I have a tougher time thinking about cool in terms of women. Jennifer Lopez is cool, as is Gwyneth Paltrow. Sally Fields is most definitely not. Debbie Reynolds is not cool, but her daughter Carrie Fisher is. Mia Farrow is way cooler than Woody Allen. Meryl Streep is above cool. Kids—and men—aspire to be cool, because (I think) it seems so safe. It's Stoic—you're so cool, you don't care about anything, nothing can hurt you. Cool can easily go too far, as when you have all the high school boys trying to outdo each other in appearing bored in class. But cool is by definition not a group thing, rather an individual thing. If you're working on fitting in, even by trying to be cool, you're not cool. People who are addicted to pleasing others, who want too much to be liked, can do well to study cool.

Mindfulness is cool, in the best sense. Mindfulness means focusing on your own experience, without distractions. It means getting past judging. Most of our judging comes from worrying about what other people will think—either the people we're involved with now or the old tapes of Mom or Dad playing in our head. Mindfulness teaches us to detach, to stand back from the stress and noise and be objective. Mindfulness, when applied to relationships, teaches us about boundaries: what things in a relationship (feelings, problems, aspirations, thoughts, responsibilities) belong to me and not you, and vice versa. People who are characterized as codependent or enabling, or trying too hard to please, are usually thought of as having loose boundaries. But I think a mindful approach to relationships takes care of boundary issues. Mindfulness leads to responsibility. Mindful awareness inevitably leads to the conclusion that I can't make you happy, I can't make you well, I can't make you stop drinking, I can't make you love me. Only you can do those things, and only I can do those things for myself. We can certainly help and support each other, but we need to be mindful of what's possible and what's not.

The World of Work

In addition to the relationships with people we find at work, we have a relationship with our work itself. Work is an object of love, an object of hate. It's often our best opportunity to feel we are doing something useful and productive. In the twenty-first century, work more than ever has the power to drive us crazy. At this time in particular, with so much job uncertainty, so many "good" jobs (both white-collar and manufacturing) disappearing overseas, with corporations being routinely revealed as corrupt, with even uncorrupted corporations unilaterally switching the deck in terms of benefits and retirement packages, with our vaunted increase in national productivity achieved by squeezing every penny's worth of work out of every employee, with a labor market dependent on illegal immigration, with corporate loyalty only to the stockholders and not to the product or the workforce, with a government that doesn't seem to want to do anything about it—it's no wonder the average employee might be feeling a little stressed.

Yet still work gives us the chance to experience some of our greatest satisfactions—strangely, by giving us the opportunity to be mindful. Mihalyi Csikszentmihalyi, a social scientist at the University of Chicago, is another researcher interested in positive psychology, the science of what makes people happy. He developed the concept of *flow,* or optimal experience. His findings are that we experience these moments not when we are passive and relaxed, but when we—body, mind, or both—are stretched and challenged in doing something difficult and worthwhile. The more time we spend in flow experiences, the better we feel about ourselves and our lives in general. Csikszentmihalyi reversed conventional wisdom by showing that most people are happier at work than at leisure.

His method was simple: He had people carry pagers, beeped them at random times, and had them describe what they were doing and rate how much they were enjoying themselves. When people were paged when they were actually working at their jobs, [3] they reported themselves as in a state of flow 54 percent of the time. But when they were at leisure, they considered themselves in flow only 18 percent of the time. For most of their leisure time, people reported themselves as bored, apathetic, dull, and mildly anxious.

Whether at work or at leisure, people who were feeling in a state of flow consider it a much more positive experience than the absence of flow. They felt happier, stronger, more creative, more active, more satisfied. These differences are highly significant, and aren't affected much by what kind of work we're doing. Some jobs were clearly more stimulating than others. People who had more autonomy were found to be more likely to be in flow more of the time

---

3 Csikszentmihalyi found that in the 1980s, when he was doing his research, people were working at their jobs only 75 percent of their time at work, which is a reasonable figure; it's probably higher now.

than clerical or assembly-line workers; but even those workers still reported feeling in flow more than twice as often at work than at leisure.

The paradox in these findings is that when people are at work, even if they are in a flow state, they're much more likely to be wishing they're somewhere else than when they're at leisure. Even though people feel happier, more stimulated, stronger, and more self-satisfied at work, they want to be at leisure. Even though people at leisure generally feel there's not much to do and are much more likely to feel bored, sad, dull, and dissatisfied, they don't wish to be at work. The reason, of course, is that we feel less freedom at work; we're working for "the man," not for ourselves. When we're at home, we're our own master, even if we can't figure out what to do with ourselves. Somehow we believe that the time we spend at work is subtracted from the time we have to enjoy our lives, even though we're enjoying ourselves much more at work. Obviously it would add to our total life satisfaction if we could modify attitudes about work somewhat—to see that time as an opportunity for happiness and achievement. A more mindful attitude in general, that has us attending to the quality of our experience deliberately, could replace Csikszentmihalyi's pagers, focusing our own attention on what circumstances make us feel good and what don't. That might help us feel more that we own our work time, that the freedom we give up temporarily while at work is more than offset by the rewards we receive.

In high school and college, and for a while after, I had my share of assembly-line and bureaucratic jobs. I saw how the workers who seemed to be happiest took pride in their work, no matter how mundane. People developed daily routines to give themselves structure and predictability. They played mind games with themselves to add to their experience of flow—daily goals, friendly competition with others, finding ways to do things better or easier. I hope that's still possible to do at Wal-Mart or McDonald's. I'm not so sure it is, because the workers are so overmanaged that they can't help feeling controlled; certainly they are robbed of the chance for initiative.

Even under the worst conditions, a more mindful attitude can enhance our experience of work. All the soccer moms I know are intensely aware that a great deal of the difference between a good day and a terrible day is their own attitude. They are in an intensely demanding position with little opportunity for the kind of feedback that tells you whether you're doing a good job or a bad job, and very little opportunity for validation—someone recognizing how hard you're trying, how stressed you're feeling. They have to be mindfully realistic about their goals, and mindfully flexible. Some days, just keeping all the kids fed and reasonably clean is all that can be accomplished, and they may need to provide their own validation for this. Their opportunities for connection with an empathic adult—another mother, their own mother, their husband—are vitally important to their sense of well-being. They need to create these opportunities for themselves, to structure them into their days.

Flow states are on the thin line between anxiety and boredom. When a task is too much for our abilities or resources, we're anxious. When a task doesn't require enough of us, we're bored. As our abilities and resources grow, the nature of the task must change if we're going to remain in flow. When we're learning something new, it's a challenge, but when we've mastered it, it's no longer a flow experience. There are other characteristics common to flow experiences:

- The most enjoyable activities are goal-directed and have rules. This applies both to work and leisure activities. There is something to be accomplished, which requires our attention and skills. Reading is more enjoyable than television because it engages our brain in more active ways. We use more of our imagination and intellect; we have to concentrate more and work harder.
- In flow states, we focus our attention on the activity itself, with little left over for distractions. We are highly involved in the task, and many of our routine worries and fears are temporarily forgotten. We forget to be self-conscious, but at the end of the activity we feel better about ourselves.
- Goals and rules are clear and well defined. Changeable or vague rules are frustrating and distracting.
- The best activities give us prompt feedback that shapes our behavior. Sports are a good example; if you miss the ball, you know that next time you should keep your eye on it. Golf and tennis are likely to remain flow activities because we are always building our sensitivity to error; at first we're happy just to hit the ball down the fairway, but as we get more skillful we can see that minor changes in stance or grip or swing make a difference in where the ball goes. My clinical work is a flow activity because I often know immediately when I've made an error with a patient, if I'm attending mindfully to his response. Activities that provide no feedback for long periods—writing a book, say—are more anxiety-provoking.
- Flow experiences give us a sense of mastery. We feel in control of a difficult situation. For this reason, many flow activities involve some sense of risk, but at the same time provide us with a set of skills that control risk.

- When we're in flow, we're so deeply focused that our sense of time changes. It can slow down or speed up. When it slows down, something that actually happens very quickly seems to take longer because we're very aware of every detail—as in how Ted Williams was said to be able to see the stitches on a pitched baseball. When it speeds up, it's because we've been so deeply immersed that we've forgotten to think about ordinary clock time.

We know a little about how flow works in the brain. Moderate and temporary stresses result in the release of dopamine in the pleasure pathway, leading to a sense of enhanced well-being. Prolonged or intense stress shuts down dopamine production. This raises a controversy regarding flow, the fact that it can be mildly addictive. The activity may bring us so much pleasure that we are drawn to it instead of to other activities that might be higher priorities. Playing golf all weekend instead of doing the taxes, for instance. Video games provide some of the characteristics of flow—they can be intensely absorbing—but they don't teach us anything or get us to think. Scientists have noticed this problem in their own research. Scientists who set out to study an important question often end up studying the trivial because it is easier to measure; and sometimes the details of measurement become so absorbing that they end up developing new methods and instruments, feeling that they are in flow, but never remembering the original point. Hence the proliferation of scientific journals.

Given all the benefits of flow in the workplace, enlightened management should be considering how to encourage it. Ellen Langer, who has done a lot of work in applying mindfulness concepts to institutional functioning, observes that the best managers create an atmosphere of "confident uncertainty." They don't want to be seen as knowing "the" answers; rather they convey the impression that finding an answer is a joint process that will usually work out well. They value collaboration and creativity over following the rules. They also reward employees for mindfulness and creativity as well as productivity. They do what they can to keep the work challenging and interesting, encouraging employees to train up to their highest level of competence, building in some immediate rewards for performance of routine work (like more breaks, or job-sharing or job-switching, or doughnuts). They make sure to be very clear about expectations, and they change the rules as infrequently as possible, refraining from the impulse to tinker with working conditions just because they've got an MBA.

Nevertheless, just as there are nasty people in the world, there are toxic work atmospheres. In an effort to get more productivity, there has been a general tendency to isolate employees from each other, with all talking and walking frowned on. Every task has been individualized, so that there is no need to collaborate or commit to team effort. People suffer from repetitive motion injuries and back pain partly because their work has become so routinized ("productive") that they don't have an excuse to go to the supply closet for a new typewriter ribbon or run down the street to get a file from a neighboring office. Cubicle culture thrives; when picturing cubicles, I'm reminded of the study, which I mentioned earlier, that found that patients recovering from gallbladder surgery recovered more quickly when their windows faced a tree rather than an airshaft. How would they have done with no window at all? How would employees do if they had a cubicle with a window one day a week?

In such conditions, employees have to take the initiative to apply mindfulness principles at work: by taking frequent stretch breaks; walking at lunch; avoiding caffeine in favor of herbal teas. Bring in a book of meditations and read a page every hour or so. Decorate the cubicle, and change the decorations often enough that they don't lose their novelty. Be sure to have pictures of loved ones. Have a plant. Don't accept invalidation from superiors. Practice assertive communication with them. Know your rights, and refuse, for instance, to work more than your contract requires. Know about harassment, abuse, and discrimination rights and resources. Find allies among the employees, people with common interests and values. Steer your conversations away from bitch sessions toward flow interests outside work: sports, hobbies, avocations, books, movies. Consider your options: a job with less pay but more room for creativity and flow.[4]

The flow studies suggest we have a real problem with leisure. Contrary to our assumptions, we generally enjoy work more than leisure time. Apparently we don't know what to do with ourselves when we're not working.

Both Csikszentmihalyi and Martin Seligman, major forces in the positive psychology movement, theorize that the resting state of the human (and

---

4 How many people do you know who've voluntarily taken a pay cut in exchange for better working conditions or more interesting work? The fact that this is so tragically rare drives home to me how tightly our economic and cultural system has us controlled.

animal) mind is one of mild anxiety. Csikszentmihalyi quotes an anthro-pologist:

> Animal experiments on the lateral hypothalamus suggest . . . that the organ-ism's chronic internal state will be a vague mixture of anxiety and desire—best described perhaps by the phrase "I want," spoken with or without an object for the verb.

Seligman argues that anxiety has been naturally selected into us. Our more content ancestors were more likely to be eaten by cheetahs, depriving us of their careless but happy genes.[5] So it's natural for us to be always alert, a little worried, not taking it for granted that we're safe. It's a smaller, more normal version of the Perpetual Stress Response.

These observations certainly seem intuitively correct. As you've learned from your mindfulness meditation practice, worries just keep bubbling up to the surface. Some days we seem powerless to control them at all; they just keep on coming relentlessly. Mild anxiety probably is our default operating mode. Add to it the disparity between what our nervous systems were designed for and the overload of stressful information we get today, and we get what we've got—people who are demoralized, confused, overwhelmed, scared without understanding why.

But since we know that there is a second operating mode, the one referred to by Csikszentmihalyi as flow, that has us feeling whatever the opposite of anx-ious is—calm, effective, confident—it seems obvious that we have to take the responsibility of learning how to save ourselves from unnecessary stress and take advantage of it. We have to enrich our own leisure time. That means we should:

• Reduce the amount of time we spend in mindless activities. Certainly it's OK to have some unstructured, lazy time. We need to rest and sleep. But apparently "recharging our batteries" doesn't happen when we do noth-ing but plop down in front of the TV.

---

5 It's time to explain that I know that cheetahs are not a natural predator of man. I picked up the image in the second chapter, with the impala's fight-or-flight response to the cheetah, and I'm stick-ing with it. Besides, even though cheetahs don't ordinarily hunt men, they still elicit *my* fight-or-flight response.

- Deliberately spend more time in activities that challenge us and enrich our lives. These are activities that walk the thin line between anxiety and boredom, that challenge our resources and abilities just enough that we feel stimulated and we add to our skills by practice.
- Some of the most stimulating of these activities are of the sports and games variety, activities that are goal-directed and have rules. Involvement with other people is also of great benefit, though apparently it has little to do with flow.
- Other avocations, to be gratifying, should give us plenty of feedback so that we quickly learn the ropes. Learning a musical instrument, for instance, or learning a foreign language; we can hear when we make mistakes. Chess practice, woodworking, fly fishing. Activities like these might be more innately gratifying than something like learning astronomy, where there is no measurement and no feedback. Still, if you're deeply interested in something like astronomy, the learning may be so innately rewarding that you don't mind the lack of feedback.
- This suggests that some adult education activities, for instance, should have homework and grades. I realize that this will turn off a segment of the market, who would just like to listen and absorb; maybe education providers need to provide both modalities.
- Reading, either literature or nonfiction, falls into the same category as learning astronomy. It's got to be innately rewarding to us. There are many ways reading enriches our lives—touching new worlds, finding new perspectives, appreciating the beauty of the language, sharing an emotional experience with the author or the characters—but we have to be sensitized to these rewards in order to experience reading as a rewarding activity.
- We need to be mindful of our values. Just because we find an activity absorbing doesn't mean it enriches our lives. We'll be better off with activities that move us toward a goal, even if it's a goal that's always remained unconscious or inchoate—to be wiser; to be more in control; to feel our experiences more. We get the joy that comes with flow and the feeling of fulfillment that comes with making a contribution or growing ourselves.
- Play is a mindful activity, a flow experience. We become fully involved, lose track of time, lose self-consciousness, experience the world from new perspectives. My mood blackened as the children grew up and I lost the

opportunity to play with them I had enjoyed so much. I had to deliberately find new ways to play. Two big, active dogs help a lot.

What we're talking about is mindfully taking responsibility and control for making ourselves happy. Perhaps we share the illusion that happiness should just happen, it should be our resting state—but all the research goes against that belief. Apparently we need to create it for ourselves. When we have relationships—with life partners or with groups—our opportunities for happiness are increased, but they don't come from just sitting around watching TV together.

Adjusting the Brain

JOSEPH Campbell, the master of myth, says this:

> The hero's journey always begins with the call. One way or another, a guide must come to say, "Look, you're in Sleepy Land. Wake. Come on a trip. There is a whole aspect of your consciousness, your being, that's not been touched. So you're at home here? Well, there's not enough of you here."

If you've gotten this far in the book, maybe it's not too audacious of me to say that I am your guide. Our culture has turned into something that discourages adventure and is afraid of insight; it values conformity over thought, things over people, show over substance. It has you working very hard and worrying a lot, but it makes you pretend you're not. It chews you up and spits you out, but you're supposed to smile about it. It's the Age of Depression, but no one asks why; instead we pop pills. If you're going to escape, you have to arm yourself. That's what this chapter is about.

If we want to survive and thrive in the world, we need to build a stable self that can stand up to stress, a self that has integrity. That's an especially good word—the most common meaning, of course, is that you can trust someone who has integrity, because they live in accordance with a moral code. They're honest, reliable, trustworthy. It's good to experience yourself as someone with those qualities; most of us who think about these things probably feel we have a good amount of that kind of integrity, but we could always use more. That's not a bad state of affairs, to be largely satisfied with ourselves but admit we could use some improvement. Integrity has other meanings, though, which may be even more important from our point of view. Integrity implies soundness; no holes in the structure, no rotting, rust, or termites—strong, incorrupt-ible, stable. Integrity also implies integration—the parts of the system are well connected to each other so that they work in a coordinated way and provide a solid structure. Finally, integrity also implies completeness. All the parts are there, nothing's missing. It's a system that can get by on its own if it needs to.

We've been talking about the need to build a *coherent autobiographical narra-tive*—a view of ourselves that is relatively stable over time, that has no holes due to unhealed trauma, that gets its sustenance through validating experi-ences with other people and the world at large. This is just another name for integrity. We have some confidence that, even under the worst stresses, our lives will go on and will not be robbed of meaning by despair. We may not re-alize that building and maintaining integrity requires constant work, because when things are going right we're not aware of the effort involved—to make ethical decisions, to be there for others who need us, to take care of our bodies. When we're good at this—*skillful*—it's largely unconscious. But it is work, and it requires skill, and if perpetual stress has you demoralized you will be very aware of the work involved to get back on your feet. And the lack of skill you seem to have.

So here in this chapter are the skills I think you need to build integrity and pull yourself up from whatever position perpetual stress has knocked you into. All along I've been promising that it's possible to rewire our own brains so that we can cope more effectively with the Perpetual Stress Response, and inciden-tally lead more fulfilling and happier lives. Now it's time to put up or shut up. Here's how to rewire the brain in twelve easy steps. I'll give you the headings, then we'll discuss each one.

How to Rewire the Brain

1. Get good at mindfulness.
2. Use mindfulness to develop a deeper awareness of your feelings.
3. Use mindfulness to recognize the limits and biases of your assumptive world.
4. Build willpower, self-control, and self-respect.
5. Control the effects of stress.
6. Be skillful about your body.
7. Learn to appreciate your symptoms.
8. Think with your whole mind.

9. Construct and reinforce your support system.
10. Learn intimacy skills.
11. Learn how to be happy.
12. Practice, practice, practice.

In order to do this, you need to give yourself an hour a day, at least five days out of seven: half to exercise, half to meditation. I'll have more to say later about how to do this.

Let's just review for a minute before we get into the details. We've said all along that our nervous systems weren't built for the twenty-first century; that almost all of us are stuck in a Perpetual Stress Response that literally wears out our brains and bodies. And on top of this our parents—and their parents, going back at least two hundred years—were being affected by their own stressors, so they were unable to provide us the kind of parenting we really need. That has left us with some weaknesses in our ability to function. The effect of perpetual stress on our individual weaknesses gives us the problems we experience today: depression, anxiety, stress-related disease, addiction, personality disorder, and the other forms of misery that seem so common and are becoming epidemic.

The promise of the new brain research and other psychophysiology research that has just been growing exponentially over the past twenty years is not that we're going to have new and better pills, though we will. The explosive new news is that experience affects the brain. The brain is not the rigid and limited dictator of our experience that we thought it was; instead, the brain is constantly growing and adapting in response to what we experience. So if we can give our brains the right kinds of experience, we can hope to *cure* all those problems we just listed. By cure I mean that the circuitry in the brain that has you depressed (or whatever) can be replaced or sidetracked so that you don't feel its effects any longer. But this is a matter of choice and necessity and circumstance. Total cure may require you to change your life more than you're willing to. You may be willing to trade off some symptoms to maintain the kind of lifestyle you want. Circumstances may make it impossible for you to recover as much as you'd like. But at least you should know what's possible, so you can make an informed choice. Even if you don't opt for a whole new brain, you can expect a great deal of relief if you learn these skills.

In *Undoing Depression* I wrote irreverently about the "skills of depression," things you've gotten good at that are not good for you—like focusing on the negative, being socially passive, keeping your anger locked down in the basement. I likened us to the cigarette smoker who has learned how to light up in a high wind, how to flick ashes without ever missing the tray, who always unconsciously knows how many are left in the pack he's carrying—little tricks that have been practiced so much they seem part of the self. But we had to learn them. We looked foolish and awkward and made ourselves sick with our first cigarettes. I suggested that we could deliberately learn new skills that would "undo" depression. That was all before I knew about the Buddhist concept of skillful action. Skillful action is a way to change your karma. The skills listed in this chapter can change your karma and your life. Instead of skills of being sick, we can learn skills of living well. But you have to learn them, and that will take practice. They will seem foolish and awkward at first, but at least they won't make you sick. Be patient with yourself and keep practicing until it feels natural and graceful to you.

Principle 1
Get Good at Mindfulness

The best way to do this is to practice a mindfulness meditation routine for a half hour every day. I *strongly* recommend you practice this until it becomes easy—follow Exercise 5 (on page 156–157) or any other method that suits you. Remember that regular meditation is known to strengthen the orbitofrontal cortex, the part of the brain that processes positive feelings and controls negative feelings, that reduces messages of fear from the amygdala. Mindfulness-Based Stress Reduction improves immune system functioning and helps with chronic pain, fibromyalgia, and eating disorders. Mindfulness-based therapy for depression proves to be more effective at preventing relapse than traditional methods.

Don't try to be the best at meditation. Don't worry about doing it the right way. Don't expect it to make you happy. Think about it as a lunch break for the mind. Sometimes it's delicious, but mostly it's just fuel and rest. The benefits aren't immediately evident, but it pays off in terms of perspective, awareness, and energy. You will get skillful at it without effort, just with practice. Even when you get good at it, it won't always feel good. In fact, some days it can be very painful, as you discover feelings that weren't on the surface. But don't let that stop you, it's something you need to go through.

In addition to learning mindfulness meditation, work on applying the values of mindful attention in your life. Here are some important skills to practice as you go through the day:

- Observe your brain as it does what it does. Don't think about what you're thinking about, think about how you think. Don't merely feel your feelings, watch what they do to you. Develop your inner mind, the one that observes your everyday mental functioning. Become a student of your mind at work. This sounds like work, but it's really easy, and will save you a great deal of *tsouris* in the long run.

- Stop judging. If you practice mindfulness meditation, you will probably notice how you are constantly judging what's in your mind. *I'm thinking about the report I have to do—that's bad, I should stop worrying. I'm having trouble focusing—damn it, I'm no good at this.* Not only in meditation, but constantly, we are evaluating and categorizing our experience. It's left-brain activity focused on consciousness itself. It's just what the brain does, but it's a destructive habit. Attaching little value judgments to things and stuffing them in mental pigeonholes deprives us of the ability to look at each thing carefully and objectively, to appreciate its uniqueness. It's an immediate, knee-jerk reaction that is just a symptom of our hypervigilance. *OK, this is good, that's bad, the next thing is neutral. I'm ready, what's next?* We don't look for the bad in the good or the good in the bad, and we just overlook the neutral altogether. What an empty, black-and-white world! We can miss all the details, and in doing so we miss out on the real stuff of living. We spoil things for ourselves—*waiting in line is such a waste of time* is an idea that will spill over and dominate the entire ten minutes you're in line, when you could be using the ten minutes to just think, or observe, or remember.

- Be present. Shift from doing to being. Be in the moment. Be still. Stop using the left brain so much. Pay attention to what's going on in all your senses right now, and work on being less distracted by the Perpetual Stress Response trying to get your attention. Being mindful of what we are doing means doing it much more effectively. The distractions will still be there when we're done.

There are, unfortunately, all those New Age clichés that are variations on this theme—*Remember be here now*—and a lot of sappy poetry to the same effect. But here I go judging. The reason why these ideas sound like clichés is that the language doesn't have a good way of conveying mystical, or transcendental, or spiritual, experience. Words communicate meanings, but there is no special meaning to what happens when we are deliberately present in the moment. Rather, what I think we experience is a heightened sense of meaning in general, a greater intensity of experience, as when Dorothy emerges after the tornado into a Technicolor world. It's as if our senses gradually improve so that we can see, hear, touch, taste—be aware of—things that went right past us before. We can look more deeply in, and see the complexities. Applying that to the self, and to our daily experience, simply leads to a richer, deeper, more meaningful life.

- Recognize stress at work in yourself. Remember that what you think is normal is not what your nervous system thinks is normal. The stress response is all-or-nothing. If you're safe from the cheetahs, there should be nothing to worry about other than where the next meal is coming from. But today, there's plenty more to worry about, and our brains and bodies are full of the hormones and neurotransmitters of stress. Our brains try to make sense of these experiences, and translate them, in our naturally self-absorbed way, into something personal. We add content to our own fears based on our assumptions about the world: *It must be my fault. No one can love me. Dad always thought I was a weakling, I guess I am. I just can't cut it.*

  Try not to take it so personally. Much of what we experience as fear is the manifestation of the stress response, not our own inadequacy. Rather, go back to Chapter 2 and challenge your assumptions about what's normal. Recognize how contemporary life works to rob us of meaning and connection, and do what you can to get them back. Don't blame yourself.

- Stop trying to boost your self-esteem. Start trying to be a good person. The only way to gain self-respect is to do the right thing as often as you can. Though we all face situations where we can't know what is the right thing, most of the time we do know. Most of the time, unfortunately, it is the more difficult thing. Be honest. Don't cheat. Don't take advantage. The Golden Rule applies.

  Virtue is a habit, argues Plato, and Buddha says it's a skill to develop. It gets easier as you keep practicing. After a while you will be a better person without knowing it, and the wrong choices won't even tempt you. They won't appear on the radar screen.

- Stop trying to be happy. Start trying to be grateful. Consumer culture for the past hundred years has been telling us that happiness is a commodity that can be bought and sold. Even more demoralizing is the implication that if we're not happy, it's our own fault, because this is certainly the best of all possible worlds. We've lost sight of the simple fact that happiness is not an end in itself, it's a result of living a certain kind of life. Essentially, that's a life that combines doing the right thing with enjoying what life has to offer. We've just talked about recognizing the right thing. Enjoying life—gratitude—is another skill to learn. Being present helps; you savor the small things more—the sunshine, the taste of coffee, a stranger's greeting. You can go further and deliberately set out to heighten awareness of good feelings. Become a connoisseur of small things. As Alice, whom you met in Chapter 4, once said, regarding a really good grilled cheese sandwich, *happiness is a lot smaller than we think.* Happiness is not a goal, it's a process, a way of living, a mind state you can learn.

Don't fall for the belief that there is something you need in order to be happy. That just gives in to the mindless "I want." It starts a search that will never end. Not that we have to overcome all wants, but we do have to realize that happiness sneaks up on us when we accept life as it is.

Authors ranging from Sarah Ban Breathnach to Martin Seligman have been stressing gratitude lately. Ban Breathnach's approach is largely a series of mindfulness reminders, and it may help to develop gratitude for small things. Seligman has developed the concept of the "gratitude visit." You think of a person in your life who has been kind or helpful to you, but whom you've never properly thanked. Then you write a detailed "gratitude letter" to that person, explaining clearly and directly what that person contributed to your life. Then you visit that person and read the testimony aloud. "According to Seligman, the ritual is powerful. 'Everyone cries when you do a gratitude visit,' he says. 'It's very moving for both people.'" No doubt it is powerful, and I think it could be a world-shaking experience for some people. But it's not only to people we should be grateful, but life itself.

- Stop trying to be smart. Start trying to be wise. In any difficult situation, find a middle path between emotions and cold logic. Do what will work, what will get you the result you need, rather than doing what you want to do or feel you have to do or feel is necessary to set the record straight. If you feel you're giving in, consider that may be the wisest thing, in these circumstances. Play by the rules. Don't get into situations where you have to justify or explain yourself; let your actions speak for themselves.
- Follow your own values. Try to spend more time each day in activities that express your core values, or that help you reach your own personal goals. Exercise 3 may have shown you how much of your day is wasted in activities that don't express your values or advance your goals. If you can learn

to mindfully plan and review your days with those factors in mind, you'll be on your way toward a much more fulfilling life. A daily mindfulness meditation—though it's not *about* reviewing or planning—will get your brain doing this unconsciously.

- Don't neglect pleasure. We've talked about the difference between pleasure (anything that makes you want to smile) and fulfillment (working toward goals that bring you lasting pride and joy). It's also true that some pleasures can be destructive to self or others, and we should avoid them. But it's important not to get the idea that somehow pleasure is cheap and meaningless. Pleasure brings spice to life. We need to smile, to laugh, to feel connected. Most pleasures are harmless and often bring joy to others as well. So play every day; find ways to have fun. You will generate endorphins, which help the immune system and block pain and, most important, enhance your ability to enjoy life in general.

  "Well-being therapy" is a novel approach to depression that seems to be more effective than traditional methods in helping people who have already recovered from their major symptoms make and consolidate further progress. Well-being therapy is essentially a cognitive-behavioral approach in which the patient, instead of focusing on troubling episodes, is encouraged to focus on times when he feels good. The therapy consists of identifying factors that interrupted the good feeling, and developing strategies for avoiding or controlling these factors. Apparently the simple act of focusing on good things rather than bad things builds greater awareness of what life has to offer.

- Wise mind and skillful action. See things as they are, not how you want them to be or how you believe they should be. Accept the reality principle. In reality, the only thing we have control over is our own behavior, and it's a continual quest to develop more control over that. Seeing things as they are, conduct yourself skillfully. Use intuition and logic, right and left brains, together.

- Free yourself from possessions, envy, greed, and mindless competition. Stop striving so much. Learn to ride the waves of craving like a skillful surfer. If we're troubled by the disparity between what we want and what we have, one approach is to get more; but the other solution, perhaps wiser, is to want less.

  This is the item I hesitate most about adding to this list, mostly because it's a very tall order. I don't expect myself to ever stop craving, to not *want* a nice car or a new plant for my garden, and you shouldn't expect yourself to stop wanting either. But so much of our lives is ruled by mindless craving that any work we do toward diminishing its effects will help us enormously. We'll have much more time left over for productive or pleasurable or relaxing activity. We won't be driven by the hormones of desire. And besides, we'll have more money, and therefore more autonomy.

- Stop running from, or denying, or trying to control, fear. That only makes you mindless. Most fears are just the Perpetual Stress Response making itself felt; the mind's experience of the fight-or-flight hormones coursing through the body. Other fears are knee-jerk reactions, the baggage of past experiences added to today's reality. Much of the time our defenses are up so high that we're not even aware that fear is motivating our mindless activity. Use mindfulness to get underneath the defenses. Face what you fear, and you'll be free. There may be some temporary pain, but it will be manageable, and you won't be a prisoner of your fear any longer.

- Notice when you're mindless. This follows from the previous point. What sends you into a mindless state? Use the Mood Journal (Exercise 2) to focus your attention. Most likely, fear is making you mindless. It may be very cleverly hidden away. But tracing it down may help you identify an old wound that is causing you great pain.

- Be mindful of your environment, and use it to remind you to be mindful. Make your surroundings as pleasant as you can, as a way of showing respect for yourself. If you have trouble concentrating or remembering, build in cues to remind yourself to be more aware—set the alarm clock, have a daily phone date with a friend, post messages to yourself. Turn off the television. Use music to amplify your mood, to calm yourself down or bring yourself up. Use music also as a focus for mindfulness: listen with full attention. Get out of the house and into nature. Expose yourself to views that will make you think out of the box. Have things that depend on you, like the plant in the nursing home (in Chapter 5). If you live alone, get a pet that will be happy to see you when you get home.

Principle 2
Use Mindfulness to Develop a Deeper Awareness of Your Feelings

We've talked about how Zen and psychoanalysis are both methods for helping us learn how to be conscious of ourselves without judging, how to be accepting of every aspect of ourselves. We need to "build a cradle for the baby"—recognize and validate our own experience in a way that has probably never been done for us. Most of us have gotten the message that some feelings are not acceptable, not polite, not to be experienced as part of the self. We've stuffed or denied or dissociated ourselves from those feelings, but the emotions underneath remain there, under the surface. They can motivate our behavior without our awareness and cause us guilt and shame that seem to come from nowhere. The chemistry from those emotions is there too, flowing into our body with no outlet, contributing to the sense of perpetual stress.

Imagine being told all you life that you have no feet. Or that feet are "dirty," repulsive, shameful. *We don't talk about those things.* You never allow yourself to be seen without socks and shoes. If you break your foot and have to go to the emergency room to get it set, everyone says you broke your arm instead. Even worse, if you do break your foot, it must be your own fault somehow.

This is how silly it is for us to deny feelings, or teach children that some feelings are shameful or wrong. Feelings are just as natural as feet, just as much a part of ourselves. Even more important, because while you can live a full life without feet, you can't live any kind of life without feelings. But because we've been trained so well that some feelings are wrong, we have to make a special effort, a mindful effort, to heighten our awareness.

- Remember to suspend judging the self. Look at your inner experience with compassionate curiosity. Be attentive and loving, but also be inquisitive: *What's going on inside?* Finding out won't hurt you at all, despite all the old fears and shames. There may be some things that will cause you some pain—old memories you'd "forgotten"—but this pain is much less than the pain you cause yourself by denying your own experience.
- Acceptance and validation. Most of what we want from others is summed up in these two words. We want to be included in the group, accepted as part of humanity, and we want to have our uniqueness recognized, our own feelings validated. But we won't get it from others if we can't give it to ourselves first. Look into yourself and your feelings mindfully, without expectations and preconceptions.
- Remember the chief paradox of feelings, that we have to experience them more fully at the same time as we consciously control their expression. This is where we have to become skillful about emotions. All our defensive systems, our character armor and our symptoms, are built from trying not to experience our own feelings. And all this is wrong-headed, based on

the false assumption that our feelings are dangerous or unacceptable. It's how we express feelings, not the feelings themselves, that can be dangerous or unacceptable. We have some ability, and we can develop more, to control how we express our feelings. Simply paying mindful attention to ourselves helps a great deal. Review "Learning to Control Emotions" in Chapter 4 for more ideas.

- Practice detachment. This is the best way to experience feelings without letting them control you. Remember the locomotive from Chapter 4—it comes roaring into the station, a huge, overwhelming experience, but we have some ability to choose whether we get on board or not. Distance yourself somewhat from mood and emotions: they are part of you, but not all of you. They won't last forever. They don't have to control your decision making; you can usually do what needs to be done despite them (and often feel better as a result).

- "Cool my head and warm my heart." Pay attention to intuition, hunches, gut feelings. Don't think too much; let your emotions inform you. We've talked about hunches and how they frequently do provide you with information from your own unconscious that you should pay attention to. We get so programmed to use our left brains, to investigate, problem-solve, *attack* that we apply this mode to all of our lives. Much of the time, especially when we're spinning our wheels, we need to stop, look, and listen: pay attention with the right brain, see the gestalt, the whole—"get" the situation as it involves ourselves and our feelings.

    Especially pay attention to first impressions of people and situations. Negative impressions are, I think, often correct amygdala reactions that there is something to be afraid of here.[1] When you have such a reaction, look into it—mindfully, objectively, carefully. Try to identify what's setting it off. Positive first impressions are also important; they may be nothing more meaningful than that you think you could have fun with this per-

---

1 I have no scientific basis for making this claim. All I have is the experience of my patients, who frequently end up regretting that they didn't follow their instincts at first—after they've been abused, or spurned, or taken to the cleaners. And of course this may be selective attention, only remembering the times when their initial apprehension proved correct and forgetting all the times it didn't. But it seems to me that I have heard this too often for it to be merely a result of that kind of bias.

son—which may be a self-fulfilling prophecy that will bring more fun into your life, not a bad thing.

- Emotions are about values, right and wrong, good and bad. In any situation that involves a moral choice, pay attention to your feelings. If you think too much, your defenses can get to work. You can rationalize doing the easy thing, or the thing that's best for you but not for others, and you won't feel bad about doing it. Or you can deny the implications, or use any other defense you want, and you won't feel bad immediately. But you'll add to your burden of unconscious guilt, add another layer to your character armor, and distort your perception of reality more. So try not to overthink ethical problems. Pay attention to what your heart, or your guts, tells you is right, because it probably is.

- Identify the stress response at work in your emotions. Don't be like the PTSD patient who doesn't recognize he has PTSD, attributing your feelings to current interactions instead of the stress response. If you're like most people nowadays, you *are* experiencing more fear and anger, guilt and shame, than you deserve or should expect to handle. And, also like most people, you defend against awareness of those feelings, so their effects emerge in disguised ways—depression, addiction, somatic symptoms. Though you have to address those problems, their impact can be lessened if you go back to the beginning and recognize that twenty-first-century life gives us great stress, though we're taught to deny it.

- Identify what makes you feel helpless, hopeless, or demoralized. What makes you choke up with sadness or frustration? What makes you feel like crying? What makes you want to yell at someone? Then be mindful of the circumstances. What's going on outside you? What's going on in your head? Use the Mood Journal (Exercise 2) to help you. Feelings like these are clues to the present and chronically endured pain, the focal problem you're always trying to resolve.

- Accept the unacceptable: lust, greed, envy, hate, murderous rage. Feelings like these are just as much a part of you as anything else. We may not be proud of it, but we can't help it, and it doesn't help to pretend it isn't there. We're social animals, and feelings about our status in the tribe, our access to the best mates to pass down our genes, are hard-wired into us. We should control how we act on these feelings, but we don't have to pretend they don't exist.

- Accept that you can want contradictory things. Wanting our parents to love us at the same time as we reserve the right to hate them is one very common example. Wanting our spouse to love us unconditionally at the same time as we attach conditions to our love is another. We can see the obvious moral inequity at work, and that may help us revise our expectations of self and others, but we won't do that unless we accept our feelings. We are capable of incredible hypocrisy, but being honest with ourselves works against that.

- Anxiety is your friend. It's your body trying to tell you something, and you ought to listen. Most likely, it's telling you that you're pushing yourself too hard, pushing yourself into something you don't want. Of course there are times when anxiety becomes the problem itself, and you may seek therapy to help you with it. But even in those circumstances a smart therapist is likely to find that you need to change your expectations of yourself, to make more room for the effects of stress.

- Anger is your friend too. Anger is telling you that someone is stepping on your toes, that something is going on that's endangering something important to you. Anger is how we're supposed to feel when our boundaries are violated. You may have gotten the message that anger is dangerous or ugly or unacceptable: not so. The people who told you that may have had something to gain from convincing you that anger is bad. In today's culture, perpetual stress may have you feeling too much anger (because there is really a lot to be angry about) and as a result you may act out your anger mindlessly, hurting those who love you. This is a real problem, and you have to get skillful about what you do with anger. But don't deny your anger; instead, pay attention to what it's telling you.

- Learn how to get out of a frenzy. There will be times when feelings are so upsetting that you may do something impulsive, something you'll regret later. Learn what helps you back off emotionally from these situations, which may be highly individual. Use my tips for controlling emotions from Chapter 4, and for getting out of a schema attack from Chapter 6. The important thing is to develop confidence that you can cool yourself down from any difficult emotional situation, because without that confidence you'll be too guarded to let yourself really experience your feelings.

Principle 3
Use Mindfulness to Recognize the Limits and Biases of Your Assumptive World

The assumptive world is our own unique set of assumptions, prejudices, perspectives, and rules for how we think reality operates. We couldn't function without one; the mere fact of organizing our memories and generalizing from them creates an assumptive world for us. But we inevitably introduce bias and distortion. If we can learn to observe skillfully how the world really seems versus how we think it should seem, we can gradually reduce much of the distortion we experience. Pay attention to your defenses and their purposes. Work on identifying your schemas. Think about how you use prejudices and categories, and how they limit your experience.

No doubt the subject that is most distorted is the self. The pressure of a Perpetual Stress Response that we don't fully recognize makes us distort our experience, displace our fears, and blame ourselves and our loved ones for unhappiness which we should recognize as inevitable. We organize our experience of ourselves into schemas, stories, recurring plotlines featuring old wounds that never heal. We develop defenses that distort reality in order to make us better or more important than we really are. We develop symptoms that express what we can't express openly. We develop character armor, a rigid shell that limits both our vision and our ability to respond flexibly to new experiences.

In order to gain mindful awareness of the limitations our assumptive world places on us, it can be helpful to:

- Develop awareness of the effects of the Perpetual Stress Response on how you see and think about reality (see Principle 5).
- At the same time, accept that your childhood experience has left its marks on you, for good and ill. This is not blaming your mother or your father, it's accepting what we know about how children's minds are formed. Parents can't help leaving their fingerprints all over their children.
- Your early years have contributed greatly to your assumptive world, influenced how your immune system functions, laid down the foundations for how you relate to others. Try to identify what of that works well for you, and what doesn't.
- Look back at your biography (Exercise 6) to identify how your world began to be distorted. Pay attention to how your fears developed. Think mindfully about how you interpreted your experience at those times.

What defenses were you learning? What did it lead you to assume about how the world works?

- Mindfully observe yourself in the present. Watch where your thoughts go when you're not paying attention—do old wounds surface? Are you ruminating about something, or rehearsing for the future? What is worrying you? Look for themes in your dreams. Look for recurring patterns in your relationships and in your jobs. Most important, just observe yourself now with compassionate curiosity. What do you find deficient about yourself?

- Ask your best friends and loved ones. Find the right opportunities, and set the ground rules: *I'm interested in understanding myself better. I'd like to hear what you'd like to say. If there was something you could tell me to change, or something I seem to keep worrying too much about, something you feel I should let go or relax about . . . I'd like to hear anything you'd like to say.* Talking with loved ones about the past can also be very enlightening: *How would you describe my parents? How did it affect you when [e.g., a certain family disaster] happened?* Be open to disconfirming information. When you learn something that doesn't click with your assumptive world, examine it mindfully.

- Look back at Exercise 10, "Injuries and Fears." It shouldn't be a surprise if, by this point, you have forgotten that exercise. That's how defenses work. You may have learned something important then, but "forgetting" clicks in to keep it from registering in your mind. But now, reviewing what you know of what hurt you and how it made you afraid—are you able to see ways you can get these to take up less room in your head? Do you feel less ashamed of them? Can you think more clearly about them?

- To the extent you can, try to identify your own defenses, using Exercise 8 and Table 2. If you think that you do something like rationalize or use selective attention, play with this idea. Mindfully observe yourself with the idea of developing your ability to spot your defenses at work, as if you were learning a new skill like playing a musical instrument. If you catch yourself at it regularly, don't feel bad or embarrassed; remember that defenses are natural. But try to look at how their use distorts or limits, or just shuts down, your experience. Imagine what giving them up would mean.

- Identify resistance at work. By that I mean your resistance to the ideas in this book. Do you keep agreeing but not doing the exercises? Do you dismiss the ideas, but keep reading? Do you believe what I say, but haven't tried mindfulness meditation yet? Are you doing what I did in college, which is to carry the book everywhere with me in the hope that something would sink in by osmosis? Those are strange, contradictory behaviors. Why do you suppose you are doing that? Could it have something to do with fear of change? If so, don't beat yourself up about it, but learn from the experience. Change is always difficult.

- As you did for defenses, try to understand yourself in terms of the schemas, character styles, or stories I listed in Chapter 6. Look at the assumptions and cognitive distortions that go with these ideas. Do you see a little of yourself anywhere? As you practice mindfulness, do it with these themes in mind. They might help you understand yourself a little better. Look at how these schemas and stories predict and control our experience of the world. Try thinking "out of the box"—in ways that are not consistent with your story of yourself—and see if it leads to different results for you.

- Mindfulness practice can help you conduct a continual, objective moral inventory—what really is your responsibility, and what is not. As you do this you must keep in mind the twin poles of excessive guilt (*everything is my fault*) and victimhood (*nothing is my fault*). It's not your fault if you're depressed or scared or ill or addicted; everything in your life up till now has led you to this point. You must learn to be more forgiving of your past mistakes, and stop blaming yourself. No one can survive today without substantial emotional scars. But, knowing what you do, it is your responsibility to do something about it now.

  Marsha Linehan's Dialectical Behavior Therapy, which we've talked about before, is based on a contradiction (hence dialectics, the resolution of opposites). Patients must accept themselves just as they are; accept their histories and current situations; learn to love and value themselves—but at the same time they must work very hard to change themselves and their environments. *You're perfect, but you have to change.* I agree. Each of us is perfect, underneath our character armor, but we have to work hard at shedding that armor.

- Learn how to comfort yourself. When you're down, in pain, in a hopeless state, overcome with fear, consider that you might be, above all else, *demoralized*. What would restore your morale? A chocolate milkshake? A brisk run? A talk with a friend? A day off? Go for it. Remember that moods are like buses—another will come along soon enough. Be patient, and distract yourself with something good while you're waiting.

Some people will have assumptive worlds so intensely affected by traumatic experiences that they need some special advice.

If you're a trauma victim:

- Get help. Get good professional help, and look for good group experiences.
- Take care of your symptoms. Sleep, eat, don't drink, don't abuse drugs, but use meds when they will help.
- Learn when you dissociate. Learn the triggers. Learn to bring yourself back.
- Relearn the signal value of emotions. Feelings are trying to tell you something important about your current experience. Before you dissociate from them, try to listen.
- Keep telling your story. Keep trying to get the feelings and the facts in sync. The goal is to reexperience the trauma nontraumatically.

If you're a chronic trauma victim:

- Follow the advice above, but pay attention to these questions:
- Be alert for how trauma has gotten into your soul. Do you end up in abusive situations now? Are you self-destructive without understanding why? Are you completely demoralized, expecting nothing, hopeless and helpless? Are you unable to want, or to feel? If yes to any of these, get yourself to very good professional help. These are the kinds of issues you might minimize and an inexperienced or inexpert clinician might miss.

Principle 4
Build Willpower, Self-Control, and Self-Respect

One thing that all the research agrees on is that the effects of stress are reduced if we believe we have some control over the stressful events. Rats' immune systems are protected if we give them something to gnaw on or a warning that the shock is coming. There are many ways we can work on getting more control and predictability in our lives:

- First, don't try to control what you can't. Remember the Serenity Prayer: *God grant me the serenity to accept the things I cannot change, the courage to change the things I can, and the wisdom to know the difference.* When faced with something you can't control, learn to be flexible. Manage your expectations and requirements. Try to find a way to be satisfied no matter how things turn out.

- Accept that self-control is limited. Often, we have enough to keep us out of serious trouble, but not enough to make us happy or proud of ourselves. The fact that it's not all-or-nothing suggests—to me, at least—that it's something we can get more of. We can develop it, like a muscle or a skill, through practice.

- Apply mindfulness to develop greater awareness of how you make—and avoid making—decisions. Decisions always involve emotions, because they're about things we care about. Do you allow yourself to experience your emotions? Purchases are an especially interesting area because we are so pressured by consumer culture to *buy*. The Hedonic Treadmill guarantees that we'll always want more; and many of us look to possessions to give us the validation and love that is otherwise missing in our lives. Can we look at these pressures and desires mindfully? We have a paradigm for making good decisions in Chapter 8. Do you follow it? Don't beat yourself up if you don't, but examine your actions sympathetically. If you can start to gain some control over mindless shopping, chances are good that you'll feel better about yourself in general.

- Control what you pay attention to. Fundamentally, this may be the only power we have over our lives. Mindfulness meditation will teach you a lot about attention, how it can be deliberately directed at or away from different subjects, except sometimes for the most pressing or obsessive issues that seem to hijack our attention. Learn to apply this ability outside the meditation situation. Practice diverting yourself from pressing but ultimately trivial desires (*A new pair of shoes would really make me feel good*). Practice directing your attention to less compelling but more meaningful subjects (*Shopping is out for today; focus on a new experience*). Not that we should do this all the time; it might take the joy out of life. But it's nice to know we can, when we need to, shut off our attention to attractive nuisances.

- Get skillful about anger. Perpetual stress has us so jazzed that it's understandable if we're crabby or want to strike out in frustration, sometimes at the nearest person. But giving in to this has many obvious negative consequences. Use your cognitive skills to learn about human communication, especially assertive communication. Remember my paradigm from Chapter 8: Attend, notice, think, decide. When someone does something that annoys you, very mindfully review what your responses might be, and choose the most skillful response. Then implement it. Then review how it worked, and learn what you might do better next time. Then do it again, and again, until it's second nature. Practicing like this lays down the new neural pathways that can become the default circuit when you're angry. You can then practice self-control without upset and effort.

- Protect your hippocampus. It's really a vital little nubbin in your brain, and it seems to be especially vulnerable to excess cortisol production. Cortisol comes with the fight-or-flight response, and its production continues if the response is not switched off. Try to develop awareness of the Perpetual Stress Response in yourself, and learn to switch it off (see Principle 5). When you can do this, the hippocampus can perform its function of consolidating memories, and you can create that coherent autobiographical narrative that we talk so much about.

- Strengthen your hippocampus. It's the only place we know of so far in the adult human brain where new nerve cells are being formed—stem cells, which can migrate to other areas of the brain and morph into their specialized function. There is good reason to believe that activities like exercise and learning, and environmental enrichment, stimulate this neurogenesis. So keep exercising, and keep challenging your brain with new learning. And be mindful of your environment. Like Ellen Langer's nursing home residents who lived longer because they were responsible for their environment, we can develop better brains by exposing ourselves to stimulation.

- Alter, avoid, accept. These are our only choices when it comes to something difficult. We can try to change it, or we can try to get away from it, or we can accept it. Don't look for a fourth choice, there isn't one. Western culture teaches us that we shouldn't accept anything without a fight, but sometimes the fight isn't worth the effort. If you're caught in the road with an eighteen-wheeler bearing down on you, avoidance is the only strategy. Don't feel badly about yourself if you can't change an unalterable situation, and don't waste time vacillating between responses. Try to make up your mind which strategy is best, and implement it as quickly and effectively as possible. Wisdom, of course, is knowing the best strategy.

- Organize yourself. Use your time and space mindfully. If control and predictability mitigate the effects of stress, here is one area where you can certainly help yourself. Go through the piles around the house, throw out what you don't need, and organize the rest. Apply mindful attention to how you spend your time, and try to spend more in high-value activities. Don't do this to pack more into your day, do it to free up time for meditation and exercise, for joy and gratification.

- Stop procrastinating. Most procrastinators tell themselves they will get to whatever it is when they feel the motivation. This is a misunderstanding of how motivation works. More often than not, if you just begin the task, then you begin to feel motivated. You get focused on the task, which is a little pleasurable, then you get interested in finishing. Procrastination is only a passive-aggressive game you play with yourself. The present you is leaving a mess that the future you will have to clean up. The future you is going to suffer self-hate and damaged self-esteem because of the actions of the present you.

People who are fighting addictions need some special words when it comes to building willpower:

If you have a soft addiction (shopping, overeating, surfing the net, etc.):

- Don't try to stop unless you mean it. You'll only demoralize yourself further with halfhearted efforts that end in failure. Carefully think about what circumstances are going to tell you you're ready, and when you're sure you're ready, go all out. Often this is an unconscious decision—you wake up one morning and decide today's the day. Pay attention to that— but if your will power is already flagging by the end of the day, just tell yourself you misread the signs, and don't waste any further effort.
- Once you decide, make it very difficult for yourself to continue with your addictive behavior. Tell all your friends you're giving it up. Tear up the credit cards, unplug the computer for a while, empty out the refrigerator. Don't tell yourself you just need willpower, because willpower is built from experience; you need all the help you can get. Removing temptation and setting yourself up with negative consequences for relapsing are very effective methods of helping.
- Enlist your support system. It's a great time to have a success team. If you don't, make sure that your existing support network knows that it's a very good time for them to be positive and encouraging, and to refrain from tempting you or helping you rationalize.

If you have a hard addiction (drugs, alcohol—any substance that will have a withdrawal effect):

- Don't try to stop unless you mean it. As above; multiple failed attempts just make it easier to fail again. And you'll wear out your support system in the process, if you haven't already.
- Don't try to fight it alone. Find a group. Find a Twelve-Step program. Find a sponsor—someone who's been through it, someone who'll be there every day for you. Use of drugs and alcohol changes you so much that you will need to construct a new self to maintain sobriety. You won't be able to do this alone.
- Warn people about withdrawal. Just give notice to your loved ones that you may have a difficult few weeks. Don't take that as license to be a jerk; do your best to control yourself, but you legitimately may need a little slack.
- Think about going away for a while. If you need to be detoxed, you should be in a supervised setting. Even if you don't absolutely need detox, there are good residential programs out in the countryside that can help you through the first difficult weeks. Being determined to white-knuckle it, to do it all on your own, is sometimes giving yourself an excuse to fail.

Principle 5
Control the Effects of Stress

- Recognize the effects of the Perpetual Stress Response at work within yourself. It's in the tension in your shoulders, neck, jaw muscles; the pains that don't go away, the gastric upset that keeps recurring. It's in the fear that makes you rigid and defensive when you don't understand why, the anger that has you snapping at people you love. Work on developing mindful awareness of the factors at work in your life that make you feel out of control, empty, and frightened—and the forces that make you pretend you're doing just fine. Look at yourself with compassionate curiosity; stop pretending, and look objectively at your life.
- Recognize that most of your conventional responses to stress only make matters worse by playing into the circularity of your problems. Depression and anxiety feed on themselves. Addictive habits or drugs reduce your self-control. Stress-related disease makes you avoid the activities that will help you feel better. Denial—lying to yourself—just makes your life more complicated. Avoidance weakens your character. *If you do nothing*

else, you can work on stopping these habits. You don't necessarily have to know what to do instead, just stop—and the vicious circle will stop—and you will be in a different position and able to think more clearly.

- Recognize that the only solution is to face perpetual stress directly, resolved to do something different about it. Give it your mindful attention and respect. Don't fall for easy solutions. Rather, take an inventory of what's overloading you, and be ready to make hard decisions. Give up trying for the impossible. Give up trying to do everything, trying to please everyone, trying to be perfect. Be more accepting of yourself as you are; recognize how stress has been handicapping you, and give yourself a break.

- Get skillful at flexibility. People who don't have to have everything just so have a little immunity from stress. Don't pin all your hopes on one horse in the race. Develop confidence that you can always land on your feet. Let yourself imagine the worst—the job moves to India, you have a health crisis, your daughter runs away with a motorcycle gang—and visualize how you will handle it. Visualize yourself coping, and don't visualize yourself falling apart. Make preparations, as much as possible, for disaster. Have some savings. Have disability insurance. Have friends who will always take you in.

- Protect yourself from popular culture. If you're a woman, don't read "women's magazines," they only make you unhappy with yourself. If you're a man, read more good fiction; it will teach you about relationships. Be careful and selective about how you get your news. Avoid exposure to advertising as much as possible. If you're going to watch television, invest in TiVo or some similar device so you can protect yourself from commercials. There's nothing at all wrong with a little escapism, whether it's silly comedy or soap operas or crime stories—but don't let it become your only source of pleasure.

- Reduce stress in every way you can. Mindfully examine every activity you do, and ask if it's a reasonable use of the time and effort you put into it. If it's not, work on ways to get it out of your schedule. Stop volunteering if you only do it to please others. Set boundaries around yourself that you can maintain. Say no when it's appropriate. Pay down your debt, and live within your means.

- Find outlets for stress. Look for activities that bring you into the "flow" state, the balance point between being stressed and being bored. Look for things that you can master, things that are creative, that get you thinking outside the box, using the other part of your brain. Take up a hobby. Learn a musical instrument, a foreign language, cabinet-making, fine cooking. Take up dancing or tai chi—it can be wonderfully integrating to get your whole body learning balance and coordination. Take up sports or games that get you your regular exercise with some people contact—riding, tennis, squash, bowling, swimming. Gardening; travel; singing. Think about what would make *you* feel good.

- Consider an adventure. After doing all the exercises in this book, you should have a pretty good idea of what's making you unhappy and overstressed. If it's truly built in to the routine of your life—your job, your family—consider chucking it all and starting over. I don't say this lightly, and I don't want you to jump impulsively from the frying pan into the fire—but if you can make concrete plans for a different life that would bring you greater freedom and not ruin the lives of those who depend on you, go for it. Open the marina on the St. John's you've always dreamed about. Sell the house in the suburbs and move to the city. Go on a spiritual journey.

- Consider activism. If what I've said in Chapter 2 about the emptiness of our culture resonates with you, do something about it. You may just start speaking up among your friends about how you really feel. You might change jobs and work for an organization that promotes cultural change. You might run for office. There's no reason to believe that the sickness in our culture can't be healed if enough people recognize it and are willing to do something about it. And of course you will feel proud of yourself for doing it.

Principle 6
Be Skillful about Your Body

"The body bears the burden," in Robert Scaer's evocative phrase, of our response to stress, trauma, abuse, invalidation. After centuries of believing that the mind doesn't affect the body, scientists are now waking up to the fact that the body and mind are the same thing, and that what we experience as mentally disturbing is also disturbing to the body. Those nonspecific illnesses, chronic pains, cranky bowels that torment so many now are the body's protest that it can't handle what we're forcing on it. Even if your body isn't protesting yet, it will. We're not designed to last much past age forty, so if we want to do it with any grace or joy, we'd better treat our body like the very valuable commodity it is.

- Treat yourself and your body with compassion, affection, and respect. Let your body warm up in the morning and relax before bedtime. Don't abuse your body by feeding it poisons or pushing it too hard. If you have a pain or a rash or an infection, or any other somatic concern, have a physician look at it, and follow the advice you get. Treat yourself like a plant: lots of water and sunlight, a regular dose of nutrients, an occasional pruning of unnecessary stress.

- Do a daily exercise routine to strengthen and stretch your body and generate endorphins. Try for a half hour or a little longer, with a warm-up period of stretching, maybe some massage of the tender points, followed by twenty or twenty-five minutes of aerobic activity, followed by some stretching and/or walking to cool down. Be present while you do this; no TV.

- Get yourself a decent aerobic exerciser for your home, if you can possibly afford it. If you can't, save up for it—it should be your next big purchase. I like my elliptical trainer. It gives me plenty of challenge but it lets me set my own pace, and it doesn't damage my knees or feet. But you may prefer a treadmill or a stationary bike or a rowing machine. Or a videotaped workout with nothing but a mat and maybe some steps. In good weather, vary your routine with some running or fast walking or swimming.

- As you're doing your workout, add a little mindfulness at the same time. Focus on the feelings in your body. Focus on integrating mind and body; visualize yourself as one big system. You don't have to *listen* to your muscles, joints, and the like because you are one big system and they're communicating all the time. The idea of listening just reinforces the myth that they are separate; instead, *attend* to them. Remember that we control what we pay attention to.

- Now you have an hour a day to give to yourself: half to meditation, half to exercise. You can do this in any pattern that suits you; most people find they like to have predictability to this routine, and it's important not to be just squeezing it in between other commitments.

- Visualize those endorphins pouring out of your pituitary gland (the olive hidden behind the thumb in Siegel's hand model of the brain) and other areas in your brain and spinal cord. Exercise gets them flowing, like water from a hand pump. Visualize how they flood your body with good feeling and pain-blocking anesthesia. Pay attention to their effects. The effects may be very subtle at first, and you may have to develop your sensitivity like a wine taster, but soon you'll be feeling them at work. Remember that endorphins have the opposite effect from opiates, which dull your sensitivity so that you always need more to get the same benefit. Instead, endorphins heighten your sensitivity so that soon you will be getting a good feeling from things that you were taking for granted—smells, tastes, people, activities that were kind of blah now become more interesting and fun. Keep those endorphins flowing.

- If you're too overweight—if it's causing health problems or restricting your activities or *really* making you feel unattractive—start a campaign to lose it. Don't call it a diet, because diets don't work; call it a new way of eating. Educate yourself about calories, carbs, and fats, and try to find a way to eat a smaller enough amount of calories that, combined with exercise, will help you lose weight. Drink a lot of water. Recruit a support system: friends who will commit to encouraging you when you're feeling down or weak. Stick with your new way of eating religiously for a month, and you should lose a few pounds, which hopefully will encourage you to keep on. Set a *realistic* goal for yourself—a delicate process—and keep at it. After the first month, if you slip, don't start thinking that you've blown your diet, with the accompanying rationalization that you might as well give up, as well as the accompanying depression and hopelessness. Instead, realize that all you've done is make a mistake. Go back to your new eating plan, and start looking at it as something you can do for the rest of your life—not as strictly as when you want to lose weight, so you can have some occasional treats—but still a lifelong commitment to yourself.

- Even if you're not overweight, educate yourself about nutrition. There are too many bad things that can happen to your body from not eating right for you to take a chance. Avoid fast food, convenience food, overprocessed food, food with too many additives (for "shelf life"), food with too much salt, food with too much fat. Eat fresh foods prepared at home or in decent restaurants. If you have unexplained symptoms like gastric upset, rashes, headaches, muscle aches, or insomnia, investigate the role of food allergies. It wouldn't hurt anything at all to have a relationship with a good nutritionist who will get to know you and your family, whom you can count on for food advice through the years. Don't count on your doctor; MDs get virtually no training in nutrition.

- If you use alcohol, use it moderately and occasionally. There is nothing good to say about regular use. Alcohol is a poison; it kills brain cells. It interferes with judgment and makes us do things we regret. Like other drugs, we habituate to it, so it takes more to get the same effect. But don't beat yourself up for occasional use. Some alcohol, especially red wine, apparently has some health benefits. Alcohol can help us in social situations, it can help us turn off the stress response, it can be a relatively harmless reward for getting through a tough day—but it can only do this occasionally. If we depend on it for these effects, it will stop working.

Principle 7
Learn to Appreciate Your Symptoms

Symptoms—physical, mental, or both—are your wise mind speaking. They're a distress signal from your overstressed bodymind (to use Candace Pert's term); something is going wrong somewhere, and we'd better pay attention. Have a little gratitude for your symptoms, because if they didn't get your attention now, things would only get worse. If you have physical or mental symptoms that are causing you distress and not responding to conventional treatment, apply your mindfulness skills to the problem. Above all, don't keep mindlessly doing more of the same of what you're doing now, because that's what has brought you to this place.

- Don't be ashamed of your symptoms; remember that all you have is burnout. The Perpetual Stress Response is an inevitable clash between contemporary living conditions and our tired old nervous systems. You've been trying to do the impossible, and there's no shame in not making it.
- At the same time as symptoms are a signal, they're also a defense. They're a disguised presentation of a problem, because we don't want to face the problem itself. Our defensive system thinks the problem is too scary to face directly. It may take a lot of mindful attention to interpret the code of the symptom.
- Start with no assumptions. Some of your assumptions have led to the state you're in now. Especially do not assume that what you think is necessary is true. Your difficulty may be coming from unexpected directions, perhaps how you interpret stress more than the stress itself. If you want to get relief you may have to make major changes in your lifestyle. That may be a scary thought, so begin work on getting your mind around it.
- Identify your hidden stressors. What do you worry about late at night? What gets you upset whenever you think about it? You may actually have to write notes to yourself because your defenses are so effective that you

forget about these things most of the time. If you're able to identify hidden stressors, bring them out of the dark and subject them to mindful attention. This in itself may take away their power. But if it doesn't, use your wise mind to figure out what to do, how to get help.

- Where does it hurt? Sometimes there is a symbolic meaning to physical symptoms. Digestive problems may mean you're trying to swallow something you shouldn't. A backache can mean you're carrying too heavy a load. Chronic fatigue can be a way of saying you're scared and overwhelmed. Breathing problems may mean someone or something is cutting off your air supply. If so, apply your mindful attention to the source of the problem, not to the symptom.
- Anxiety simply means we're scared, but not usually of the thing that *seems* to be scaring us. My height phobia was never about heights, it was about a fear of destroying myself (among other things). If you have an anxiety problem, stop and look objectively at your life. Are you pushing too hard? Are you trying to do the impossible, make everyone love you, make everyone safe? Are you afraid of your own anger, so afraid you can't even recognize it?
- PTSD has to be recognized for what it is, not an easy process because the stress seems to be coming from your present life. If you're having nightmares or flashbacks, or if you're dissociating, or if your loved ones don't understand why you're acting strange, look mindfully at your life for past trauma. If that's what it is, you need to get professional help. You also need to develop your ability to look at yourself with compassionate curiosity and see the trauma as what it is, a terrible injustice that happened to you, something so terrible that you've tried to pretend it didn't happen or didn't affect you. Stop pretending.
- Depression is nature's way of telling you to give up; the bodymind recognizes that we're not getting anywhere, so it goes into shutdown mode. In the process you've generated so much stress that you've burned out your endorphin system, and now you can't feel good at all. Back off, look at your whole life situation mindfully, and be prepared to start over. Find a good therapist, and try to rekindle hope in yourself that things can change.
- Addictions—both hard and soft—are about feeling empty, unloved, and overwhelmed. Besides conquering your addiction, you're going to have to

figure out how to limit your stress and get your own needs met. Mindfulness in itself will help you feel better, but you're going to have to be patient—not an easy thing when you've gotten used to instant gratification. Work on developing pride about being patient.

- "Personality disorders" are supposed to be symptom free, but you know if all your relationships are a mess, if you can never seem to get what you want, if you drive people crazy or keep shooting yourself in the foot. If this is you, slow down, stand back, and look at your behavior objectively. Remember that the essence of neurosis is to keep on doing the same thing but expecting a different result. You're probably going to need to find a good therapist to help you sort it out. As you try, mindfully look at your own defenses in action, and work on letting your guard down.
- Educate yourself about your condition. Remember that the truth is probably somewhere between rabble-rousing hysteria and "doctor knows best." Use your wise mind to help you identify reliable, truthful information. Don't look for what you want to hear or what confirms your assumptions. Look for practical advice, anything that helps empower you to do something about the situation.
- Apply Schwartz's four Rs to any symptom: *Relabel, reattribute, refocus, revalue.* Relabel your symptom as a faulty circuit in the brain, something that grew there as the best solution you could work out the first time this problem came up. Reattribute the distress you feel to the faulty circuit at work—no matter how real or compelling it feels, it's not the truth. Things are not as bad as they seem, they're being distorted by your bad wiring. Refocus your attention from the distress to any behavior that helps you adapt to or tolerate the situation, or distracts you from it. Go for a walk, read the paper, play some music, call a friend. Finally, revalue your symptoms and life as a whole. If these symptoms, which seemed so real, are just the result of a glitch in the brain, perhaps you should be more mindful about how you experience reality. Revalue your values, this time with more freedom from stress, fear, and compulsion.
- If you have unexplained physical symptoms, ask your doctor who he would send his mother to with this condition. Go to that person. These things we're talking about are at the cutting edge of medicine. Don't settle for average care.
- At the same time as you get the best care you can, don't expect too much.

Don't give the power to make you well to your doctor, but reserve it for yourself. Take medications as prescribed, unless you have bad side effects. If they don't seem to be helping, discuss with your doctor taking a medication holiday to see if they really are effective. Meanwhile, keep on implementing all these principles and see if the symptoms don't recede in importance.

- Find a therapist. Chances are you won't be able to get past this without the help of an objective but caring third party. See my guidelines in Chapter 7 for how to find a good one.
- Work on acceptance that you may have a chronic illness. No, it's not fair, but there's nothing you can do about that. People usually don't make a complete recovery from the things we're talking about in this book. That doesn't mean they'll never feel good again. What you can do is be proactive in making sure you make the most complete recovery you can, and work on learning how to limit the illness's impact on your life.

Principle 8
Think with Your Whole Mind

As you practice mindfulness, pay attention to both sides of your brain, the holistic, impressionistic, "emotional" voice and the linear, historical, "logical" voice. Don't think about them in terms of right or wrong, black or white—remember we're not judging. Appreciate that they see the world in two very different ways, and be grateful for the advantage that gives you. Remember that, as a result of the Perpetual Stress Response, the emotional brain is scared and hypervigilant. The logical brain, though, is overdeveloped like a body builder, constantly trying to interpret more data than it was designed for and respond to stresses never before experienced in the history of humanity. As if that weren't enough, it's always trying to quiet or reassure or dismiss the slightly hysterical left brain.

But, as they say about paranoia, just because you're hysterical doesn't mean there's nothing to be alarmed about. The left brain is giving us vital information that we'd better not dismiss. It's aware of danger before consciousness is. It knows who we can trust and who we can't before we can say why. It knows when we're safe. We make our best judgments when we can use both sides of the brain, intuition informing logic, rationality checking instinct.

I described a simple process for making decisions in Chapter 8; the main steps:

- *Attend.* Pay attention to what's going on. Focus your attention on the decision at hand. Mentally define its boundaries, and don't pay attention to what's irrelevant. Look at things mindfully, objectively, curiously. Don't get hung up on details, but don't push any awareness aside.
- *Notice.* Let your awareness expand to the whole picture. How many choices are there? Who besides me has an interest in the outcome? How should I value their interests? What do I know, and what am I only guessing at? When I'm guessing, can I find out more so I don't have to guess?
- *Think.* What will be the likely outcome of the different choices you have? Visualize each scenario as it plays out tomorrow, next week, next year. Which will make you happiest? Proudest? What happens if you don't decide? Is there an external deadline? Should you make a deadline for yourself?
- *Decide.* Having considered the likely outcomes, which is best for you and the other parties concerned? You have to consider the degree of uncertainty attached to any scenario; clearly the best choice is the one that is most certain *and* has the greatest value for all participants. But sometimes the choice that has the greatest value is less certain than others. Then it becomes a risk analysis. What's at stake if you're wrong? Can you afford it? If there's a lot at stake, perhaps you have to go with a more certain choice that is of only moderate value.

There are other considerations in how you think and make decisions:

- Make decisions you're proud of. This is a good way to use gut feelings as a check on pure logic. You probably shouldn't choose something you'd be ashamed to tell your mother about, even if it seems like a great idea at the time. If you're forced to choose between the lesser of two evils—whether to lay off Joe or Jack—you're in a very stressful system, and you should probably be working to get out of it or improve it.
- Educate yourself. This should be a lifelong task. It's not enough to be smart, you have to be knowledgeable as well. Read a good newspaper regularly, and consider it your duty as a citizen to be informed about current affairs. Read books on subjects you'd like to know more about. Attend adult education classes. Put yourself around people who have something to teach you. Be curious about the world, and learn to trust your own judgment. Don't take anybody's word for it.

- Don't make hasty decisions under stress. Sometimes under stress we feel an imperative to make a decision in the belief that doing so will reduce the stress we feel. Resist that temptation. Decisions made in these circumstances usually backfire, with long-term negative consequences. Learn techniques to buy time for yourself to think. If someone is pressuring you, there is nothing wrong with saying *I'm going to sleep on it*. If you're getting that much pressure, you should be suspicious.

Sometimes we get stuck thinking too much, and it can help to do something so that we change our perspective. Barbara Sher, in her valuable little book *I Could Do Anything if I Only Knew What It Was,* has this to say about the values of taking action:

- Action helps you think. Even action in the wrong direction is informative.
- Action raises your self-esteem. You're a success every time you face down fear. Acting "as if" you know what you're doing teaches you skills; you have to remember that everything new feels awkward and difficult at first.
- Good luck happens when you're in action. Doing something—anything—increases the likelihood that good things will happen to you.
- Action brings you in better communication with your guts—your self, your inner desires.
- Action exposes your resistances. Some sense of danger prevents you from action, but unless you take action, you may never know what the danger is.

Principle 9
Construct and Reinforce Your Support System
American society has had a bias in favor of autonomy over interdependency. We've been led to believe that the ideal person is the John Wayne character in the movies—completely able to take care of himself, not needing any support from others, in fact suspicious and uncomfortable with closeness. It's about time we got over that. People who are connected to others live longer, happier, more productive lives and have fewer health problems than people who are isolated. In fact, people who are isolated, far from being the strong, silent, independent type, run the risk of becoming both strange and estranged unless they take steps to maintain relationships with the rest of the world.

Relationships go both ways. As much as we get from the support of others, we also get a lot from what we do to provide support for others. The next point focuses on the values of intimate relationships; here we're going to attend to the network of connections you build with the rest of the world. Consider the following values of your relationships:

- Creating meaning. If we lack a formal religious belief, we face the problem of the apparent randomness of existence, and the question of the purpose of our own. The shallowness of contemporary culture reduces us all to shoppers and happiness-seekers, but happiness is not an acquisition. Relationships give purpose: to be fruitful, to be helpful, to make a difference in the lives of others. As a side effect, they give us opportunities for happiness.
- Encouraging creativity. It's difficult to see things differently if we only interact with ourselves. Opening ourselves up to others' points of view gives us the opportunity to see how much our assumptive world has constricted our vision. The support and encouragement of others can motivate us to take risks we would otherwise avoid. We can do things as a group we'd never do alone: sing for an audience, get up and dance, march on Washington.
- Developing empathy. When we get to know someone's emotional life, and let them in on our own, we get the opportunity to check out and correct our assumptions about emotions. Contrary to our most basic assumption, not everyone feels the same way we do about the same experience. Realizing this, we may challenge our own feelings, find that they are more complex than we assumed. It can shake up our little world, a good thing. We also develop our skills in understanding others, something we can always get better at.
- Sharing information. We can't read everything, be informed about everything of interest or importance. Having a network of friends who know your interests is like having a group of readers at your service, people who are in contact with the world, interested in finding out for you what you need to know.
- Sharing emotional experience. When we participate with others in emotional experiences, from watching a ball game to watching a disaster, we have an instant connection. The more we do this, the deeper the connection. Having other people who've shared some of our experiences makes our experiences more real, somehow, and richer because we hear from others nuances and details that have not registered on ourselves.
- Seeing the self through others' eyes. Not only does it keep us humble, it

gets under our defenses. When we learn that we're not fooling people, we can give up trying to pretend.

- Play. It's pretty hard to play alone. But we need play in our lives. Laughter stimulates endorphins and makes life much easier to take. I love to play with my dogs, and that kind of play is good for me too, but it's not enough. We need to have people involved to get the full benefit of play. Jokes can break up an impacted bad mood. Wit can make us see the farcical side of our biggest worries. Spending a few hours playing a board game can help us de-stress as effectively as anything else we can do.

- Fruitfulness. We gain in self-respect and stress tolerance when we feel we are contributing something to others. We get the opportunity to be kind and generous, to live up to our best image of ourselves. We feel we are capable of having an impact on life, something that may be unfortunately too rare for many of us in today's culture. We don't have to be glamorous, we don't have to be a celebrity, we don't have to be an All-Star; we can just be ourselves, and still be important to someone. What a wonderful opportunity!

- Building community. We can build a home for ourselves—something we never knew we missed—through developing a network of relationships. The Perpetual Stress Response has us full of fear, always looking for danger, hypervigilant and worn out. Having people who make us feel that we're loved, respected, and cared for can help us let down our guard. It's a very old, primitive feeling of safety that goes back to sharing a cave with the rest of the clan. Feeling accepted, feeling validated, turns down the fear valve and lets us drain the tension from our bodies.

Principle 10
Learn Intimacy Skills

Be patient with your relationships. Intimacy always involves conflict. We want to be loved, but we fear being smothered at the same time. We want to respect our partner, but we want to have our own way. We want commitment, but we want freedom too. That's just the way we're built, and we can't change it. Being really close to someone—lover, parent, child, sibling, good friend—is always going to have its headaches, but it also provides us with the richest, most joyful and fruitful experiences we will ever have. In order to preserve the opportunity for those experiences, we have to be mindful of how we are in relationships, how we feel, how we communicate.

In order to maintain and deepen intimacy, we have to do a few things:

- Express love. Let our loved ones know our feelings. Loosen up and act on your feelings. Give a hug or a kiss when the spirit moves you, and let it move you often. Smile. Be interested in their experience. Bring home gifts; it's magical to show someone you were thinking about them while apart.
- Be thoughtful and considerate. Some of my patients, from neglectful families, have never had the experience of someone being interested in them, curious about what's on their minds, wanting to help and protect them. When they find it for the first time, it's scary, it feels like too much, it feels like a drug that is way too powerful. That's what being thoughtful and considerate can do for your loved ones, even if they're comfortable with it—what a gift!
- Express appreciation. Recognize effort and achievement. Practice noticing what your loved ones do; get out of your own head and apply your mindfulness skills to others. Being grateful, as we've already said, is good for you in a hundred ways. Expressing gratitude is also very good for the recipient. Show that you notice when someone has done something beyond the call of duty. On the other hand, practice not noticing the little slips and errors that come just because someone is tired or mindless. You can help them be more mindful; that's a thousand times better than reminding them about wiping their feet.
- Practice empathy. Help your loved ones express themselves. Tell them how you think they're feeling, and check it out against their reality. It will help your communication enormously, and it will also improve your empathic abilities. It's another area where practice can really make a difference.
- Reveal yourself. Let your loved ones know what you're thinking and feeling. It can feel like a tremendous gift, especially if you're someone who is typically buttoned up and self-sufficient. Just talk about what's going on inside your head. Let your guard and your defenses down.

There are some other skills we need to learn in order to resolve conflicts with loved ones:

- Demonstrate mindful concern about your partner's experience. You don't have to agree that she's right in order to validate that you understand how she feels. By trying to understand her feelings, you get important clues about how this conflict developed, and how communication problems might have contributed to it.

- Employ healthy listening and communication. Be mindful about how you listen and what you say. In the midst of conflict, nonverbal communication can be misleading. You may be upset, but it gets interpreted as angry. So repeat the message you're receiving back to the sender: *I understand that you mean* . . . And don't rely on your nonverbals to accurately frame your meaning. Provide the frame verbally: *I'm really uncomfortable with all this conflict, but the only thing I'm really mad at you about is* . . . Use your assertiveness skills from Chapter 10 to make sure you are being direct. If you're not sure how you feel, say so.
- Adopt a problem-solving approach. Take our decision-making process from Chapter 8 and apply it to the present situation, and invite your partner to join you. This helps frame the conflict as a problem for you to solve together, rather than a dispute about who's to blame. It also helps to define and limit the problem, so that you can both be sure you're talking about the same thing.
- Don't amplify problems; don't raise the ante. Emotions are contagious. If someone's angry in the room, we're likely to catch the anger. The same goes for fear, or happiness for that matter, but we're talking about unpleasant feelings now. Remember to be mindful of your internal state, and even if you're feeling provoked, resist the temptation to provoke back. You'll be proud of yourself in the morning, and the conflict will get resolved faster.

There are a few things we can do to add depth and connection to our relationships:

- Share plans and dreams. Plan your vacations together. Plan your retirement together. But don't let it end there; talk about your values, about wishes you might consider silly or fantastic. Let yourself go in the blue sky of daydreaming. It's a gift to others to let them into your interior world. Of course, you also have to return the favor, and be interested in what your loved one wants. Don't be afraid to say what you want, and what your fears or doubts might be.
- Have partners in adventure. Encourage each other to take risks—to learn ballroom dancing or mountain climbing together. Go off on a trip without the usual reservations and firm schedules. Encourage each other to play,

to get silly, to compromise your dignity. It strengthens your bond and enriches your life.

- Have partners in learning too. Encourage each other to stretch your minds. Share your knowledge with each other. Get out of the house and go to adult ed together—preferably not taking the same subject. Keeping your mind limber is more and more important as our life spans extend so far beyond what nature intended for us.

Then there are our relationships with God, nature, and the rest of the world:

- Treat yourself, and others, with mindful attention and compassionate curiosity. Bias yourself toward affection and caring. Perpetual stress has us seeing others as potential threats, ourselves as deficient and vulnerable. Try to correct for that by consciously going in the other direction. Consider that strangers are really a blank screen that you project your internal world onto. If strangers are always scary, or untrustworthy, consider what that says about what's going on inside you.
- On the other hand, look at the people you spend time with. If there are some whose visits you dread, who you are always glad to see leave, then shake up the relationship. Talk compassionately and directly with them about what you think is wrong and what you'd like to see changed. If they listen, the relationship might improve. If they're offended, so be it. Life is too short to spend time with people who make you feel uncomfortable.
- We have a relationship with nature, too, or at least we should. We need to recognize how the world outside affects us—the weather, the sun, the physical surroundings. It can make us feel loved, or safe, or at home, or hated, or unimportant. We need to construct our lives so that we spend more time in nature feeling loved, safe, and at home—to deliberately place ourselves in settings where we can experience those feelings more.
- God is also a relationship. You have feelings for God; almost no one is indifferent. Those who say they are indifferent are usually angry or contemptuous, and that's a problem. It suggests there's a bitterness in your soul that will hurt you. You may want to drag that out and give it your mindful attention. If you're afraid of God, that also suggests a problem. On the other hand, if you have positive or benign feelings, that suggests you're getting yourself into a good place.

There are other relationship skills that have to do with setting limits. You don't want to have a deeper relationship with the kinds of people who generate these problems:

- Don't let people push you around. Don't be a people-pleaser. Don't try to be liked.
- Learn how to identify when you're being manipulated, and what to do about it.
- Learn how to identify and protect yourself from controllers, sadists, passive-aggressive obstructionists, and other difficult people.
- Don't go along with the crowd. There's a fine line between a crowd and a mob, and a mob can do some pretty horrible things. Be skeptical of the infectious enthusiasm you sometimes get in groups.

Principle 11
Learn How to Be Happy

Our brain does not simply store our experiences. Each experience changes the brain, structurally, electrically, chemically. The brain becomes the experience. In order to break free from the stress cycle, we need to feed our brains and bodies with experiences of mastery, creativity, and joy. Our minds—the way we think about things—have tremendous power to help us rebuild and rewire our brains, power that we too often ignore or use self-destructively. But we can use that power constructively, to build autonomy, competence, and relatedness, and help ourselves step off the stress cycle forever.

When you go to bed and turn out the light, try to think of three good things that happened during the day. Three things that brought you joy, or made you proud, or helped you relax, or just made you smile. Chances are that you will find yourself remembering small things. I have no scientific studies to rely on, but I believe that making a practice of this will gradually boost endorphin levels and make us feel better in general. It will certainly enhance our appreciation of what we've got.

One of the best ways we can *change our minds* is by relearning how to play. Most of us, thankfully, had some opportunity to play as children, because play comes naturally when you're young. Play is about fantasy, about pretending, about using our brains to get good at physical activity. Play generates endorphins, those happy little hormones that make us smile.

Attitude has tremendous power to change our experience; work can be play.

As I sit in my office, cataloging references for this book, stepping back from the content and tinkering with the outline, trying to discover new patterns and meanings, I'm taken back to my childhood fantasies: kneeling in the dust with Howard Carter as he peers into Tutankhamen's tomb, seeing wonderful things inside; standing beside Sherlock Holmes in his laboratory, identifying the ash of a Trichinopoly cigar; following the map to buried treasure with Jim Hawkins and Long John Silver. Just as I was then comforting myself from too much awareness of mysterious conflicts in my family by identifying with heroes and solving imaginary mysteries, so do I now insulate myself a little from the bigger mysteries of adulthood by expanding my knowledge of what I know something about and passing it on to others. And I enjoy it just as much as I did when I was ten.

But play is not the only route to happiness. There are other ways to bring joy to life, and joy is not the only element of happiness. Fulfillment is equally, if not more, important. Joy is right here and now, a laugh, a smile. Fulfillment is the attainment of our dreams. It's a quiet joy, with pride mixed in.

Let's look at getting more joy into our lives first, then return to the subject of fulfillment.

Joy through play:

- Play increases mindfulness. It demands risk taking and involvement; if it could be done mindlessly, it would not be play anymore.
- In fact, being around young children makes you mindful, because you spend time seeing the world through their fresh eyes, without much of your assumptive world to distort things.
- Play depends on incongruity and loss of dignity. It causes us to take ourselves less seriously.
- It's pretend, it has you acting like someone else, so again it gives you a different perspective on the world. It teaches you empathy, the capacity to think like others.
- Play teaches us flexibility—it allows us to practice what it's like to be a child, an elder, the opposite sex. Flexibility is essential in a world that changes so quickly.
- Play and humor coalesce a crowd of individuals into a group sharing an experience. We all want to feel as if we are a part of the group.
- Humor is a mature defense, a healthy adaptation to stress. We can express forbidden feelings through jokes or wit.

- Lenore Terr, a child therapist, writes of "traumatic play"—repeating an experience over and over again in safety, in order to develop a sense of mastery and file the trauma away—which may be behind our fascination with suspense movies and ghost stories.

Joy through other means:

- Sensual gratification. The body knows what it likes; we're wired that way. Sex, smells, tastes, drugs. Unfortunately, these things depend on novelty for much of their effectiveness, so we quickly habituate to them. In order to preserve their ability to bring us joy, it's necessary to space them out, savor them, and figure out ways to surprise yourself (usually with the assistance of a loved one).
- Joy comes from many little things, as well, like a really good grilled cheese sandwich. We need to practice being mindful of these things, like tastes, smells, smiles, views. The first shoots coming up in the spring. The first really ripe tomato of August. A voice on the phone. A memory of someone we loved. We need to practice paying attention; the more we do it, the easier it gets.
- Music can touch us emotionally, and in doing so it makes us more mindful; it speaks directly to the right brain, waking it up and getting it to pay attention. Music can bring us great pleasure. I challenge anyone, even the most die-hard opera haters, to listen to Mozart's "Marriage of Figaro" and not smile.
- Fireworks: a neglected pleasure, in the United States too often relegated to one day a year. I can't analyze fireworks, they just make us happy.
- Humor lowers our defenses; laughing, we can be caught off guard. Humor turns the world upside down, making the serious funny, unstuffing stuffed shirts and puncturing pomposity. These things all add to mindfulness.

Fulfillment:

- Fulfillment is my term for the mix of pride and pleasure we feel as we bring a challenging project to fruition, read a good book, or watch as our children or other people we help along the way grow and thrive. Though there are elements of joy in fulfillment, they are clearly different things.

- Here are some other experiences that may help us reach fulfillment: catching a fish, developing a new skill, getting a promotion we deserve, becoming spiritually awakened in a church service, realizing that we've had an impact on others' lives, leaving a legacy to the future, having your book be a best-seller. There is usually a sense that we've done something difficult, even if it's only reading a book, and usually a sense that the experience has had an impact on ourselves, or others, or the world.

- Flow is a component of fulfillment. The project has demanded our attention, has been just challenging enough to keep us engaged without getting discouraged. It walks that thin line between boredom and anxiety. It makes us feel strong, active, creative, satisfied. But remember the dangers of flow, and hence of gratification: the activity may be so absorbing that we lose sight of the fact that it may be meaningless in itself. We may be attracted to projects that promise flow rather than projects that will make more of a contribution but are more challenging. There is a value system inherent in the concept of fulfillment; fulfilling activities accomplish something useful or good.

- Pride is also a component of fulfillment. We've done something difficult, something that adds to our self-respect. We've made a mark on the world, a contribution to society or the future. We've satisfied an ambition.

- When we feel fulfilled, we've developed our skills. We've practiced something until we got it right. Perhaps fulfillment entails laying down new brain circuitry, and perhaps our brain is aware of that somehow. It feels stronger, like a muscle after exercise.

- Fulfillment also entails doing something creative, which helps grow the brain. Putting information together in new ways, making new connections, seeing hidden patterns, understanding connections that were hidden, expressing ourselves in new or more effective ways—these elements of creativity are inherently pleasurable.

Integrity:

Here's something I'm slipping in unannounced. We have to talk a little about death.

We all face death. For some, it is a source of great conscious fear. For the rest of us, the fear may not be so conscious, but it's probably always there in the background. It's ultimately unthinkable; I don't think we can really get our minds around the idea that our consciousness will end. That's why belief in an afterlife of some sort is so appealing. When tragedy strikes in our lives, when we've been victimized by people we've trusted or hurt by simple random fate, if we lack a belief in cosmic justice or a divine plan we can give in to despair.

When we lived in a simpler age, in closer harmony with nature, linked together in kinship groups, we saw birth and death around us all the time. It might have been easier then to feel that death was not such a big deal. After a certain number of years, you began to grow tired, not able to keep up, and you prepared yourself for death, knowing that you would live on at least in the memories and gene pool of your group. And there were rituals with death, almost always suggesting that there was an afterlife: death was a journey, and you were buried with tools and totems to help you on your way. Now it seems like we try to deny death, and maybe we shouldn't.

Integrity, writes Judith Herman, "is the capacity to affirm the value of life in the face of death, to be reconciled with the finite limits of one's own life and the tragic limits of the human condition, and to accept these realities without despair. Integrity is the foundation upon which trust in relationships is originally formed, and upon which shattered trust may be restored. The interlocking of integrity and trust in caretaking relationships completes the cycle of generations and regenerates the sense of human continuity which trauma destroys." Integrity comes, I think, from being fulfilled, from having enough experiences of having an impact, of having created something. Perhaps from having created a self that can be resilient yet solid, that can remain curious and caring right up to the last days.

Facing death with integrity is the last gift we can give our children. Consider the Buddhist "middle way." Neither cling to nor reject what life has to offer. Savor it, but be prepared to let go.

Principle 12
Practice, Practice, Practice
Here's some tough talk: All through this book I've tried to help you understand your problems and see what is good for you. Very little is your fault; the problems have mostly to do with the vulnerabilities you grew up with and the effect of perpetual stress on them. But you still have to live with yourself as you are. The only choice you have is to practice what's good for you, right now, in the present moment. Choice is not in the past or the future. But if you practice now, it will get easier in the future. If you don't, it won't. That's your choice. That's your free will in action.

Life has been difficult, and will remain so. We've adapted to some difficulties, but now some of our adaptations have become problems, constricting our ability to feel, to think, to be creative. We can choose to practice the skills that will help us be ready for what the rest of life throws at us, that will help us shed some of our constricting adaptations and be more flexible. We need to keep in mind that practicing today makes tomorrow easier. Each time we learn a new skill, we are creating connections in the brain; each time we practice, we reinforce and strengthen those connections.

- You have to give yourself an hour a day (all right, you can have one day off a week) for meditation and physical fitness. For many readers, that's going to seem like too much to ask right off the bat. I recognize that some people are extraordinarily busy and that this demand is legitimately difficult—mothers with young children; people with long commutes; business travelers; the people who hold down two or three part-time jobs to get by. But you have to find a way; there's no shortcut.
- Consider the time a gift to yourself, rather than a subtraction from the rest of your life. Joseph Campbell says we need a sacred space and a sacred time. Give yourself these things. Find a time—it may mean getting up an hour early, staying up an hour later; it may be first thing in the morning, or when the kids get off to school, or lunch hour in the office. Build a routine, and learn to cherish it. It won't be long before you feel deprived when you miss it and you wonder how you ever got along without it.
- You're not going to get overnight results from meditation or other means of cultivating mindfulness. We're trying to change the structure of your brain, develop new pathways to replace the default circuits you've taken a lifetime to develop. Remember that Kabat-Zinn takes eight weeks to teach Mindfulness-Based Stress Reduction. Remember that it took three months of practice for the jugglers to develop that tiny mental muscle that was visible in PET scans. Be patient with yourself. Make a commitment to a solid month of daily exercise and meditation. After that you should be feeling enough change to convince yourself that it's worthwhile to go on, so do that: go on practicing. What you feel after the first month is only a taste of how much things can change.
- Meditation and exercise are not enough. I can see people who will jump into these routines but will only be going through the motions. You have to learn to apply mindfulness in every waking moment. You have to never

see things the same old way again. It means developing a new sense, one that monitors how you are paying attention. It will take time.

- The Perpetual Stress Response has been at work on your body and nervous system almost all your life. You won't master it overnight. Take encouragement from small changes. Your blood pressure may decrease. You might sleep a little better. You might notice you're thinking a little more clearly. Something that would have upset you might not anymore. Appreciate these little victories.

- Remember that extinction of responses—learning not to fear something we used to, for instance—is not forgetting but is laying down new circuitry in the brain. Learning something new results in changes in brain structure scientists can actually see. As you're practicing, it may help to visualize these processes at work.

- Practice makes everything easier next time. We start out any new thing feeling awkward and unskillful—typing, skiing, playing tennis. We don't remember, but walking and running, eating with silverware, and blowing our noses were awkward and difficult too. Nobody showed us, except by example, how to express and control our feelings, so we got a lot of it wrong. Now in order to change our emotional responses, it's not sufficient to *understand* how to do it, or to *know* what to do. It's not sufficient to *get* mindfulness, you have to *do* mindfulness. It's only with practice that we can make that knowledge a part of ourselves, a new circuit in the brain, something that feels normal and natural to us.

- Practicing mindful living by making new choices—taking time for ourselves, cultivating healthy relationships, taking care of our bodies, facing our fears, developing creativity—will seem phony and forced at first. It will feel like we are pretending, trying to be someone we are not. It can feel like a betrayal of our basic nature. But I hope I've made clear by now that our nature is highly malleable; that what feels like "me" is the result of a gradual accretion of habits, some healthy, some not. It's quite possible to change "me," that basic nature, and to make of ourselves what we want, something stronger and more resilient, someone able to recognize and overcome the effects of perpetual stress, someone loving, wise, productive, and healthy. I'm going to be working on it for the rest of my life, and I hope you will too.

How to Find Further Help

HERE I'm consolidating some links, references, and resources which I think can be very helpful in achieving relief from the Perpetual Stress Response. This book covers a lot of territory, and of necessity can't provide all the detail every reader will need to achieve recovery. I encourage you to look further. Be inquisitive and adventurous, and find out more about what feels just right to you.

Meditation

I am only a beginner at meditation. There are many methods, some quite Western, some deeply rooted in Buddhism. I encourage you to experiment with different approaches. Look for an instructor in your area. Join a group. Get away for a weekend mindfulness retreat. Here are some resources that are worth exploring:

- www.buddhanet.net, which has hundreds of Buddhist texts, commentaries on them, and instructional guides available for free downloading.
- www.accesstoinsight.org, which itself is a well-organized guide to Theravada Buddhism (the southern tradition, as opposed to Chinese and Japanese forms) and also has many texts and articles available for downloading.
- The Community of Mindful Living (www.iamhome.org) follows the teachings of the Vietnamese monk Thich Nhat Hanh. Among other things, the website provides a list of meditation groups (*sanghas*) all over the world.
- The Google string "Society"/"Religion and Spirituality"/"Buddhism" will take you to thousands more resources on the Internet. You can even locate

the nearest Zen master (each of whom seems to have his or her own website!) through "Society"/"Religion and Spirituality"/"Buddhism"/"Lineages"/"Zen"/"Masters and Teachers."

- As we've said, Jon Kabat-Zinn's books (*Full Catastrophe Living* and *Wherever You Go, There You Are*) and tapes are very helpful for many people: www.mindfulnesstapes.com.
- Thich Nhat Hanh has a very popular book called *The Miracle of Mindfulness.* I find even more accessible *Mindfulness in Plain English,* by Bhante Henepola Gunaratana.
- Finally, *Mindfulness in the Marketplace,* edited by Alan Hunt Badiner, will make you a more mindful consumer.

Help for Anxiety Disorders

These books present reliable information and advice about anxiety:

- *Calming Your Anxious Mind,* by Jeffrey Brantley. New Harbinger, 2003.
- *Painfully Shy: How to Overcome Social Anxiety and Reclaim Your Life,* by Barbara Markway and Gregory Markway. Thomas Dunne Books, 2003.
- *Coping with Anxiety: 10 Simple Ways to Relieve Anxiety, Fear, and Worry,* by Edmund J. Bourne and Lorna Garano. New Harbinger, 2003.
- *The Anxiety and Phobia Workbook,* by Edmund J. Bourne. New Harbinger, 2000.
- *Anxiety, Phobias, and Panic,* by Reneau Z. Peurifoy. Warner Books, 1995.
- *Anxiety and Its Disorders,* by David H. Barlow. Guilford Press, second edition, 2001. (Unlike the others, this is a professional book, included here because it is the best authoritative guide.)

Help for Depression

These books present reliable information and advice about depression:

- *Undoing Depression: What Therapy Can't Teach You and Medication Can't Give You,* by Richard O'Connor. Berkley Books, 1999. How depression gets deep into your psyche and what we must do to "undo" its effect.
- *Breaking the Patterns of Depression,* by Michael Yapko (Also Yapko's *Hand-Me-Down Blues,* about how to keep depression from spreading in families.)

Yapko presents the clinical wisdom about depression in a clear and understandable way, making it clear that it doesn't come from nowhere. A
great advantage of this book is the one hundred–plus exercises he gives to
help you get out of your own assumptive world.

- *A Zen Path Through Depression,* by Philip Martin. HarperSanFrancisco,
  2000. Especially relevant in the context of mindfulness.
- *Feeling Good: The New Mood Therapy,* by David Burns. Avon, 1999.
  Cognitive-behavioral therapy explained in self-help terms.
- *How You Can Survive When They're Depressed,* by Anne Sheffield. Crown,
  1999. Sheffield has written several good books for loved ones of depressed
  people.
- *I Don't Want to Talk About It: Overcoming the Secret Legacy of Male Depres-
  sion,* by Terrence Real. Scribner, 1998.
- *The Noonday Demon: An Atlas of Depression,* by Andrew Solomon. Scribner,
  2002. A very comprehensive, very personal look at the subject.
- *Active Treatment of Depression,* by Richard O'Connor. Norton, 2001. Meant
  primarily for the professional, it describes a systems approach to the subject.
- *Darkness Visible: A Memoir of Madness,* by William Styron. Vintage, 1992.
  Styron was among the first public figures to reveal his struggle with de-
  pression. This is a beautiful, powerful book.
- *An Unquiet Mind,* by Kay Redfield Jamison. Vintage, 1997. For bipolar dis-
  order: a nationally recognized research psychiatrist talks about her experi-
  ence of the disease.
- *The Depression Workbook,* by Mary Alice Copeland and others. New Har-
  binger, second edition, 2002.
- *Ending the Depression Cycle,* by Peter J. Bieling and Martin M. Antony. New
  Harbinger, 2003.

Help for PTSD

These books present reliable information and advice about PTSD:

- *Trauma and Recovery,* by Judith Herman. Basic Books, 1997. A dense but
  complete and moving overview of the subject. The *New York Times* called it
  one of the most important psychiatric works since Freud.
- *The Body Remembers,* by Babette Rothschild. Norton, 2000. The somatic effects of psychological trauma.

- *Traumatic Stress: The Effects of Overwhelming Experience on Mind, Body, and Society,* by Bessel van der Kolk and others (editors). A comprehensive professional guide to the subject.
- *The PTSD Workbook,* by Mary Beth Williams and others. New Harbinger, 2002.
- *Parenting from the Inside Out: How a Deeper Self-Understanding Can Help You Raise Children Who Thrive,* by Daniel Siegel and Mary Hartzell. J.P. Tarcher, 2003. An excellent resource for trauma survivors who are raising children.

Help for Personality Disorders

These books present reliable information and advice about personality disorders:

- *Cognitive-Behavioral Treatment of Borderline Personality Disorder,* by Marsha Linehan. Guilford, 1992. A dense professional book, but absolutely the best.
- *I Hate You, Don't Leave Me: Understanding the Borderline Personality,* by Jerold J. Kreisman and Hal Straus. Avon, 1991.
- *Stop Walking on Eggshells,* by Paul T. Mason, Randi Krieger, and Larry J. Siever. New Harbinger, 1998.
- *Lost in the Mirror: An Inside Look at Borderline Personality Disorder,* by Richard A. Moskovitz. Taylor, 2001.
- *The Drama of the Gifted Child,* by Alice Miller. Basic Books, revised edition, 1996. The origins of narcissism.
- *Treating the Self: Elements of Clinical Self Psychology,* by Ernest Wolf. Guilford Press, 1988. The most accessible introduction to Kohut's treatment of narcissism.

Help for Addictions

I'm not going to recommend any books to help with recovery from addictions. In general, anything published by the Hazelden Foundation or New Harbinger books will be worthwhile, but I don't know the literature well enough to make specific recommendations. Besides, the field is fragmented, as are the problems. You ought to be able to find something that addresses your particular situation, whether it's giving up drinking or being in a relationship with an addict. There are many books, I see, that present alternatives to Alcoholics Anonymous for substance abuse. Though I know there are many people who have stopped drinking without AA, I'm skeptical. It's a proven method, and a good way to live your life; seeking alternatives carries the whiff of denial to me.

I do have one recommendation when it comes to getting free from alcohol or any other hard drug: consider going away for a while. There are thousands of good residential programs out there, and most health insurance policies will cover your stay for a few weeks. The first weeks are indeed the most difficult; and if you've tried on your own but failed, or if you're just afraid of trying, check yourself into a good program. You'll get a lot of emotional support during a very rough time, and you'll be introduced to the tools you need to maintain your recovery.

Then you have to be prepared to face a daily decision about living without your addiction. The drugs you've taken have changed your brain, and it will be a long time before you find a new "normal." You will need a lot of support, and you should seek it out. You will have to cut yourself off from people who don't want you to be sober. All this will be a lot easier if you allow yourself to join a Twelve-Step program. But don't let the fact that it's going to be a daily battle scare you too much. It doesn't mean you won't be able to feel good. If you go about it the right way, you can find some help for the problems that made you want to get high in the first place; then you can start to feel better than you've ever felt.

References

Abramson, L. Y., M. E. Seligman, and J. E. Teasdale. 1978. Learned helplessness in humans: Critique and reformulation. *Journal of Abnormal Psychology* 87:49–74.

Ackerman, K. D., R. Heyman, B. S. Rabin, B. P. Anderson, P. R. Houck, E. Frank, and A. Baum. 2002. Stressful life events precede exacerbations of multiple sclerosis. *Psychosomatic Medicine* 64:916–920.

Ader, R. 2003. Psychoneuroimmunology. In *The biopsychosocial approach: Past, present, and future*, edited by R. M. Frankel, T. E. Quill, and S. H. McDaniel. Rochester, NY: University of Rochester Press.

Ader, R., N. Cohen, and D. Bovbjerg. 1982. Conditioned suppression of humoral immunity in the rat. *Journal of Comparative and Physiological Psychology* 3:517–521.

Adler, N. E., E. S. Epel, G. Castellazzo, and J. R. Ickovics. 2000. Relationship of subjective and objective social status with psychological and physiological functioning: Preliminary data in healthy white women. *Health Psychology* 19 (6):586–592.

Adolphs, R., D. Tranel, and A. R. Damasio. 1998. The human amygdala in social judgment. *Nature* 393:470–474.

Afari, N., and D. Buchwald. 2003. Chronic fatigue syndrome: A review. *American Journal of Psychiatry* 160:221–236.

Agency for Health Care Policy and Research. 1993. Clinical practice guideline: *Depression in Primary Care*: vol. 1. Detection and diagnosis. Washington, DC: United States Department of Health and Human Services, Public Health Service.

Ahern, J., S. Galea, H. Resnick, D. Kilpatrick, M. Bucuvalas, J. Gold, and D. Vlahov. 2002. Television images and psychological symptoms after the September 11 terrorist attacks. *Psychiatry: Interpersonal and Biological Processes* 65 (4):289–300.

Ainsworth, M.D.S., M. D. Blehar, E. Waters, and S. Wall. 1978. *Patterns of attachment: A psychological study of the strange situation*. Hillsdale, NJ: Lawrence Erlbaum and Associates.

Alexander, F., and T. Benedek. 1987. *Psychosomatic medicine*. New York: Norton.

Alloy, L. B., and L. Y. Abramson. 1979. Judgment of contingency in depressed and nondepressed students: Sadder but wiser? *Journal of Experimental Psychology: General* 108(4):441–485.

———. 1988. Depressive realism: Four theoretical perspectives. In *Cognitive processes in depression*, edited by L. B. Alloy. New York: Guilford.

Altemus, M., M. Cloitre, and F. S. Dhabhar. 2003. Enhanced cellular immune response in women with PTSD related to childhood abuse. *American Journal of Psychiatry* 160 (9):1705–1707.

American Association of Suicidology. 1997. Some facts about suicide and depression [Brochure]. Washington, DC: American Association of Suicidology.

American Psychiatric Association. 1994. *Diagnostic and statistical manual of mental disorders DSM-IV)*. Washington, DC: American Psychiatric Association.

American Psychological Association. The costs of failing to provide appropriate mental health care. http://www.apa.org/practice/failing.html.

Anderson, M., K. N. Ochsner, B. Kuhl, J. Cooper, C. Robertson, S. W. Gabriel, G. H. Glover, and J.D.E. Gabrieli. 2004. Neural mechanisms underlying the suppression of unwanted memories. *Science* 303:232–235.

Andrews, G. 1996. Comorbidity and the general neurotic syndrome. *British Journal of Psychiatry* 168 (suppl. 30):76–84.

Badiner, A. H., editor. 2002. *Mindfulness in the marketplace*. Berkeley, CA: Parallax Press.

Baker, C. B., M. T. Johnsrud, M. L. Crismon, R. A. Rosenheck, and S. W. Woods. 2003. Quantitative analysis of sponsorship bias in economic studies of antidepressants. *British Journal of Psychiatry* 183:498–506.

Ballenger, J. C., J.R.T. Davidson, Y. Lecrubier, D. J. Nutt, R. B. Lydiard, and E. A. Mayer. 2001. Consensus statement on depression, anxiety, and functional gastrointestinal disorders. *Journal of Clinical Psychiatry* 62 (suppl. 8):48–51.

Ban Breathnach, S. 1995. *Simple abundance*. New York: Warner.

Bargh, J. A. 1990. Auto-motives: Preconscious determinants of social interaction. In *Handbook of motivation and cognition*, edited by T. Higgins and R. M. Sorrentino. New York: Guilford.

———. 1992. Being unaware of the stimulus vs unaware of its interpretation: Why subliminality per se does matter to social psychology. In *Perception without awareness*, edited by R. Bornstein and T. Pittman. New York: Guilford.

Barkley, R. A. Revised edition, 2000. *Taking charge of ADHD*. New York: Guilford.

Barlow, D. A. 1988. *Anxiety and its disorders*. New York: Guilford.

Barsky, A. J., and J. F. Borus. 1999. Functional somatic syndromes. *Annals of Internal Medicine* 130 (11):910–921.

Bartholomew, K., M. J. Kwong, and S. D. Hart. 2001. Attachment. In *Handbook of personality disorders*, edited by W. J. Livesley. New York: Guilford.

Basch, M. F. 1988. *Understanding psychotherapy: The science behind the art*. New York: Basic Books.

Bateson, G. 1972. *Steps to an ecology of mind*. New York: Ballantine Books.

Beardslee, W. R. 1998. Prevention and the clinical encounter. *American Journal of Orthopsychiatry* 68 (4):521–533.

Beardslee, W. R., S. Swatling, L. Hoke, P. C. Rothberg, P. van de Velde, L. Focht, and D. Podorefsky. 1998. From cognitive information to shared meaning: Healing principles in prevention intervention. *Psychiatry* 61:112–129.

Beardslee, W. R., E. M. Versage, and T. R. Gladstone. 1998. Children of affectively ill parents: A review of the past 10 years. *Journal of the American Academy of Child and Adolescent Psychiatry* 37 (11):1134–1141.

Beck, A. T. 1976. *Cognitive Therapy and the Emotional Disorders.* New York: New American Library.

Beck, A. T., A. J. Rush, B. F. Shaw, and G. Emery. 1979. *Cognitive therapy of depression.* New York: Guilford Press.

Bennett-Goleman, T. 2001. *Emotional alchemy: How the mind can heal the heart.* New York: Harmony Books.

Benson, H. 1975. *The relaxation response.* New York: Morrow.

Benson, H., and T. P. McCallie. 1979. Angina pectoris and the placebo effect. *New England Journal of Medicine* 300:1424–1429.

Benson, H., and M. Stark. 1996. *Timeless healing: The power and biology of belief.* New York: Fireside.

Benson, H., and E. M. Stuart. 1992. *The wellness book.* New York: Fireside.

Berndt, E. R., L. M. Koran, S. N. Finkelstein, A. J. Gelenberg, S. G. Kornstein, I. M. Miller, M. E. Thase, G. A. Trapp, and M. B. Keller. 2000. Lost human capital from early-onset chronic depression. *American Journal of Psychiatry* 157:940–947.

Berne, E. *Games people play.* 1964. New York: Ballantine Books.

Berridge, K. C. 1999. Pleasure, pain, desire, and dread: Hidden core processes of emotion. In *Well-being: The foundations of hedonic psychology,* edited by D. Kahneman, E. Diener, and N. Schwartz. New York: Russell Sage Foundation.

Bishop, S. R. 2002. What do we really know about mindfulness-based stress reduction? *Psychosomatic Medicine* 64:71–83.

Blatt, S. J., C. A. Sanislow, D. C. Zuroff, and P. A. Pilkonis. 1996. Characteristics of effective therapists: Further analyses of data from the NIMH Treatment of Depression Collaborative Research Program. *Journal of Consulting and Clinical Psychology* 64:1276–1284.

Blatt, S. J., D. C. Zuroff, D. M. Quinlan, and P. Pilkonis. 1996. Interpersonal factors in brief treatment of depression: Further analyses of the NIMH Treatment of Depression Collaborative Research Program. *Journal of Consulting and Clinical Psychology* 64:162–171.

Bradshaw, J. 1990. *Bradshaw on: The family.* New York: Health Communications.

Brandchaft, B., and R. Stolorow. 1984. The borderline concept: Pathological character or iatrogenic myth? In *Empathy II,* edited by J. Lichtenberg, M. Bornstein, and D. Silver. Hillsdale, NJ: Analytic Press.

Bremner, J. D. 2002. *Does stress damage the brain?* New York: Norton.

Bremner, J. D., L. Staib, D. Kalupek, S. M. Southwick, R. Soufer, and D. S. Charney. 1999. Neural correlates of exposure to traumatic pictures and sound in Vietnam combat veterans with and without post-traumatic stress disorder (PTSD): A positron emission tomography study. *Biological Psychiatry* 45:806–816.

Bremner, J.D., M. Vythilingam, E. Vermetten, S.M. Southwick, T. McGlashan, A. Nazeer, S. Khan, L.V. Vaccarino, R. Soufer, P.K. Garg, C.K. Ng, L.H. Stab, J.S. Duncan, and D.S. Charney. 2003. MRI and PET study of deficits in hippocampal structure and function in women with childhood sexual abuse and posttraumatic stress disorder. *American Journal of Psychiatry* 160:924–932.

Brickman, P., D. Coates, and R. Janoff-Bulman. 1978. Lottery winners and accident victims: Is happiness relative? *Journal of Personality and Social Psychology* 36 (8):917–27.

Broadbent, E., K.J. Petrie, P.G. Alley, and R.J. Booth. 2003. Psychological stress impairs early wound repair following surgery. *Psychosomatic Medicine* 65:865–869.

Brooks, D. 2001. *Bobos in paradise: The new upper class and how they got there.* New York: Simon and Schuster.

Brosnan, S.F., and F.B.M. de Waal. 2003. Monkeys reject unequal pay. *Nature* 425:297–299.

Brown, J.D., and M.A. Marshall. 2002. Great expectations: Optimism and pessimism in achievement settings. In *Optimism and pessimism: Implications for theory, research, and practice,* edited by E.C. Chang. Washington, DC: American Psychological Association.

Brown, W.A. 1998. The placebo effect. *Scientific American* (January): 90–95.

Burns, D.D. Revised edition, 1999. *Feeling good: The new mood therapy.* New York: Avon Books.

Buss, D.M. 2000. The evolution of happiness. *American Psychologist* 55 (1):15–21.

Camí, J., and M. Farré. 2003. Drug addiction. *New England Journal of Medicine* 349 (10):975–986.

Campbell, J. 1995. *Reflections on the art of living: A Joseph Campbell companion,* selected and edited by Diane K. Osbon. New York: Harper Perennial.

Carlson, E.A. 1998. A prospective longitudinal study of disorganized/disoriented attachment. *Child Development* 69:1970–1979.

Carlson, L.E., M. Speca, K.D. Patel, and E. Goodey. 2003. Mindfulness-based stress reduction in relation to quality of life, mood, symptoms of stress, and immune parameters in breast and prostate cancer outpatients. *Psychosomatic Medicine* 65:571–581.

Carney, C.P., L. Jones, R.F. Woolson, R. Noyes, and B.N. Doebbeling. 2003. Relationship between depression and pancreatic cancer in the general population. *Psychosomatic Medicine* 65:884–888.

Carter, J. Revised edition, 2003. *Nasty people.* New York: McGraw-Hill.

Caudill, M.A. Revised edition, 2002. *Managing pain before it manages you.* New York: Guilford.

Cavada, C., and W. Schultz. 2000. The mysterious orbitofrontal cortex. Foreword. *Cerebral Cortex* 10:205.

Centers for Disease Control, 2003. Chronic disease overview. http://www.cdc.gov/nc cdphp/overview.htm.

———, 2004. Chronic fatigue syndrome. http://www.cdc.gov/ncidod/diseases/cfs/info.htm

Champagne, F., and M.J. Meaney. 2001. Like mother, like daughter: Evidence for nongenomic transmission of parental behavior and stress responsivity. *Progress in Brain Research* 133:287–302.

Chödrön, P. 2000. *When things fall apart*. Boston: Shambhala.

Christakis, D. A., F. J. Zimmerman, D. L. DiGiuseppe, and C. A. McCarty. 2004. Early television exposure and subsequent attentional problems in children. *Pediatrics* 113(4):708–713.

Ciccone, D. S., and B. H. Natelson. 2003. Comorbid illness in women with chronic fatigue syndrome: A test of the single syndrome hypothesis. *Psychosomatic Medicine* 65:268–275.

Cohen, S., D. A. Tyrell, and A. P. Smith, 1993. Negative life events, perceived stress, negative affect, and susceptibility to the common cold. *Journal of Personality and Social Psychology* 64 (1):131–140.

Cole-King, A., and K. G. Harding. 2001. Psychological factors and delayed healing in chronic wounds. *Psychosomatic Medicine* 63(2):216–220.

Collins, C., and F. Yeskel. 2000. Boom for whom? Economic apartheid in America. http://www.tompaine.com/features/2000/08/01/4.html.

Collins, W. A., E. E. Maccoby, L. Steinberg, E. M. Hetherington, and M. H. Bornstein. 2000. Contemporary research on parenting: The case for nature and nurture. *American Psychologist* 55 (2):218–232.

Conlin, M. 2003. Unmarried America. *Business Week* (October 20).

Cooper, G. 2003. Clinician's digest: The roots of borderline personality disorder. *Psychotherapy Networker* (January/February):15–16.

Costello, E. J., S. N. Compton, G. Keeler, and A. Angold. 2003. Relationships between poverty and psychopathology. *Journal of the American Medical Association* 290:2023–2029.

Csikszentmihalyi, M. 1990. *Flow: The psychology of optimal experience*. New York: HarperCollins.

———. 1993. *The evolving self*. New York: HarperCollins.

Cushman, P. 1995. *Constructing the self, constructing America: A cultural history of psychotherapy*. Cambridge, MA: Perseus.

Dallman, M. F., N. Pecoraro, S. F. Akana, S. E. la Fleur, F. Gomez, H. Houshyar, M. E. Bell, S. Bhatnapar, K. D. Laugero, and S. Manalo. 2003. Chronic stress and obesity. A new view of "comfort food." *Proceedings of the National Academy of Sciences* 100 (20):11696–11701.

Damasio, A. R. 1994. *Descartes' error: Emotion, reason, and the human brain*. New York: Grosset/Putnam.

———. 1999. *The feeling of what happens: Body and emotion in the making of consciousness*. New York: Harcourt Brace.

Dateline NBC. 2003. Drug giant accused of false claims. (July 11).

Davidson, R. J. 2000. Affective style, mood, and anxiety disorders: An affective neuroscience approach. In *Anxiety, depression, and emotion*, edited by R. J. Davidson. New York: Oxford University Press.

Davidson, R. J., J. Kabat-Zinn, J. Schumacher, M. Rosenkranz, et al. 2003. Alterations in brain and immune function produced by mindfulness meditation. *Psychosomatic Medicine* 65:564–570.

Davis, M., E. R. Eshelman, and M. McKay. Fifth edition, 2000. *The relaxation and stress reduction workbook.* Oakland, CA: New Harbinger Publications.

Davison, K. P., J. W. Pennebaker, and S. S. Dickerson. 2000. Who talks? The social psychology of illness support groups. *American Psychologist* 55 (2):205–217.

DivorceMagazine.com. http://divorcemag.com/statistics/statsWorld.shtml.

Dörner, D. 1989; translated by R. and R. Kimber. *The logic of failure.* Cambridge, MA: Perseus Books.

Dowrick, S. 1991. *Intimacy and solitude.* New York: W. W. Norton.

Draganski, B., C. Gaser, V. Busch, G. Schuierer, U. Bogdahn, and A. May. 2004. Neuroplasticity: Changes in grey matter induced by training. *Nature* 427:311–312.

Edwards, V. J., G. W. Holden, V. J. Felitti, and R. F. Anda. 2003. Relationship between multiple forms of childhood maltreatment and adult mental health in community respondents: Results from the Adverse Childhood Experiences Study. *American Journal of Psychiatry* 160 (8):1453–1460.

Eich, E., I. A. Brodkin, J. L. Reeves, and A. F. Chawla. 1999. Questions concerning pain. In *Well-being: The foundations of hedonic psychology,* edited by D. Kahneman, E. Diener, and N. Schwartz. New York: Russell Sage Foundation.

Eisenberger, N. I., M. D. Lieberman, and K. D. Williams. 2003. Does rejection hurt? An fMRI study of social exclusion. *Science* 302:290–292.

Ekman, P. 2003. *Emotions revealed.* New York: Times Books.

Elkin, I., M. T. Shea, J. T. Watkins, S. D. Imber, S. M. Sotsky, J. F. Collins, D. R. Glass, P. A. Pilkonis, W. R. Leber, J. P. Dockerty, S. J. Fiester, and M. B. Parloff. 1989. NIMH treatment of depression collaborative research program: General effectiveness of treatments. *Archives of General Psychiatry* 46:971–982.

Emery N. J., J. P. Capitanio, W. A. Mason, C. J. Machado, S. P. Mendoza, and D. G. Amaral. 2001. The effects of bilateral lesions of the amygdala on dyadic social interactions in rhesus monkeys (Macaca mulatta). *Behavioral Neuroscience* 115(3):515–544.

Engel, G. L. 1959. "Psychogenic" pain and the pain-prone patient. *American Journal of Medicine* 26:899–918.

———. 1977. The need for a new medical model: A challenge for biomedicine. *Science* 196:129–136.

———. 1980. The clinical application of the biopsychosocial model. *American Journal of Psychiatry* 137 (5):535–544.

Epstein, M. 1998. *Going to pieces without falling apart.* New York: Broadway Books.

Epstein, R. M., T. E. Quill, and I. R. McWhinney. 1999. Somatization reconsidered: Incorporating the patient's experience of illness. *Archives of Internal Medicine* 159:215–222.

Eriksson, P. S., E. Perfilieva, T. Bjork-Eriksson, A. Alborn, C. Nordborg, D. A. Peterson, and F. H. Gage. 1998. Neurogenesis in the adult human hippocampus. *Nature Medicine* 4 (11):1313–1317.

Evans, F. B. 1996. *Harry Stack Sullivan: Interpersonal Theory and Psychotherapy.* New York: Routledge.

Ewing, R., T. Schmid, R. Killingsworth, A. Zlot, and S. Raudenbush. 2003. Relationship between urban sprawl and physical activity, obesity, and morbidity. *American Journal of Health Promotion* (September/October):47–57.

Fava, G. A., C. Rafanelli, M. Cazzaro, S. Conti, and S. Grandi. 1998. Well-being therapy: A novel psychotherapeutic approach for residual symptoms of affective disorders. *Psychological Medicine* 28 (2):475–480.

Fava, G. A., and C. Ruini. 2003. Development and characteristics of a well-being enhancing psychotherapeutic strategy: Well-being therapy. *Journal of Behavior Therapy and Experimental Psychiatry* 34 (1):45–63.

Fawzy, F. I., N. Cousins, N. W. Fawzy, M. E. Kemeny, R. Elashoff, and D. Morton. 1993. A structured psychiatric innovation for cancer patients: I. Changes over time and methods of coping and affective disturbance. *Archives of General Psychiatry* 47:720–725.

Felitti, V. J. 2001. Reverse alchemy in childhood: Turning gold into lead. *Family Violence Prevention Fund Health Alert* 8 (1):1–8.

Felitti, V. J., R. F. Anda, D. Nordenberg, D. F. Williamson, A. M. Spitz, V. Edwards, M. P. Koss, and J. S. Marks. 1998. Relationship of childhood abuse and household dysfunction to many of the leading causes of death in adults: The Adverse Childhood Experiences (ACE) study. *American Journal of Preventive Medicine* 14 (4):245–258.

Fields, H. 1987. *Pain.* New York: McGraw-Hill.

Flack, W. F., B. T. Litz, and T. M. Keane. 1998. Cognitive-behavioral treatment of warzone–related posttraumatic stress disorder: A flexible, hierarchical approach. In *Cognitive-behavioral therapies for trauma,* edited by V. M. Follette, J. I. Ruzek, and F. R. Abueg. New York: Guilford.

Focht-Birkerts, L., and W. R. Beardslee. 2000. A child's experience of parental depression: Encouraging relational resilience in families with affective illness. *Family Process* 39:417–434.

Fonagy, P., T. Leigh, R. Kennedy, G. Matoon, H. Steele, M. Target, M. Steele, and A. Higgitt. 1995. Attachment, borderline states and the representation of emotions and cognition in self and other. *Emotion, cognition, and representation,* edited by D. Cicchetti and S. L. Toth. 371–414. Rochester, NY: University of Rochester Press.

Fortes, C., S. Farchi, F. Forastiere, N. Agabiti, R. Pacific, P. Zuccaro, C. A. Perucci, and S. Ebrahim. 2003. Depressive symptoms lead to impaired cellular immune response. *Psychotherapy and Psychosomatics* 72 (5):253–260.

Fosha, D. 2000. *The transforming power of affect.* New York: Basic Books.

———. 2003. Dyadic regulation and experiential work with emotion and relatedness in trauma and disorganized attachment. In *Healing trauma: Attachment, mind, body, and brain,* edited by M. F. Solomon and D. J. Siegel. New York: Norton.

Frank, J. D. Revised edition, 1974. *Persuasion and healing.* New York: Schocken Books.

Frankel, R. M., T. E. Quill, and S. H. McDaniel. 2003. Introduction to the biopsychosocial approach. In *The biopsychosocial approach: Past, present, and future,* edited by R. M. Frankel, T. E. Quill, and S. H. McDaniel. Rochester, NY: University of Rochester Press.

Frasure-Smith, N., F. Lespérance, M. Juncau, M. Talajic, and M. G. Bourassa. 1999. Gender, depression, and one-year prognosis after myocardical infraction. *Psychosomatic Medicine* (61):26–37.

Frederick, S., and G. Loewenstein. 1999. Hedonic adaptation. In *Well-being: The foundations of hedonic psychology,* edited by D. Kahneman, E. Diener, and N. Schwartz. New York: Russell Sage Foundation.

Freud, S. 1916. On transience. In *The standard edition of the complete psychological works of Sigmund Freud* (14):305–307. New York: W. W. Norton, 2000.

Fullerton, C. S., R. J. Ursano, and L. Wang. 2004. Acute stress disorder, posttraumatic stress disorder, and depression in disaster or rescue workers. *American Journal of Psychiatry* 161 (8):1370–1376.

Gabbard, G. O. 2000. A neurologically informed perspective on psychotherapy. *British Journal of Psychiatry* 177:117–122.

Gage, F. H. 2000. Mammalian neural stem cells. *Science* 287:1433–1438.

George, C., N. Kaplan, and M. Main. 1996. Adult attachment interview. Unpublished protocol. Department of Psychology, University of California, Berkeley.

Geracioti, T. D., D. G. Baker, N. E. Ekhator, S. A. West, K. K. Hill, A. B. Bruce, D. Schmidt, B. Rounds-Kugler, R. Yehuda, P. E. Keck, and J. W. Kasckow. 2001. CSF norepinephrine concentrations in posttraumatic stress disorder. *American Journal of Psychiatry* 158:1227–1230.

Giedd, J., J. Blumenthal, N. Jeffries, F. Castellanos, H. Liu, A. Zijdenbos, T. Paus, A. Evans, and J. Rapoport. 1999. Brain development during childhood and adolescence: A longitudinal MRI study. *Nature Neuroscience* 2 (10):861–863.

Gilligan, J. 1996. *Violence: Our deadly epidemic and its causes.* New York: Putnam.

Goffman, E. 1971. *Relations in public: Microstudies of the public order.* New York: Harper Colophon.

Goldapple, K., Z. Segal, C. Garson, M. Lau, P. Bieling, S. Kennedy, and H. Bayberg. 2004. Modulation of cortical-limbic pathways in major depression. *Archives of General Psychiatry* 61 (1):34–41.

Goldenberg, D. L., K. H. Kaplan, M. G. Nadeua, C. Brodeur, S. Smith, and C. H. Schmid. 1994. A controlled study of a stress-reduction, cognitive-behavioral treatment program in fibromyalgia. *Journal of Musculoskeletal Pain* 2:53–66.

Goldenson, R. E., editor. 1984. *Longman Dictionary of Psychology and Psychiatry.* New York: Longman.

Goleman, D. 1995. *Emotional intelligence.* New York: Bantam.

———. 2003a. *Destructive emotions: How can we overcome them? A scientific dialogue with the Dalai Lama.* New York: Bantam.

———. 2003b. Finding happiness: Cajole your brain to lean to the left. *New York Times* (February 4):F5.

Goodwin, R., and M. Olfson. 2001. Treatment of panic attack and risk of major depressive disorder in the community. *American Journal of Psychiatry* 158 (7):1146–1148.

Goodwin, R., and M. B. Stein. 2002. Generalized anxiety disorder and peptic ulcer disease among adults in the United States. *Psychosomatic Medicine* 64:862–866.

Goozner, M. 1998. Are Americans working harder—or just more? *Chicago Tribune* (June 22):1.

Gottman, J. M., and L. F. Katz. 1990. Effects of marital discord on young children's peer interaction and health. *Developmental Psychology* 25:373–381.

Greenberg, P. E., L. E. Stiglin, S. N. Finkelstein, and E. R. Berndt. 1993. The economic burden of depression in 1990. *Journal of Clinical Psychiatry* (11):405–418.

Gruber, A. J., J. I. Hudson, and H. G. Pope. 1996. The management of treatment-resistant depression in disorders on the interface of psychiatry and medicine. *Psychiatric Clinics of North America* 19 (2):351–369.

Gunaratana, Bhante Henepola. 2002. *Mindfuless in plain English.* Boston: Wisdom Publications.

Gündel, H., A. López-Sala, A. O. Ceballos-Baumann, J. Deus, N. Cardoner, B. Marten-Mittag, C. Sorano-Mas, and J. Pujol. 2004. Alexithymia correlates with the size of the right anterior cingulate. *Psychosomatic Medicine* 66:132–140.

Gunderson, J. G., D. Bender, S. Sanislow, S. Yen, J. B. Rettew, R. Dolan-Sewell, I. Dyck, L. C. Morey, T. H. McGlashan, M. T. Shea, and A. E. Skodol. 2003. Plausibility and possible determinants of sudden "remissions" in borderline patients. *Psychiatry: Interpersonal and Biological Processes* 66 (2):111–119.

Guthrie, E. 2000. Psychotherapy for patients with complex disorders and chronic symptoms. *British Journal of Psychiatry* 177:131–137.

Hallowell, E. M., and J. J. Ratey. *Driven to distraction.* New York: Pantheon.

Harlow, H., and M. Harlow. 1962. Social deprivation in monkeys. *Scientific American* 207:136–146.

Harris, G. 2003. Debate resumes on the safety of depression's wonder drugs. *New York Times* (August 7):A1.

Hebb, D. O. 1949. *The organization of behavior.* New York: John Wiley and Sons.

Hedges, L. 1992. *Interpreting the countertransference.* New York: Jason Aronson.

Heim, C., J. Newport, S. Heit, Y. P. Graham, M. Wilcox, R. Bonsall, A. H. Miller, and C. B. Nemeroff. 2000. Pituitary-adrenal and autonomic responses to stress in women after sexual and physical abuse in childhood. *Journal of the American Medical Association* 284 (5):592–597.

Henwood, D. 1997. Visa not welfare. *Bad Subjects 32,* April, 28–29. http://eserver.org/bs/32/henwood.html.

Herman, J. 1992. *Trauma and recovery.* New York: Basic Books.

Herman, S., J. A. Blumenthal, M. Babyak, P. Khatri, W. E. Craighead, K. R. Krishnan, and P. M. Doraiswamy. 2002. Exercise therapy for depression in middle-aged and older adults: Predictors of early dropout and treatment failure. *Health Psychology* 21 (6):553–563.

Herrmann, C., S. Brand-Driehorst, B. Kaminsky, E. Leibing, H. Staats, and U. Ruger. Diagnostic groups and depressed mood as predictors of 22 month mortality in medical inpatients. *Psychosomatic Medicine* (60):570–577.

Hesse, E., M. Main, K. Y. Abrams, and A. Rifkin. 2003. Unresolved states regarding loss or abuse can have "second generation" effects: Disorganization, role inversion, and frightening ideation in the offspring of traumatized, non-maltreating parents. In *Healing trauma: Attachment, mind, body, and brain,* edited by M. F. Solomon and D. J. Siegel. New York: Norton.

Hoffman, I. Z. 1998. *Ritual and spontaneity in the psychoanalytic process.* Hillsdale, NJ: Analytic Press.

House, J. S. 2001. Social isolation kills, but how and why? *Psychosomatic Medicine* 63 (2):273–274.

Hudson, J. I., M. S. Hudson, L. F. Pliner, D. L. Goldenberg, and H. G. Pope. 1985. Fibromyalgia and major affective disorder: A controlled phenomenology and family history study. *American Journal of Psychiatry,* 142 (4):441–446.

Hyams, K. C. 1998. Developing case definitions for symptom-based conditions: The problem of specificity. *Epidemiologic Reviews* 20 (2):148–156.

International Labour Organization. 2003. Press release. (September 1) http://www.ilo. org/public/english/bureau/inf/pr/2003/40.htm.

Johnson, S. 2004. *Mind wide open.* New York: Scribner.

Josephs, L. 1995. *Character and self-experience.* Northvale, NJ: Jason Aronson.

Judd, L. I., H. S. Akiskal, J. D. Maser, P. J. Zeller, J. Endicott, W. Coryell, M. P. Paulus, J. L. Kunovac, A. C. Leon, T. J. Mueller, J. A. Rice, and M. B. Keller. 1998. A prospective 12-year study of subsyndromal and syndromal depressive symptoms in unipolar major depressive disorders. *Archives of General Psychiatry* 55:694–700.

Kabat-Zinn, J. 1982. An outpatient program in behavioral medicine for chronic pain patients based on the practice of mindfulness meditation: Theoretical considerations and preliminary results. *General Hospital Psychiatry* 4:33–47.

———. 1990. *Full catastrophe living: Using the wisdom of your body and mind to face stress, pain, and illness.* New York: Delacorte.

———. 1994. *Wherever you go, there you are: Mindfulness meditation in everyday life.* New York: Hyperion.

Kabat-Zinn, J., M. D. Massion, J. Kristeller, L. G. Peterson, K. E. Fletcher, L. Pbert, W. R. Lenderking, and S. F. Santorelli. 1992. Effectiveness of a meditation-based stress reduction program in the treatment of anxiety disorders. *American Journal of Psychiatry* 149:936–943.

Kabat-Zinn, J., E. Wheeler, T. Light, A. Skillings, M. J. Scharf, T. G. Cropley, D. Hosmer, and J. D. Bernhard. 1998. Influence of a mindfulness-based stress reduction intervention on rates of skin clearing in patients with moderate to severe psoriasis undergoing phototherapy UVB and photochemotherapy PUVA. *Psychosomatic Medicine* 50:625–632.

Kaplan, J. R., S. B. Manuck, T. B. Clarkson, F. M. Lusso, D. M. Taub, and E. W. Miller. 1983. Social stress and atherosclerosis in normocholesterolemic monkeys. *Science* 220:733–735.

Karen, R. 1992. Shame. *The Atlantic* (February):40–70.

———. 1994. *Becoming attached.* New York: Warner Books.

Katon, W. R., L. Richardson, P. Lozano, and E. McCauley. 2004. The relationship of asthma and anxiety disorders. *Psychosomatic Medicine* 66:349–355.

Keller, M. B., and D. L. Hanks. 1994. The natural history and heterogeneity of depressive disorders. *Journal of Clinical Psychiatry* 55 (suppl. 9A.):25–31.

Kenrick, D. T., S. L. Neuberg, K. L. Zierk, and J. M. Krones. 1994. Evolution and social cognition: Contrast effects as a function of sex, dominance, and physical attractiveness. *Personality and Social Psychology Bulletin* 20:210–217.

Kessler, R. C., K. A. McGonagle, S. Zhao, C. B. Nelson, M. Hughes, S. Eshleman, H.-U. Wittchen, and K. S. Kendler. 1994. Lifetime and 12-month prevalence of DSM-III-R psychiatric disorders in the United States: Results from the National Comorbidity Study. *Archives of General Psychiatry* 51:8–19.

Kessler, R. C., C. B. Nelson, K. A. McGonagle, J. Liu, M. Swartz, and D. G. Blazer. 1996. Comorbidity of DSM-III-R major depressive disorder in the general population: Results from the US National Comorbidity Study. *British Journal of Psychiatry* 18 (suppl. 30):17–30.

Kessler, R. C., A. Sonnega, E. Bromet, M. Hughes, and C. B. Nelson. 1995. Posttraumatic stress disorder in the National Comorbidity Survey. *Archives of General Psychiatry* 52:1048–1060.

Kiecolt-Glaser, J. K., L. McGuire, T. F. Robles, R. Glaser. 2002. Psychoneuroimmunology: Psychological influences on immune function and health. *Journal of Consulting and Clinical Psychology* 70 (3):537–547.

Kirkpatrick, D. D. 2000. Inside the happiness business. *New York Magazine* (May 15).

Kirsch, I., T. J. Moore, A. Scoboria, and S. S. Nicholls. 2002. The emperor's new drugs: An analysis of antidepressant medication data submitted to the U.S. Food and Drug Administration. *Prevention and Treatment* 5 (article 23). http://journals.apa.org/prevention/volume5/pre0050023a.html.

Klein, D. N., K. A. Norden, T. Ferro, J. B. Leader, K. L. Kasch, L. M. Klein, J. E. Schwartz, and T. A. Aronson. 1998. Thirty-month naturalistic follow-up study of early-onset dysthymic disorder: Course, diagnostic stability, and prediction of outcome. *Journal of Abnormal Psychology* 1072:338–348.

Klein, D. N., J. E. Schwartz, S. Rose, and J. B. Leader. 2000. Five-year course and outcome of dysthymic disorder: A prospective, naturalistic follow-up study. *American Journal of Psychiatry* 157 (6):931–939.

Klein, D. N., J. E. Schwartz, N. J. Santiago, D. Vivian, C. Vocisano, L. G. Castonguay, B. Arnow, J. A. Blalock, R. Manber, J. C. Markowitz, L. P. Riso, B. Rothbaum, J. P. McCullough, M. E. Thase, F. E. Borian, F. W. Miller, and M. B. Keller. 2003. Therapeutic alliance in depression treatment: Controlling for prior change and patient characteristics. *Journal of Consulting and Clinical Psychology* 71 (6):997–1006.

Kohut, H. 1971. *The analysis of the self.* New York: International Universities Press.

———. 1977. *The restoration of the self.* New York: International Universities Press.

Konner, M. 1990. Human nature and culture: Biology and the residue of uniqueness. In *The boundaries of humanity,* edited by J. J. Sheehan and M. Sosna. Berkeley: University of California Press.

Koran, L. M., H. W. Chuong, K. D. Bullock, and S. C. Smith. 2003. Citalopram for compulsive shopping disorder: An open-label study followed by double-blind discontinuation. *Journal of Clinical Psychiatry* 64 (7):793–798.

Kornfield, J. 2000. *After the ecstasy, the laundry.* New York: Bantam Books.

Kramer, P. 1997. *Listening to Prozac.* New York: Penguin.

Kraut, R., M. Patterson, V. Lundmark, S. Kiesler, T. Mukopadhyay, and W. Scherlis. 1998. Internet paradox. *American Psychologist* 53 (9):1017–1031.

Kristeller, J. L., and and C. B. Hallett. 1999. An exploratory study of a meditation-based intervention for binge eating disorder. *Journal of Health Psychology* 4:357–363.

Kubey, R., and M. Csikszentmihalyi. 2002. Television addiction is no mere metaphor. *Scientific American* (February).

Kuhn, T. Third edition, 1996. *The structure of scientific revolutions.* Chicago: University of Chicago Press.

Kulka, R. A., W. E. Schlenger, J. A. Fairbank, R. L. Hough, B. K. Jordan, C. R. Marmar, and D. S. Weiss. 1990. *Trauma and the Vietnam war generation: Report of findings from the national Vietnam veterans readjustment study.* New York: Brunner/Mazel.

Kutz, I., J. Leserman, C. Dorrington, C. Morrison, J. Borysenko, and H. Benson. 1985. Meditation as an adjunct to psychotherapy. *Psychotherapy and Psychosomatics* 43:209–218.

Lamott, A. 1994. *Bird by bird: Some instructions on writing and life.* New York: Anchor Books.

Lancet, The 1989. Investigation of failed low-back surgery. Unsigned editorial. 1 (8644):939–40.

Lane, R. E. 2000. *The loss of happiness in market democracies.* New Haven: Yale University Press.

Langer, E. J. 1989. *Mindfulness.* Reading, MA: Addison-Wesley.

Langer, E. J., and M. Moldoveanu. 2000. The construct of mindfulness. *Journal of Social Issues* 56: 1–9.

Lanius, R. A., P. C. Williamson, M. Densmore, E. Boksman, R. W. Neufeld, J. S. Gati, and R. S. Menor. 2004. The nature of traumatic memories: A 4-T fMRI functional connectivity analysis. *American Journal of Psychiatry* 161:36–44.

Larimer, M. E., R. S. Palmer, and G. A. Marlatt. 1999. Relapse prevention: An overview of Marlatt's cognitive-behavioral model. *Alcohol Research and Health* 23:151–160.

LeDoux, J. 1996. *The emotional brain: The mysterious underpinnings of emotional life.* New York: Touchstone.

———. 2002. *Synaptic self: How our brains become who we are.* New York: Viking.

Leff, J., S. Vearnals, C. R. Brewin, G. Wolff, B. Alexander, E. Asen, D. Dayson, E. Jones, D. Chisholm, and B. Everitt. 2000. The London depression intervention trial. *British Journal of Psychiatry* 177:95–100.

Lett, H. S., J. A. Blumenthal, M. A. Babyak, A. Sherwood, T. Strauman, C. Robins, and M. F. Newman. 2004. Depression as a risk factor for coronary artery disease: Evidence, mechanisms, and treatment. *Psychosomatic Medicine* 66:305–315.

Levenstein, S. 2000. The very model of a modern etiology: A biopsychosocial view of peptic ulcer. *Psychosomatic Medicine* 62: 176–185.

Lewinsohn, P. M., W. Mischel, W. Chaplin, and R. Barton. 1980. Social competence and depression: The role of illusory self-perceptions. *Journal of Abnormal Psychology* (89):203–212.

Lewis, M., and D. Ramsay. 2002. Cortisol response to embarrassment and shame. *Child Development* 73:1034–1045.

Linehan, M. 1992. *Cognitive-behavioral treatment of borderline personality disorder.* New York: Guilford.

———. 1993. *Skills training manual for treating borderline personality disorder.* New York: Guilford.

Liotti, M., H. S. Mayberg, S. McGinnnis, S. L. Brannan, and P. Jerabek. 2002. Unmasking disease-specific cerebral blood flow abnormalities: Mood challenge in patients with remitted unipolar depression. *American Journal of Psychiatry* 159:1830–1840.

Lopez, F. G., and K. A. Brennan. 2000. Dynamic processes underlying adult attachment organization: Toward an attachment theoretical perspective on the healthy and effective self. *Journal of Counseling Psychology* 47 (3):283–300.

López, J. C. 2003. Two ways to look after your hippocampus. *Nature Reviews: Neuroscience* 4:939.

Luborsky, L. 1984. *Principles of psychoanalytic psychotherapy.* New York: Basic Books.

Luhrmann, T. M. 2000. *Of two minds: The growing disorder in American psychiatry.* New York: Knopf.

Luthar, S. S., and K. D'Avanzo. 1999. Contextual factors in substance use: A study of suburban and inner-city adolescents. *Developmental Psychopathology* 11 (4):845–867.

Magid, B. 2002. *Ordinary mind: Exploring the common ground of Zen and psychotherapy.* Boston: Wisdom Publications.

Maguire, E. A., D. G. Gadian, I. S. Johnsrude, C. D. Good, J. Ashburner, R. S. Frackowiak, and C. D. Frith. 2000. Navigation-related structural change in the hippocampi of taxi drivers. *Proceedings of the National Academy of Sciences* 97 (March 14):4398–4403.

Main, M. 1996. Introduction to the special section on attachment and psychopathology: 2. Overview of the field of attachment. *Journal of Consulting and Clinical Psychology* 64 (2):237–243.

Main, M., and J. Solomon. 1990. Procedures for identifying infants as disorganized/disoriented during the Ainsworth Strange Situation. In *Attachment in the preschool years,* edited by M. T. Greenberg, D. Cicchetti, and E. M. Cummings. Chicago: University of Chicago Press.

Malan, D. H. 1979. *Individual psychotherapy and the science of psychodynamics.* London: Butterworths.

Mann, J. 1973. *Time-limited psychotherapy.* Cambridge: Harvard University Press.

Mann, J., and R. Goldman. 1982. *A casebook in time-limited psychotherapy.* New York: McGraw-Hill.

Marinoff, L. 2000. *Plato, not Prozac.* New York: Perennial Books.

Marlatt, G. A., and J. R. Gordon. 1985. *Relapse prevention: Maintenance strategies in the treatment of addictive behaviors.* New York: Guilford.

Martin, D. J., L. Y. Abramson, and L. Alloy. 1984. The illusion of control for self and others in depressed and nondepressed college students. *Journal of Personality and Social Psychology* (46):125–136.

Marvel, M. K., R. M. Epstein, K. Flowers, and H. B. Beckman. 1999. Soliciting the patient's agenda: Have we improved? *Journal of the American Medical Association* (281):283–287.

Marvin, R., G. Cooper, K. Hoffman, and B. Powell. 2002. The Circle of Security Project: Attachment-based intervention with caregiver-preschool child dyads. *Attachment and Human Development* 4 (1):1–31.

Mayberg, H. S., J. A. Silva, S. K. Brannan, J. L. Tekell, R. K. Mahurin, S. McGinnis, and P. A. Jerbek. 2002. The functional neuroanatomy of the placebo effect. *American Journal of Psychiatry* 159 (5):728–737.

Mazure, C. M., M. L. Bruce, P. K. Maciejewski, and S. C. Jacobs. Adverse life events and cognitive-personality characteristics in the prediction of major depression and antidepressant response. *American Journal of Psychiatry* 1576:896–903.

McDougall, J. 1989. *Theaters of the body: A psychoanalytic approach to psychosomatic illness.* New York: Norton.

McEwen, B. S., with E. N. Lasley. 2002. *The end of stress as we know it.* Washington, DC: Dana Press/Joseph Henry Press.

McGrath, E., and G. P. Keita. 1990. *Women and depression: Risk factors and treatment issues. Final report of the American Psychological Association's National Task Force on Women and Depression.* Washington, DC: American Psychological Association.

McLeer, S. V., E. Deblinger, M. S. Atkins, E. B. Foa, and D. L. Ralphe. 1988. Posttraumatic stress disorder in sexually abused children. *Journal of the American Academy of Child and Adolescent Psychiatry* 27:650–654.

Meadows, E. A., and E. B. Foa. 1998. Intrusion, arousal, and avoidance: Sexual trauma survivors. In *Cognitive-behavioral therapies for trauma,* edited by V. M. Follette, J. I. Ruzek, and F. R. Abueg. New York: Guilford.

Mechanic, D. 1995. Sociological dimensions of illness behavior. *Social Science and Medicine* 419:1207–1216.

Melmed, R. N. 2001. *Mind, body, and medicine: An integrative text.* New York: Oxford University Press.

Miller, M. C. 2001. The benefits of positive psychology. *Harvard Mental Health Letter* (December 31).

Mitchell, S. 1984. The problem of the will. *Contemporary Psychoanalysis* 20 (2):257–265.

———. 1993. *Hope and dread in psychoanalysis.* New York: Basic Books.

———. 2000. *Relationality.* Hillsdale, NJ: Analytic Press.

Morris, W. N. 1999. The mood system. In *Well-being: The foundations of hedonic psychology,* edited by D. Kahneman, E. Diener, and N. Schwarz. New York: Russell Sage Foundation.

Murray, L., and D. Lopez. 1996. The global burden of disease: A comprehensive assessment of mortality and disability from disease, injuries, and risk factors in 1990 and projected to 2020. World Health Organization, World Bank, Harvard University.

Musselman, D. L., A. H. Miller, M. R. Porter, A. Manatunga, F. Gao, S. Penna, B. D. Pearce, J. Landry, S. Glover, J. S. McDaniel, and C. B. Nemeroff. 2001. Higher than normal plasma interleukin-6 concentrations in cancer patients with depression: Preliminary findings. *American Journal of Psychiatry* (158):1252–1257.

Myers, D. G. 1992. *The pursuit of happiness.* New York: Avon Books.

———. 2002. *Intuition: Its powers and perils.* New Haven, CT: Yale University Press.

Nathanson, D. L. 1992. *Shame and pride: Affect, sex, and the birth of the self.* New York: Norton.

Nemeroff, C. B. 2002. Comorbidity of mood and anxiety disorders: The rule, not the exception? *American Journal of Psychiatry* 159 (1):3–4.

Nesse, R. M. 2000. Is depression an adaptation? *Archives of General Psychiatry* 57 (1):14–20.

Nesse, R. M., and K. C. Berridge. 2004. Psychoactive drug use in evolutionary perspective. In D. T. Kenrick and C. L. Luce. *The functional mind: Readings in evolutionary psychology.* Boston, MA: Pearson.

Nesse, R. M., and G. C. Williams. 1994. *Why we get sick.* New York: New York Times Books.

Nhat Hanh, Thich. 1999. *The miracle of mindfulness.* Boston: Beacon Press.

Norem, J. K. 2001. *The positive power of negative thinking.* New York: Basic Books.

Norris, F. H., and K. Kaniasty. 1995. Received and perceived social support in times of stress: A test of the social support deterioration deterrence model. *Journal of Personality and Social Psychology* 64:723–39.

Notzon, F. C., Y. M. Komarov, S. P. Ermakov, C. T. Sempos, J. S. Marks, and E. V. Sempos. 1998. Causes of declining life expectancy in Russia. *Journal of the American Medical Association* 279:793–800.

Noyes, R., S. P. Stuart, D. R. Langbehn, R. L. Happel, S. L. Longley, B. A. Muller, and S. J. Yagla. 2003. Test of an interpersonal model of hypochondriasis. *Psychosomatic Medicine* 65:292–300.

Nudo, R. J., G. W. Milliken, W. M. Jenkins, and N. M. Merzenich. 1996. Use-dependent alterations of movement representations in primary motor cortex of adult squirrel monkeys. *Journal of Neuroscience* (January 16):785–780.

Nussbaum, M. C. 2001. *Upheavals of thought: The intelligence of emotions.* New York: Cambridge University Press.

O'Connor, R. 1997. *Undoing depression: What therapy doesn't teach you and medication can't give you.* New York: Little, Brown.

———. 2001. *Active treatment of depression.* New York: Norton.

Ohayon, M. M., and A. F. Schatzberg. 2003. Using chronic pain to predict depressive morbidity in the general population. *Archives of General Psychiatry* 60:39–47.

Ornish, D. 1993. *Eat more, weigh less.* New York: HarperCollins.

Ornstein, R. E. 1972. *The psychology of consciousness.* San Francisco: W. H. Freeman.

———. 1997. *The right mind.* New York: Harcourt Brace.

Parsons, T. 1964. *Social Structure and Person.* New York: Free Press.

Paykel, E. S., J. Scott, J. R. Teasdale, A. L. Johnson, A. Garland, R. Moore, A. Jenaway, P. L. Cornwall, H. Hayhurst, R. Abbot, and M. Pope. 1999. Prevention of relapse in major depression by cognitive therapy. *Archives of General Psychiatry* 56:829–835.

Payson, H. 2002. Personal communication.

Pert, C. 1997. *Molecules of emotion: The science behind mind-body medicine.* New York: Simon and Schuster.

Peterson, C., and L. M. Bossio. 2002. Optimism and physical well-being. In *Optimism and pessimism: Implications for theory, research, and practice,* edited by E. C. Chang. Washington, DC: American Psychological Association.

Phillips, M. L. 2003. Understanding the neurobiology of emotion perception: Implications for psychiatry. *British Journal of Psychiatry* 182:190–192.

Pink, D. 2003. The 3rd annual year in ideas: Gratitude visits. *New York Times Sunday Magazine* (December 14).

Pinel, J. P. J., S. Assanand, and D. R. Lehman. 2000. Hunger, eating, and ill health. *American Psychologist* 55:1105–1116.

Plomin, R. 1990. *Nature and nurture: An introduction to human behavioral genetics.* Pacific Grove, CA: Brooks/Cole.

Polanyi, K. 2001. *The great transformation.* Boston, MA: Beacon Press.

Poonai, N., M. M. Antony, K. E. Binkley, P. Stenn, R. P. Swinson, P. Corey, F. S. Silverman, and S. M. Tarlo. 2000. Carbon dioxide inhalation challenges in idiopathic environmental intolerance. *Journal of Allergy and Clinical Immunology* 105:358–363.

Posener, J. A., L. Wang, J. L. Price, M. H. Gado, M. A. Province, M. I. Miller, C. M. Babb, and J. G. Csernansky. 2003. High-dimensional mapping of the hippocampus in depression. *American Journal of Psychiatry* 160:83–89.

Posner, M. I., M. K. Rothbart, N. Vizueta, K. N. Levy, D. E. Evans, K. M. Thomas, and J. F. Clarkin. 2002. Attentional mechanisms of borderline personality disorder. *Proceedings of the National Academy of Sciences* 99 (25):16366–16370.

Putnam, F. W., and P. K. Trickett. 1997. Psychobiological effects of sexual abuse: A longitudinal study. In *Psychobiology of Posttraumatic Stress Disorder,* edited by R. Yehuda and A. C. McFarland. New York: New York Academy of Sciences.

Ratey, J. J. 2001. *A user's guide to the brain.* New York: Pantheon Books.

Ray, P. H. 1997. The emerging culture. *American Demographics* (February 1997). Available at www.demographics.com. (Accessed Sept. 28, 2003.)

Reibel, D. K., J. M. Greeson, G. C. Brainard, and S. Rosenzweig. 2001. Mindfulness-based stress reduction and health-related quality of life in a heterogeneous patient population. *General Hospital Psychiatry* 23 (4):183–192.

Reich, W. Third edition, 1980. *Character analysis,* translated by V. R. Cafagno. New York: Noonday Press.

Resick, H. S., D. G. Kilpatrick, B. S. Dansky, B. E. Saunders, and C. L. Best. 1993. Prevalence of civilian trauma and posttraumatic stress disorder in a representative national sample of women. *Journal of Consulting and Clinical Psychology* 61:984–991.

Reuters. 2004. Summit: U.S. executive pay still out of control. (February 18) http://www.reuters.com/newsArticle.jhtml.

Rich, A. 1978. *The dream of a common language.* New York: W. W. Norton.

Ridley, M. 2003. *Nature via nurture.* New York: HarperCollins.

Rieff, P. 1966. *The triumph of the therapeutic: Uses of faith after Freud.* Chicago: University of Chicago Press.

Robinson, J. 2003. *Work to live: The guide to getting a life.* New York: Berkley Books.

Roelofs, K., G. P. F. Keijsers, K. A. L. Hoogduin, G. W. B. Näring, and F. C. Moene. 2002.

Childhood abuse in patients with conversion disorder. *American Journal of Psychiatry* 159:1908–1913.

Roisman, G. I., E. Padrón, L. A. Sroufe, and B. Egeland. 2002. Relationships and interactions: Earned-secure attachment status in retrospect and prospect. *Child Development* 73 (4):1204–1219.

Rosenkranz, M. A., D. C. Jackson, K. M. Dalton, I. Dolski, C. D. Ruff, B. H. Singer, D. Moller, N. H. Kalin, and R. J. Davidson. 2003. Affective style and in vivo immune response: Neurobehavioral mechanisms. *Proceedings of the National Academy of Sciences* 100 (19):11148–11152.

Rosvold, H. E., A. F. Mirsky, and K. H. Pribram. 1954. Influence of amygdalectomy on social behavior in monkeys. *Journal of Comparative and Physiological Psychology* (47):173–178.

Rothbaum, B. O., E. B. Foa, T. Murdock, D. S. Riggs, and W. Walsh. 1992. A prospective examination of post-traumatic stress disorder in rape victims. *Journal of Traumatic Stress* 5:455–475.

Rotundo, E. A. 1993. *American manhood: Transformations in masculinity from the revolution to the modern era.* New York: Basic Books.

Roudinesco, E. 2001. *Why psychoanalysis?*, translated by R. Bowlby. New York: Columbia University Press.

Rowan, A. B., D. W. Foy, N. Rodriguez, and S. Ryan. 1994. Posttraumatic stress disorder in a clinical sample of adults sexually abused as children. *Child Abuse and Neglect* 18:51–61.

Roy-Byrne, P., N. Afari, S. Aston, M. Fischer, J. Goldberg, and D. Buchwald. 2002. Chronic fatigue and anxiety/depression: A twin study. *British Journal of Psychiatry* 180:29–34.

Rubin, T. I. 1975. *Compassion and self-hate.* New York: Touchstone.

Rufus, A. 2003. *Party of one: The loners' manifesto.* New York: Marlowe and Co.

Ryan, R. M., and E. L. Deci. 2000. Self-determination theory and the facilitation of intrinsic motivation, social development, and well-being. *American Psychologist* 55 (1):68–78.

Ryff, C. D., and B. H. Singer. 2003. The role of emotion on pathways to positive health. In *Handbook of Affective Sciences,* edited by R. J. Davidson, K. R. Scherer, and H. H. Goldsmith. Oxford, England: Oxford University Press.

Rymer, R. 1994. *Genie: A scientific tragedy.* New York: Penguin.

Safran, J. 1998. *Widening the scope of cognitive therapy.* Northvale, NJ: Jason Aronson.

———, editor. 2003. *Psychoanalysis and Buddhism.* Somerville, MA: Wisdom Publications.

Safran, J., and Z. Segal. 1996. *Interpersonal process in cognitive therapy.* New York: Jason Aronson.

Sapolsky, R. M. 1996. Why stress is bad for your brain. *Science* 273:749–750.

———. Revised edition, 1998. *Why zebras don't get ulcers: An updated guide to stress, stress-related diseases, and coping.* New York: W. H. Freeman.

———. 1999. The physiology and pathophysiology of unhappiness. In *Well-being: The foundations of hedonic psychology,* edited by D. Kahneman, E. Diener, and N. Schwarz. New York: Russell Sage Foundation.

———. 2002. Foreword. In B. S. McEwen, *The end of stress as we know it.* Washington, DC: Joseph Henry Press.

———. 2003. Taming stress. *Scientific American* 289 (3):86–95.

Sarno, J. E. 1998. *The mindbody prescription: Healing the body, healing the pain.* New York: Warner.

Scaer, R. C. 2001. *The body bears the burden: Trauma, dissociation, and disease.* New York: Haworth Press.

Scheier, M. F., K. A. Matthews, J. F. Owens, R. Schulz, M. W. Bridges, G. J. Magovern, and C. S. Carver. 1999. Optimism and rehospitalization after coronary artery bypass graft surgery. *Archives of Internal Medicine* 159(8):829–835.

Schliefer, S. J., S. E. Keller, M. Camerino, J. C. Thornton, and M. Stein. 1983. Suppression of lymphocyte stimulation following bereavement. *Journal of the American Medical Association* 250 (3):374–377.

Schor, J. B. 1998. *The overspent American.* New York: Basic Books.

Schore, A. N. 1994. *Affect regulation and the origin of the self: The neurobiology of emotional development.* Hillsdale, NJ: Erlbaum.

———. 2003a. *Affect dysregulation and disorders of the self.* New York: Norton.

———. 2003b. *Affect regulation and the repair of the self.* New York: Norton.

Schwartz, B. 2004. *The paradox of choice: Why more is less.* New York: HarperCollins.

Schwartz, J. 2004. Always on call and anxious, employees pay with health. *New York Times,* Sept. 5, A1.

Schwartz, J., and S. Begley. 2002. *The mind and the brain: Neuroplasticity and the power of mental force.* New York: HarperCollins.

Schwartz, J. M., P. W. Stoessel, L. R. Baxter, K. M. Martin, and M. E. Phelps. 1996. Systematic changes in cerebral glucose metabolic rate after successful behavior modification treatment of obsessive-compulsive disorder. *Archives of General Psychiatry* 53: 109–113.

Searles, H. F. 1960. *The nonhuman environment.* New York: International Universities Press.

Segal, Z. V., J. M. G. Williams, and J. D. Teasdale. 2002. *Mindfulness-based cognitive therapy for depression.* New York: Guilford.

Segerstrom, S. C., and G. F. Miller. 2004. Psychological stress and the human immune response: A meta-analytic study of 30 years of inquiry. *Psychological Bulletin* 130: 601–630.

Seligman, M. 1990. *Learned optimism: How to change your mind and your life.* New York: Free Press.

———. Revised edition, 1992. *Helplessness: On depression, development, and death.* New York: W. H. Freeman and Co.

———. 1994. *What you can change and what you can't.* New York: Fawcett.

———. 2002. *Authentic happiness.* New York: Free Press.

Servan-Schreiber, D. 2003. *The instinct to heal.* Emmaus, PA: Rodale.

Servan-Schreiber, D., N. R. Kolb, and G. Tabas. 2000. Somatizing patients: Part I. Practical diagnosis. *American Family Physician* 61: 1073–1078.

Servan-Schreiber, D., G. Tabas, and N. R. Kolb. 2000. Somatizing patients: Part II. Practical management. *American Family Physician* 61:1423–1428.

Shapiro, D. 1965. *Neurotic styles.* New York: Basic Books.

———. 2000. *Dynamics of character.* New York: Basic Books.

Shapiro, F. 1989. Efficacy of the eye movement desensitization procedure in the treatment of traumatic memories. *Journal of Traumatic Stress* 2:199–223.

Shapiro, S. L., G. E. Schwartz, and G. Bonner. 1998. Effects of mindfulness-based stress reduction on medical and premedical students. *Journal of Behavioral Medicine* 21:581–599.

Sharpe, M., K. Hawton, S. Simkin, C. Surawy, A. Hackmann, I. Klimes, T. Peto, D. Warrell, and V. Seagroatt. 1996. Cognitive behaviour therapy for the chronic fatigue syndrome: A randomised controlled trial. *British Medical Journal* 312:22–26.

Sheline, Y. I., M. H. Gado, and H. C. Kraemer. 2003. Untreated depression and hippocampal volume loss. *American Journal of Psychiatry* 160 (8):1516–1518.

Sher, B. 1994. *I could do anything if I only knew what it was.* New York: Dell.

Showalter, E. 1997. *Hystories: Hysterical epidemics and modern media.* New York: Columbia University Press.

Siegel, D. J. 2001. *The developing mind.* New York: Guilford.

———. 2003. An interpersonal neurobiology of psychotherapy: The developing mind and the resolution of trauma. In *Healing trauma: Attachment, mind, body, and brain,* edited by M. F. Solomon and D. J. Siegel. New York: Norton, 2003.

Siegel, D. J., and M. Hartzell. 2003. *Parenting from the inside out.* New York: Jeremy Tarcher.

Slaby, A., and L. F. Garfinkel. 1994. *No one saw my pain: Why teens kill themselves.* New York: Norton.

Solomon, A. 2001. *The noonday demon: An atlas of depression.* New York: Scribner.

Solomon, D. A., M. B. Keller, A. C. Leon, T. I. Mueller, P. W. Lavori, M. T. Shea, W. Coryell, M. Warshaw, C. Turvey, J. D. Maser, and J. Endicott. 2000. Multiple recurrences of major depressive disorder. *American Journal of Psychiatry* 1572:229–233.

Solomon, M. F., and D. J. Siegel, editors. *Healing trauma: Attachment, mind, body, and brain.* New York: Norton, 2003.

Speca, M., L. E. Carlson, E. Goodey, and M. Angen. 2000. A randomized, wait-list controlled clinical trial: The effect of a mindfulness meditation-based stress reduction program on mood and symptoms of stress in cancer outpatients. *Psychosomatic Medicine* 62:613–622.

Spiegel, D. 1996. Cancer and depression. *British Journal of Psychiatry* 168 (suppl. 30):119–116.

Spiegel, D., J. R. Bloom, H. C. Kraemer, and E. Gottheil. 1989. Effect of psychosocial treatment on survival of patients with metastatic breast cancer. Lancet 14:888–891.

Spollen, J. J., and D. Gutman. 2003. The interaction of depression and medical illness. *Medscape.* http://www.Medscape.com/viewarticle/457165.

Stern, D. N. 1985. *The interpersonal world of the infant.* New York: Basic Books.

———. 1995. *The motherhood constellation.* New York: Basic Books.

Sternberg, E. 2001. *The balance within: The science connecting health and emotions.* New York: W. H. Freeman.

Stevens, D. E., K. R. Merikangas, and J. R. Merikangas. 1995. Comorbidity of depression and other medical conditions. In *Handbook of depression* (2nd ed.), edited by E. E. Beckham and W. R. Leber. New York: Guilford.

Stimmel, B. 1997. *Pain and its relief without addiction: Clinical issues in the use of opioids and other analgesics.* New York: Haworth.

Striegel, R. H., F. Dohm, K. M. Pike, D. E. Wilfley, and C. G. Fairbairn. 2002. Abuse, bullying, and discrimination as risk factors for binge eating disorder. *American Journal of Psychiatry* 159:1902–1907.

Strupp, H. H., and J. L. Binder. 1984. Psychotherapy in a new key: A guide to time-limited dynamic psychotherapy. New York: Basic Books.

Sullivan, H. S. 1968. *The interpersonal theory of psychiatry.* New York: Norton.

Surowiecki, J. 2002. Boom and gloom. *The New Yorker* (November 11):76.

Surtees, P. G., N. W. J. Wainwright, K. Khaw, and N. E. Day. 2003. Functional health status, chronic medical conditions, and disorders of mood. *British Journal of Psychiatry* 183:299–303.

Swanson, L. 2001. Neurobiological substrates of emotion. Paper presented at Neurobiology of Emotion in Psychosomatic Medicine, March 6, conference sponsored by American Psychosomatic Society and NIH Office of Behavioral and Social Science Research.

Tannen, D. 1990. *You just don't understand: Women and men in conversation.* New York: Ballantine Books.

———. 2001. *I only say this because I love you.* New York: Random House.

Taylor, S. E. 1989. *Positive illusions: Creative self-deception and the healthy mind.* New York: Basic Books.

Teasdale, J. D. 1999a. Emotional processing, three modes of mind and the prevention of relapse in depression. *Behavior Research and Therapy* 37 (suppl. 1):53–77.

———. 1999b. Metacognition, mindfulness and the modification of mood disorders. *Clinical Psychology and Psychotherapy* 6:146–155.

Teasdale, J. D., R. G. Moore, H. Hayhurst, M. Pope, S. Williams, and Z. V. Segal. 2002. Metacognitive awareness and prevention of relapse in depression: Empirical evidence. *Journal of Consulting and Clinical Psychology* 70 (2):275–287.

Teasdale, J. D., Z. Segal, and J. M. G. Williams. 1995. How does cognitive therapy prevent depressive relapse, and why should attentional control mindfulness training help? *Behavior Research and Therapy* 33:25–39.

———. 2003. Mindfulness training and problem formulation. *Clinical Psychology: Science and Practice* 10:157–160.

Teasdale, J. D., Z. Segal, J. M. G. Williams, V. A. Ridgeway, J. M. Soulsby, and M. A. Lau. 2000. Prevention of relapse/recurrence in major depression by mindfulness-based cognitive therapy. *Journal of Consulting and Clinical Psychology* 68:615–623.

Terr, L. 1999. *Beyond love and work: Why adults need to play.* New York: Simon and Schuster.

Thase, M. E. 1999a. How should efficacy be evaluated in randomised controlled trials of treatments for depression? *Journal of Clinical Psychiatry* 60 (suppl. 4):23–31.

———. 1999b. The long-term nature of depression. *Journal of Clinical Psychiatry* 60 (suppl. 4):3–35.

Timimi, S., and E. Taylor. 2004. In debate: ADHD is best understood as a cultural construct. *British Journal of Psychiatry* 184:8–9.

Tomkins, S. S. 1962. *Affect/imagery/consciousness: Volume 1. The positive affects.* New York: Springer.

Trungpa, C. 2002. *The myth of freedom and the way of meditation.* Boston: Shambhala.

Ulrich, R. S. 1984. View through a window may influence recovery from surgery. *Science* 224:420–421.

U.S. Bureau of Justice Statistics, EOY 2002. http://www.ojp.usdoj.gov/bjs/prisons. htm.

U.S. Department of Health and Human Services. 1999. *Mental health: A report of the Surgeon General.* Rockville, MD: U.S. Department of Health and Human Services, Substance Abuse and Mental Health Services Administration, Center for Mental Health Services, National Institutes of Health, National Institute of Mental Health.

———. 2002. Substance Abuse and Mental Health Services, Results: 2002 National Survey on Drug Use and Health. Online: www.drugabusestatistics.samhsa.gov/nhsda/2k2nsduh/results/2k2results.

U.S. General Accounting Office, 2003. Youth Illicit Drug Use Prevention, GAO-03-172R. www.gao.gov/new.items/d03172r.pdf.

U.S. House of Representatives, Committee on Government Reform. 2003. Politics and science: Prescription Drug Advertising. Online: http://democrats.reform.house.gov/features/politics_and_science/example_prescription_drug_advertising.htm.

U.S. Public Health Service. 1999. *The Surgeon General's call to action to prevent suicide.* Washington, DC: U.S. Department of Health and Human Services.

———. 2001. *The Surgeon General's call to action to prevent and decrease overweight and obesity.* Washington, DC: U.S. Department of Health and Human Services.

Vaillant, G. E. 1993. *The wisdom of the ego.* Cambridge, MA: Harvard University Press.

van der Kolk, B. A. 1996. The body keeps the score: Approaches to the psychobiology of posttraumatic stress disorder. In *Traumatic stress: The effects of overwhelming experience on mind, body, and society,* edited by B. A. van der Kolk, A. C. McFarlane, and L. Weisaeth. New York: Guilford.

———. 2002. In terror's grip: Healing the ravages of trauma. *Cerebrum* 4:34–50. New York: The Dana Foundation.

van der Kolk, B. A., J. C. Perry, and J. L. Herman. 1991. Childhood origins of self-destructive behavior. *American Journal of Psychiatry* 148:1665–1671.

Van Houdenhove, B., E. Neerinckx, R. Lysens, H. Verkommen, L. Van Houdenhove, P. Onghena, R. Westhovens, and M. B. D'Hooghe. 2001. Victimization in fibromyalgia and chronic fatigue syndrome in tertiary care: A controlled study on prevalence and characteristics. *Psychosomatics* 42:21–28.

Vedhara, K., P. D. Bennett, S. Clark, S. L. Lightman, S. Shaw, P. Perks, M. A. Hunt, J. M. Philip, D. Tallon, P. J. Murphy, R. W. Jones, G. K. Wilcock, and N. N. Shanks. 2003. Enhancement of antibody responses to influenza vaccination in the elderly following a cognitive-behavioural stress management intervention. *Psychotherapy and Psychosomatics* 72 (5):245–252.

Von Korff, M., and G. Simon. 1996. The relationship between pain and depression. *British Journal of Psychiatry* 168 (suppl. 30):101–108.

Vythilingam, M., C. Heim, J. Newport, A. H. Miller, L. Anderson, R. Bronen, M. Brummer, L. Staib, E. Vermetten, D. S. Charney, C. B. Nemeroff, and J. D. Bremner. 2002. Childhood trauma associated with smaller hippocampal volume in women with major depression. *American Journal of Psychiatry* 159 (12):2072–2080.

Wachtel, P. L. 1994. Cyclical processes in personality and psychopathology. *Journal of Abnormal Psychology* 1031:51–54.

———. 1997. *Psychoanalysis, behavior therapy, and the relational world*. Washington, DC: American Psychological Association.

Wagner, A. W., and M. W. Linehan. 1998. Dissociative behavior. In *Cognitive-behavioral therapies for trauma*, edited by V. M. Follette, J. I. Ruzek, and F. R. Abueg. New York: Guilford.

Wagner, U., S. Gais, H. Haider, R. Verleger, and J. Born. 2004. Sleep inspires insight. *Nature* 427:352–355.

Walker, E. A., D. Keegan, G. Gardner, M. Sullivan, D. Bernstein, and W. J. Katon. 1997. Psychosocial factors in fibromyalgia compared with rheumatoid arthritis: II. Sexual, physical, and emotional abuse and neglect. *Psychosomatic Medicine* 59:572–577.

Wallerstein, J. S., and S. Blakeslee. 1989. *Second chances: Men, women, and children a decade after divorce*. New York: Ticknor and Fields.

Waters, R. 2004. Kids, meds, and suicide. *Psychotherapy Networker* (January/February):19–20.

Wegner, D. M. 1994. Ironic processes of mental control. *Psychological Review* 101 (1):34–52.

Wegner, D. M., R. Erber, and S. Zanakos. 1993. Ironic processes in the mental control of mood and mood-related thought. *Journal of Personality and Social Psychology* 65 (6):1093–1104.

Wegscheider-Cruse, S. 1989. *Another chance: Hope and health for the alcoholic family*. New York: Science and Behavior Books.

Weissman, J. S., D. Blumenthal, A. J. Silk, K. Zapert, M. Newman, & R. Leitman. 2003. Consumers' reports on the health effects of direct-to-consumer drug advertising. *Health Affairs* web exclusive, W3-84, Feb. 26.

Wessely, S., C. Nimnuan, and M. Sharpe. 1999. Functional somatic syndromes: One or many? *The Lancet* 354:936–939.

Willman, D. 2003. Stealth merger: Drug companies and government medical research. *Los Angeles Times* (December 29):1.

Wolf, A. E. Revised edition, 2002. *Get out of my life, but first could you drive me and Cheryl to the mall?* New York: Farrar, Straus, and Giroux.

Woodruff-Borden, J., C. Morrow, S. Bourland, and S. Cambron. 2002. The behavior of anxious parents: Examining mechanisms of transmission of anxiety from parent to child. *Journal of Clinical Child and Adolescent Psychology* 31:364–74.

World Markets Research Centre. 2002. Press release: US are the world's biggest spenders on healthcare—but there is trouble ahead. Available online: http://www.wmrc.com/pc_press_releases.html.

Wulsin, L. R., and B. M. Singal. 2003. Do depressive symptoms increase the risk for the onset of coronary disease? A systematic quantitative review. *Psychosomatic Medicine* 65:201–210.

Young, J. 1994. *Reinventing your life.* New York: Plume Books.

Zanarini, M. C., F. R. Frankenburg, J. Hennen, and K. R. Silk. 2003. The longitudinal course of borderline psychopathology: A 6-year prospective follow-up of the phenomenology of borderline personality disorder. *American Journal of Psychiatry* 160:274–283.

Notes

Chapter 1

p. 11 *Depression and anxiety make physical wounds heal more slowly:* Cole-King and Harding, 2001.

p. 11 *Social isolation is as great a mortality risk as smoking:* House, 2001.

p. 11 *Stress increases susceptibility to the common cold:* Cohen, Tyrell, and Smith, 1991.

p. 11 *Psychotherapy results in brain changes visible on PET scans:* Schwartz and Begley, 2002.

p. 11 *When placebos work, they do so by changing brain chemistry:* Mayberg et al., 2002.

p. 11 *The brains of London cabdrivers are enlarged and enriched:* Maguire et al., 2000.

p. 11 *Serotonin levels in baboons varies with social status:* Sapolsky, 1998.

p. 11 *Stroke victims can . . . reprogram their brains:* Schwartz and Begley, 2002.

p. 12 *In the last days of the twentieth century, that truth was proved false:* Eriksson et al., 1998.

p. 12 *stem cells, which have the potential to replace any specialized cell in the brain:* Gage, 2000. Gage goes on to say, in his understated way, "The observation of stem cells in the adult nervous system has not been adequately integrated into our ideas of the function of the adult brain" (p. 1444).

p. 12 *Practicing a task seals the connections between the new cells and the existing ones:* LeDoux, 2002.

p. 12 *Depression is now ten times as prevalent as it was just a generation ago:* Seligman, 2002. He is comparing current data to 1960.

p. 12 *17 percent of us suffer from anxiety:* U.S. Department of Health and Human Services, 1999.

p. 12 *Ninety million Americans live with a chronic health problem:* Centers for Disease Control, 2003.

p. 12 *stress-related diseases like chronic fatigue syndrome:* Stimmel, 1997.

p. 14 *more than half of patients with major depression also meet the formal diagnostic criteria for an anxiety disorder:* Kessler et al., 1994; Kessler, et al., 1996.

p. 15 *anxiety/depression is one of the most common reasons why people visit their MDs:* Stevens, Merikangas, and Merikangas, 1995.

p. 17 *depression is the second biggest public health problem in the world:* Murray and Lopez, 1996.

p. 17 *matching Russia as the country with the highest rate of incarceration:* U.S. Bureau of Justice Statistics, 2002. Despite the fact that changes in drug laws account for much of the growth in prison population, many would argue that a high proportion of those behind bars must be, ipso facto, antisocial.

p. 19 *We're caught in a vicious circle:* The importance of the vicious circle in maintaining psychological problems is especially well described by Paul Wachtel: Wachtel, 1994, 1997.

p. 21 *Eight out of ten of the most commonly used medications in the United States treat conditions directly related to stress:* Servan-Schreiber, 2003.

Chapter 2

p. 24 *"We do not ride on the railroad":* Henry David Thoreau, *Walden; or, Life in the Woods.* 1854. Available online at www.bartleby.com.

p. 24 *our conventional meaning of stress . . . wasn't part of the vocabulary fifty years ago.* Sternberg, 2001, describes Selye's role in the popularization of the "stress" concept.

p. 25 *an animal's responses to stress:* Robert Sapolsky's wonderful book *Why Zebras Don't Get Ulcers* (1998) is my primary source for understanding the physiology of the stress response. Sapolsky is a fascinating individual who spends half the year studying baboons in Kenya and half lecturing at Stanford. His autobiography, *A Primate's Memoir,* is an engrossing, funny, and moving account of a scientist's life.

p. 25 *It may "learn helplessness":* See Seligman, 1992, for a thoughtful discussion of learned helplessness research, which has proven to be highly meaningful in understanding human depression and trauma.

p. 26 *"Allostatic load":* McEwen, 2002.

p. 28 *Some philosophers are calling this the "age of depression":* e.g., Roudinesco, 2001.

p. 28 *R. E. Lane's massive* Loss of Happiness in Market Democracies: Lane, 2000.

p. 30 *In 1976, the richest 10 percent of Americans controlled:* Collins and Yeskel, 2000.

p. 30 *CEOs in the United States . . . were earning:* Reuters, 2004.

p. 30 *By most measures, our national health ranks seventeenth among developed countries,* World Markets Research Centre, 2002.

p. 31 *the average American workweek has increased:* Goozner, 1998. For a more comprehensive account of changes in American working conditions, see Joe Robinson's *Work to Live: The Guide to Getting a Life* (Berkley Books, 2003).

p. 31 *Americans were working more hours than the workforce in any European country, and equal to the Japanese:* International Labour Organization, 2003.

p. 31 *the average life expectancy for men dropped:* Notzon et al., 1998.

p. 31 *In 2004, it was estimated that workplace stress costs the U.S. economy more than $300 billion each year.* Schwartz, 2004.

p. 31 *Four out of ten Americans work largely at evenings, weekends, night shifts, or staggered shifts:* Schwartz, 2004.

p. 32 *Americans . . . take less vacation time off than they earn:* Robinson, 2003.

p. 32 *in 1997, indebtedness equaled 95 percent of income:* Henwood, 1997.

p. 34 *The divorce rate is currently about 49 percent:* DivorceMagazine.com.

p. 34 *they're poorer, more stressed, and feel guiltier after the divorce:* This conclusion is from Wallerstein and Blakeslee, 1989. There's a certain amount of controversy about the effects of divorce, with advocates not wanting to accept the real damage that is done to children and adults. Judith Wallerstein has documented the effects by following the same families over twenty-five years. Her recent books with Sandra Blakeslee (*The Unexpected Legacy of Divorce,* 2001, and *What About the Kids?* 2003) should be required reading.

p. 34 *bombarded with images of highly attractive members of the opposite sex:* Kenrick et al., 1994.

p. 34 *Suburban sprawl:* Ewing et al., 2003.

p. 34 *trend in frequent visiting with neighbors:* From Lane, 2002, p. 104. Original data in National Opinion Research Center, General Social Survey.

p. 35 *each hour per day of television watching increases a child's risk of ADHD by 9 percent:* Christakis et al., 2004.

p. 36 *According to the Department of Health and Human Services estimates:* U.S. Dept. of Health and Human Services, 2002.

p. 36 *The DARE antidrug education program doesn't work:* GAO-03-172R Youth Illicit Drug Use Prevention www.gao.gov/new.items/d03172r.pdf

p. 36 *Affluent teens have higher rates of anxiety disorder and substance abuse than inner-city kids:* Luthar and D'Avanzo, 1999.

p. 36 *incidence of depression and suicide in children:* These depressing statistics on youth depression and suicide are from Slaby and Garfinkel, 1994; American Association of Suicidology, 1997; and U.S. Public Health Service, 1999.

p. 37 Figure 4, "Chasing Comfort," is based on data from Schor, 1998.

p. 37 *The Hedonic Treadmill was first described:* The famous article in question is Brickman, Coates, and Janoff-Bulman, 1978.

p. 38 *Later research has tended to confirm these findings:* Frederick and Loewenstein, 1999.

p. 38 *the pain of losing outweighs the joy of acquiring:* Surowiecki, 2002. Barry Schwartz's *The Paradox of Choice: Why More Is Less* explains these phenomena in a clear and readable way, and goes into much greater detail than I can here about the effects of our contemporary cognitive overload.

p. 38 *Barry Schwartz gives another example:* Schwartz, 2004.

p. 39 *heavy viewers actually enjoy their TV watching* less *than light viewers:* Kubey and Csikszentmihalyi, 2002.

p. 41 *"Consumers 'know,' without being told or convinced, that they are not adequate"*: Cushman, 1995, p. 85.

p. 43 *$2.5 billion was spent on direct-to-consumer advertising:* Weissman et al. 2003.

p. 44 *the FDA . . . published a report in 2003 distorting its own research:* This is documented on the website of Rep. Henry Waxman's committee on government reform, U.S. House of Representatives, 2003.

p. 44 *"Individuals ceased to be thought of as public citizens"*: Cushman, 1995, p. 67.

p. 45 *Doctors are paid . . . for attending industry-sponsored promotions of their drugs that are held in places like Yankee Stadium and yacht cruises:* These are among the abuses described in a *Dateline NBC* feature, July 11, 2003.

p. 45 *43.6 million uninsured: Christian Science Monitor,* January 26, 2004.

p. 46 Figure 6 *Percentage of Americans who say they trust the government "most of the time":* From Lane, 2000, p. 199. Source: National Election Studies.

p. 47 *"The ideal man, then, was pleasant, mild-mannered, and devoted to the good of the community"*: Rotundo, 1993.

p. 47 *"Victorian-era doctors, especially psychiatrists, explained [the] psychological disorders . . . of their female patients . . . through biologically based theories"*: Cushman, 1995, p. 102.

p. 48 *"a self that embodies the absences, loneliness, and disappointments of life as a chronic, undifferentiated emotional hunger"*: Cushman, 1995, p. 79.

p. 48 *"On the eve of the third millennium"*: Roudinesco, 2001.

p. 49 *Those who participated in the rescue and cleanup efforts are likely to bear permanent emotional scars.* A recent study of disaster workers after an airplane crash shows much higher rates of PTSD and depression as much as 13 months after the crash. Fullerton, Ursano, & Wang, 2004.

p. 49 *"To defeat an enemy that lurks in the shadows and seeks relentlessly for some small crack through which to slip their evil designs—such a victory requires the vigilance of every American."* This is on the "Home and Community" page of the Department of Homeland security website." http://www.dhs.gov/dhspublic/display?theme= 32.

p. 50 *All it takes to damage the immune systems of rats and stop the production of nerve cells in their brains is a few weeks of confinement.* McEwen, 2002.

p. 50 *Depressive realism:* This is a phenomenon that's been a focus of attention in psychology for the past twenty-five years. People with depression are able to see some things more objectively than the nondepressed. The nondepressed seem to function by creating happy little illusions about their ability to influence events. For instance, if you tell people their behavior in the lab (pushing a button or flipping a lever) will influence the outcome of an event that is in reality random (like rolling dice), the depressed people will tell you there's something wrong with your experiment while the nondepressed will go on happily pushing their buttons. Unfortunately for them, depressed people are less objective when it comes to themselves: they consistently underrate their own performance, popularity, intelligence, and so on when compared to others. Lauren Alloy is chiefly responsible for discovering and exploring the phenomenon (see

Alloy and Abramson, 1988), but Julie Norem's *The Positive Power of Negative Thinking* (Basic Books, 2001) is-up-to-date and also a provocative read.

p. 51   *"In Western societies we are seeing an unbelievable growth in the little world of bonesetters, wizards, clairvoyants, and mesmerists,"* Roudinesco, 2001.

p. 52   *the effects on us of the loss of opportunity to be part of nature haven't been taken seriously:* Searles, 1960.

p. 54   *research is needed on the effects of chronic stress or psychosocial stress:* Swanson, 2001.

p. 54   *We are not "blank slates":* See Stern, 1985, 1995, for the most respected and comprehensive review of innate differences and the intricacies of the mother-infant dyad.

p. 54   *Introversion (shyness):* LeDoux, 2002, p. 30.

p. 54   *Positive affectivity (bubbliness):* Seligman, 2002, p. 33.

p. 55   *General intelligence:* Ridley, 2003; Plomin, 1990.

p. 55   *The so-called Big Five character traits:* Ridley, 2003.

p. 55   *Activity level and conservatism:* Both figures are from Plomin, 1990.

p. 56   *biological siblings separated at birth . . . end up being parented more alike than adopted siblings in the same household do:* Collins et al., 2000.

p. 56   *children with that vulnerability [to depression] who are raised by uninvolved or critical parents are more likely to develop the illness than children raised by supportive and interested parents:* Gabbard, 2000.

p. 56   *we've identified over twenty-five hundred connections [between the hypothalamus and the cerebral cortex], and no one knows what they all mean:* Swanson, 2001.

p. 59   *George Engel and his followers have been calling for a general reform of Western medicine:* Engel's 1977 paper, "The need for a new medical model: A challenge for biomedicine" (*Science* 196: 129–136) is cited whenever anyone suggests that contemporary medicine needs a more "holistic" approach, but the actual implementation of his recommendations has barely begun.

p. 60   *there is a great deal of neurasthenia in China:* David Mechanic's 1995 article on the cultural expression of disease, especially depression, is "Sociological dimensions of illness behavior" in *Social Science and Medicine* 419: 1207–1216.

p. 60   *Two-thirds of patients in primary care now have unexplained physical symptoms:* Epstein, Quill, and McWhinney 1999.

p. 60   *David Mechanic . . . relates how a distinguished physician could find no help:* Mechanic, 1995.

Chapter 3

p. 66   *"The brain does not mechanically store the information that it acquires":* Ratey, 2001, p. 343; emphasis added.

p. 67   *There are currently fifty-three known neurotransmitters:* Ratey, 2001, p. 17

p. 67   *Serotonin, dopamine, epinephrine (adrenaline), and norepinephrine are called variously neuromodulators or neurotransmitters:* LeDoux, 2002; McEwen, 2002.

p. 67   *Each neuron connects with about 10,000 others:* Siegel, 2003.

p. 68   *"Neurons that fire together, wire together":* Hebb, 1949.

p. 69 *In a delightful recent study, researchers taught twelve volunteers to juggle:* Draganski et al., 2004.

p. 69 *Children born with cataracts who don't have them removed:* Ridley, 2003.

p. 69 *children like Genie:* Rymer, 1994.

p. 69 *the brain continues developing new cells, circuits, and structures:* Geidd et al., 1999.

p. 70 *Daniel Siegel makes it easy to visualize:* Siegel and Hartzell, 2003.

p. 70 *the different basic emotional responses . . . are due to the activation of characteristic pathways:* LeDoux, 1996.

p. 72 *the hippocampus is significantly reduced in size in people with PTSD:* Bremner, 2002, p. 46; *new antidepressants apparently help the hippocampus reverse the process and increase in size:* Sheline, Gado, and Kraemer, 2003.

p. 72 *placebos . . . are often very effective with stress-related conditions:* Brown, 1998.

p. 72 *The hippocampus is one area where we know that new neuronal stem cells are formed:* This groundbreaking discovery was the result of a lifetime of dedicated research on the nervous system by Peter Eriksson. The discovery was reported in Eriksson et al., 1998.

p. 72 *mother's attentiveness means that more neurons survive:* López, 2003.

p. 73 *face evaluation is disrupted, with a bias toward interpreting others' expressions as sad:* Phillips, 2003.

p. 73 *under repeated stress, the neurons in the amygdala sprout new branches:* Sapolsky, 2003.

p. 73 *Some have called this the "high road," and the direct amygdala-body connection the "low road":* LeDoux, 1996.

p. 73 *"emotional hijacking"—when our emotions control our actions without input from the thinking brain:* Goleman, 1995, p. 13.

p. 73 *Vietnam veterans with PTSD, shown movies of wartime, are hijacked down the low road:* Bremner et al., 1999.

p. 74 *the right and left sides of the brain differ slightly in function:* This discussion draws heavily on Ornstein, 1997.

p. 75 *Some people with right hemisphere damage can speak perfectly well but cannot dress themselves:* Ornstein, 1972, p. 53.

p. 76 *Rats, like humans, do their sequential processing in the left brain:* Ornstein, 1997, p. 15.

p. 76 *it is the right hemisphere that is the seat of the unconscious:* Schore, 2003b, p. 34.

p. 77 *[The OFC] is the repository of Bowlby's internal working model . . ., or what I call the assumptive world:* Schore, 2003b, p. 45.

p. 77 *The right portion of the OFC . . . functions as an executive control system for the entire right brain:* Schore, 2003b, p. 42.

p. 77 *"The orbitofrontal cortex is involved in critical human functions . . . that are crucial in defining the 'personality' of an individual."* Cavada and Schultz, 2000, p. 205. Taken from Schore, 2003b, p. 42.

p. 78 *when trauma interferes with the connection, a stable and coherent conception of the self cannot be fully developed:* Siegel, 2003, p. 15; Siegel and Hartzell, 2003, p. 245.

p. 78   *The OFC's responsiveness to neurotransmitters . . . may be permanently reduced:* Schore, 2003a, p. 34.

p. 78   *These effects are likely caused by the excess production of stress hormones such as cortisol, which can kill nerve cells:* Siegel, 2003, p. 17.

p. 78   *it's not just trauma, but constant everyday stress, that can activate the low road more and more often:* Siegel and Hartzell, 2003, p. 179.

p. 79   *Davidson tested an advanced Buddhist monk . . . and found that he had the greatest difference between left and right lobe activity of anyone yet tested:* Goleman, 2003a.

p. 80   *"In a fight-or-flight scenario, epinephrine [adrenaline] is the one handing out the guns.":* Sapolsky, 2003.

p. 80   *Cortisol also impacts the immune system:* Sternberg, 2001, pp. 110–111. Also see Bremner, 2002, p. 6–7.

p. 80   *small wounds took an average of nine days longer to heal among people taking care of a loved one with Alzheimer's:* Kiecolt-Glaser et al., 2002.

p. 80   *Bruce McEwen and his colleagues have demonstrated the effects of continuing stress on lab rats:* McEwen, 2002.

p. 81   *sugar and other comfort foods . . . put a brake on the chronic stress response:* Dallman et al., 2003.

p. 81   *stress hormones interfere with the production of growth hormones and insulin:* Sapolsky, 1996.

p. 82   *Monkeys under social stress are likely to die from excess cortisol secretion:* Ibid.

p. 82   *People with PTSD are more likely to smoke:* Bremner, 2002, p. 10.

p. 82   *Men in combat training have lower testosterone levels:* Sternberg, 2001, p. 118.

p. 82   *When cortisol is more or less at a constant level, our rhythms are disrupted and we have insomnia:* McEwen, 2002, p. 25.

p. 83   *Attachment research:* Robert Karen has a fascinating book called *Becoming Attached,* which tells the history of attachment research at least through 1994. Also see Main, 1996, and Hesse et al., 2003.

p. 84   *Harry Harlow . . . was demonstrating that infant monkeys sought something more than food from their mothers:* This groundbreaking research was published as Harlow and Harlow, 1962.

p. 84   *Ainsworth and her colleagues determined that infants could be reliably classified into three groups:* Ainsworth et al., 1978.

p. 84   *Later researchers identified a fourth group:* Main and Solomon, 1990.

p. 86   *Children who are securely attached are more curious about the world:* Fosha, 2003, p. 226.

p. 86   *Many hypochondriacs are found to be ambivalently or anxiously attached:* Noyes et al., 2003.

p. 86   *avoidant children tended to become victimizers as adolescents; ambivalent children tended to become victims:* Karen, 1994, p. 198.

p. 86   *Disorganized infants seem to be, as adults, at highest risk for mental illness and violence:* Siegel, 2003; Hesse et al., 2003; Main, 1996.

p. 86   *a relationship with another caregiver can provide that secure attachment that the child needs:* Fonagy et al., 1995.

p. 87   *mothers can be rather easily helped to provide a more secure attachment:* Marvin et al., 2002.

p. 87   *programs designed to help the child express his feelings about the parent's illness:* Focht-Birkerts and Beardslee, 2000.

p. 87   *The amount of stress a female rat is exposed to during pregnancy . . . can alter the structure and function of that fetal rat's hippocampus in adulthood:* Sapolsky, 2003.

p. 87   *Caregivers who themselves are coping with the aftereffects of trauma or unresolved grief are most likely to be unable to provide appropriate attunement to the needs of a frightened child:* Hesse et al., 2003.

p. 87   *An analysis of videotaped interactions of parents helping children with a homework task:* Woodruff-Borden et al., 2002.

p. 87   *imprinting . . . "a very rapid form of learning that irreversibly stamps early experience upon the developing nervous system":* Schore, 1994, p. 118.

p. 87   *mother's and infant's heartbeats become synchronous:* Fosha, 2003, p. 227.

p. 88   *"coherent autonoetic narrative":* This rather abstruse term comes from Siegel, 2003 pp. 27–28.

p. 88   *"an internal working model":* Fosha, 2003. p. 229.

p. 88   *what Siegel calls the self-as-perceived-by-the-other:* Siegel, 2003.

p. 89   *the effects of wealth on children's mental health:* Costello et al., 2003.

p. 90   *Allan N. Schore . . . has published an enormous and groundbreaking body of work tracing the connections between infant attachment, brain development, and adult mental health:* See Schore, 1994, 2003a, 2003b.

p. 91   *A study of four groups of women:* Heim et al., 2000.

p. 91   *A study of male combat veterans with PTSD:* Geracioti et al., 2001.

p. 91   *Bremner and his study group have consistently found that both the left and right hippocampus are significantly reduced in size:* Bremner, et al. 2003.

p. 91   *A study comparing sexually abused girls to nonabused controls:* Putnam and Trickett, 1997.

p. 91   *Childhood abuse and neglect apparently interfere with the growth of GABA calming fibers:* Siegel and Hartzell, 2003.

p. 91   *adults with borderline personality disorder respond to purely cognitive tasks with more anxiety and confusion than other people do:* Cooper, 2003; Posner et al., 2002.

p. 92   *infant rats who receive more licking and grooming from their mothers are less fearful and more intelligent as adults, have better immune systems, and are more attentive mothers themselves:* Champagne and Meaney, 2001.

p. 92   *Adverse Childhood Experiences (ACE) study:* Felitti, 2001; Felitti et al., 1998; Edwards et al., 2003.

p. 93   *In the general population of women, the incidence of childhood sexual abuse has been found to range from 22 to 37 percent:* McGrath and Keita, 1990.

p. 94   *Rats and other animals, separated at birth from their mothers for just a few minutes at a time, have their stress responses compromised:* Sternberg, 2001.

p. 94   *Babies from Romanian orphanages:* Sternberg, 2001, p. 148.

p. 96 *A study of more than 200 individuals who had responded to a major plane crash:* Fullerton, Ursano, and Wang, 2004.

p. 96 *In the hippocampus, stress interferes with long-term potentiation, damaging neurons and making it more difficult to put memories of the stressful situation away:* Sapolsky, 2003.

p. 97 *A recent study shows very clearly that in PTSD patients traumatic memories are stored in the right brain, the emotional, no-boundaries brain:* Lanius et al., 2004.

p. 98 *[The PTSD patient] thinks these symptoms are caused by present events:* van der Kolk, 2002.

p. 98 *Childhood sexual abuse seems to result in problems with dissociation more often than physical abuse:* Wagner and Linehan, 1998.

p. 104 *A huge NIMH-funded study of psychotherapy for depression:* The summary report of this study is Elkin et al., 1989.

p. 104 *The degree to which the patients experienced their therapists as empathic, caring, open, and sincere at the end of the second session significantly predicted outcome at termination:* Blatt et al., 1996. For more recent confirmation and a thoughtful discussion of the effects of the patient-therapist relationship, see Klein et al., 2003.

p. 104 *Analytic leaders like Steven Mitchell and Irwin Hoffman:* Mitchell, whose untimely death was a great loss, was a prolific writer; among his best are Mitchell, 1993 and 2000; Hoffman has only one book in print, but it is a classic: Hoffman, 1998.

p. 106 *Cognitive theorists like Jeremy Safran and Zindel Segal:* Among their many publications I recommend Safran, 1998, 2003; Safran and Segal, 1996; Segal, Williams, and Teasdale, 2002.

p. 106 *The language of psychoanalysis and psychotherapy—the id, the ego, the self, selfobjects, object relations, defenses, drives—can begin to be translated into the structures and functions of the brain:* Schore makes this goal explicit in 2003a, p. 110, but it is of course the whole direction of his monumental work.

p. 106 *I feel like Keats:* John Keats, "On First Looking Into Chapman's Homer," 1817.

Chapter 4

p. 110 *There is a famous passage in Catch-22:* Joseph Heller, *Catch-22*. Simon and Schuster reprint, 1996.

p. 110 *Paul Ekman, who has spent a lifetime studying emotions, has finally settled a long debate, showing that emotional expressions (face and body language) are the same across all human cultures:* Ekman, 2003; the quote is from p. 4.

p. 112 *Martha Nussbaum's* Upheavals of Thought *is a massive philosophical treatise on the role of emotions in thinking:* Nussbaum, 2001.

p. 112 *The amygdala makes instantaneous assessments of strangers' faces:* LeDoux, 2002.

p. 113 Emotions *are our innate response to a novel situation;* moods, *on the other hand, reflect an assessment of our resources or motivation to handle the situation:* Morris, 1999.

p. 114 *Daniel Goleman has a good example of how this works for fear:* Goleman, 1995, p. 54.

p. 114 *LeDoux discusses a pair of experiments by social psychologist John Bargh:* LeDoux, 1996, p. 62. The experiments are in Bargh, 1990, 1992.

p. 115 *Daniel Stern has been studying the interactions of mothers and infants for more than thirty years:* See Stern, 1985, 1995.

p. 115 *"Associated experiences and behavioral systems may thus never be fully defined as part of the infants' sense of self":* Safran and Segal, 1996, p. 63. Italics in original.

p. 116 *"negative emotion-phobic":* Linehan, 1992.

p. 116 *"Children in an abusive environment develop extraordinary abilities to scan for warning signs of attack":* This quote is from Judith Herman's powerful and groundbreaking *Trauma and Recovery* (1992, p. 99), which we will be returning to many times.

p. 120 *"Learned Helplessness":* This discussion is largely based on Seligman, 1990, though I have also drawn on some of his other publications.

p. 121 *Seligman and his colleagues introduced the concept of attributional style:* Abramson, Seligman, and Teasdale, 1978.

p. 123 *Shame is thought to start out as an adaptive response of the infant whose cries for its mother go unheeded:* Karen, 1992.

p. 123 *the brain registers rejection the same way it registers physical pain:* Eisenberger, Lieberman, and Williams, 2003.

p. 123 *the experience of shame elicits a higher cortisol response to stress:* Lewis and Ramsay, 2002.

p. 124 *As Marsha Linehan observes, when our feelings are consistently invalidated, we can do one of three things:* Linehan, 1993, p. 52.

p. 124 *"a stone, a leaf, an unfound door":* This is the epigram to Thomas Wolfe's *Look Homeward, Angel* (1929).

p. 125 *"To be self-aware is to retrieve from long-term memory our understanding of who we are and place it in the forefront of thought":* LeDoux, 2002, p. 28.

p. 126 *The right brain contains a dictionary of nonverbal behavior, allowing us to unconsciously respond to emotional cues from others:* Schore, 1994, p. 42.

p. 126 *The orbitofrontal cortex operates on an unconscious level, generating the unconscious biases that guide our behavior before conscious knowledge does:* Schore, 2003b, p. 45.

p. 129 *Some have suggested, though, that instead of the specific techniques, what is really effective about cognitive therapy is that all the techniques are teaching you to recognize upsetting thoughts and feelings as mental events (expressions of emotions), not as "the truth":* See Teasdale et al., 2002.

p. 129 *When we become used to the idea that upsetting thoughts and feelings are simply replays of the same old tape, we may even get bored with the tape:* Segal, Williams, and Teasdale, 2002.

p. 129 *Learning to live with emotions as a responsible adult requires a paradoxical strategy, as Marsha Linehan and many others have pointed out:* Linehan, 1992, p. 45.

p. 133 *"Learning to Control Emotions":* These suggestions are a distillation of a lot of reading and my own clinical and personal experience; but the last four points specifically are from Linehan, 1992, p. 46, citing Gottman and Katz, 1990.

p. 134 *As Jimmy Connors said, "I hate to lose more than I like to win."* Cited in Buss, 2000.

p. 134 *Earlier research showed that amygdalectomy in dominant monkeys resulted in their al-*

most immediate reduction to the lowest position in the pecking order: Rosvold, Mirsky, and Pribram, 1954.

p. 134   *Newer research is suggesting that removal of the amygdala results in an almost complete loss of the fear response:* Emery et al. 2001.

p. 134   *Patients whose amygdalae have been removed can't differentiate between "trustworthy" and "untrustworthy" facial expressions:* Adolphs, Tranel, and Damasio, 1998.

p. 135   *"Unconscious Feelings."* This research was discussed by Swanson, 2001.

p. 136   *Men who've had the fear center—the amygdala—in their brains removed have the highest self-esteem in creation:* Damasio, 1999.

p. 137   *Irwin Hoffman, an analyst who gets right to the point, believes that the basic anxiety is fear of death:* Hoffman, 1998.

p. 137   *Buddhism looks at Western attempts to fill (by consuming) or cure (by finding the right pill) or explain away (with a psychological explanation) the emptiness as wasted effort:* Epstein, 1998.

p. 138   *Mark Epstein relates how the Buddha and Freud both understood the fear of death:* Epstein, 1998, p. 45.

p. 138   *One of Freud's short essays relates a beautiful mountain walk with two friends:* Freud, 1916.

p. 138   *"It is possible to cultivate a mind that neither clings nor rejects, and . . . in so doing we can alter the way in which we experience both time and our selves":* Epstein, 1998, p. 62.

p. 138   *the recent finding that Buddhist monks may be the happiest people on earth:* Goleman, 2003a.

p. 141   *Daniel Goleman and the Dalai Lama and others have talked of reducing "destructive" emotions—principally anger:* Goleman, 2003a.

p. 142   *monkeys also have a sense of justice:* Brosnan and de Waal, 2003.

p. 143   *the heart of an anger-prone individual must work harder to achieve the increased blood flow that the stress response commands:* McEwen, 2002, p. 83.

p. 146   *Robert Karen gives a gut-wrenching example:* This is from a superb article Karen published in *The Atlantic* (Karen, 1992).

Chapter 5

p. 149   *Practicing mindfulness has been shown to affect how the brain deals with emotions, especially in the prefrontal cortex (PFC):* Bennett-Goleman, 2001, p. 34.

p. 150   *mindfulness teaches how "to observe oneself without the usual judgment or criticism":* This quote is from my friend Hope Payson, 2002.

p. 150   *"we've been trying to bake the cake with all the ingredients but sugar":* Ibid.

p. 152   *[The relaxation response] was first described by Herbert Benson:* Benson, 1975.

p. 152   *RR has any number of positive benefits:* All reported in Benson and Stark, 1996.

p. 153   *Benson's "generic" technique:* Benson and Stark, 1996, p. 136.

p. 154   *He has described mindfulness in famously succinct terms: "paying attention in a particular way: on purpose, in the present moment, and nonjudgmentally":* Kabat-Zinn, 1994.

p. 154 *Kabat-Zinn and others have had very promising results using the program (with some special adaptations, depending on the problem) with all sorts of issues:* See Segal, Williams, and Teasdale, 2002; Kabat-Zinn, 1982; Kabat-Zinn et al., 1992; Kristeller and Hallett, 1999; Kabat-Zinn et al., 1998; Goldenberg et al., 1994; Kutz et al., 1985; Speca et al., 2000; Shapiro, Schwartz, and Bonner, 1998.

p. 154 *Studies new in 2003 showed that MBSR produced brain changes associated with positive moods and an improved immune response among healthy volunteers, and it decreased stress symptoms and improved immune response in cancer patients:* Davidson et al., 2003; Carlson et al., 2003.

p. 154 *Though some of these studies have been criticized for small sample sizes and lack of control groups:* Bishop, 2002.

p. 154 *The application of mindfulness meditation techniques to depression is being investigated by Segal, Williams, and Teasdale, with very encouraging results:* Segal, Williams, and Teasdale, 2002.

p. 155 *The authors are cautious to suggest that MBSR is not likely to be a generic technique that can be effectively applied to a broad range of psychological problems:* Teasdale, Segal, and Williams, 2003.

p. 158 *The area of the brain devoted to the "reading finger" of Braille readers is much larger than that for their other fingers:* Schwartz and Begley, 2002.

p. 158 *Most human problems are examples of vicious circles in action:* Wachtel, 1997.

p. 160 *The fundamental difference between Buddhism and the secular Western view of man is succinctly described by Mark Epstein:* Epstein, 1998. p. 19.

p. 160 *From a Buddhist perspective, Cartesian dualism—the belief that there is a self separate from our physical bodies—is itself a defense:* Magid, 2002, p. 45.

p. 160 *A standard introductory Buddhist text:* Trungpa, 2002, p. 2.

p. 161 *Mindlessness is being controlled by categories:* These ideas are from Langer, 1989, pp. 15–18.

p. 162 *In Goleman's terms, emotional intelligence refers to several related abilities:* Goleman, 1995, p. 43.

p. 163 *Ellen Langer's approach to mindfulness comes from a non-Buddhist tradition and is concerned with how our environment facilitates (or hinders) a mindful attitude:* Langer, 1989; Langer and Moldoveanu, 2000.

p. 163 *For her, "the subjective 'feel' of mindfulness is that of a heightened state of involvement or being in the present":* Langer, 1989.

p. 163 *In one famous experiment, she gave a group of nursing home residents a plant for their rooms:* Langer and Moldoveanu, 2000, p. 2.

p. 164 *Jeffrey Schwartz . . . performed a revolutionary feat in 1996 by demonstrating that psychotherapy results in changes in the brain visible on PET scans:* Schwartz et al., 1996. A more recent demonstration that psychotherapy for depression also results in brain changes can be found in Goldapple et al., 2004.

p. 166 *Marsha Linehan's Dialectical Behavior Therapy (DBT) is a highly structured and detailed program for treating borderline personality disorder, borrowing from many sources:* Linehan, 1992, 1993.

p. 167   *"Watch your thoughts coming and going, like clouds in the sky"*: All quotations in this section are from Linehan, 1993, pp. 111–113.

p. 168   *Another approach that incorporates mindfulness skills is the Relapse Prevention Therapy of Marlatt and Gordon:* Marlatt and Gordon, 1985; Larimer, Palmer, and Marlatt, 1999.

p. 168   *The advice of the Stoic philosophers—Value only that which no one can take from you— may sound appealing, especially to those who have been hurt a lot:* See Lou Marinoff's interesting book, *Plato, Not Prozac* (2000), for a more extended discussion on this point and on the value of another ancient form of mindfulness—the introspective life.

p. 169   *"Extinction is an active learning process, a repatterning of new memory over an old one that takes place in the smartest brain area of all, the prefrontal cortex"*: McEwen, 2002, p. 38.

p. 169   *Focusing attention on a specific task, like paying attention to color, or movement, results in increased electrical activity and increased blood flow in the brain areas that correspond to color and movement:* Schwartz and Begley, 2002, p. 333.

p. 170   *Richard Davidson, a leading brain researcher based at the University of Wisconsin, has documented that the brain has a set point for mood:* Davidson, 2000.

p. 171   *the Buddhist monk was in the happiest state yet found:* This is reported in Goleman, 2003a, 2003b.

p. 171   *Davidson and Jon Kabat-Zinn have been able to show that a mindfulness training program with healthy volunteers results in shifts in PFC activity to the left, as well as improved moods and motivation, after only eight weeks:* Goleman, 2003b; Davidson et al., 2003.

p. 172   *Magid puts it in a nutshell: "the common goal of Zen and psychoanalysis is putting an end to the pursuit of happiness"*: Magid, 2002, p. 82. Emphasis in the original.

p. 172   *Epstein has an observation that fits the theme of this book: "The traditional view of therapy as building up the ego simply does not do justice to what people's needs actually are"*: Epstein, 1998, p. 31.

p. 173   *After the ecstasy, the laundry, in Jack Kornfield's phrase:* Kornfield, 2000.

p. 174   *Even the most comprehensive research studies on how therapy works have left us with more questions than answers:* See, for example, Blatt, Sanislow et al., 1996; Blatt, Zuroff et al., 1996.

p. 174   *[Schore's] theory is that therapy helps the patient by providing the same kind of synchrony that the child had with its mother, and that results in the same kinds of changes in the right brain that the mother-infant bond creates:* Schore, 2003b.

p. 175   *As Jerome Frank observed long ago, most patients are, more than anything else, demoralized:* Frank, 1974.

p. 175   *Thoughts can come to seem more like transient mental events than imperatives or absolutes:* Teasdale et al., 2002.

p. 175   *As far as I know, no one has written about this effect of antidepressants:* The exception is Peter Kramer, in *Listening to Prozac* (1997). Although dated now in its medical information, it is still the most thought-provoking exploration of the implications of these drugs for what we think of as personality and character.

Chapter 6

p. 178   *"The crucial thing to live for is the sense of life in what you are doing, and if that is not there, then you are living according to other peoples' notions of how life should be lived."* This quotation, and the next few Campbell citations, are all from *Reflections on the Art of Living,* selected and edited by Diane K. Osbon; Campbell, 1995, p. 73.

p. 178   *Endorphins (the body's own morphine, the source of good feelings) are present in the most primitive vertebrates:* Pert, 1997.

p. 179   *"the land of people doing what they think they ought to do or have to do is the waste-land."* Campbell, 1995, p. 72.

p. 183   *"In order to be able to function, everyone must impose an order and regularity on the welter of experiences impinging upon him":* Frank's definition of the assumptive world is in *Persuasion and Healing* (1974).

p. 183   *the concept of explanatory (or attributional) style in cognitive-behavioral therapy:* Seligman, 1990; Abramson, Seligman, and Teasdale, 1978.

p. 183   *the cognitive distortions that have been so well documented by Aaron Beck and others:* Beck et al., 1979.

p. 183   *Thomas Kuhn's concept of the paradigm in science:* Kuhn, 1970.

p. 184   *Medicine discouraged trying to teach them to use the affected limb because it was seen as pointless—until people started to realize that other areas of the brain could take over for the affected area if the patient were encouraged to use the limb.* This calamity of mindlessness is documented in Schwartz and Begley, 2002, p. 191.

p. 190   *"The defense is what hurts":* From Epstein, 1998, p. 176.

p. 194   *The walls we put up for protection have become a prison instead:* Magid, 2002, p. 41.

p. 195   *Exercise 8: "Identifying Defenses":* This is based on an exercise in Barbara Sher's provocative book, *I Could Do Anything if I Only Knew What It Was* (1994).

p. 196   *Table 2: "Defense Mechanisms":* These definitions are from my 2002 book, *Active Treatment of Depression,* and from *Longman Dictionary of Psychology and Psychiatry* (R. E. Goldenson, editor, 1984).

p. 200   *Table 3: "Mature Defenses":* Except for acceptance, these are taken from Vaillant, 1993.

p. 200   *Character analysis:* See Reich, 1980; Josephs, 1995; Shapiro, 1965, 2000.

p. 201   *"We no longer have any problems. That is, we no longer divide our life into the good parts and the problematic parts; there is simply life, one moment after another":* From Magid, 2002, p. 50. Emphasis in the original.

p. 202   *James Mann, a uniquely gifted therapist, referred to these scenarios as* "the present and chronically endured pain": Mann, 1973; Mann and Goldman, 1982.

p. 205   *Harry Stack Sullivan, the influential but abstruse American psychoanalyst:* See Sullivan, 1968, and Evan, 1996.

p. 205   *People divide experiences into those that belong to the self, and those that don't—these instead belong to the "not me":* Safran, 1998, p. 5.

p. 205   *Researchers have been able to demonstrate that schemas have some demonstrable effects:* This research is summarized in Safran, 1998, pp. 5–6.

p. 206   *Jeffrey Young, an influential writer and therapist following in the cognitive-behavioral tradition of Aaron Beck, uses the term "lifetrap," which he says is the same as "schema":* Young, 1994.

p. 207   *A study of 180 borderline patients found that more than 10 percent made dramatic improvements over a period of two years:* Gunderson et al., 2003.

p. 208   *Table 4: Young's Lifetraps:* From Young, 1994.

p. 210   *Table 5: "Character Styles—Impact on the Assumptive World":* Character styles are based on Lawrence Josephs, *Character and Self-Experience* (1995).

p. 214   *Tara Bennett-Goleman's notion of "schema attacks"—the emotional hijacking that occurs when something triggers one of our old tapes:* Bennett-Goleman, 2001, p. 107.

p. 218   *Daniel Siegel's hypothesis in* The Developing Mind *is that we build a coherent autobiographical narrative:* Siegel, 2001.

p. 219   *Narrative can be understood to mean the "story beneath the story" that we live out on a daily basis:* This discussion again comes from Payson, 2002.

p. 228   *Descartes' Error, Skinner's Fumble.* In 1994, Antonio Damasio, a respected neurological researcher, published *Descartes' Error,* a book which has become a minor classic of the mind-body field. Descartes' error, in Damasio's view, was the split between the body and mind known as *dualism.* Dualism took on the strength of a paradigm in Western medicine and philosophy, an underlying assumption so taken for granted that it was rarely challenged and its negative effects were rarely noticed.

When French philosopher René Descartes (1596–1650) developed the concept of dualism—the idea that mind, soul, or psyche exists independently of the body, and that although the mind can move the body, the body cannot touch the mind—he was trying to resolve a conflict between science and the church, which felt itself threatened by scientific materialism. Materialism proposed that everything about nature, including the inner workings of man, could be investigated scientifically and ultimately reduced to its basic material components. Descartes postulated that the mind, or the soul, was not of material substance and therefore could never be subjected to scientific inquiry. This accomplished his main purpose, which was to permit scientists to go on with their inquiries without too much interference from the church. But it had a great many of those unforeseen negative consequences—the effects on our understanding of health have been described in this book—which seem to haunt the history of ideas.

Meanwhile, materialism flourished. As scientists were more and more successful at demonstrating the physical basis for phenomena, including the human nervous system, there was more support for the materialist view taken by philosophers like Hobbes and Marx, that nothing exists but the material world. After the Russian scientist Ivan Pavlov demonstrated that much of behavior could be explained by a mindless process of learning the connection between stimulus and response, the American psychologist B. F. Skinner (1904–1990) took materialism to the extreme. Skinner and other psychologists, known as behaviorists, made it uncomfortable for any psychologist to talk about concepts such as mind, thought, feeling, or will. Instead, all human actions were assumed to be the result of conditioning, the simple connection of a response to a stimulus. When I went to school, this view so dominated academia that I chose to pursue social work rather than psychology. Fortunately for psychology, Skinner's extreme position has largely been replaced by cognitive-behavioral theory, which believes that there is a mind and that it does influence behavior. Unfortunately for psychiatry, there is a new materialist trend toward explaining all behavior as a function of neuronal connections and chemical messengers.

The mind-body problem still remains. How can we explain how mental events, like thoughts, affect behavior? How does something that doesn't seem to have a physical existence make physical objects move? I'm not even going to try to tackle that here, rather just assume with the rest of the commonsense world that it happens somehow. But we are still left with some problems that are very important when we're trying to figure out how to live our lives free of stress and all the symptoms that it gives us: What about free will and responsibility? To what extent are we responsible for our behavior, even behavior that we feel compelled to perform, like addictions or obsessive-compulsive rituals? How do we explain how the mind and body interact to create symptoms that have a physical manifestation and seem to be not under our control at all—like back pain or chronic fatigue? Does the mind have a role to play in recovery? How does what happens to us in the world get into our minds and become experienced as symptom pictures we can't shake—like depression and anxiety? Do we have to change the world to get better?

p. 228   *The bottom line, which I share with Stephen Mitchell and others, is that it's a mistake to view free will as an either-or:* Mitchell, 1984.

Chapter 7

p. 233   *Ellen Langer argues forcefully that categorical thinking is essentially mindless—it blinds us to differences between things in the category, and to similarities between things in different categories:* See Langer, 1989.

p. 235   *Shyness is probably the personality trait that is most heavily influenced by genetics— about 50 percent:* LeDoux, 2002, p. 30.

p. 235   *The specific form of the symptoms, though, may be, as Jeffrey Schwartz and others have suggested, due to a specific faulty circuit in the brain that doesn't turn off the anxiety response when we know, rationally, that there is no danger:* Schwartz and Begley, 2002.

p. 236   *With enough stress, dendrites in the hippocampus begin to shrivel up; with more, the nerve cells themselves begin to die. Vietnam vets and victims of child abuse have shrunken hippocampi:* LeDoux, 1996, p. 242.

p. 238   *Preparedness theory suggests that our brains are evolutionarily wired to be afraid of some things (snakes, spiders, heights, perhaps being the center of attention when we're not full of serotonin) that were dangerous to our ancestors:* See LeDoux, 1996, p. 237.

p. 239   *Benzodiazepines (minor tranquilizers like Xanax or Klonopin) are the drug of choice. They not only relax muscles, they also inhibit the amygdala's ability to turn on the sympathetic nervous system—the fight-or-flight response:* Sapolsky, 2002.

p. 239   *Anxiety is linked to what epidemiologists blithely call "excess mortality"—early death, primarily from cardiovascular disease and suicide:* Barlow; 1988.

p. 239   *One study of alcoholics found that 33 percent of them had severe, crippling agoraphobia or social phobia, and another 35 percent had milder versions of the same things:* See Barlow, 1988, p. 15.

p. 239   *In the National Comorbidity Study it was found that a much smaller proportion (19 percent) of people who received treatment for panic disorder developed major depression than those who did not receive treatment (45 percent):* Goodwin and Olfson, 2001.

p. 240   *Benzodiazepines have natural receptor sites in the brain, which when stimulated release the inhibiting neurotransmitter GABA:* LeDoux, 1996, p. 262.

p. 242   *Depression is second only to heart disease in its health impact worldwide:* The World Bank/WHO study is Murray and Lopez, 1996.

p. 242   *the cost of treatment of depression, increased mortality, and loss of productivity was estimated at $44 billion a year:* Greenberg et al., 1993.

p. 242   *Nationally, there are approximately thirty thousand suicides annually, as compared to twenty thousand homicides:* American Association of Suicidology, 1997.

p. 243   *One person in five will suffer an episode of major depression during his or her lifetime, and one person in five is suffering from some form of depression at any given moment:* Agency for Health Care Policy and Research [AHCPR], 1993.

p. 243   *Health economists equate the disability caused by major depression with that of blindness or paraplegia:* Murray and Lopez, 1996.

p. 243   *For each group born since 1900, the age of onset of depression has gotten younger, and the lifetime risk has increased. If current trends continue, the average age of onset for children born in the year 2000 will be twenty years old:* Thase, 1999b.

p. 243   *The chances of developing major depression at some point in your life are estimated at about 22 percent for women, 10 percent for men:* The disparity between men and women is controversial. My own opinion is that women are somewhat more likely to experience major depression than men, but that the incidence in men is underreported because the diagnosis is biased against women. There is a much more detailed discussion in *Active Treatment of Depression:* O'Connor, 2001.

p. 246   *A twelve-year follow-up of 431 patients who had sought treatment for a major depressive episode found that although they remained in major depression about 15 percent of the time, still only 41 percent of their time was spent symptom-free:* Judd et al., 1998.

p. 246   *Most patients have a combination of symptoms that could be considered either anxiety or depression, depending on rather small changes in emphasis:* Andrews, 1996.

p. 246   *Major studies have found that anxiety and depression are likely to be found together at rates from 51 to 68 percent of the time:* These are reviewed in O'Connor, 2001.

p. 246   *Medicine and psychiatry are increasingly agreeing that the two conditions are, if not the same, at least siblings:* See, for example, Nemeroff, 2002.

p. 246   *It may be that anxiety is the initial response to too much stress—our panicky attempts to escape an inescapable situation—while depression represents the damage done to the nervous system, and the mind, when the stress goes on too long:* Sapolsky, 2002.

p. 246   *In developing countries, young people have higher rates of depression than older folks:* Nesse and Williams, 1994.

p. 247   *Getting depressed—which means to cease activity, become lethargic, and conserve energy—may be adaptive for the species if it gets us to retreat in the face of danger or overwhelming obstacles:* The idea of depression as adaptation is well argued in Nesse, 2000.

p. 247   *In a four-year study of nursing home residents, those who were assessed as most depressed at the outset had the greatest impairment of the immune response as time went on:* Fortes et al., 2003.

p. 248   *Depressive symptoms appear to be a significant risk factor for heart attack:* Wulsin and Singal, 2003.

p. 248   *Depression is significantly associated with higher death rates following heart attack, for both sexes, controlling for all other health and social variables:* Frasure-Smith et al., 1999.

p. 248   *Depression is associated with increased mortality for the general hospital population, across all diagnostic groups, not only cardiac cases. Patients with depression visit their MDs more frequently, are operated on more frequently, and have more nonpsychiatric emergency room visits than the general population:* Herrmann et al., 1998.

p. 248   *a survey of almost twenty thousand Europeans found that 17 percent had chronic pain and 4 percent had major depression; but of those with depression, 40 percent also had chronic pain:* Ohayon and Schatzberg, 2003.

p. 248   *The damage to the hippocampus caused by prolonged stress probably accounts for the difficulty concentrating, learning, and remembering that is frequently seen with depression:* Sapolsky, 2002.

p. 248   *There is reliable evidence that long-term depression is associated with an overall decrease in size of the hippocampus by 10 to 20 percent:* See Sheline, Gado, and Kraemer, 2003; Vythilingam et al. 2002, Sapolsky, 2002.

p. 248   *In laboratory animals, treatment with antidepressants has been shown to help the hippocampus regain its ability to generate new nerve cells:* Sapolsky, 2003.

p. 248   *A recent study showed that treatment with either Paxil or cognitive-behavioral therapy results in improved blood flow to the hippocampus, perhaps leading to repair:* Goldapple et al., 2004.

p. 248   *repeated episodes of depression result in shrinkage of the brain overall:* Posener et al., 2003.

p. 248   *depression results in specific changes in brain activity that remain as a vulnerability when sad or stressful events occur to patients who have recovered:* Liotti et al., 2002.

p. 249   *One way the feedback loop gets disrupted is that, in infants and children who are under severe stress, the neuroreceptors for CRF diminish in size and number:* See Pert, 1997, p. 270; Sternberg, 2001; also LeDoux, 2002.

p. 250   *In one study, it was found that men with early-onset (before age twenty-two) major depression were only half as likely to marry and form intimate relationships as men with late-onset (or no) depression. Women with early-onset depression were only half as likely to obtain a college degree as their female counterparts, and their future annual earnings could be expected to be 12 to 18 percent lower:* Berndt et al., 2000.

p. 250 *"The news that depression is a chemical or biological problem is a public relations stunt," says Andrew Solomon:* Solomon, 2001, p. 399.

p. 251 *Antidepressants have been vastly oversold, sometimes by extremely aggressive marketing techniques:* Kirkpatrick, 2000, is a justifiably indignant and well-documented exposé of the lies and distortions in antidepressant marketing.

p. 251 *We now recognize that as many as 50 percent of drug-industry sponsored studies are never published:* Thase, 1999a.

p. 251 *A recent review comparing drug industry-sponsored research to independent research has shown that industry sponsorship creates a significant bias among the researchers— and almost all research on antidepressants is industry-sponsored:* Baker et al., 2003.

p. 251 *Another recent review created a firestorm of controversy within the professional community by going to the FDA armed with the Freedom of Information Act and finding out that, in all the research the drug companies had submitted to the FDA to get license to manufacture the new antidepressants, their drugs were only slightly more effective than placebo—but the FDA never pointed this out to the public:* Kirsch et al., 2002.

p. 251 *Concerns have again surfaced about the safety of these medications with children:* Waters, 2004. As of this writing, the British Committee on Safety of Medicines has banned use of antidepressants in children (except for Prozac, which has demonstrated some benefits), saying there are no documented benefits and there are documented risks of suicide and violence. The U.S. Food and Drug Administration, only after great public outcry, put a warning label on antidepressants, suggesting that they only be used in youth under careful consideration.

p. 251 *The outlook for complete recovery using the treatment methods that have been researched and demonstrated to be "effective" is bleak—because they measure recovery at the end of the three-month treatment period:* See O'Connor, 2001; Judd et al., 1998; Keller and Hanks, 1994; Solomon et al., 2000; Thase, 1999b.

p. 252 *In one study which followed people over five years, only half of patients with dysthymia recovered, and of those half relapsed. Many developed major depression:* Klein et al., 2000.

p. 252 *if you have one episode of major depression, your odds of having another are 50 percent; if you have three episodes, your odds of having more are 90 percent:* Thase, 1999b.

p. 252 *Several studies of older adults have found that brisk exercise three times a week was at least as effective as Zoloft in the short term, and that adults who continued their exercise program had a significantly greater chance of avoiding future depressive episodes:* These studies are summarized in Herman et al., 2002.

p. 252 *In one study, couples therapy was more effective than medication over a two-year period, and it also reduced overall health-care costs:* Leff et al., 2000.

p. 252 *Drug money funds research—and has even tainted the National Institutes of Health:* Willman, 2003.

p. 253 *Mindfulness-Based Cognitive Therapy:* Segal, Williams, and Teasdale, 2002.

p. 258 *"The chronic hyperarousal and intrusive symptoms of post-traumatic stress disorder fuse with the vegetative symptoms of depression, producing . . . the 'survivor triad' of insomnia, nightmares, and psychosomatic complaints":* Herman, 1992, p. 94.

p. 258 *Because the emotional impact of the trauma is separated from memories of it, she keeps reexperiencing the trauma, as nightmares, flashbacks, or pain; but he thinks these symptoms are caused by present events:* van der Kolk, 2002.

p. 258 *Pat Barker's profound and powerful trilogy:* This is the "Regeneration Trilogy": *Regeneration, The Eye in the Door, The Ghost Road,* all available from Plume in paperback.

p. 259 *almost half of all veterans suffering from PTSD had served time in jail at least once; almost 40 percent of all serving veterans developed alcohol problems; there were also high rates of depression, anxiety disorders, eating and psychophysiological disorders, and borderline personality disorders:* Kulka et al., 1990.

p. 259 *"Trauma-spectrum disorders": PTSD, dissociative disorders, borderline personality, adjustment disorder:* Bremner, 2002.

p. 259 *In the U.S. general population, the lifetime prevalence of PTSD is estimated at 7.8 percent:* Kessler et al., 1995.

p. 259 *Almost all women have symptoms of PTSD immediately following sexual assault:* Rothbaum et al., 1992; Meadows and Foa, 1998.

p. 259 *More than 30 percent will continue to have symptoms during their lifetime:* Resick, et al., 1993.

p. 259 *between 10 and 15 percent of women are estimated to have an experience of date or spousal rape:* McGrath and Keita, 1990.

p. 259 *Similar rates of PTSD are seen among children who have been sexually abused:* McLeer et al., 1998.

p. 259 *. . . and in adult women who were sexually abused as children:* Rowan et al., 1994.

p. 259 *Helplessness to change the outcome may make the difference between acute PTSD and normal stress reactions:* van der Kolk, 2002.

p. 260 *Survivors of Hurricane Hugo in the Carolinas in 1989:* Morris, 1999, p. 180.

p. 260 *In PTSD, the qualitative difference between emotions seems to disappear, and everything is evaluated as a threat:* van der Kolk, 1996.

p. 260 *while an increase in norepinephrine levels in normal people improves concentration, learning, memory, and decision making, in PTSD patients just the opposite happens:* Bremner, 2002, p. 89.

p. 261 *In a review of the cognitive-behavioral efficacy research, Meadows and Foa concluded that "prolonged exposure" (PE) therapy is the most efficacious treatment method for acute PTSD:* Meadows and Foa, 1998.

p. 261 *many PTSD victims have developed such ingrained adaptations to their fears that this approach is not possible, and treatment consists of replacing unhealthy adaptations . . . with healthier ones:* Flack, Litz, and Keane, 1998.

p. 262 *Chronic trauma syndrome:* Herman, 1992.

p. 263 *In the ACE study of seventeen thousand . . . people, 22 percent reported childhood sexual abuse:* Felitti, 2001, Felitti et al., 1998; Edwards et al., 2003.

p. 263 *The moment that one partner abuses a child, and the other partner doesn't do anything, that child becomes an orphan:* This dramatic but accurate image is from an April 14, 2000, lecture by van der Kolk.

p. 264   *"Long after their liberation, people who have been subjected to coercive control bear the psychological scars of captivity":* Herman, 1992, p. 94.

p. 267   *New psychiatrists are being trained to think of personality disorders as "the patients you don't like, don't trust, don't want":* Luhrmann, 2000, p. 115. This book is a fascinating and frightening sociological analysis of modern American psychiatry, focusing especially on the fault line between those who still want to practice psychotherapy and those who are dedicated to the pharmaceutical model.

p. 269   *Allan Schore's thinking is that both borderline and narcissistic personality disorders are manifestations of brain circuitry that failed to develop optimally during the first two years of life:* Schore, 1994, 2003a.

p. 269   *Attachment researchers have found some links between adult borderline personality and ambivalent or avoidant attachment in infancy:* Bartholomew et al., 2001.

p. 270   *Children who were classified as disorganized, followed into adolescence, have been found to have high overall psychopathology, with apparent predilections for violence:* Carlson, 1998; Hesse et al., 2003.

p. 271   *Judith Herman reports that 81 percent of her borderline patients had histories of severe childhood trauma:* Herman, 1992.

p. 271   *Van der Kolk reports that only 13 percent of his borderline patients did not report childhood trauma:* van der Kolk, 2002.

p. 271   *a study of psychiatric inpatients with a history of sexual abuse: 44 percent had never talked to anyone about the experience before:* Linehan, 1992, p. 54.

p. 272   *Self psychologists long ago argued that if you treated borderline patients well enough, you couldn't distinguish them from narcissistic patients:* Brandchaft and Stolorow, 1984.

p. 272   *Heinz Kohut had already shown that narcissistic patients, previously thought untreatable, were in fact quite treatable if you just took their needs seriously:* Kohut, 1971.

p. 272   *some borderlines, at least, recover naturally—something that is not supposed to happen at all—when their social environment changes:* Gunderson et al., 2003.

p. 272   *There is a radical strain in psychoanalytic circles today, suggesting that there is no such thing as personality at all: that the individual doesn't exist except in a social context:* For more on this refreshing change, and how it's changing practice, see Magid, 2002; Hoffman, 1998; Mitchell, 2000.

p. 273   *James Gilligan, who has spent his professional life as a psychiatrist in the Massachusetts penal system:* His powerful book is *Violence: Our Deadly Epidemic and Its Causes* (1996).

p. 273   *Marsha Linehan's Dialectical Behavior Therapy (DBT) for borderlines is full of her dedicated refusal to judge her patients:* Linehan, 1992.

p. 276   *Long-term use [of addictive drugs] produces alterations in the brain that increase vulnerability to relapse and maintain craving even months or years after the last use. Nerve cells in the dopamine and opioid systems are damaged:* Camí and Farré, 2003.

p. 276   *We know that there is a purely hereditary link for alcoholism among men, but we don't know much about the heritability of abuse for other drugs:* Camí and Farré, 2003.

p. 280 *Mihalyi Csikszentmihalyi, the author of* Flow *and a leading researcher into what makes us happy, discovered inadvertently that television watching shares some special qualities with addictive drugs:* Kubey and Csikszentmihalyi, 2002.

p. 282 *In order to achieve the kind of reliability necessary to pass the tests of scientific evidence, CBT researchers have done what medication researchers have also done, which is to concentrate on efficacy rather than effectiveness:* Guthrie, 2000.

p. 282 *"The first principle of recovery is the empowerment of the survivor":* Herman, 1992, p. 133.

Chapter 8

p. 289 *In research on depression, those patients who are most perfectionistic tend to have the worst outcomes:* Elkin et al., 1989.

p. 293 *The cognitive therapists working with depression introduced the concept of attributional style. They have produced a large body of research showing that people with depression make common assumptions:* Summarized in Alloy and Abramson, 1988.

p. 299 *Aaron Beck first described what he called "automatic thinking"—our natural tendency to react to events with little evaluations, barely conscious—and noticed how in depression so many of the automatic thoughts were negative:* Beck, 1976; Beck et al., 1979.

p. 301 *As David Burns notes, often the mere act of counting a habit like this will result in a reduction in its frequency:* Burns, 1999.

p. 302 *Depressed people forget about positive feedback, while nondepressed people forget about negative feedback:* These and the subsequent cognitive distortions of depression were first described in Alloy and Abramson, 1988.

p. 302 *As people recover from depression, they begin to overestimate themselves again:* Lewinsohn et al., 1980.

p. 305 *In the traditional analytic view, consciousness and will were largely treated as irrelevant; that is, as epiphenomena of unconscious processes:* See, e.g., Shapiro, 2000.

p. 305 *much of our decision making seems to consist of snap judgments, decisions we make on the basis of instinct or emotion. The right brain steps in a few milliseconds later to create rationalizations for our decisions:* Myers, 2002.

p. 306 *Daniel Wegner has developed a theory of "ironic processes" of mental control, which suggests that it is largely stress that guarantees we will sabotage ourselves at the worst possible time:* See Wegner, 1994; Wegner, Erber, and Zanakos, 1993.

p. 307 *Women who are exposed to repeated images of other women who are unusually attractive—as in, say, reading women's magazines—feel less attractive themselves, and their self-esteem is diminished. The same is true for men who read descriptions of dominant and influential men:* Buss, 2000.

p. 307 *Some time ago, a researcher studied the effects of television access in three small Canadian communities that were just receiving cable for the first time. She found that, after the introduction of television, both adults and children became less creative at problem solving, less able to stick to tasks, and less tolerant of unstructured time:* This research is described in Kubey and Csikszentmihalyi, 2002.

p. 308 *When we deliberately try to suppress memories of a recent event, we make it less likely that the event will be stored in long-term memory. The prefrontal cortex is activated in suppression, while the hippocampus is deactivated, just the reverse of the remembering process:* Anderson et al., 2004.

p. 311 *Hemingway famously said "What is moral is what you feel good after, and what is immoral is what you feel bad after":* Ernest Hemingway, *Death in the Afternoon.* 1932; Vintage, 2000.

p. 312 *What matters more than absolute wealth is perceived wealth:* Myers, 1992, p. 39.

p. 313 *When people are told that the "correct" button-pressing pattern will turn on a light, but the light actually goes on at random intervals, depressed people soon realize that the button and the light are not connected:* Alloy and Abramson, 1979.

p. 313 *Nondepressed people think that others like them, even if they don't; depressed people think that others don't like them, even if they do:* Martin, Abramson, and Alloy, 1984.

p. 313 *Aaron Beck described these as false assumptions:* Beck, 1976.

p. 315 *"What I do at this point, as the panic mounts and the jungle drums begin beating and I realize that the well has run dry and that my future is behind me and I'm going to have to get a job only I'm completely unemployable":* This is from Lamott, 1994, p. 17; her little book, besides being funny and memorable, will forever change the way you practice procrastination; she'll make you too self-conscious of your foolishness to put up with yourself.

p. 316 *Silvan Tomkins, the most widely respected theorist of emotions, only identified three basic positive emotions:* Tomkins, 1962.

p. 317 *When infants are socially isolated, deprived of the attachment connection with their mother, they experience a permanent reduction in the number of endorphin receptors:* Schore, 1994, p. 438.

p. 318 *Breathing helps with labor pains by flooding one with endorphins, which kill pain as well as making us feel happy:* Pert, 1997.

p. 318 *Martin Seligman . . . has a distinction between* pleasures, *which are roughly equivalent to my joys, and* gratifications, *which are activities that engage us fully in a state of flow:* Seligman, 2002.

Chapter 9

p. 323 *"Most of us will live long enough and well enough to get seriously ill with a stress-related disease":* Sapolsky, 2002.

p. 324 *optimists' wounds heal more quickly than those of pessimists:* Scheier et al., 1999.

p. 324 *Monkeys who are far down in the pecking order have more atherosclerosis and are less fertile:* Kaplan et al., 1983.

p. 324 *Women who view their social status as higher than average sleep better, have lower resting cortisol levels, more efficient hearts, and less abdominal fat:* Adler et al., 2000.

p. 324 *Pessimistic, anxious, and depressed people, besides enjoying life less, have poorer health. They have higher blood pressure, their immune systems are less effective, and they recover more slowly and less completely from surgery:* Miller, 2001.

p. 324 *One study of over twenty thousand individuals suggested that the net effect on physical health of chronic anxiety or depression was the equivalent of feeling twelve years older than your age:* Surtees et al., 2003.

p. 325 *people who are hopeful have better health after heart transplants, recover more quickly from bypass surgery, have less anginal pain, do better and live longer with HIV treatment, and have generally better-functioning immune systems:* Ryff and Singer, 2003.

p. 325 *Study after study shows that restricting intake to 30 to 70 percent less than free eating results in improvements in longevity, immune response, etc.:* Pinel, Assanand, & Lehman, 2000.

p. 325 *We're designed to graze, an eating style that leaves us healthier and makes much more efficient use of food:* Ornish, 1993.

p. 326 *twice as many adults and three times as many adolescents overweight now as in 1980:* U.S. Public Health Service, 2001.

p. 326 *Overweight people are less likely to be hired, and they earn less money than thin people:* Ornish, 1993.

p. 327 *Low-fiber, high-fat, and high-sodium diets increase risk for heart disease, colon cancer, and high blood pressure. Obesity increases risk of degenerative joint disease:* Caudill, 2002.

p. 327 *An overload of stress hormones interferes with our ability to store fat, sending more of it directly to the abdomen (as does alcohol: if you want to lose a beer belly, stop drinking):* Ornish, 1993.

p. 327 *sugar and other comfort foods are known to interfere with the Perpetual Stress Response, but of course they add to our weight and damage our health:* Dallman et al., 2003.

p. 327 *Scientists know that diets don't work:* See Seligman's 1994 book *What You Can Change and What You Can't* for some unpopular but realistic news.

p. 330 *Patients with depression visit their MDs more frequently, are operated on more frequently, and have more nonpsychiatric emergency room visits than the general population:* Herrmann et al., 1998.

p. 330 *Anxiety and depression somehow result in wounds healing more slowly:* Cole-King and Harding, 2001.

p. 330 *50 to 70 percent of visits to primary care physicians are for psychologically related complaints:* American Psychological Association.

p. 330 *I began to wonder what people like Candace Pert, not a New Age mystic but a tough-minded research scientist, meant when they said things like "the body is the unconscious mind":* Pert, 1997, p. 141.

p. 330 *"I like to speculate that what the mind is is the flow of information as it moves among the cells, organs, and systems of the body":* Pert, 1997, p. 185. Emphasis added.

p. 331 *"The biochemicals of emotion are . . . the messengers carrying information to link the major systems of the body into one unit that we can call the bodymind":* Pert, 1997, p. 189.

p. 331 *Neither the primary care physician nor the specialist wants to tell the patient directly what everyone thinks: that the symptoms are the result of stress, more emotional than physical in origin:* Servan-Schreiber, Kolb, and Tabas, 2000.

p. 332   *When few or no emotions are permitted into the "me," children grow into alexithymic adults—who have few or no words for feelings, who indeed experience almost no feelings:* Melmed, 2001, p. 10.

p. 332   *John Sarno, a respected back pain specialist, and others have commented on the irony of our aversion to the term [psychosomatic]:* Sarno, 1998, p. 40.

p. 332   *In one study, subjects were given the hypnotic suggestion to rid themselves of warts only on one side of their bodies. Nine of fourteen were able to do just that:* Cited in Langer, 1989, p. 192.

p. 335   *There are several types of cells, which serve important roles in the immune response:* This discussion is based on Benson and Stuart, 1992, p. 335.

p. 336   *Careful research has shown that the initial immune response to stress is to direct those white blood cells to where they will be needed most, organs like the skin and lymph nodes:* McEwen, 2002, p. 99.

p. 337   *A major review of the literature on stress and the immune system published in 2004 bears that out:* Segerstrom and Miller, 2004.

p. 337   *Too much cortisol (and other glucocorticoids) . . . causes shrinkage of the thymus gland, where new T cells and B cells are formed. It makes the T and B cells already in the system less responsive to messages from other cells about foreign invaders. And, most impressive, too much cortisol kills immune cells:* Sapolsky, 1998, p. 133.

p. 337   *People who had an anxious or ambivalent attachment relationship with their mother turn out, as adults, to be more likely to report symptoms and seek medical attention than securely attached or dismissing patients:* Bartholomew, Kwong, and Hart, 2001.

p. 337   *infant rats who get licked and groomed more by their mothers are smarter and less fearful as adults, have stronger immune systems, and are more attentive mothers themselves:* Champagne and Meaney, 2001.

p. 337   *a child who is not "handled" very much has lower levels of immune cells in the bloodstream. This leads to increased activity by the infant's pituitary and adrenal systems, resulting in increasing levels of stress hormones (ACTH and cortisol) in the bloodstream:* Schore, 1994, p. 433.

p. 338   *Allan Schore feels enough confidence to state definitively: "The infant's attachment relationship with the mother permanently influences the development of the individual's future immune capacities":* Schore, 1994, p. 436.

p. 338   *When the child is left under stress, stress hormones kill, among other things, the cells that produce T cells, and T cell disturbances are seen in autoimmune diseases like rheumatoid arthritis, MS, and lupus. Continuing stress in adult life means overproduction of cortisol and adrenaline, which interfere with the ability of T and B cells to reproduce:* Benson and Stuart, 1992, p. 352.

p. 338   *It's possible that the baby who was invasively traumatized goes on to develop rashes, allergies, or diarrhea as a way of communicating "stay away from me," while the baby who was neglected develops pain, weakness, or another debility as a way of saying "take care of me":* See McDougall, 1989, p. 42.

p. 338   *disturbances in attachment result in nerve cells never fully developing in that same orbitofrontal cortex that is thought to be so important in developing a healthy self-concept.*

This same area controls ACTH and corticosteroid (stress hormones again) levels in the brain. The same area has been implicated in gastric ulcer, bulimia, and hypertension: Schore, 1994, p. 442.

p. 339   *people with PTSD as a result of childhood trauma have disturbances in the body's two main stress-response systems: the hypothalamic-pituitary-adrenal (HPA) axis and the sympathoadrenomedullary system. As a result, the individual with PTSD suffers from difficulty regulating the immune system:* McEwen, 2002.

p. 339   *One difficulty is an out-of-proportion inflammatory response:* Altemus, Cloitre, and Dhabhar, 2003.

p. 339   *People who are unemployed or socially isolated are more likely to develop colds than other people. Marital strife and bereavement can weaken the immune system:* McEwen, 2002, p. 93.

p. 339   *Patients who report greater stress levels before surgery have slower wound healing and impaired immune responses in the wound:* Broadbent et al., 2003.

p. 339   *People with cancer who form strong bonds with each other through group treatment will generally live longer than those who keep to the periphery:* Sternberg, 2001, p. 156.

p. 339   *Caregivers of Alzheimer's patients improved their immune response after a simple eight-week stress management program:* Vedhara et al., 2003.

p. 339   *Patients with cancer who learn relaxation and cognitive therapy also have an improved immune response:* Benson and Stuart, 1992, p. 354.

p. 339   *The brain has receptors for the immune system–signaling molecule, interleukin:* Pert, 1997, has a vivid account of the scientific race to find the connections between the brain and immune system.

p. 340   *Robert Ader and Nick Cohen at the University of Rochester gave mice saccharine at the same time as an anticancer drug that suppresses the immune system:* Ader, Cohen, and Bovbjerg, 1982.

p. 340   *Later, Ader and his colleagues were able to show that the immune system can also be strengthened by learning:* Ader, 2003, p. 101.

p. 340   *spouses of patients who died from breast cancer were found to have reduced lymph cell production. It reached its lowest ebb about two months after the patient's death and returned to normal gradually over the next year:* Schliefer et al., 1983.

p. 340   *Our own belief in our ability to control the stresses that we experience (not our actual ability, our belief in our ability) dramatically affects our neuroendocrine functioning in ways that can have an important impact on immune functioning:* Taylor, 1989, p. 108.

p. 340   *Robert Ader and other researchers are concerned that their discoveries in psychoneuroimmunology have been adopted and bastardized by people who claim to teach us to control our immune systems through various New Age techniques—fads in nutrition, in psychotherapy, in hypnosis, even in meditation—without any documentation at all that their methods are effective. As Ader says, these people often represent an "antiscientific, anti-intellectual, and anti-establishment" viewpoint:* Ader, 2003, p. 103.

p. 341   *Eighty-five percent of exacerbations of multiple sclerosis are caused by psychological stress, though there is such a long latency period—an average of two weeks—that most patients probably do not feel the connection:* Ackerman et al., 2002.

p. 342   *Two recent review articles discuss many of the conditions I have been calling nonspecific illnesses, under different names: functional somatic syndromes and symptom-based conditions:* Barsky and Borus, 1999; Hyams, 1998.

p. 344   *These conditions often respond to placebo. People with these illnesses often react defensively to that news, because they feel they are being told it's all in their heads. On the contrary: this is a very important clue to the real nature of these problems:* See Brown, 1998, for an enlightening discussion of the implications of the placebo response.

p. 345   *"Doctors, of course, typically feel the need to direct, interrupt, or cut off":* Mechanic, 1995.

p. 345   *Treatment with antidepressants alone has been shown to be at least partially effective for six of the most difficult-to-treat nonspecific illnesses:* Gruber, Hudson, and Pope, 1996.

p. 345   *Most patients with fibromyalgia also suffer from depression, and treatment with antidepressants and/or cognitive psychotherapy has been demonstrated to be effective in relieving the physical symptoms:* Hyams, 1998.

p. 345   *People with rheumatoid arthritis—another painful, chronic condition with an unpredictable course—are no more likely to suffer depression than the general population, while those with fibromyalgia almost all have depression:* Hudson et al., 1985.

p. 346   *Chronic fatigue syndrome is characterized by fatigue bad enough to interfere with the activities of daily living, which is not relieved by bed rest and has no obvious other cause. To meet the formal diagnostic criteria, the patient should have the condition for at least six months. Secondary symptoms often reported include sore throat, tender lymph nodes, weakness, muscle or joint pain, impaired memory or concentration, insomnia, and severe fatigue after exertion:* Centers for Disease Control 2004.

p. 346   *A problem with diagnosis is that healthy individuals often experience pain when a doctor presses on the same "tender points":* Hyams, 1998.

p. 346   *Many studies have documented that a great many patients with fibromyalgia also meet the criteria for chronic fatigue syndrome, and also meet the criteria for multiple chemical sensitivity and other functional conditions:* Ciccone and Natelson, 2003.

p. 346   *It's quite likely, to me at least, that many if not all these conditions are simply different names for the same thing, some underlying condition that has not been formally named but is the body's reaction to the Perpetual Stress Response:* This idea is explored in Barsky and Borus, 1999, and Wessely, Nimnuan, and Sharpe, 1999.

p. 346   *In both conditions, it turns out that the hormonal stress responses are out of balance (CRF-ACTH-adrenaline-steroids):* Sternberg, 2001, p. 103.

p. 347   *The most encouraging results come from applications of cognitive behavior therapy and graded exercise programs:* Afari and Buchwald, 2003.

p. 347   *An ad for one popular book on the condition claimed "This book reveals that a devastating infectious disease is reaching epidemic proportions while government researchers ignore the evidence and the shocking statistics":* Cited in Showalter, 1997.

p. 347   *A study of twins with chronic fatigue syndrome found that there was little genetic linkage; instead, the twin with CFS was likely to be depressed or be suffering other psychological distress:* Roy-Byrne et al., 2002.

p. 347   *Treatment with antidepressant medications, both SSRIs and the older tricyclics, is just about as effective for chronic fatigue syndrome as it is for major depression:* This point is elaborated in O'Connor, 2001.

p. 347   *Cognitive-behavioral therapy, added to medical care, results in satisfactory outcomes for a much higher proportion of patients:* Sharpe, et al., 1996.

p. 347   *A study compared child and adult abuse and victimization patterns among three groups: those with chronic fatigue syndrome or fibromyalgia (CFS/FM); those with rheumatoid arthritis or multiple sclerosis; and a matched group of healthy controls:* Van Houdenhove et al., 2001.

p. 347   *Another study comparing fibromyalgia with rheumatoid arthritis patients found that the fibromyalgia patients had much higher rates of both childhood and adult victimization, particularly adult physical assault:* Walker et al., 1997.

p. 347   *One study compared reactions to inhaling increasing concentrations of carbon dioxide (which can induce panic reactions) among patients with IEI, patients with panic disorder, and healthy controls. While only 5 percent of the healthy controls reported panic symptoms, the overwhelming majority of IEI and panic disorder patients did; meanwhile there were no differences between groups in heart rate, breathing rate, and other physical measures:* Poonai et al., 2000.

p. 348   *"They are conscious of having failed to meet their own expectations or those of others, or of being unable to cope with some pressing problem":* From Frank, 1974, p. 314.

p. 349   *Flabby muscles hurt more than fit muscles:* Margaret Caudill's informative book *Managing Pain Before It Manages You* (2002) brought this interesting fact to my attention.

p. 349   *In 1983, two Australian researchers reported that they consistently found a bacterium,* Helicobacter pylori, *in the autopsied stomachs of people with ulcers:* Sapolsky, 1998, p. 66.

p. 350   *the more symptoms of generalized anxiety disorder you have, the more likely you are to have an ulcer:* Goodwin and Stein, 2002.

p. 350   *there's been a substantial decline in research into the stress component [of ulcer]:* Levenstein, 2000.

p. 350   *It seems highly likely that patients with IBS have developed a specific neural pathway between the brain and the gut that makes the brain highly sensitive to any abdominal discomfort, and the gut ready to respond to any stress with the chemicals that produce diarrhea and other IBS symptoms:* Ballenger et al., 2001.

p. 350   *As with other nonspecific illnesses, there is often a history of physical or sexual abuse [with IBS]:* Frankel, Quill, McDaniel, 2003, p. 21.

p. 350   *A recent review article concluded that, while the incidence of panic disorder is between 1 and 3 percent in the general adult population, it ranges from 7 to 24 percent among asthmatics:* Katon et al., 2004.

p. 351   *Franz Alexander, a respected psychoanalyst, wrote of the psychosomatic component of diseases such as irritable bowel, ulcer, arthritis, and asthma:* Alexander and Benedek, 1987.

p. 351   *We now know that nerve cells from the brain have long extensions that reach deep into the body, into the guts and the heart:* McEwen, 2002, p. 78.

p. 351 *the same parts of the brain that control the stress response play an important role in inflammatory diseases such as arthritis and are implicated in depression as well:* Sternberg, 2001.

p. 351 *treating rats that are susceptible to arthritis with CRF—the hypothalamic stress hormone we discussed in Chapter 7—reduces their vulnerability to the disease:* Sternberg, 2001.

p. 351 *"Modern society—through the media, the glamorization of medicine, the sensationalism and fear-mongering of disease—gives them new prototypes."* Quoting from myself here: O'Connor, 2001.

p. 353 *Depressed patients with cancer have higher than normal immune system abnormalities:* Musselman et al., 2001, p. 1252.

p. 353 *Depression appears to be linked to higher risk for pancreatic cancer; but this seems to be a unique association among all the types of cancer, one for which no one has any explanation:* Carney et al., 2003.

p. 353 *depression does seem to slightly increase the risk for all cancers, probably because it affects the immune system:* Spollen and Gutman, 2003.

p. 353 *Psychotherapy for depression among cancer patients has been shown to result in longer survival time:* Spiegel, 1996.

p. 353 *Some research on cancer patients reinforces the idea that psychotherapy and meaningful supportive relationships can influence brain functioning:* Gabbard, 2000.

p. 353 *Spiegel and his colleagues reported a controlled study in which sufferers from metastatic breast cancer were randomly assigned to group psychotherapy or a control group. Those in group psychotherapy lived an average of eighteen months longer than the controls:* Spiegel et al., 1989.

p. 353 *the death rate was lower, and remissions were longer, among members of the support group than in the control group. This impact was highly significant even though the support group lasted a mere six weeks:* Fawzy et al., 1993.

p. 354 *the fight-or-flight response releases adrenaline and norepinephrine, which can increase blood pressure, increase cholesterol, and cause more rapid blood clotting:* McEwen, 2002.

p. 354 *One study of 192 high-risk patients found that after four years, those who had been taught about the relaxation response and stress management techniques had significantly lower rates of cardiac disease:* Benson and Stuart, 1992, p. 376.

p. 354 *People with depression are twice as likely as others to develop coronary artery disease:* Lett et al., 2004.

p. 354 *Depressive symptoms are also a risk factor for heart attack, almost as great risk factor as smoking:* Wulsin and Singal, 2003.

p. 354 *Depression after a heart attack increases risk of death—from 6 percent to 20 percent, eighteen months after the attack:* Spollen and Gutman, 2003.

p. 354 *Further research has suggested that the real factor that makes type A's vulnerable to heart disease is overt hostility:* Benson and Stuart, 1992, p. 375.

p. 355 *60 percent of pain sufferers are reluctant to take analgesics, partly because analgesics are only effective in about 50 percent of cases:* Stimmel, 1997.

p. 355 *There is no generally accepted pain mechanism theory:* Stimmel, 1997.

p. 355 *BDNF levels in the hippocampus are reduced in depressed patients:* Sapolsky, 1998.

p. 356 *one study of over a thousand patients with angina found that 85 percent reported their pain relieved by medications that were later proven to be ineffective:* Benson and Mc-Callie, 1979.

p. 356 *Another study of ten years' worth of patients recovering from gallbladder surgery at a particular hospital found that the patients who could see trees from their windows requested significantly less pain medication, got along better with the nurses, and had shorter hospital stays than those whose windows faced an airshaft:* Ulrich, 1984; cited in Sapolsky, 1998.

p. 356 *the same neurotransmitters, serotonin and norepinephrine, that seem to be implicated in depression also play a critical role in pain modulation:* Fields, 1987.

p. 356 *One study of psychological complaints shared by chronic pain patients found that the patients scored significantly higher on all the symptoms:* Von Korff and Simon, 1996.

p. 356 *If you take a dozen X rays of healthy backs and a dozen of painful backs and shuffle them together, many orthopedists couldn't tell which is which:* My own faithful and patient back specialist, Evan Rashkoff, MD, tells me this is true.

p. 357 *Seventy percent of back pain patients have no apparent injury:* Eich et al., 1999.

p. 357 *As many as 90 percent of back pain patients don't have a definitive diagnosis; there is a poor correlation between symptoms and objective findings:* Stimmel, 1997.

p. 357 *Surgery on the back is performed eight times more frequently in the United States than in Great Britain, which should make us question the value of surgery:* The Lancet, 1989.

p. 357 *The general wisdom is that if there is no definitive physical finding—tumor, fracture, nerve damage—aspirin and ibuprofen are as effective as anything else for pain relief:* Stimmel, 1997.

p. 358 *Acupuncture also gets its analgesic effect from release of endorphins, though the mechanism is not quite clear:* Sapolsky, 1998.

p. 358 *People who exercise regularly seem to enjoy the little things in life more: relationships, tastes, other sensory pleasures:* Servan-Schreiber, 2003.

p. 359 *Andrew Solomon has pointed out that, in depression, there is no such thing as a placebo:* Solomon, 2001.

p. 359 *both pain and depression reinforce negative self-focusing, which may magnify symptoms of both. Surprisingly, the intensity of pain does not seem to be a predictor of depression, but interference with activities and diffusion of pain does:* Von Korff and Simon, 1996.

p. 361 *"The prescription of a dependency-producing drug to relieve pain and allow adequate function is not only appropriate but extremely beneficial. Such a person should not be considered to be addicted any more than a diabetic would be considered addicted to insulin":* Stimmel, 1997, pp. 55–56.

p. 361 *Physicians consistently prescribe inadequate doses of narcotic analgesics at too infrequent intervals, regardless of the actual cause of the pain:* Stimmel, 1997.

p. 362 *Accident victims and people who have become disabled through illness generally return to their former levels of happiness once they have accepted their condition:* Brickman, Coates, and Janoff-Bulman, 1978.

p. 362 *It's easier for us to accept the pain and limitation caused by a condition we can understand than it is when the diagnosis is mushy—a bulging disk, muscle spasms, tension headaches. It's easier to adapt when we know bad news for certain: a sudden, permanent loss rather than gradual deterioration:* Frederick and Lowenstein, 1999, p. 315.

Chapter 10

p. 365 *loneliness is as great a risk factor for early death as is cigarette smoking:* House, 2001.

p. 366 *In Goleman and Ekman's research with the Dalai Lama, they discovered incidentally that monks who are adept at mindfulness meditation are extremely good at reading other people's emotional messages:* Goleman, 2003a.

p. 367 *my favorite example, from* The Great Gatsby: F. Scott Fitzgerald, *The Great Gatsby.* New York: Charles Scribner's Sons, 1925.

p. 367 *Deborah Tannen, whom I consider simply the greatest authority at analyzing communication, has this vignette in her book* I Only Say This Because I Love You: Tannen, 2001, p. xviii.

p. 369 *"The core experiences of psychological trauma are disempowerment and disconnection from others":* Herman, 1992, p. 133.

p. 371 *Many theorists and researchers have organized their approach to treatment with this [the triangle of insight; the link between past trauma, presenting problem, and transference problem] as one of the main assumptions:* For example, Strupp (Strupp and Binder, 1984); Malan, 1979; Luborsky, 1984; Mann, 1973.

p. 372 *Daniel Siegel talks about the attunement between two brains that facilitates the natural healing, integrating force of the one:* Siegel, 2003, p. 32.

p. 372 *When the response from the therapist, or the parent, or the intimate partner, is validating, the neural representations of the self-as-perceived-by-the-self and the self-as-perceived-by-the-other are in agreement; they are* coherent: Siegel and Hartzell, 2003, p. 83.

p. 374 *Tannen is perhaps best known for her observation that men and women speak different languages—or at least use the same language very differently:* Tannen, 1990.

p. 374 *one difference not explained by hormones is that women seem to have the left and right hemispheres better integrated:* Johnson, 2004.

p. 379 *There is a particular way that couples get into vicious circles of oppositional behavior that is referred to as, of all things, complementary schismogenesis:* This is from Tannen, 2001, borrowing the term from the anthropologist and philosopher Gregory Bateson.

p. 380 *"As in a distorting mirror, we see our spouse's defensive system as the ideal solution to our problem; but the spouse, inside that suit of armor, is only too aware of its chinks and weaknesses, and is looking at our armor as what he needs":* O'Connor, 1997.

p. 384 *The model for resolving the content of the conflict is the dialectic, as revived by Linehan:* Linehan, 1992, 1993.

p. 388 *The judge in the Microsoft antitrust case said, "If they don't admit they did wrong before, how do we know they won't keep doing it?":* Tannen, 2001, p. 109.

p. 389 *The effect on mortality is roughly the same as that of smoking:* House, 2001.

p. 389 *We're getting near the point where more people in the United States live alone than live in families:* Conlin, 2003.

p. 391 *Sher developed the concept of the success team, simply a group of people who have made a commitment to help each other achieve their goals:* Sher, 1994. There is lots of information about success teams on her website, www.barbarasher.com.

p. 391 *One study found that greater Internet use was associated with less communication with other household members, a reduction in size of the social network, and an increase in depression and loneliness:* Kraut et al., 1998.

p. 392 *A poem by Adrienne Rich:* Rich, 1978; cited in Dowrick, 1991.

p. 397 *These are just plain nasty people (to borrow Jay Carter's term):* Carter, 2003.

p. 398 *My psychiatric dictionary just says it [manipulation] is "behavior designed to control or exploit others to gain special consideration or advantage":* Goldenson, 1984.

p. 400 *Living as part of a kinship network is known to reduce the incidence of domestic violence, and it probably has the same effect on child abuse and incest:* Buss, 2000.

p. 404 *Mihalyi Csikszentmihalyi, a social scientist at the University of Chicago, is another researcher interested in positive psychology, the science of what makes people happy:* Csikszentmihalyi, 1990.

p. 407 *Prolonged or intense stress shuts down dopamine production:* Sapolsky, 2003.

p. 407 *Ellen Langer, who has done a lot of work in applying mindfulness concepts to institutional functioning, observes that the best managers create an atmosphere of "confident uncertainty":* Langer, 1989, p. 145.

p. 408 *patients recovering from gallbladder surgery recovered more quickly when their windows faced a tree rather than an airshaft:* Ulrich, 1984.

p. 409 *"Animal experiments on the lateral hypothalamus suggest . . . that the organism's chronic internal state will be a vague mixture of anxiety and desire—best described perhaps by the phrase 'I want,' spoken with or without an object for the verb":* Csikszentmihalyi, 1993, quoting Konner, 1990.

p. 409 *Seligman argues that anxiety has been naturally selected into us:* Seligman, 1994.

Chapter 11

p. 412 "The hero's journey always begins with the call." Campbell, 2001.

p. 415 *Mindfulness-Based Stress Reduction improves immune system functioning and helps with chronic pain, fibromyalgia, and eating disorders:* Kabat-Zinn, 1990.

p. 415 *Mindfulness-based therapy for depression proves to be more effective at preventing relapse than traditional methods:* Segal, Williams, and Teasdale, 2002.

p. 418 *Authors ranging from Sarah Ban Breathnach to Martin Seligman have been stressing gratitude lately:* Ban Breathnach, 1995; Seligman, 2002.

p. 418 *According to Seligman, the ritual is powerful. "Everyone cries when you do a gratitude visit," he says. "It's very moving for both people":* Pink, 2003.

p. 419 *"Well-being therapy" is a novel approach to depression that seems to be more effective* than traditional methods in helping people who have already recovered from their major symptoms make and consolidate further progress: Fava et al., 1998; Fava and Ruini, 2003.

p. 434 "The body bears the burden," in Robert Scaer's evocative phrase, of our response to stress, trauma, abuse, invalidation: Scaer, 2001.

p. 442 Barbara Sher, in her valuable little book I Could Do Anything if I Only Knew What It Was has this to say about the values of taking action: Sher, 1994.

p. 449 Play increases mindfulness. It demands risk taking and involvement; if it could be done mindlessly, it would not be play anymore: Langer, 1989, p. 44.

p. 449 Lenore Terr, a child therapist, writes of "traumatic play"—repeating an experience over and over again in safety, in order to develop a sense of mastery and file the trauma away: Terr, 1999.

p. 452 Integrity, writes Judith Herman, "is the capacity to affirm the value of life in the face of death, to be reconciled with the finite limits of one's own life and the tragic limits of the human condition, and to accept these realities without despair": Herman, 1992, p. 154.

Index

Page numbers in *italic* indicate illustrations; those in **bold** indicate tables.

THE GAME OF
WORDS

*To the Reader**

> I'll never **** as ***'* own kissing kin,
> As none who **** this puzzle book can doubt.
> Still, I am pleased you worked my **** in,
> And hope you work it out.

* The missing words: *Pose*; *Poe's*; *opes*; *epos*.

THE
GAME OF
WORDS

WILLARD R. ESPY

GROSSET & DUNLAP
A National General Company
Publishers   *New York*

51 MADISON AV

10010

First American Edition 1972
Published simultaneously in Canada
Printed in the United States of America

First published in Great Britain by Wolfe Publishing Ltd

ISBN: 0-448-01196-4
Library of Congress Catalog Card Number: 73-183017

ACKNOWLEDGEMENTS

The author would like to thank publishers, agents and authors for permission to reprint the following material:

The Daily Telegraph for *Intercom in Nasakom* by Towyn Mason (from *The Daily Telegraph* 24 Dec. 1967).

Cleveland Amory, David M. Glixon and the *Saturday Review* for extracts from 'Our Gray Nashnul Pastime' and 'Your Literary I.Q.'. Copyright 1970 *Saturday Review*, Inc.

A. D. Peters and Company for *Hush, Hush* from *The Best of Beachcomber* by J. B. Morton (published by William Heinemann Ltd. and reprinted by permission of A. D. Peters and Company).

Methuen and Co. Ltd. for *How I Brought The Good News From Aix To Ghent* from *Horse Nonsense* by W. C. Sellar and R. J. Yeatman.

Mrs. Anne Wolfe for *The British Journalist* from *The Uncelestial City* by Humbert Wolfe, and *When Lads Have Done With Labour* from *Lampoons* by Humbert Wolfe.

Patrick Ryan for an extract from *Blood* (first published in *New Scientist*).

Penguin Books Ltd. for conundrums from *Word Play* by Hubert Phillips.

Nicolas Bentley and The Bodley Head Ltd. for clerihews from *Clerihews Complete* by E. C. Bentley.

Little, Brown and Co. for an extract from 'The Cliché Expert Testifies on Love' from *A Pearl In Every Oyster* by Frank Sullivan. Copyright 1935 by Frank Sullivan; originally published in *The New Yorker*.

Sydney ('Steak') T. Kendall for extracts from *Up The Frog* (Wolfe Publishing Ltd.).

The Society of Authors as the literary representatives of the Estate of A. E. Housman, and Jonathan Cape Ltd. publishers of *A.E.H.* by Laurence Housman, for *The Elephant, Or The Force Of Habit* and *When Adam Day By Day* by A. E. Housman.

Alfred A. Knopf, Inc. and Routledge & Kegan Paul Ltd. for an extract from *The American Language* by H. L. Mencken.

The Society of Authors as the literary representative of the Estate of James Joyce and The Viking Press, Inc. for an extract from *Finnegan's Wake* by James Joyce. Copyright 1939 by James Joyce; copyright (c) renewed 1967 by George Joyce and Lucia Joyce.

Doubleday & Company, Inc. and Putnam & Company Ltd for extracts from *Fractured French* by Fred Pearson II and Richard Taylor. Copyright 1950 by Fred Pearson II and Richard Taylor.

The New Yorker and Howard Moss for *Geography: A Song* by Howard Moss. (c) 1968 The New Yorker Magazine, Inc.

Mary Ann Madden for double dactyls from *New York Magazine* (now published in *Thank You for the Giant Sea Tortoise* by The Viking Press, Inc. Edited by Mary Ann Madden. (c) 1971).

Justin Richardson for *High-Life Low-Down* from *Verse Come Verse Served* (published by Hugh Evelyn Ltd. London). (c) Justin Richardson, 1966.

Peter Dickinson for *I Arise From Dreams Of Steam Publishing*. Copyright Peter Dickinson.

A. P. Watt & Son Ltd. for *I Can't Think What He Sees In Her* by A. P. Herbert. (Originally published in *Punch*.)

CONTENTS

Introduction

ANY fair-minded person must concede that words are not tools of communication in the way that, say, frowns and kisses are. In childhood we communicate by screaming, chuckling, sticking fingers into eyes and pulling hair. Our parents communicate with us by suckling, hugging, changing diapers, spanking and sending us to bed without our suppers.

A few years later teachers communicate with us by putting gold stars after our names, or standing us in corners. We answer by turning our hair into blackberry bushes and, these days, knocking the teachers down and stomping them.

In college, we communicate by locking the president in his office and bombing the library. The president communicates by calling in the constabulary, who communicate by means of truncheons, Mace, tear gas and, occasionally, gunfire. The meaning of these exchanges is perfectly understood by everyone involved, though an observer would not be able to recognise any words at all in the din, except for a continuous chant of 'Motherf——', which does not count, since it does not appear in either Webster's or the *Oxford English Dictionary*.

By the time we marry and settle down we are locked for life into the Manichean fallacy. Everything we do not like about the world is the result of someone's deliberate evildoing. So we have no reason for verbal expression. One does not hold a dialogue with the wicked; and as for the good (that is, those who are on our side) one communicates very satisfactorily simply by grunting.

13

The working man communicates with his boss by striking, arriving late, getting messages wrong, disarranging the cards in the computer and forgetting to flush the toilet. The boss talks back by flaunting a Cadillac or Mercedes-Benz, taking winter holidays and having no money left over for a Christmas bonus.

Politicians communicate by waving their arms, shaking their fists and glaring into the television camera. Nations communicate by stockpiling, and at times using, napalm, atom bombs, submarines, missiles and poison gas.

These forms of communication outrank words because they are far more effective. Sticks and stones may break my bones, but words will never hurt me. Promises are pleasant, but diamonds are a girl's best friend. Speak softly, but carry a big stick. I'll brave the thunder if you'll brave the lightning.

The pretence that words make a difference in human affairs is one of the oldest and dirtiest tricks of English teachers and the ruling classes. Long before we emerged from our caves it had become clear that if one man could fool another one into arguing instead of throwing a rock, he—the first man, that is—had it made. Marie Antoinette did not say, 'Let them eat cake'. She said, 'Keep them talking'. When people stop talking, they are becoming dangerous.

This granted, you may wonder why I have written a book not only made up of words (it is really very difficult to avoid them in writing), but actually *about* words. The reason is simple: I have nothing whatever to communicate, and words are the best means of non-communication I know.

You will notice, though, that I do not treat them as equals, but as pets, to be stroked or kicked according to their desert and my whim. Go thou and do likewise. Housebreak your words while they are still too young to know better. When you take one for its exercise, curb it, or the neighbours will become angry. Be considerate but firm. Teach your words to sit, lie, stay, fetch. Reward them for obedience and cleverness with a dog biscuit or, in the case of catty words, with a sardine.

You may be one of those persons whom words frighten. If so, never let them know it. The instant you shrink back, they will rush at you and take a piece out of your trouser leg. Thereafter, they will ignore your commands.

But if they respect you, they will like you, and if they like you, there is nothing in their power that they will not do for you.

For a few rare people they not only roll over and play dead, but walk on their hind legs. For an even tinier number, they soar up to Heaven and play angel, or God himself.

This book is a friendly salute to the utterly unimportant Game of Words. Since you will go on playing this game, willy-nilly, as long as you live, you may as well learn to relax and enjoy it. I offer you, as a starter, a share in some of the wordplay *I* have enjoyed, from pig Latin to palindromes (horrible stuff, some of it), and some of the word games I have played (always badly), from *Bouts Rimés* to Guggenheim. You can take it from there.

Do not try to arrive at a deep reason for my helter-skelter inclusion of light verses by other writers. They are here simply as wordplay which happened to strike my fancy.

My own effusions aside, everything you will find here is lost, strayed or stolen from some other pasture. 'When you steal from one author,' says Wilson Mizner, 'it is plagiarism; when you steal from many, it is research.' This book is research.

But please do not think it lacks serious purpose. It is a reminder to you of something the world seems to be fast losing, and for lack of which we all may perish. That something is irrelevance. If Alexander Woolcott had not been there before me, my title would have been 'While Rome Burns'. *The Game of Words* is uniquely useful because you cannot put it to any good use whatever, except perhaps as a horrible example. On irrelevance I give myself high marks.

Elsewhere I make acknowledgement to the many writers and publishers who graciously acceded to my thievery. Here I wish to express special gratitude to Louise, my wife, who located many of the sources I have used. I also owe a debt to the long-defunct magazine *Notes and Queries*, which I was able to consult at the British Museum. Many of the language oddities represented here first came to my attention in its pages.

My thanks also to two Victorian gentlemen: William Dobson, an Englishman, and C. C. Bombaugh, an American. Both spent the best and, no doubt, happiest part of their lives locating and preserving obscure and outrageous examples of wordplay. Often, indeed, their findings overlapped. Mr. Dobson wrote *Literary Frivolities* and *Poetical Ingenuities* in the 1880s. At about the same time, Mr. Bombaugh was writing *Gleanings for the Curious from the Harvest Fields of Literature*, which Dover Publications reissued in 1961 as *Oddities and Curiosities of Words and Literature*, with

Martin Gardner as editor. I have shamelessly ghouled both graves.

Finally, I hope the following pages may provide you with a few hours' irrelevant entertainment, and perhaps tempt you to do a little wordplaying of your own. Words may be an inferior means of communication, but they are fun.

W. R. E.

THE GAME OF
WORDS

For Alexander, Elliott, Jeremy, and Medora the Sixth,
with this special note for the last:

> I christened my daughter Medora,
> She christened her daughter the same.
> Medorable, dorable daughters;
> Medorable, durable name.

'The question is,' said Alice, 'whether you *can* make words mean so many different things.'

'The question is,' said Humpty Dumpty, 'which is to be master—that's all.'

LEWIS CARROLL

A, B, C, D, J, K, M, P, Q and Z Shall Overcome, with a Little Help from L

Some 794 letters make up the words for the numbers from one through to ninety-nine. Among them all, I notice, there are only two *l*'s. In an effort to determine the significance of this blatant alphabetical discrimination, I checked the frequency of the other letters in the same set of words. How many *a*'s are there? None! How many *b*'s? None! How many *c*'s? None! How many *d*'s? None! Clearly, first-grade arithmetic is a club which arbitrarily excludes some of the finest letters in the alphabet. Where is *j*? *k*? *m*? *p*? *q*? *z*? All outside looking in.

I maintain that *l* is not being permitted to make anything like its full contribution to our understanding of arithmetic. And just imagine what might be accomplished for a better world, without racism, poverty, pollution, or war, by a full infusion of *a*, *b*, *c*, *d*, *j*, *k*, *m*, *p*, *q*, and *z*! Why not give these deserving, disadvantaged letters a chance, instead of spending all that money on sending a man to the moon?

ABC Language

ABCD GOLDFISH

Abey takes one side of the following argument. Who takes the other side is not recorded:

> AB C D goldfish!
> L M N O goldfish!
> O S A R 2 goldfish.

Abey also figures in a provocative line which has come without explanation down the years:

> AB C D FEG!

He appears as a greengrocer in the following:

> AB, F U NE X?
> S V F X.
> F U NE M?
> SV F M.
> OK L F M N X.

The following ABC communication is part rebus:

> YY U R
> YY U B
> I C U R
> YY 4 me.

One solves by treating YY as two Ys.

The same system is at work in:

> If U eat TT
> I shall have TT U.

To write in ABC, begin by listing all digits and letters that have the approximate sound of words. Cheat by counting, for instance, D or Z for *the*, E for *he*, F for *if* and *have*, L for *hell*, M for *am*, *him* and *them*, N for *an*, *Ann*, and *in*, S for *is*, *as*, *ass*, and *yes*, V for *we*, X for *eggs*, and so on. ME is *Emmy*, MU *emu*. You now have a vocabulary in ABC about the size of a bushman's, though less practical. I hope it serves you well.

LAMENT OF A 4SAKN LOVER

U 4N female K9's son,
U KG CD flea,
My heart CCCC its hope's DK;
Your AAAA on my QT may
Have B10 me, I C.

U C me 2 N N8 worth
Be W, no less;
Your MT BD glances bore
My II; had I IIIIIIIII more,
They'd bore me 2 XS.

Y 1 should fall 4 U S hard
4 NE 1 2 C;
Your PP never fit U L;
N this, N all, I U XL;
Yet o's left 4 me.

With NRG and EZ skill,
U 1 1 I love well.
I NV U that 1 B9,
U 4N S, and hourly pine
4 U 2 B N L.

W. R. E.

ANSWER

You foreign female canine's son,
You cagey, seedy flea,
My heart foresees its hope's decay;
Your forays on my cutie may
Have beaten me, I see.

You see me to in innate worth
Be double you, no less;
Your empty, beady glances bore
My two eyes; had I ten eyes more,
They'd bore me to excess.

Why one should fall for you is hard
For anyone to see;
Your toupees never fit you well;
In this, in all, I you excel;
Yet nothing's left for me.

With energy and easy skill,
You won one I love well.
I envy you that one benign,
You foreign ass, and hourly pine
For you to be in Hell.

Acronyms

An acronym is a word formed of the initials of other words. WASP, for instance, is an acronym for 'white Anglo-Saxon Protestant'—an odd notion, since it is hard to conceive of a non-white Anglo-Saxon Protestant. Were there such, a black one would be a BASP; a red one a RASP; a yellow one a YASP.

Tantum Ergo, meaning 'So great, therefore', a familiar expression to Roman Catholics, is an acronym for the words of the last two stanzas of a hymn sung when the Eucharist is borne in procession.

Posh, for 'elegant, luxurious', is probably short for 'polished', but some say is an acronym for 'Port Out, Starboard Home', the preferred ship accommodations for the families of nineteenth-century civil servants on their way to and from India.

The common opinion that SOS is an acronym for 'Save our ship' is incorrect; it is simply three call letters of the Morse code, the quickest and simplest that can be transmitted by one in distress.

Equally unfounded is the legend that *cabal*, meaning a 'conspiratorial group', is an acronym for Clifford–Ashley–Buckingham–Arlington–Lauderdale, a clique of cabinet ministers under Charles II. They probably conspired no more than others of their ilk. *Cabal* actually derives from Hebrew *cabala*, 'an occult theosophy, full of hidden mysteries'. The first letters of the ministers' names just happened to fit.

World War II saw the rise of such acronyms as WAC (in the United States, Woman's Army Corps); loran (long range navigation); sonar (sound navigation ranging); and radar (radio detecting and ranging).

Technically, a combination of initials does not become an acronym until it is accepted as a word in its own right. Loosely, however, the term acronym is applied to any series of first letters of the words in a given phrase, even when these letters do not themselves form accepted words. I give you two sets of such informal acronyms, the first drawn from nursery rhymes and the second from Shakespeare.

Nursery rhyme acronyms

1. Omhwttctghpdab
2. Dddmsj
3. Twalmahhalg
4. Wwwrttt
5. Ssmapgttf

Shakespearean acronyms

1. Tbontbtitq
2. Ftniw
3. Arbaonwsas
4. Nitwoodmgsbtsoy
5. Ahahmkfah
6. Orrwatr

ANSWERS

Nursery rhyme acronyms

1. Old Mother Hubbard went to the cupboard to get her poor dog a bone.
2. Diddle diddle dumpling my son John.
3. There was a little man and he had a little gun.
4. Wee Willy Winkie runs through the town.
5. Simple Simon met a pieman going to the fair.

Shakespearean acronyms

1. To be or not to be, that is the question.
2. Frailty, thy name is woman.
3. A rose by any other name would smell as sweet.
4. Now is the winter of our discontent made glorious summer by this sun of York.
5. A horse! a horse! my kingdom for a horse!
6. O Romeo, Romeo! Wherefore art thou Romeo?

INITIALLY SPEAKING

The substitution of initials for familiar word combinations goes on apace. This may not always be a service. Sometimes the initials take longer to say, if not to write, than the words themselves. Often, too, they lose their meaning as the expressions for which they stand lose their currency. It is doubtful whether our grandchildren will instantly identify an R.L.S., F.D.R., G.B.S., or J.F.K.* Many of the following phrases are products of World War II that are already fading from memory.

* Robert Louis Stevenson; Franklin Delano Roosevelt; George Bernard Shaw; John Fitzgerald Kennedy.

Others, however, are so common that we know what the initials mean even if we do not know the words they stand for. See how many you can identify.

1. A1, A.A.A.S., A.B.C., A.D., AFL-CIO, AID, A.M., ANZAC, AP, ARC, AWOL.
2. BBC, B.E., B.I.S., B.L.E., C.I.A., C.I.D., C.I.F., C.O.
3. COD, CORE, C.P.A., C.S.C., CSC, C.S.O., D.S.C., D.S.T., D/W, ENE, E.E.C., E.R.V.
4. FBI, F.O.B., FM, G.H.Q., G.P.O., H.M.S.
5. i.e., I.N.S., IOU, I.Q., KO, K.P., L.C.L., L.C.M., LP, LSD.
6. MC, MP, Nato, N.C.O., NEA, N.F., N.G., N.S.P.C.C., N.A.A.C.P., O.B.E., O.D., O.G., O.K.
7. P.A.U., P.D.Q., P.M., P.O.D., P.S., P.T.A., Q.E.D., Q.M.C., QT, R.A.F., R.A.A.F., RFD.
8. R.I.P., R.O.T.C., R.S.V.P., Scuba, SHAPE, snafu, SOB, S.R.O., SWALK, TB, TNT, TV, TVA, VC, V.D., V.I.P., W.B., WC, YMCA.

ANSWERS

1. First rate (at Lloyd's); American Association for the Advancement of Science; Argentina, Brazil, and Chile; Anno Domini; American Federation of Labor-Congress of Industrial Organizations; Agency for International Development; *ante meridian* (before noon); Australian and New Zealand Army Corps; Associated Press; American Red Cross; Absent Without Official Leave.
2. British Broadcasting Corporation; bill of exchange; Bank for International Settlements; Brotherhood of Locomotive Engineers; Central Intelligence Agency; Criminal Investigation Department; Cost, Insurance and Freight; Commanding Officer (or conscientious objector).
3. Cash (or collect) on delivery; Congress of Racial Equality; Certified Public Accountant; Conspicuous Service Cross; Civil Service Commission; Chief Signal Officer; Distinguished Service Cross; Daylight Saving Time; dock warrant; east-northeast; European Economic Community; English Revised Version (of the Bible).
4. Federal Bureau of Investigation; free on board; Frequency Modulation; General Headquarters; General Post Office; Her Majesty's Ship.
5. That is; International News Service; I owe you; intelligence quotient; knockout; kitchen police; less than carload lots; lowest, or least, common multiple; long-playing; lysergic acid diethylamide.

INTERCOM IN NASAKOM

The poem below appeared in the *Sunday Telegraph* on December 24, 1967. The author did not explain his acronyms, but most of them are familiar to any newspaper reader.

'Euratom!' cried Oiccu, sly and nasa,
'I'll wftu in the iscus with my gatt.'
'No! No!' the Eldo pleaded, pale with asa.
'My unctad strictly nato on comsat.'

The Oiccu gave a wacy little intuc,
He raft and waved his anzac oldefo.
'Bea imf!' he eec, a smirk upon his aituc,
And smote the Eldo on his ganefo.

The Eldo drew his udi from its cern,
He tact his unicet with fearless fao.
The Oiccu swerved but could not comintern;
He fell afpro, and dying moaned, 'Icao!'

The moon came up above the gasbiindo,
The air no longer vip with intercom.
A creeping icftu stirred the maphilindo
And kami was restored to Nasakom.

'O kappi gum!' the fifa sang in cento,
'O cantat till the neddy unficyp.'
The laser song re-echoed through the seato,
As the Eldo radar home to unmogip.

Towyn Mason

INITIALLY SPEAKING—*Answers*

6. Master of ceremonies; Military Police; North American Treaty Organization; noncommissioned officer; National Editorial Association (also Newspaper Enterprise Association and National Education Association); no funds (banking); no good; National Society for the Prevention of Cruelty to Children; National Association for the Advancement of Colored People; Officer (of the Order) of the British Empire; officer of the day (also overdraft, or overdrawn); officer of the guard; all right. (*Continued overleaf*)

Acrostic Verses

Poets, particularly when in love, are apt to conceal messages in their verses. In the simplest such code the first letters of the lines, taken together, form a complete word or sentence, but most frequently a name. Or the poet may use the first letter of the first line, the second letter of the second line, and so on; or the first letter of the first word of the first line, the second letter of the second word of the second line . . . the combinations are limited only by ingenuity. If he uses the last letter of the last word of each line, the result is not an acrostic but a *telestich*.

Admirers of the French actress Rachel once presented her with a diadem, so arranged that the initials of the name of each stone in the proper order formed both her name and the initials of some of her principal roles, thus:

Ruby	Roxana
Amethyst	Amenaide
Cornelian	Camille
Hematite	Hermione
Emerald	Emilie
Lapis lazuli	Laodice

INITIALLY SPEAKING—*Answers*

7. Pan American Union; pretty damned quick; *post meridian* (afternoon; also prime minister and post mortem); Post Office Department; postscript; Parent-Teacher Association; *quod erat demonstrandum* (which was to be proven); quartermaster corps; quiet; Royal Air Force; Royal Australian Air Force; Rural Free Delivery.

8. *Requiescat in pace* (rest in peace); Reserve Officers Training Corps; *répondez s'il vous plaît* (please reply); S(elf) C(ontained) U(nder-water) B(reathing) A(pparatus); Supreme Headquarters, Allied Powers, Europe; situation normal all fouled up; son of a bitch; standing room only; sealed with a loving kiss; tuberculosis; trinitro-toluene, or trininitrotoluol; television; Tennessee Valley Authority; Viet Cong (or Victoria Cross); venereal disease; very important person (one given priority for transportation in World War II); waybill; water closet; Young Men's Christian Association.

Here is a brief sampling of acrostic verses:

I

Beauty to claim, among the fairest place,
Enchanting manner, unaffected grace,
Arch without malice, merry but still wise,
Truth ever on her lips as in her eyes;
Reticent not from sullenness or pride,
Intensity of feeling but to hide;
Can any doubt such being there may be?
Each line I pen, points, matchless maid, to thee!

Planche's *Songs and Poems*

2

Cursèd, ugly moustache; I forgot
That it was bound to not
Tickle only my kissee, but *me*—
Frequently, frequently me.

W. R. E.

3

Unite and untie are the same—so say you.
Not in wedlock, I ween, has the unity been
In the drama of marriage, each wandering *goût*
To a new face would fly—all except you and I
Each seeking to alter the *spell* in their scene.

Author unknown

ANSWERS

1. The first letters of each line: BEATRICE.
2. The first letters of the first and second words of each line: CUT IT OFF.
3. Unless you are sharper than many, this one fooled you. It is both an acrostic and a telestich. The opening letters of the lines form UNITE; the closing letters, UNTIE.

Additives

An infinite variety of words can be created by adding words or letters to existing words or letters or, contrariwise, subtracting. Here are some examples:

1. Add a tree to *h*; may your sloop answer to its.
2. Drop the *n* from gun; add a home for swine; better hold on to your hat.
3. Drop the *t* from count; add effort; it has less pollution than the city.
4. Add a tree to *s*; often mine needs stiffening.
5. Drop the final *l* from bell and add to cook in hot fat, not ordinarily in a church tower.
6. Take your dog in your automobile, and you have a floor covering.
7. Add a tree to *b*, and it shows you are no longer a youth; but you can't do much about it.

ANSWERS

1. Helm	4. Spine	7. Balder
2. Gusty	5. Belfry	
3. Country	6. Carpet	

'C'?

By adding *c*'s to the entries below, you will create complete sentences. The numbers indicate how many *c*'s are required.

1. ANELONERTEDESAPADESSUHAOMPLISHINALULA BLEINDISRETIONSIRREONILEABLETOIVIHARATE R (17).
2. AORDINGTOSIKHOLERITYOONSTHEALORIAPAIT YOFONOTIONSINONRETEROKSISRYPTIANDHAOT I (21).
3. LUKLUKLUKAKLEDTHEORNEREDHIKTOTHEROW INGOKSUHONUPISENEISSARELYONEIVABLE (23).
4. OURAOPHONOUSOUSINLARAOLLETSINALULABLE ARETIONSOFATIINOHINHINAASTLES (16).

28

ANSWERS

1. Cancel concerted escapades. Such accomplish incalculable indiscretions irreconcilable to civic character.
2. According to sick choleric tycoons, the caloric capacity of concoctions in concrete crocks is cryptic and chaotic.
3. 'Cluck, cluck, cluck!' cackled the cornered chick to the crowing cock. 'Such concupiscence is scarcely conceivable.'
4. Our cacophonous cousin Clara collects incalculable accretions of cacti in Cochin China castles.

'HE HATH SUFFERED A C CHANGE . . .'

There is one lone *c* in my passage below; it requires many. Put a *c* before each capitalised word except those that begin the sentences, and the message will clear up.

The Optic Reed has a Haste Harm. It Hose, one assumes, not to be Lever; it neither Heats the Ripple, nor Hides the Razed sinner for his Rude Rime; it is not Old. Then Leave to it; ere thy grave Loses, thou mayst find here the Hart to the Rest thou Ravest to Limb.

ANSWER

The Coptic creed has a chaste charm. It chose, one assumes, not to be clever; it neither cheats the cripple, nor chides the crazed sinner for his crude crime; it is not cold. Then cleave to it; ere thy grave closes, thou mayst find here the chart to the crest thou cravest to climb.

All 26 Letters of the Alphabet

EZRA VII, 21

This is supposed to be the only verse of the Bible that contains every letter of the alphabet; but it does not. It lacks *j*, a latecomer on the alphabetical scene.

And I, even I Artaxerxes the king, do make a decree to all the treasurers which are beyond the river, that whatsoever Ezra the priest, the scribe of the law of the God of heaven, shall require of you, it be done speedily.

29

All 26 Letters in Four Lines
MALE CHAUVINIST

Though I enjoy the zeal of Women's Lib,
It's quite a comfort knowing Adam's rib
Is long re-fixed, and waits there in reserve
Should God opine the first one's ceased to serve.

W. R. E.

All 26 Letters in Two Lines
PEACE IN OUR TIME

God be his judge: that passive, zealous Quaker
Who first yields Country: Kindred next; then Maker.

W. R. E.

EACH LETTER USED ONCE

It is not particularly difficult to write a four-line, or even a two-line, verse containing all the letters of the alphabet. Try cutting back to a one-line sentence, though, and the difficulty waxes. And anyone who tries to compose a sensible line which contains each of the 26 letters of the alphabet only once has his work cut out for him. Here is how various forgotten puzzlers have crept up on the goal:

> A quick brown fox jumps over the lazy dog. (33)
> Pack my bag with five dozen liquor jugs. (32)
> Quick wafting zephyrs vex bold Jim. (29)
> Waltz, nymph, for quick jigs vex Bud. (28)

Augustus DeMorgan, a nineteenth-century mathematician, reached the 26-letter goal through a ruse: he substituted *u* for *v* and *i* for *j*. (In alphabetic genealogy, *u* descends from *v* and *j* from *i*.) The result was:

> I, quartz pyx, who fling muck beds.

Others emulated him, but so far nobody has been able to squeeze in the *v* or the *j*. Some examples:

> Dumpy Quiz, whirl back fogs next.
> Get nymph; quiz sad brow; fix luck.
> Export my fund! Quiz black whigs.

It is hard to accept the impossibility of composing a sensible line which contains every letter of the alphabet once and only once. There are 403,000,000,000,000,000,000,000,000 possible combinations of those 26 letters; surely *some* of them should make sense.

ALPHABETICAL ADVERTISEMENT

TO WIDOWERS AND SINGLE GENTLEMEN.—WANTED by a lady, a SITUATION to superintend the household and preside at table. She is Agreeable, Becoming, Careful, Desirable, English, Facetious, Generous, Honest, Industrious, Judicious, Keen, Lively, Merry, Natty, Obedient, Philosophic, Quiet, Regular, Sociable, Tasteful, Useful, Vivacious, Womanish, Xantippish, Youthful, Zealous, &c. Address X. Y. Z., Simmond's Library, Edgware-road.

The Times, 1842

ALPHABETICAL LOVER

Cervantes wrote that the whole alphabet is required of every good lover, and proceeded to list the qualities he had in mind. For some reason, though, he left out *u* and *x*. 'Understanding' would have been a good choice for *u*, it seems to me. So would 'useful'. As for *x*, there is nothing wrong with 'xenial', meaning 'hospitable'.

Make your own alphabetical list of the qualities you expect of a lover, and see how often you agree with Cervantes.

ANSWERS

Agreeable, bountiful, constant, dutiful, easy, faithful, gallant, honourable, ingenious, just, kind, loyal, mild, noble, officious,* prudent, quiet, rich, secret, true, valiant, wise, young, zealous.

---

* This word has gone downhill with the years. It once meant 'disposed or eager to serve or do kind offices'.

AN ANIMAL ALPHABET

Alligator, beetle, porcupine, whale,
Bobolink, panther, dragon-fly, snail,
Crocodile, monkey, buffalo, hare,
Dromedary, leopard, mud-turtle, bear,
Elephant, badger, pelican, ox,
Flying-fish, reindeer, anaconda, fox,
Guinea-pig, dolphin, antelope, goose,
Humming-bird, weasel, pickerel, moose,
Ibex, rhinoceros, owl, kangaroo,
Jackal, opossum, toad, cockatoo,
Kingfisher, peacock, anteater, bat,
Lizard, ichneumon, honey-bee, rat,
Mocking-bird, camel, grasshopper, mouse,
Nightingale, spider, cuttle-fish, grouse,
Ocelot, pheasant, wolverine, auk,
Periwinkle, ermine, katydid, hawk,
Quail, hippopotamus, armadillo, moth,
Rattlesnake, lion, woodpecker, sloth,
Salamander, goldfinch, angleworm, dog,
Tiger, flamingo, scorpion, frog,
Unicorn, ostrich, nautilus, mole,
Viper, gorilla, basilisk, sole,
Whippoorwill, beaver, centipede, fawn,
Xantho, canary, polliwog, swan,
Yellowhammer, eagle, hyena, lark,
Zebra, chameleon, butterfly, shark.

Author unknown

32

GEMINI JONES

At several times the speed of light,
Astronaut Gemini Jones took flight,
Buzzing about, now to, now from,
All the constellations of God's kingDOM:

Acrux, Ras Algethis, Tarf, Acanar;
Benetnasch, Kitalpha, Salm, Giansar;
Castor, Herculis, Skat, Ursae Majoris,
Delta, Kids, Adib, Cor, Ursae Minoris;
Electra, Draconis, Polaris, Mizar;
Furud, Australis, Pleione, Dog Star;
Gomeisa, Ed Asich, Schedar, Sulafat,
Hamal, Kaus Australis, Aldhaf'ra, Skat;
Izar, Sagittirri, Spica, Merope;
Juga, Giansar, Homam, Asterope;
Kitalpha, Mekbuda, Yed Posterior,
Lesath, Vinddemistrix, Zaurak, Yed Prior;
Mintaka, Porrima, Rasalas, Wasat,
Nashiri, Presepe, Taygete, Andrat;
Orionis, Alcyone, Pegasi, Alya,
Pherkad, Nair al Zurak, Al Chiba, Alscha;
Rastaban, Suzlocin, Canopis, Mwnkar,
Seginis, Algenib, Alphecca, Schedar;
Talitha, Taygete, Ruchbah, Scheat, Kochab,
Unuk al H, Piscium, Altair, Arkab;
Vega, Peiadum, Graffies, Leonis,
Wezen, Tarized, Virginis, Draconis;
Yildun, Angetenar, Kaus Borealis;
Zaurak, Antares, Alula Australis:

Buzzing about, now to, now from,
All the constellations in God's kingDOM.

W. R. E.

Alliteration

Alliteration—what the *Encyclopaedia Britannica* calls 'the jingle of like beginnings', by contrast with Milton's definition of rhyme as 'the jingling sound of like endings'—is everywhere in English. Early English poetry, indeed, had no rhyme, but was held together entirely by a pattern of alliteration, as in these lines from Beowulf:

> . . . then friendship he awaited,
> Waned under the welkin, in worship throve,
> Until each one of those outdwelling
> Over the whale-road, must hearken to him,
> Gold must give him; that was a good king.

Piers Plowman was an alliterist:

> In a somer seson when soft was the sonne,
> I shope me in shroudes as I a shepe were.
>
> A depe dale benethe, a dongeon there-inne,
> With depe dyches and derke and dredful of sight.

So was Chaucer:

> But of the fyr and flaumbe funeral
> In which my body brennen shal to glede.

Some familiar alliterative lines:

Shakespeare:

> After life's fitful fever.
> Full fathom five thy father lies.

Coleridge:

> The fair breeze blew, the white foam flew,
>   The furrow followed free;
> We were the first that ever burst
>   Into that silent sea.

Tennyson:

> Fly o'er waste fens and windy fields.

Swinburne, famous for his alliterative poetry, sometimes parodied himself:

34

From the depth of the dreamy decline of the dawn through a notable number of nebulous noonshine.

We alliterate without noticing it, as we breathe. 'Like Louise?' I might exclaim; 'I love that lady!'. Many expressions continue to be the small change of our small talk simply because of the way they trip off the tongue.

Some of these are defined below—see if you can identify them.

1. In good shape, generally referring to one who has been through a misadventure.
2. Through good and bad.
3. New and fresh; neat and trim.
4. Neither one thing nor another.
5. Friends and relatives.
6. Without attachments that impede freedom of action.
7. Uncivilised; rough in manner.
8. Most important.
9. Meticulous in what does not matter, careless in what does.
10. Completely extinct.

ANSWERS

1. Safe and sound.
2. Through thick and thin; through weal or woe; through fair or foul.
3. Spick and span.
4. Neither fish, flesh, nor fowl.
5. Kith and kin.
6. Footloose and fancy free.
7. Wild and woolly.
8. First and foremost.
9. Penny wise, pound foolish.
10. Dead as a doornail (or dodo).

SPANKER

The advertisement below for the sale of a horse appeared in a Manchester paper in 1829.

SPANKER:
The Property of O—— D——

Saturday, the 16th September next, will be sold, or set up for sale, at Skibbereen:

A strong, staunch, steady, sound, stout, safe, sinewy, service-able, strapping, supple, swift, smart, sightly, sprightly, spirited, sturdy, shining, sure-footed, sleek, smooth, spunky, well-skinned, sized, and shaped sorrel steed, of superlative symmetry, styled SPANKER; with small star and snip, square-sided, slender-shouldered, sharp-sighted, and steps singularly stately; free from strain, spavin, spasms, stringhalt, staggers, strangles, surfeit, seams, strumous swellings, scratches, splint, squint, scurf, sores, scattering, shuffling, shambling-gait, or sickness of any sort. He is neither stiff-mouthed, shabby-coated, sinew-shrunk, saddle-backed, shell-toothed, skin-scabbed, short-winded, splay-footed, or shoulder-slipped; and is sound in the sword-point and stifle-joint. Has neither sick-spleen, sleeping-evil, snaggle-teeth, sub-cutaneous sores, or shattered hoofs; nor is he sour, sulky, surly, stubborn, or sullen in temper. Neither shy nor skittish, slow, sluggish, or stupid. He never slips, strips, strays, starts, stalks, stops, shakes, snivels, snaffles, snorts, stumbles, or stocks in his stall or stable, and scarcely or seldom sweats. Has a showy, stylish switch-tail, or stern, and a safe set of shoes on; can feed on stubble, sainfoin, sheaf-oats, straw, sedge, or Scotch grass. Carries sixteen stone with surprising speed in his stroke over a six-foot sod or a stone wall. His sire was the Sly Sobersides, on a sister of Spindleshanks by Sampson, a sporting son of Sparkler, who won the sweepstakes and subscription plate last session at Sligo. His selling price is sixty-seven pounds, sixteen shillings and sixpence sterling.

VERSE BY GERARD MANLEY HOPKINS

No poet loved wordplay more than Gerard Manley Hopkins; nor did any alliterate more angelically. Almost any Hopkins line will serve as an example; I lift three from *Henry Purcell*:

The thunder-purple seabeach, plumed purple-of-thunder,
If a wuthering of his palmy snow-pinions scatter a colossal smile
Off him, but meaning motion fans fresh our wits with wonder.

These are from the more familiar *Pied Beauty*:

Glory be to God for dappled things—
For skies of couple-colour as a brindled cow;
For rose-moles all in stipple upon trout that swim;
Fresh-firecoal chestnut-falls; finches' wings;

Landscape plotted and pieced—fold, fallow, and plough;
    And all trades, their gear and tackle and trim.

All things counter, original, spare, strange;
    Whatever is fickle, freckled (who knows how?)
        With swift, slow; sweet, sour; adazzle, dim;
He fathers-forth whose beauty is past change:
        Praise him.

THE SIEGE OF BELGRADE

It is a shame that no-one seems to know who wrote this, one of
the cleverer examples of alphabetical alliteration. (The author
couldn't work in the *j*, though.)

An Austrian army, awfully arrayed,
Boldly, by battery, besieged Belgrade;
Cossack commanders cannonading come—
Dealing destruction's devastating doom;
Every endeavour, engineers essay,
For fame, for fortune—fighting furious fray:—
Generals 'gainst generals grapple—gracious God!
How honours Heaven, heroic hardihood!
Infuriate,—indiscriminate in ill,
Kindred kill kinsmen,—kinsmen kindred kill!
Labour low levels loftiest, longest lines—
Men march 'mid mounds, 'mid moles, 'mid murderous mines:
Now noisy, noxious, noticed nought
Of outward obstacles opposing ought:
Poor patriots, partly purchased, partly pressed;
Quite quaking, quickly quarter, quarter quest,
Reason returns, religious right redounds,
Suwarrow stops such sanguinary sounds.
Truce to thee, Turkey—triumph to thy train!
Unjust, unwise, unmerciful Ukraine!
Vanish vain victory, vanish victory vain!
Why wish ye warfare? Wherefore welcome were
Xerxes, Ximenes, Xanthus, Xaviere?
Yield! ye youths! ye yeomen, yield your yell!
Zeono's, Zapater's, Zoroaster's zeal,
And all attracting—arms against acts appeal.

America Speaks

There are almost as many varieties of spoken American as there are of speaking Americans. In the *Saturday Review*, Cleveland Amory presents a common, or field, variety in an account called 'Our Gray Nashnul Pastime', signed Jim Barnett and submitted by James Bonnell. After an introduction listing the major league baseball teams (in one league the Allanna Brays, the Pissburgh Pyruss, the Los Angeles Dahjers, the Sane Louis Carnals, the Monreal Espos and the Cincinnaai Res; in the other, the Ballimore Orioles, the Washinton Senaturs, the Deetroy Tigers, the Cleeland Indians, and the Minnesota Twins) the story, which I judge to be jotted down from a television announcer's report, begins:

Each mannijer signs the car showing his lineup for the day and joins the daily huddle arown home plate to learn the groun rules . . .

(As the batteen order appears before us on the screen, we are told that certain named players are in leff, senner an rye feels. Others are at the traditional spots of firss, secun an thirr base, an shorestop.)

The pisher no longer goes inna wineup, but a stresh. The firss pish is stry one, followed by ball one. Then stry two, ball two, ball three—the full cown. The ba—er fouls one inna the stanns an the cown remains aa three an two. Finally he flies deep to the senner feeler who makes a long run anna fine runnen catch up againssa wall, beyonna warneen track.

Another ba—er goes to one an one, then pulls one downa leff feel line, where the feeler plays it offa wall an fires to secun. But the ba—er, with a hook sly, slies in safely at secun with a double. He calls for time while he duss off his suit, or at leass his pans.

The game moves along. It develops into a real pishers ba—l.

The nex ba—er grouns to shore, anna runner on firss slies inna secun, to break up the du-ul play.

Three weeks from necks Sa–arday is Ole Timers' day, so get your tickus early at onea the many convenion box offices. Come ow an see baseball's grays, including several memmers of the Hall a Fame.

Anagrams

ANAGRAM EXERCISE

Not only does the quatrain below contain three unrelated sets of anagrams, but one anagram combination is broken into two words. Start solving by rhyming 'commend it'.

> My *******'s low, my ***** is high,
> A ***** with little to commend it;
> Of ******, ****** few have I;
> I ***** **.

But on second thought, I am more interested in pointing out the elegance of the verse than in making the solution difficult for you. So if you wish to take the easy way out, play with any one of the three variants below without looking at the others. Solving one solves them all.

> My *******'s low, my taste is high,
> A state with little to commend it.
> Of specie, pieces few have I;
> I ***** **.

Or

> My stipend's low, my ***** is high,
> A ***** with little to commend it.
> Of specie, pieces few have I;
> I spend it.

Or

> My stipend's low, my taste is high,
> A state with little to commend it.
> Of ******, ****** few have I;
> I spend it.

W. R. E.

39

ANAGRAMS from *Punch*

Drinking Song

He **** for gold,
As I for ale;
I've **** of this:
Of that has he.
For me a kiss
**** Holy Grail;
He'd go cuckold
To **** a fee.
Yet, ****! I wist
(And I'd **** bail)
He'd pay fourfold
To be like me.

W. R. E.

ANSWER: Opts, pots, tops, spot, stop, post.

Highland Fling

Sweet Molly MacDougal, in labour,
Warned her sister, 'It hurts like a *****.
Sin ***** a high price,
So a girl should think twice
What she ***** on the ***** for a neighbour.'

W. R. E.

ANSWER: Sabre, bears, bares, braes.

I Hope to Meet my Bartender Face to Face

'Twould much ****** you to me if, when I
Have ****** my fatal moment, and must die,
You'd share one well ****** drink, and pray there are
Some more to come across that final bar.

W. R. E.

ANSWER: Endear, neared, earned.

40

History Revisited: *The Mayflower*

********* and repainting and refitting,
Rescraping, -calking, -binding and -bowspritting,
They patched the little vessel, with the notion
Of ********* oppression . . . and the ocean.
When she was shipshaped, holystoned and gleaming,
Aboard the pilgrim ********* came *********.

W. R. E.

ANSWER: Remasting, mastering, emigrants, streaming.

Minatory Note to my Unborn Son

Asleep in your ******** pad,
You dream of future joys ********.
Don't be in such a hurry, lad;
******** bills are monumental.

W. R. E.

ANSWER: Prenatal, parental, paternal.

Ugly Does as Handsome Is

Though flowers need tending to survive,
While weeds get on alone,
The *****'s loved by all alive,
While ***** are loved by none.
Man ***** the horse above the mule,
Although the mule is abler;
At pretty girls we ***** and drool,
Though ugly ones are stabler.
   I say through *****, I wish I could
   Be much more handsome, and less good.

W. R. E.

ANSWER: Aster, tares, rates, stare, tears.

We Mean a Lot to Each Other

When I am ******* and in bliss,
While Death my mortal clay *******
Beneath some ******* stone, I'll miss
The softer parts of my remains.
My bones will last, but who *******
Will **** ** * do liver, brains,
And other organs best unsaid?
I'll miss my vitals when I'm dead.

W. R. E.

ANSWER: Sainted, detains, stainèd, instead, tend as I.

I HATE YOU, JOHN RIDDS
A Tirade in Five Bursts

BURST THE FIRST

I hate my neighbour, ***** John Ridds,
As superegos hate their ids.
If e'er he turns his back, then zip!
I'll smite that neighbour, ***** and hip;

And, laughing as he lies *****,
***** John Ridds beneath the dirt.

My loathing has the mass, the *****,
The permanence of planet Earth.
Dear reader, you've a ***** to know
Why I despise this fellow so.

42

BURST THE SECOND

My ****** hangs upon a ******
So stout that none can shear it:
John ever ******, where I dread;
He shames my ****** of spirit.

John's big and bold; he ******* nought
From wave or wind or weather.
But I am small and ill begot,
And frightened by a *******.

A ******* John is to the end,
While I equivocate;
If battles are in store, my friend,
I'd rather pull my *******.

When John's besieged and sorely pressed,
He most delights in being.
In fact, he's ******* quite his best
Precisely when I'm *******.

And since I run from **** of fray,
I **** you, John, because you stay.

BURST THE THIRD

The fair sex scorn me for my *****;
While John, *preux chevalier*,
In matters amorous, one hears,
***** better every day.

While I can barely foist my kisses
On spinster aunts and cousins,
John's ******** with a hundred misses,
And ******** with dozens.

Now why, ******, should such as he
Win hearts and hands ****** to me?

43

Do not ***** that I pronounce
John Ridds a paragon;
I am, in all that really counts,
A ***** man than John.

True, John is ******, good to touch,
A natural for pairing;
It's not his girls I ****** so much,
But rather his not sharing.

John's ******* lies in hoarding beauties
As misers hoard their winnings.
He's overloaded with his duties,
And I deserve my *******.

The *** truth is, I hate John for
Excelling me in love and ***.

So here I sit, my **** before,
And brood, as embers cool;
If John were wood, how I'd adore
To throw him on for ****.

If God ******, I'll toll the bell
Some morning for John Ridds;
And as he's sliding down to Hell,
I'll gladly ****** the skids.

But if to Heaven he's conveyed,
I'll picket, jeer, and carp;
And when the angels' ***** are played,
I'll pray that John's plays *****.

W. R. E.

ANSWERS

Burst the First: Hight, Thigh; Inert, Inter; Girth, Right
Burst the Second: Hatred, Thread, Dareth, Dearth; Feareth, Feather;
Fighter, Freight; Feeling, Fleeing; Heat, Hate
Burst the Third: Fears, Fares; Flirting, Trifling; Indeed, Denied
Burst the Fourth: Infer, Finer; Rugged, Grudge; Sinning, Innings; Raw,
War
Burst the Fifth: Flue, Fuel; Agrees, Grease; Harps, Sharp

MILTON, THOU SHOULD'ST BE RE-VERSING
AT THIS HOUR

W. S. Gilbert wrote:

> If this young man expresses himself
> In terms too deep for *me*,
> Why, what a singularly deep young man
> This deep young man must be!

Unplumbable depths are the hallmark of some present-day
poets. The reversal verse below is simple by comparison with
theirs; every word is a real and common one. If you don't care for
it this way, turn each word around and you will get the second
version.

> won ma I
> a keels, gums, live rail, am?
>   on,
> ton I. I garb ton, reel ton, lever ton.
>   o,
> snug yam time tips; slag era diva; a eros lived yam knits;
>   tub I,
>   on dam flow
> ward laud drawer:
> I flog, I peels. ogre,
>   I ma ton deliver,
> tub trams.

W. R. E.

(ANSWER OVERLEAF)

45

ANSWER

now am I
a sleek, smug, evil liar, ma?
                                no,
not I. I brag not, leer not, revel not.
                                        o,
guns may emit spit; gals are avid; a sore devil may stink;
    but I,
            no mad wolf,
draw dual reward,
I golf, I sleep. ergo,
                    I am not reviled,
but smart.

REVERSE VERSES

Each of the couplets below defines two words, the first the reverse
of the second in spelling but otherwise unrelated to it. Guess the
words.

I

Without her I know that there wouldn't be me;
Turn her around, she's a word from 'to be'.

2

Detractors will say I'm too greedy by far;
Turn me around, I'm an opera star.

3

If I bore you by boasting and putting on airs,
Turn me around, and I'm something one wears.

4

A tinker's is worthless, it's often opined,
But worse turned around, for it's out of its mind.

5

It's used on your luggage to fasten about;
Turn it around, and your clothes may fall out.

6

Its meaning is kingly, a word to revere;
Turn it around, and it's rather small beer.

7

A river will do this, though shallow, though deep;
Turn it around, and it likes eating sheep.

W. R. E.

ANSWERS

1. Ma, am
2. Avid, diva
3. Brag, garb
4. Dam, mad

5. Strap, parts
6. Regal, lager
7. Flow, wolf

WHAT'S IN A NAME?

The following names have all given birth to well-known anagrams. If you don't recall the anagrams off-hand, you may enjoy anagramming the names yourself before looking at the time-honoured transpositions which follow.

1. Horatio Nelson
2. Adolf Hitler
3. Henry Wadsworth
   Longfellow

4. Florence Nightingale
5. Robert Louis Stevenson
6. Dante Gabriel Rossetti
7. Oliver Wendell Holmes

ANSWERS

1. Honor est a Nilo.
2. Hated for ill.
3. Won half the New World's glory.
4. Flit on, cheering angel!

5. Our best novelist, señor!
6. Greatest idealist born.
7. He'll do in mellow verse.

Anguish Languish

LADLE RAT ROTTEN HUT

Professor Howard Chace, Department of Romance Languages, Miami University, Oxford, Ohio, had a hobby of reducing folk tales to what he called 'Anguish Languish' by replacing all the words of the story with others, similar in sound but unrelated in meaning. The following example of his art appeared in *Word Study*, May 1953.

Wants pawn term dare worsted ladle gull hoe lift wetter murder inner ladle cordage honor itch offer lodge dock florist. Disc ladle gull orphan worry ladle cluck wetter putty ladle rat hut, end fur disc raisin pimple caulder ladle rat rotten hut. Wan moaning rat rotten hut's murder colder inset: 'Ladle rat rotten hut, heresy ladle basking winsome burden barter an shirker cockles. Tick disc ladle basking tudor cordage offer groin murder hoe lifts honor udder site offer florist. Shaker lake, dun stopper laundry wrote, end yonder nor sorgum stenches dun stopper torque wet strainers.'

'Hoe-cake, murder,' resplendent ladle rat rotten hut, end tickle ladle basking an sturred oft. Honor wrote tudor cordage offer groin murder, ladle rat rotten hut mitten anomalous woof.

'Wail, wail, wail,' set disc wicket woof, 'evanescent ladle rat rotten hut! Wares or putty ladle gull goring wizard ladle basking?'

'Armor goring tumor groin murder's,' reprisal ladle gull. 'Grammars seeking bet. Armor ticking arson burden barter end shirker cockles.'

'O hoe! Heifer blessing woke,' setter wicket woof, butter taught tomb shelf, 'Oil tickle shirt court tudor cordage offer groin murder. Oil ketchup wetter letter, an den—O bore!'

Soda wicket woof tucker shirt court, end whinney retched a cordage offer groin murder, picket inner widow an dore debtor port oil worming worse lion inner bet. Inner flesh disc abdominal woof lipped honor betting adder rope. Zany pool dawn a groin murder's nut cup an gnat gun, any curdle dope inner bet.

Inner ladle wile ladle rat rotten hut a raft attar cordage an ranker dough ball. 'Comb ink, sweat hard,' setter wicket woof, disgracing is verse. Ladle rat rotten hut entity bet rum end stud buyer groin murder's bet. 'Oh grammar,' crater ladle gull, 'Wart bag icer gut! a nervous sausage bag ice!' 'Butter lucky chew whiff,

48

doling,' whiskered disc ratchet woof, wetter wicket small. 'Oh grammar, water bag noise! A nervous sore suture anomalous prognosis!' 'Buttered small your whiff,' inserter woof, ants mouse worse wadding. 'Oh grammar, water bag mousey gut! A nervous sore suture bag mouse!'

Daze worry on forger nut gull's lest warts. Oil ofter sodden throne offer carvers an sprinkling otter bet, disc curl an bloat Thursday woof ceased pore ladle rat rotten hut an garbled erupt.

Mural: Yonder nor sorghum stenches shud ladle gulls stopper torque wet strainers.

DARN BODY OAT MEAL STREAM

Darn body oat meal stream,
Wear a first mate shoe,
Ouija eyesore blue
Dresden gingham, too.
It was there anew
Thatch a loft me too.
You were sixteen,
Marvel itch Queen,
Darn body oat meal stream!

Dave Morrah

APPLESAUCE

The Apple which the Snake supplied
Arrived complète, with Worm inside.
Child, shun this Sequence of the Snake:
First Fruit, then Worm, then Belly-Ache.

W.R.E.

49

Animal Noise

The cry of a cat's a ****,
And an **** is the **** of a hog;
And a *** is the **** of a cow,
And a **** is the *** of a dog;

And a ***** is the **** of a horse,
And a *******'s an elephant's *****;
And the ******** of lions are *****,
And the **** of a donkey's a ****;

And the **** of a duck is a *****,
And the ***** of a snake is a ****;
And if that doesn't take you aback,
You may be confounded by this:

The **** of a sheep is a ***,
And a hyena's *** is a *****;
And the ***** of a babe is a ****,
And the **** of a . . . say a . . . giraffe
  Is so small
    It is nothing
      Nothing at all.

W. R. E.

ANSWER

The cry of a cat's a meow,
And an oink is the meow of a hog;
And a moo is the oink of a cow,
And a bark is the moo of a dog;

And a neigh is the bark of a horse,
And a trumpet's an elephant's neigh;
And the trumpets of lions are roars,
And the roar of a donkey's a bray;

And the bray of a duck is a quack,
And the quack of a snake is a hiss;
And if that doesn't take you aback,
You may be confounded by this:

The hiss of a sheep is a baa,
And a hyena's baa is a laugh;
And the laugh of a babe is a waah,
And the waah of a . . . say a . . . giraffe
   Is so small
      It is nothing
         Nothing at all.

Animal Offspring

A cow has a ****, but the **** of a mare
Is a ****, and a *** is the **** of a bear;
A **** is the *** of a deer, while the ****
Of a beaver's a ******, and, carrying on,
The *** of a sheep is a ****, and the ****
Of a wolf is a *****, while the ***** of madame
Is a ****, and the **** of a dog is a ***,
And I thought for awhile this would wind the thing up,
But the *** of a goat is a ***, and, Mon Dieu!
A ****'s the *** of a kangkangaroo.

               W. R. E.

ANSWER

A cow has a calf, but the calf of a mare
Is a foal,* and a cub is the foal* of a bear;
A fawn is the cub of a deer, while the fawn
Of a beaver's a kitten, and, carrying on,
The kit of a sheep is a lamb, and the lamb
Of a wolf is a whelp, while the whelp of Madame
Is a babe, and the babe of a dog is a pup,
And I thought for awhile this would wind the thing up,
But the pup of a goat is a kid, and, Mon Dieu!,
A joey's the kid of a kangkangaroo.

* Or colt.

As I Lay Dying

You are asked to develop an appropriate deathbed statement for past or present notables. (The *New Statesman* performed the same service for beasts. The flea, for instance, said, 'And now for Abraham's bosom'; the ostrich, 'Where's that sand?'; the Phoenix, 'It's my wish to be cremated'.)

Some last words of record:

The British statesman Henry Labouchere, noting the flaring of the oil lamp beside the bed where he lay dying, said, 'Flames? Not yet, I think.'

Hugh Latimer, the Protestant martyr, told Nicholas Ridley, Bishop of London, as the lighted fagots touched their pyres: 'Be of good comfort, Master Ridley, and play the man. We shall this day light such a candle, by God's grace in England, as I trust shall never be put out.'

Louis XIV: 'When I was King . . .'

Lady Mary Wortley Montagu: 'It has all been very interesting.'

William Palmer, the poisoner, told to step out on the gallows trap: 'Are you sure it's safe?'

Anna Pavlova: 'Get my swan costume ready.'

Heinrich Heine: 'God will pardon me—it's his profession.'

A. E. Housman (after being cheered by his doctor with a risqué story): 'Yes, that's a good one and tomorrow I shall be telling it on the Golden Floor.'

Disraeli (asked whether he would like Queen Victoria at his deathbed): 'Why should I see her? She will only want to give a message to Albert.'

Auguste Comte, the positivist: 'What an irreparable loss!'

Michael Restuzhev-Ryumin, the Russian revolutionary whose first rope broke at his hanging: 'Nothing succeeds with me. Even here I meet with disappointment.'

Anne Boleyn, approaching the guillotine: 'The executioner is, I believe, very expert; and my neck is very slender.'

Buffalo Bill (William Frederick Cody), on being told his remaining time was short: 'Well, let's forget about it and play high five.'

Thoreau, asked if he had made his peace with his God: 'I was not aware that we had ever quarrelled.'

W. C. Fields: 'On the whole, I'd rather be in Philadelphia.'

Nero's mother, to the assassins sent by her son: 'Smite my womb!'

P. T. Barnum: 'How were the circus receipts today at Madison Square Garden?'

Clarence Walker Barron, publisher of the *Wall Street Journal*: 'What's the news?'

Clifton Fadiman has suggested deathbed utterances for the notables listed below. To make sure you know how As I Lay Dying should be played, write down your own last words for each of these men and women. Then see how yours compare with Mr. Fadiman's.

1. Gypsy Rose Lee, ecdysiast.
2. Henry Luce, founder of *Time* and *Life*.
3. Sam Goldwyn, cinema producer.
4. Mary Baker Eddy, founder of Christian Science.

ANSWERS

1. Gypsy Rose Lee: 'Are those wings detachable?'
2. Henry Luce: 'It's time, life.'
3. Sam Goldwyn: 'I never thought I'd live to see the day.'
4. Mary Baker Eddy: 'Impossible!'

AUTHOR'S QUERY

William Cole, in *Pith and Vinegar*,* asked who wrote the couplet which follows. As far as I know, he has received no reply. If you send me the answer, it will put me one up on William Cole.

> Do you love me or do you not?
> You told me once but I forgot.

*Simon and Schuster, New York

B

Basic English

'What is the difference between visiting a man and going to see
him, extracting a tooth and taking it out, forbidding a person solid
food and saying he may not have it, preparing a meal and getting
one ready, retiring at 10 and going to bed at that hour, rising at 7
and getting up then, dispatching a message and sending one,
maintaining silence and keeping quiet, assisting your friends and
helping them, commenting on something they do and making an
observation about it, enlisting in one of the services and joining up,
occupying a house and living in it, concentrating on your work
and putting your mind to it?'

The question is put by Mr. I. A. Richards and Miss Christine
Gibson, advocates of Basic English, a simplified form of the
language. Anyone reasonably proficient in English can master the
basics of Basic English in a few days, or even a few hours, though
it is not clear why one should. But to a person born to any of
the other 1700 languages in the world, Basic affords perhaps the
easiest possible entry to English.

There are only 850 words to learn. As one might suspect, many
of these become portmanteau words; *seat*, for instance, is used for
such particular kinds of seats as settees, couches, settles, thrones,
stalls, divans, hassocks, tripods, taborets, and woolsacks. This
Liberty Hall does not make for precision of speech.

Still, if you know Basic you can make yourself understood
wherever English is spoken, and there is nothing to stop you
from adding less basic words as you go along.

One of the reasons Basic is easy to learn is that it has only
sixteen verbs: *come, get, give, go, keep, let, make, put, seem, take,*

be, do, have, say, see, and *send.* These may be combined with *may, will,* and a number of prepositions.

I have given here only a very sketchy idea of the way Basic works. It would not be surprising, though, if you could figure out the rest for yourself. Below is a Basic English exercise. If your answers agree with those which follow the exercise, you don't need to take the course.

1. When we *enter* a room, we——.
2. When we *leave* it, we——.
3. If an army *advances*, it——.
4. If an army *retreats*, it——.
5. If a man *hurries*, he——.
6. If he *dawdles*, he——.
7. If you *ascend* steps, you——.
8. In *descending*, you——.
9. If a man *precedes* another, he——.
10. If he *follows* him or *pursues* him, he——.
11. If you *forget* a thing, it——.
12. If you *recollect* it, it——.
13. If you *visit* someone, you——.
14. If you *inherit* money, you——.
15. When the sun *rises*, it——.
16. When it *sets*, it——.
17. If it *disappears* behind a cloud, it——.
18. If it *reappears*, it——.

ANSWERS

1. come *or* go into it.
2. go out.
3. goes forward.
4. goes back.
5. goes quickly.
6. goes slowly.
7. go up them.
8. come down.
9. goes before him.
10. goes after him.
11. goes out of your mind.
12. comes back to you.
13. go to see him *or* go to his house.
14. come into it.
15. comes up.
16. goes down.
17. goes under it, *or* out of view.
18. comes out again.

HOW COMMON CAN YOU GET?

Ten English words, according to advocates of Basic English, make up a full fourth part of all our reading. When you have guessed which ones they are, check your list with the one given below.

ANSWER

The ten most frequent words in English are *the, of, and, to, a, in, that, it, is, I*.

Beasts at Bay

CREATURES IN COUPLETS

1 There's a word that holds a cat, and means a social class;
2 There's a word that holds a cow, and means a silly ass.
3 One that holds a goat's a mighty giant, David's menace.
4 One that holds a dog was once a magistrate in Venice.

5 There's a word that holds a horse, and means an incubus;
6 One that holds a bear, and bore me, you, him, her, and us;
7 One that holds a lion is a medal oversize;
8 One that holds a seagull means to lock up, penalise.

9 One that holds a kind of fish, a kind of pattern, too;
   I must stop this game before I use up all the zoo.

W. R. E.

ANSWERS

1. Caste.
2. Clown.
3. Goliath.
4. Doge.
5. Nightmare.
6. Forebear.
7. Medallion.
8. Intern.
9. Herringbone.

TALE OF THE NAKED RABBI

If the night had not been so dark, the two unfortunate rabbis whose adventures are related below would have found a number of animals concealed in the haunted wastes they were traversing —one, in fact, to a line. Once you have located the first beast, you should have no trouble flushing out the others.

1	Two naked rabbis, one black night,
2	Not local folk, but strangers,
3	Called on a German for a light.
4	One said, 'O God, such dangers!
5	In such black ink a journey ne'er
6	Was planned till now, or taken;
7	Drab ruins ring me everywhere;
8	'Neath each stele, phantoms waken.
9	Would that wide Erie flowed e'en now
10	Betwixt those shapes and me!
11	They made a most terrific row;
12	One sobbed and wailed, on key.
13	And one would sigh, or seem to sigh,
14	And one would yell amain,
15	And one, with blust'ring oath and cry,
16	Would grab, bite, kick, and pain.
17	Dear God! It rushes to attack!
18	I struck it ten times three;
19	A spirit moans, while striking back,
20	"I'm vile—O, pardon me!"
21	Th' avowal rustles to an end;
22	What rout or final victory befell
23	This naked rabbi and his friend
24	'Twould take a sadder, wiser pen to tell.

W. R. E.

(ANSWERS OVERLEAF)

1. Bison. 2. Calf. 3. Onager. 4. Dog. 5. Kinkajou. 6. Wasp. 7. Bruin.
8. Elephant. 9. Deer. 10. Ape. 11. Crow. 12. Donkey. 13. Horse. 14.
Llama. 15. Goat. 16. Rabbit. 17. Stoat. 18. Kitten. 19. Asp. 20. Leopard.
21. Walrus. 22. Trout. 23. Snake. 24. Serpent.

TROJAN HORSE WORDS

Some creatures slip into words as slyly as the Trojan horse
slipped into Troy. Each of the phrases below holds a clue to a
word in which another word is hidden.

1. Alas for this beautiful vanishing heron!
2. Such an insect might blow its own horn.
3. Poor Fido! In the soup!
4. Who, a-hunt by night? Who?
5. When hunted it hasn't sense enough to do what it's part of.
6. At the farthest end from the squeal is the whole hairstyle.
7. Not a bully, anyhow.
8. Even the Augean stables never stank like this.

ANSWERS

The container	The contained
1. Regret	Egret
2. Bugle	Bug
3. Chowder	Chow
4. Prowl	Owl
5. Scoot	Coot
6. Pigtail	Pig
7. Coward	Cow
8. Maremma	Mare

Berlitz School

Say 'Donkey field mice' to a Viennese, and he will think you
speak excellent German; for that is the Viennese pronunciation
of 'Danke viel mals', 'Thank you very much'.

Charles F. Berlitz, on an opposite tack, once published a list of foreign words that sound like English. Some of these international homonyms are the subjects of the verses below.

I

'Good day,' said I to Jap chauffeur.
'Ohio,' was his sequitur.
I thanked him for the motor ride;
'Don't touch my moustache, sir,' he cried.
'You're wanting manners, man,' said I;
He deeply bowed, and said, 'High, high.'
I said, 'My mother is in town.'
'Ha ha,' said he. I knocked him down.

2

How 'how' resounds in every nation!
How different its interpretation!
In Hawaiian, 'how' 's 'to smoke';
'Greetings' 'tis to redskin bloke;
'Aristocrat' to Japanese;
'Good' to neighbouring Chinese.
To a German in a twit
It's imperative for 'hit'.

3

'I beg a Mere lighthearted Sin,'
Said I to Moscow maid;
'Peace be to you and me,' said she,
'But no Son, I'm afraid.'
'A Brat you are to treat me so!'
I cried out angrily;
'I'll be your sister,' she replied,
'A Brother I can't be.'
'My brother's name is Bill,' I said;
'He was?' said she to me.
'I call him Billy,' I went on.
'They were? How nice!' said she.

W. R. E.

(ANSWERS OVERLEAF)

ANSWERS

1. The name of the American state means 'good morning' in Japanese. 'You are welcome' is *'Do itashimash'te'*—as near as makes no difference to 'Don't touch my moustache'. 'High, high,' is 'No, no'. 'Ha ha' is 'mother'.
2. Self-explanatory.
3. 'Mere' in Russian means 'peace' or 'world'; 'sin' means 'son'; 'brat' means 'brother'; 'Bill' means 'was'; 'Billy' means 'were'.

IMPERIAL ENGLISH

The English-speaking peoples may (or may not) be losing rank in the councils of the mighty, but their language continues to spread. Sometimes, to be sure, it is hard to recognise; one has to think a moment before realising that 'Oossmaheel' is simply the Puerto Rican way of pronouncing 'U.S. mail'. The Puerto Ricans have similarly turned the baseball term 'home run' into 'jonron'. The Japanese call the afternoon rush hour 'rushewawa'.

'Le week-end' is one of hundreds of English expressions that have slipped past the guard of the wary and indignant French. I note, for instance, that French engineers working on the faster-than-sound Concorde aircraft say 'broque' for 'broke'. A fashion advertisement in Germany says, 'Was ist IN, was ist OUT?' another, 'Auf in den Winter mit Country Boots'! Politicians in the western countries accept unchanged such Anglo-American words and phrases as appeasement, escalation, rollback, comeback and 'no comment'.

*

BUSTS AND BOSOMS

Busts and bosoms have I known
Of various shapes and sizes,
From grievous disappointments
To jubilant surprises.

Author unknown

*

Bogus is to Borghese as Phoney is to Forney

Some of the best stories about word origins suffer from the minor disadvantage of being lies. Among these bogus, phoney reports are those on *bogus* and *phoney*.

Bogus is allegedly a corruption of Borghese, the name of a man who in the nineteenth century made a good thing of drawing cheques on fictitious banks. His name, according to the story, came to be used as a description of any such worthless bills.

At about the same time, one Mr. Forney was happily selling fake jewellery to buyers who knew no better. Again, *phoney* is said to be corrupted from his name.

Messrs. Borghese and Forney may well have existed, but at best their names could only have reinforced words already in existence. *Bogus* comes from an old dialectal term in south-west England, *tankerabogus*, 'a goblin'. (Its tail end survives in *bogey*.) As to *phoney*, it is a corruption of the British underworld term *fawny*, in turn a corruption of Irish *fainne*, meaning 'finger-ring' —hence ring-switching and cheating in general.

While Borghese and Forney were playing their games, a man named Colonel Booze was distilling whisky and selling it in a bottle bearing his name. For this reason, it is said, *booze* came to mean hard liquor. But again, his name can only have reinforced an existing word: *booze* goes back to Middle English *bousen*, 'to carouse'.

Corsair may have become a common word because so many privateers lurked in the harbours of Corsica, the French island in the Mediterranean; but this common tradition does not alter the fact that the true origin of the word is Latin *correre*, 'to run'.

Gibberish is probably a corruption of *jabber*. Yet it was once called 'the mystic language of Geber, used by chymists', by no less a lexicographer than Samuel Johnson. The Geber he referred to was Jabir ibn Hayyan, an eighth-century alchemist who is reputed to have written more than 2000 books. The likely explanation is that other medieval alchemists borrowed his name to give authority to their works.

Blazer is often credited to the captain of H.M.S. *Blazer*, who ordered his officers to spruce up by wearing blue jackets with metal buttons. But probably the name simply refers to the blazing colour of the jacket.

Thomas Costain says in one of his novels that a man named Blanket, famous as a weaver of fine wools, dwelt long ago in Britain, and gave his name to the common bedcover. Actually, 'blanket' is simply an anglicisation of French *blanc*, 'White'. Once more, I do not rule out the possibility that Mr. Blanket gave the term currency by association; if he had been Mr. White, we might today be calling blankets 'whites'.

Tom Stoppard, in *Lord Malquist and Mr. Moon*, says: 'In the 13th century Sir John Wallop so smote the French at sea that he gave a verb to the language. But there must be less energetic ways of doing that.' But as far as I can learn, Sir John exists only in Mr. Stoppard's mind. *Wallop* comes from an old French word meaning 'gallop'.

My friend Irwin Shapiro once told me with a straight face that *pumpernickel* was named for Napoleon's horse. According to Irwin, the Emperor was offered a piece of this dark, sourish rye bread by a peasant while on one of his recurrent military expeditions in Eastern Europe. He tasted it, made a face, and gave the bread to his horse, Nicole, with the comment, 'Bon pour Nicole'. Hence, by corruption, *pumpernickel*. The true story is even odder. The bread gets its name because it is so hard to digest. The word is early New High German *Pumpern*, 'a fart', + *Nickel*, 'the devil': 'the devil's fart'.

Marmalade is traced by some to *Marie malade*, 'sick Mary'. The reason given is that this jam, then a rarity, was among the few foods that Mary, Queen of Scots, could hold on her stomach during an illness. The true source, though, is Greek *melimelon*, 'sweet apple'.

Russell Baker, a tongue-in-cheek newspaper columnist, once attributed the word *pragmatism* to Giovanni Pragma, whom he described as a nineteenth-century Florentine councilman and bungler. When I raised an eyebrow, he insisted that the provenance was authentic, coming to him by way of his friend Nino, who manages a trattoria in Washington, D.C. He wrote that Nino would be glad to confirm the derivation for me in person if I would first buy him a bottle of Bollo to loosen his tongue.

If the lexicographers take Mr. Baker seriously, you may find in some future *OED* a definition starting like this:

prag.ma-tism (prag'ma-tizm), n. [G. Pragma, It. statesman.] A philosophy holding that the truth is pre-eminently to be tested by the practical consequences of belief . . .

Burlesque and Parody

A parody is a comic imitation of a serious poem, and a burlesque is a particularly ludicrous form of parody.

The English seem to take special pleasure in parodies, perhaps because so many Englishmen had to write compositions after the manner of classical poets when in public school.

HUSH, HUSH

Hush, hush,
Nobody cares;
Christopher Robin
Has
    Fallen
        Down-
           Stairs.

'Beachcomber' (J. B. Morton)

THE TENTH DAY OF CWTHMAS

On the tenth day of Cwthmas,* the Commonwealth brought to me
Ten Sovereign Nations
Nine Governors General
Eight Federations
Seven Disputed Areas
Six Trust Territories
Five Old Realms
Four Present or Prospective Republics
Three High Commission Territories
Two Ghana-Guinea Fowl

  One Sterling Area
  One Dollar Dominion
  One Sun That Never Sets
  One Maltese Cross
  One Marylebone Cricket Club
  One Trans-Arctic Expedition

And a Mother Country up a Gum Tree.

from *The Economist*

---

* Contraction of 'Commonwealthmas'.

HOW I BROUGHT THE GOOD NEWS FROM AIX TO GHENT

(*or Vice Versa*)

I sprang to the rollocks and Jorrocks and me,
And I galloped, you galloped, we galloped all three.
Not a word to each other: we kept changing place,
Neck to neck, back to front, ear to ear, face to face:
And we yelled once or twice, when we heard a clock chime,
'Would you kindly oblige us, *is that the right time?*'
As I galloped, you galloped, he galloped, we galloped, ye
    galloped, they two shall have galloped: *let us trot.*

I unsaddled the saddle, unbuckled the bit,
Unshackled the bridle (the thing didn't fit)
And ungalloped, ungalloped, ungalloped, ungalloped a bit.
Then I cast off my buff coat, let my bowler hat fall,
Took off both my boots and my trousers and all—
Drank off my stirrup-cup, felt a bit tight,
And unbridled the saddle: it still wasn't right.

Then all I remember is, things reeling round,
As I sat with my head 'twixt my ears on the ground—
For imagine my shame when they asked what I meant
And I had to confess that I'd been, gone and went
And *forgotten* the news I was bringing to Ghent,
Though I'd galloped and galloped and galloped and galloped
    and galloped
And galloped and galloped and galloped. (Had I not would
    have been galloped?)

ENVOI

So I sprang to a taxi and shouted 'To Aix!'
And he blew on his horn and he threw off his brakes,
And all the way back till my money was spent
We rattled and rattled and rattled and rattled and rattled
And rattled and rattled—
And eventually sent a telegram.

    Walter Carruthers Sellar
    and Robert Julian Yeatman

OH, POE!

Few poets are more tempting to parodists than Edgar Allen Poe, described by James Russell Lowell as 'three-fifths genius, two-fifths fudge'. Here is a happy take-off by Bret Harte:

> But Mary, uplifting her finger,
>   Said, 'Sadly this bar I mistrust—
>   I fear that this bar does not trust.
> Oh, hasten—oh, let us not linger—
>   Oh, fly—let us fly—ere we must!'
> In terror she cried, letting sink her
>   Parasol till it trailed in the dust,—
> In agony sobbed, letting sink her
>   Parasol till it trailed in the dust,—
>   Till it sorrowfully trailed in the dust.
>
> Then I pacified Mary and kissed her,
>   And tempted her into the room,
>   And conquered her scruples and gloom;
> And we passed to the end of the vista,
>   But were stopped by the warning of doom,—
> By some words that were warning of doom.
>   And I said, 'What is written, sweet sister,
>   At the opposite end of the room?'
> She sobbed as she answered, 'All liquors
>   Must be paid for ere leaving the room.'

*

THE BRITISH JOURNALIST

> You cannot hope
>   To bribe or twist
> (Thank God!) the British
>   Journalist;
> But, seeing what
>   The man will do
> Unbribed, there's no
>   Occasion to.

Humbert Wolfe

*

PARODIES BY LEWIS CARROLL

As a boy I always had the feeling there was something that just escaped me about the verses in *Alice and Wonderland* and *Through the Looking-Glass*. Probably I had read in passing the verses that inspired them, and sensed some indefinable reminiscence in the lines. A parody cannot be effective—as a parody, that is—if the original has been forgotten. Since most of the originals from which Mr. Carroll worked *have* been forgotten, the 'Alice' verses have become immortal not as burlesques, but as nonsense.

Below are some stanzas of verse familiar to every Victorian child, followed by excerpts from Lewis Carroll's takeoffs.

1. Dr. Isaac Watts: *Against Idleness and Mischief*

> How doth the little busy bee
>   Improve each shining hour,
> And gather honey all the day
>   From every opening flower! ...
>
> In works of labour or of skill,
>   I would be busy too;
> For Satan finds some mischief still
>   For idle hands to do ...

1A. *Lewis Carroll's rendition*

> How doth the little crocodile
>   Improve his shining tail,
> And pour the waters of the Nile
>   On every golden scale!
>
> How cheerfully he seems to grin,
>   How neatly spreads his claws,
> And welcomes little fishes in
>   With gently smiling jaws!

2. Robert Southey: *The Old Man's Comforts and How He Gained Them*

> 'You are old, Father William,' the young man cried;
>   'The few locks which are left you are grey;
> You are hale, Father William—a hearty old man:
>   Now tell me the reason, I pray.'

66

'In the days of my youth,' Father William replied,
  'I remembered that youth would fly fast,
And abused not my health and my vigour at first,
  That I never might need them at last . . .'

2A. *Lewis Carroll's rendition*

'You are old, Father William,' the young man said,
  'And your hair has become very white;
And yet you incessantly stand on your head—
  Do you think, at your age, it is right?'

'In my youth,' Father William replied to his son,
  'I feared it might injure the brain;
But now that I'm perfectly sure I have none,
  Why, I do it again and again . . .'

3. Jane Taylor: *The Star*

Twinkle, twinkle, little star
How I wonder what you are!
Up above the world so high,
Like a diamond in the sky.

3A. *Lewis Carroll's rendition*

Twinkle, twinkle, little bat!
How I wonder what you're at!
Up above the world you fly,
Like a teatray in the sky.

*

BLOOD

A scientific humourist named Patrick Ryan makes the following comments on blood:

To the human mind there is more to blood than its mere chemical content. . . . For example, blood must essentially be thicker than water, impossible to get out of stones, indelible in its staining. . . . When apparent on heads, it should leave them unbowed; and should have the capacities to combine formidably with toil, tears and sweat; and to attain boiling-point when its host faces frustration.

WHEN LADS HAVE DONE WITH LABOUR

When lads have done with labour
In Shropshire, one will cry,
'Let's go and kill a neighbour,'
and t'other answers 'Aye!'

So this one kills his cousins,
and that one kills his dad;
And, as they hang by dozens
at Ludlow, lad by lad,

Each of them one-and-twenty,
all of them murderers,
The hangman mutters: 'Plenty
even for Housman's verse.'

Humbert Wolfe

WISE SAWS AND MODERN INSTANCES
(OR POOR RICHARD IN REVERSE)

Saw, *n.* A trite popular saying, or proverb. (Figurative and colloquial.) So called because it makes its way into a wooden head. The following are examples of old saws fitted with new teeth.

A penny saved is a penny to squander.
A man is known by the company that he organises.
A bad workman quarrels with the man who calls him that.
A bird in the hand is worth what it will bring.
Better late than before anybody has invited you.
Example is better than following it.
Think twice before you speak to a friend in need.
What is worth doing is worth the trouble of asking somebody to
   do it.
Least said is soonest disavowed.
He laughs best who laughs least.
Speak of the Devil and he will hear about it.
Of two evils choose to be the least.
Strike while your employer has a big contract.
Where there's a will there's a won't.

Ambrose Bierce

68

C

Chain Verse

A curious literary form, in which little of note has been accomplished, is the chain verse—an arrangement in which the last word or phrase of each line becomes the beginning of the next. Here is such a one:

AD MORTEM

The longer life, the more offence;
The more offence, the greater pain;
The greater pain, the less defence;
The less defence, the greater gain—
    Wherefore, come death, and let me die!

The shorter life, less care I find,
Less care I take, the sooner over;
The sooner o'er, the merrier mind;
The merrier mind, the better lover—
    Wherefore, come death, and let me die!

Come, gentle death, the ebb of care;
The ebb of care, the flood of life;
The flood of life, I'm sooner there;
I'm sooner there—the end of strife—
The end of strife, that thing wish I—
    Wherefore, come death, and let me die!

                Author unknown

Charades

1. I am a word of 12 letters.
My 12, 4, 7, 2, 5 is an Eastern beast of burden.
My 1, 8, 10, 9 is a street made famous by Sinclair Lewis.
My 11, 3, 6 is past.
My whole is a person suffering from delusions of greatness.

2. I am a word of 11 letters.
   My 7, 3, 8, 4, 5 is what the little girl did when her cat died.
   My 9, 10, 6, 2 is an obscuring smudge.
   My 1, 11 is an abbreviation for that is.
   My whole is as little as it can get.

3. I am a word of 11 letters.
   My 4, 9, 5 is worn on the head.
   My 10, 9, 1, 11 is a narrow road.
   My 11, 2, 3, 4, 5 is a number.
   My 8, 6, 7 is a spirit.
   My whole is an excellent songster.

ANSWERS: 1. Camel, Main, ago; megalomaniac.
2. Cried, blur, i.e.; irreducible.
3. Hat, lane, eight, gin; nightingale.

The following three charades are by Hubert Phillips.

1

My first wears my second; my third might be
What my first would acquire if he went to sea.
Put together my one, two, three
And the belle of New York is the girl for me.

2

No hard decode. And, in this case,
A solid answer you can claim.
It has (I'm told) a different face
For every letter of its name.

3

Execration perhaps—though it seems very wrong
On request to the dog to oblige with a song.

ANSWERS

1. Manhattan.
2. Dodecahedron (a 12-sided solid; anagram of 'no hard decode').
3. Cur-sing.

A CENTURY OF CHARADES

William Bellamy's *Century of Charades*,* a book of an even hundred unsolved charade verses, appeared in 1894. It was followed a year later by another book, *Open Sesame*,† also in rhyme, which gave the solutions. But the second book was not by Mr. Bellamy—it was by Harland H. Ballard, whom Bellamy had never so much as laid eyes on.

I give three of the Bellamy charades below.

I

My first endured a hundred years,
    A progeny of logic and of wit;
My last the faro banker fears,
    King Solomon was not arrayed like it.
My whole, dear reader, you'll divine
    When you peruse this book of mine.

2

No longer for the Roman dame
    My second from my first is brought;
Where once the Roman legions fought
    No terror has the Roman name.
My whole is master of the soil,
And reaps in peace the fruits of toil.

3

A product of coniferous trees,
    A hardy toiler of the seas;
These make when joined and matched
    A Russian scratched.

I make this statement wholly on
The authority of Napoleon.

(ANSWERS OVERLEAF)

---

* Riverside Press, Cambridge, 1894.
† Colonial Press, Boston, 1895.

ANSWERS (by Ballard)

1

Have you heard of the wonderful 'one-hoss *shay*',
    That ran a century to a day,
Then stopped and shivered as if af*raid*?
    Aha! But I've answered the first *charade*.

2

No galleys now bring *myrrh* from *far*
    To stately dames of Rome;
Where Caesar drove his conquering car
    Now stands the *farmer*'s home.

3

Tar is the blood of pine trees, shed
    To save the gallant *tar*.
Napoleon had cause to dread
    The '*Tartars*' of the Tsar.

CHARISMA AT THE OCTAGONAL ROUND TABLE

When I to tell a Howler thirst,
I soften up my Hearers first,
And get them in a Laughing Mood,
For otherwise they might be Rude,
And say to Wait till after Lunch,
Or drown my Punch line in the Punch.
I offer to hang up their Hats,
Put out their Dogs and walk their Cats.
I pour Martinis in their Beers,
And tickle them behind the Ears.
And when I have that little band
Right in the Hollow of my Hand,
I spring my Masterpiece of Wit. . . .
They never see the point of it.

W. R. E.

My first last line for 'Charisma' read: 'and laugh until they think I'll split'. Was I wrong in substituting 'They never see the point of it'?

72

Chronograms

In the days when Roman numerals for the Year of Our Lord were more common than they are now, they were occasionally used in wordplay. XL, for instance, in sound is *excel*, in sense 'forty'. MIX is both *mix* and 1009. Holofernes is indulging in this sort of word game when he says in *Love's Labour's Lost*:

> If sore be sore, then L to sore makes fifty sores;
>   O sore L!
> Of one sore I an hundred make, by adding but one more L.

'This kind of wit,' Addison wrote in *The Spectator*, 'appears very often on modern medals, especially those of Germany, when they represent in the inscription the year in which they were coined. Thus we see on a medal of Gustavus Adolphus the following words—*'ChrIstVs DuX ergo triVMphVs'*. If you take the pains to pick the figures out of the several words and range them in their proper order, you will find they amount to MDCXVVVII, or 1627, the year in which the medal was stamped; for, as some of the letters distinguish themselves from the rest and overtop their fellows, they are to be considered in a double capacity, both as letters and as figures.'

It is said that Michael Stifelius, a Lutheran minister at Wirtemberg, predicted that the world would end on October 3, 1533, at ten o'clock. He had figured this out by analysing John xix, 37—'They shall look on Him whom they pierced.' The Latin of this is *Videbvnt In qvem transfixervnt*, which the good divine rendered *VIDebVnt In qVeM transfIXerVnt*, making MDXVVVVIII, or 1533. How he arrived at the day, month and hour is not revealed. At any event, that year, month, day, and hour did arrive, and as Stifelius was preaching to the congregation, a violent storm arose, convincing many that the prophecy was coming true. Fortunately for us, but perhaps unfortunately for Stifelius, the rage in the sky passed quickly, only to reappear in the hearts of the congregation, who dragged Stifelius from his pulpit and thrashed him.

One more note, and I think we shall have had enough of chronograms:

The death of Queen Elizabeth gave rise to the line
    'My Day Closed Is In Immortality'

The initial letters, in order, are MDCIII, or 1603, the year she died. A perfect chronogram, but I doubt whether by exhuming it I have resurrected the art.

Clerihews

Before the first world war, an English journalist named Edmund Clerihew Bentley developed the novel verse form which bears his middle name. A clerihew is an irreverent, unscanned rhyming quatrain upon a fanciful biographical theme, always beginning with the name of its subject. For instance:

> Sir James Jeans
> Always says what he means;
> He is really perfectly serious
> About the Universe being Mysterious.

The four men listed below are among the subjects of Mr. Bentley's sly attentions. Try writing your own clerihews about them; then compare your proficiency with Mr. Bentley's.

1. Alfred de Musset
2. George the Third

3. John Stuart Mill
4. Sir Christopher Wren

ANSWERS

1

Alfred de Musset
Used to call his cat Pusset.
His accent was affected.
This was to be expected.

2

George the Third
Ought never to have occurred.
One can only wonder
At so grotesque a blunder.

3

John Stuart Mill
By a mighty effort of will
Overcame his natural bonhomie
And wrote 'Principles of Practical Economy'.

4

Sir Christopher Wren
Said 'I am going to dine with some men.
If anyone calls
Say I am designing St. Paul's.'

Clichés, Platitudes and Proverbs

The other day a book reviewer wrote of a novelist: 'If she can think of a handy epithet that will do the work, she appropriates it, even if it *is* worn by time. Damsels are fair, waves are mountainous, doom imminent, chases merry, vows silent and people are in a brown study. Correspondence is regular, and is maintained, too; problems are turned over in the mind, rooms tastefully furnished; hope soars and death's breath is icy.'

He was having at the cliché, as common a target for erudite attack as the pun. 'A cliché,' says Partridge, 'is an outworn commonplace; a phrase (or virtual phrase) that has become so hackneyed that scrupulous speakers and writers shrink from it because they feel that its use is an insult to the intelligence of their auditor or audience, reader or public . . . They range from fly-blown phrases (*explore every avenue*) through soubriquets that have lost all point and freshness (*the Iron Duke*) to quotations that have become debased currency (*cups that cheer but do not inebriate*), metaphors that are now pointless, and formulas that have become mere counters (*far be it from me to . . .*).'

All very well. Yet Partridge's own 'fly-blown phrase' is next door to being a cliché. Not, perhaps, for the purposes of literature, but certainly for those of everyday intercourse, I suggest that the job is rather to be clear than to be brilliant. Clichés, for most of us, including fine writers, are like old clothes, useful for everyday, even if we hastily change when we see the rector approaching the house.

If there is a fault of language worse than a cliché, and I can think of several, it is a tortured effort to *avoid* a cliché. The results are less often funny than embarrassing. Most of us, in the first place, do not have the kind of facility that is required for verbal gymnastics; or, even if we have, we are not going to make the effort twenty-four hours a day, any more than the world's fastest runner is going to do hundred-yard sprints all day long. We are not so stupid.

Agreed that most clichés have long lost their lustre (if they are supposed to shine) or their cutting edge (if they are supposed to be sharp). Yet they have endured because no better statement of the case has come along. When one does, it will become a cliché in its turn.

The poem below is built around a series of proverbs so hackneyed that I suspect you will scarcely notice that key words are missing. But does that make the poem itself hackneyed? Bosh!

THE LADDY WHO LIVED BY THE BOOK

O sad is the story of Reginald Rory, a laddy who lived by the book;
If the longest way round was the ******** *** ****, why, the
longest way Reginald took.
No chickens he counted before they were *******, nor yet wasted
his tears on spilt ****,
Nor lopped with his shears at a lady pig's ears as a way to make
purses of ****.

His best monologue was 'Love me love my ***,' although once in
awhile he'd exclaim,
'It isn't the winning or ****** that counts, but the manner of
playing the ****.'
He ran the good **** and he fought the good *****, and he
thought an extremely good think;
He often led horses to *****, but never insisted they *****.

Well, all roads lead to **** as their ultimate home, and our
Reginald's led him there too;
And he well understood that in Rome it is good to do as the
good ****** **.
When he found they cohabit as fast as a rabbit, he resolved to
leave no stone ********
To match their example; he tried a free sample, and got himself
horribly burned.

Moral:
One *should* sometimes **** a gift horse in the *****, inasmuch as
to *** is but human.
He wouldn't have trusted a ***** bearing gifts, but he thought
the Greek girl was a Roman.

W. R. E.

ANSWER

Shortest way home; hatched; milk; silk; dog; losing; game; race; fight;
water; drink; Rome; Romans do; unturned; look; mouth; err; Greek.

THE CLICHÉ EXPERT TAKES THE STAND

The best evidence that the cliché is indestructible is that it has withstood even the assaults of Frank Sullivan, who all his life has been fouling clichés in their own nests and hoisting them by their own petards. For *The New Yorker* he created Mr. Arbuthnot, the cliché expert, who was regularly grilled in the pages of the magazine along the lines below.

Q. Mr. Arbuthnot, as an expert in the use of the cliché, are you prepared to testify here today regarding its application in topics of love, sex, matrimony and the like?

A. I am.

Q. Very good. Now, Mr. Arbuthnot, what's love?

A. Love is blind.

Q. Good. What does love do?

A. Love makes the world go round.

Q. Whom does a young man fall in love with?

A. With the Only Girl in the World.

Q. They are then said to be?

A. Victims of Cupid's darts.

Q. And he?

A. Whispers sweet nothings in her ear.

Q. Describe the Only Girl in the World.

A. Her eyes are like stars. Her teeth are like pearls. Her lips are ruby. Her cheek is damask, and her form divine.

Q. Haven't you forgotten something?

A. Eyes, teeth, lips, cheek, form—no, sir, I don't think so.

Q. Her hair?

A. Oh, certainly. How stupid of me. She has hair like spun gold.

Q. Very good, Mr. Arbuthnot. Now will you describe the Only Man?

A. He is a blond Viking, a he-man, and a square-shooter who plays the game. There is something about him that rings true, and he has kept himself pure and clean so that when he meets the girl of his choice, the future mother of his children, he can look her in the eye.

Q. How?

A. Without flinching.

Q. Now, Mr. Arbuthnot, when the Only Man falls in love, madly, with the Only Girl, what does he do?

A. He walks on air.

Q. Yes, I know, but what is it he pops?

A. Oh, excuse me. The question, of course.

Q. Than what do they plight?

A. Their troth.

Q. Mr. Arbuthnot, your explanation of the correct application of the cliché in these matters has been most instructive, and I know that all of us cliché-users here will know exactly how to respond hereafter when, during a conversation, sex—when sex—ah—

A. I think what you want to say is 'When sex rears its ugly head', isn't it?

Q. Thank you, Mr. Arbuthnot. Thank you very much.

A. Thank *you.*

Cockney

FRAMED IN A FIRST-STOREY WINDER

Framed in a first-storey winder of a burnin' buildin'
Appeared: A Yuman Ead!

Jump into this net, wot we are 'oldin'
And yule be quite orl right!

But 'ee wouldn't jump . . .
And the flames grew Igher and Igher and Igher.
(Phew!)

Framed in a second-storey winder of a burnin' buildin'
Appeared: A Yuman Ead!

Jump into this net, wot we are 'oldin'
And yule be quite orl right!

But 'ee wouldn't jump . . .
And the flames grew Igher and Igher and Igher
(Strewth!)

Framed in a third-storey winder of a burnin' buildin'
Appeared: A Yuman Ead!

Jump into this net wot we are 'oldin'
And yule be quite orl right!
Honest!

And 'ee jumped . . .
And 'ee broke 'is bloomin' neck!

Anonymous

EPITAPH ON A MARF

Wot a marf 'e'd got,
Wot a marf.
When 'e was a kid,
Goo' Lor' luv'll
'Is pore old muvver
Must 'a' fed 'im wiv a shuvvle.

Wot a gap 'e'd got,
Pore chap,
'E'd never been known to larf,
'Cos if 'e did
It's a penny to a quid
'E'd 'a' split 'is face in 'arf.

Anonymous

RHYMING SLANG

In my childhood, 'See you later alligator' was considered the height of wit. If we had thought to condense the expression to plain 'alligator', we should have been using something like rhyming slang.

In this light-hearted Cockney locution, the speaker substitutes a rhyming word or phrase for the one that is meant. 'Fire' becomes 'Anna Mariah'; 'stairs', 'apples and pears'; 'tram', 'baa-lamb'; 'ticket', 'bat and wicket', and so on. To make matters still more difficult for the uninitiated, the rhyming expressions are often condensed, so that the rhyme itself disappears. Thus, a man may say, 'You'd 'ardly Adam it; 'is trouble's going to have another Gawdfer.' Here 'Adam' is short for 'Adam and Eve', 'trouble' for 'trouble and strife', and 'Gawdfer' for 'God forbid'. The intended words are 'believe', 'wife', and 'kid'. In 'Shut yer north, yer a Dunlop', further complications are introduced: 'North' is the opposite of 'south', which rhymes with 'mouth'; 'Dunlop' is a kind of tyre, which rhymes with 'liar'. So: 'Shut your mouth, you're a liar.'

Rhyming slang was developed by London pickpockets and vagabonds in the nineteenth century to outwit the police. The following examples are from the book *Up the Frog*, by Sydney ('Steak') T. Kendall.

1. Up the *apples and pears* to *lemon squash* me *Ramsgate Sands*.
2. D'yer want any *fisherman's daughter* wiv yer *pimple and blotch*?
3. 'E's only got one *mince pie* and 'e's as *Mutt an' Jeff* as anyfink.
4. I've got to take the *cock sparrer* up the *Dolly Varden* fer some *rosebuds*.
5. Shove this *saucepan lid* in your *sky rocket*.

(The shorthand versions of the foregoing expressions would be considerably more difficult to translate. They are: 1. Up the apples to lemon me Ramsgates; 2. D'yer want any fisherman's wiv yer pimple?; 3. 'E's only got one mince and 'e's mutt'n as anyfink; 4. I've got to take the cock sparrer up the Dolly for some roses; and, 5. Shove this saucepan in yer sky.)

ANSWERS

1. Upstairs to wash my hands.
2. Do you want any water with your Scotch?
3. He's only got one eye and he's as deaf as anything.
4. I have to take the barrow up to Covent Garden for some potatoes (spuds).
5. Shove this quid in your pocket.

UP THE FROG

I was taking the cherry 'og for a ball o' chalk up the frog and toad the other night, when I met a China plate o' mine. We 'ad a few dicky birds an' then 'e suggested we 'ad a tumble dahn the sink together.

Well, instead of going into the Red Lion, we went into the first rub-a-dub we comes to. I sez 'what are you going to 'ave?' 'E sez, 'I'll 'ave a drop o' pig's ear,' so I gets a pint o' pig's ear for 'im an' I 'ad a drop of needle and pin, just for a start.

We got chatting an' one fing led to anuvver when we 'ears the Guv'nor calling 'Time, gents please!'

I could 'ardly Adam and Eve it that we 'ad bin at it so long. So I gets an Aristotle of In-and-out for the plates and dishes, picks up the cherry 'og an' orf we Scarpa Flow.

As it's so 'Arry Tate I gets on a trouble an' fuss, an' when I gets 'ome, I find the plates 'n' dishes is out 'avin' a butcher's 'ook round the rub-a-dubs for me and the cherry 'og. So I gets up the apples and pears an' into the ol' Uncle Ned and when she comes in, there I am wiv me loaf o' bread on the weeping willow, readin' the linen draper. She starts a few early birds but I don't want no bull and cow, so I turns over an' in a couple o' cock linnets I'm Bo-Peep.

Sydney T. Kendall

ANSWER

I was taking the dog for a walk up the road the other night, when I met a mate of mine. We had a few words and then he suggested we had a drink together.

Well, instead of going into the Red Lion, we went into the first pub we came to.

I said, 'What are you going to have?' He said, 'I'll have a drop of beer,' so I got a pint of beer for him and I had a drop of gin, for a start.

We got chatting and one thing led to another, when we hear the landlord calling, 'Time, Gents, please!'

I could hardly believe that we had been at it for so long, so I got a bottle of stout for the missus, picked up the dog and off we go.

As it's so late I got on a bus and when I got home, I found the missus is out having a look round the pubs for me and the dog. So I got upstairs and into bed, and when she came in, there I was with my head on the pillow, reading the paper.

She started having a few words but I didn't want a row, so I turned over, and in a couple of minutes I was asleep.

Colourful Words

The opening letters of each of the words defined below spell a colour, which may or may not have anything to do with the meaning of the whole word.

1. A disease
2. A flower
3. A goblin
4. An insect
5. A keep
6. Lessen
7. An old man
8. Used in school
9. A weapon

ANSWERS

1. Pinkeye
2. Bluebell
3. Brownie
4. Bluebottle
5. Dungeon
6. Reduce
7. Greybeard
8. Blackboard
9. Bayonet

Controlling the Language Explosion

I have an acquaintance who is writing quite an important paper on the threat of unbridled population growth, which he calls 'pollulution': very clever, and I can see why he finds the word irresistible. But are all these new words really necessary?

Why do so many people worry about the population explosion, and so few about the language explosion? Words, like people, when they multiply too fast, crowd into slums, lose their innocence in the hour of their birth, and decay before they have time to mature. Charles W. Ferguson points out that Dr. Samuel Johnson's *Dictionary*, published in 1755, contained but 58,000 words; Noah Webster's, in 1828, offered 70,000; and the current Webster's *Unabridged* carries well over 600,000, with another 400,000 technical terms waiting in the wings. Professor Albert H. Marckwardt of the University of Michigan adds that the next two centuries may see an increase of the total English vocabulary to more than two million words.

There is probably no author in the language from whose works, however voluminous, as many as 10,000 words could be collected. Few of us use as many as 5000 in conversation. Our dictionaries are bulked out with words that are useless save to the specialist, and not always to him. As Bombaugh remarks, 'What man in his senses would use zythepsary for a brewhouse, and zymologist for a brewer; would talk of a stormy day as procellous and himself as madefied; of his long-legged son as increasing in procerity but sadly marcid; of having met with such procacity from such a one; of a bore as a macrologist; of an aged horse as macrobiotic; of important business as moliminous, and his daughter's necklace as moniliform; of some one's talk as meracious, and lament his last night's nimiety of wine at that dapatical feast, whence he was taken by ereption?'

The language explosion has become ridiculous. I suggest an end to sentimentality. Let us begin throwing unwanted words out into the snow to perish, as the Spartans did with their girl babies.

Better still, let us carry out a verbal vasectomy on all writers, excepting only two or three dozen selected poets. I should be tempted to include even them, but the ones I have excepted are long dead.

Crossing Jokes

David Frost, the television interviewer, has a speciality called 'crossing jokes'. He puts two names together to get a third. If you can solve the crossing jokes below, he may invite you to appear on his programme. Then again he may not. Anyhow, here are the three jokes.

1. Cross a cowboy with a gourmet and you get a . . .
2. Cross Jimmy Durante with an employment agency and you get a . . .
3. Cross a zebra with an ape-man and you get . . .

ANSWERS: 1. Hopalong Casserole. 2. Nose job.
3. Tarzan Stripes Forever.

Cryptograms

A cryptogram being merely a coded message, it can scarcely be considered a literary form; a sonnet would have to be written in the clear before it could be encoded. Still, cryptograms do pop up in books and stories, especially when international hanky-panky is involved. The following substitution cipher is from Poe's *The Gold-Bug*:

'53##+305))6*;4826)4#.)4#);806*;48+8%60))85;1#(;:#*8+83(88)5*+;46(;88*96*?;8)*#(;485);5*+2:*#(;4956*2(5*—4)8%8*;4069285);)6+8)4##;1(#9;48081;8;8#1;48+85;4)485+528806*81(#9;48;(88;4(#?34;48)4#;161;:188;#?;'

William LeGrand, who solved the cryptogram in Poe's story, started with the knowledge that by far the most common letter in English is e, followed in order, as he thought, by a o i d h n r s t u y c f g l m w b k p q x z. (*The World Book Encyclopaedia* agrees on the primacy of e, but puts the other letters in quite a different order: t r i n o a s d l c h f u p m y g w v b x k q j z. Poe forgot the letters j and v altogether.)

The most common character in the cryptogram was 8, which appeared thirty-three times. LeGrand therefore concluded that 8 represented e.* He next listed each set of three characters ending in 8. The most frequent of these trios was ;48. LeGrand assumed that these represented the word 'the.' He now had three of his letters—e, t, and h—as well as an indication of the beginning and end of several words. Continuing in this fashion, he soon arrived at his solution. I trust that you, building on the clues already given (and bearing in mind that Poe treats #), +1, 92, :3 and—. as single characters) can do as well. In any event, you will find the solution on the next page.

Morse code is a form of cryptogram; so is journalistic cable-ese; so is shorthand. Francis Bacon developed a substitution cipher in which each letter of the alphabet is represented by five letters, each of which is either a or b. Thus the letter a becomes aaaaa; b, aaaab; c, aaaba; and so on. You can attain the same result by substituting for a and b a long and short straw, a circle and triangle, or any other symbol you find convenient.

In a substitution cipher the letters of the message remain in their proper order. In a transposition cipher they are rearranged.

---

* If the man who wrote the puzzle had held down his e's deliberately, or even omitted them, as in a lipogram, the solution would have been more difficult, though far from impossible.

There is nothing to prevent the cryptogrammer from employing both transposition and substitution in the same code, or piling one substitution on another. For me, however, the most elementary substitution code is quite difficult enough to riddle. The expert will solve these two at a glance:

1. NW SHQW EVHOWP OSHUBWR YA STBS WDEVYRTQW LJPWU WQWUC YJW YA KSW GUTPBWR VWHPTJB AUYI KSW KYNJ NSWJ NW UWOWTQW NYUP AUYI CYL NW NTVV GVYN KSWI LE HJP KSLR TRYVHKW KSW OTKC AYU ALKLUW IWRRHBWR NW NTVV LRW KSW JWN OYPW.

2. BAY BQ WKY XOHMYHV KYHY RV GCRWY O LBBM VBHW BQ QYIIBX R OT VCHY WKOW KY XRII KYIU TY WB YVNOUY RQ R NOA LHYOVY KRV UOIT XRWK QRQWE GCRM RQ EBC NOA HORVY WKY NOVK IYW TY JABX OAM R VKOII OHHOALY QBH KRT WB LYW RW QHBT EBC.

ANSWERS

The '*Gold-Bug*' cryptogram reads:

'A good glass in the bishop's hostel in the devil's seat forty-one degrees and thirteen minutes northeast and by north main branch seventh limb east side shoot from the left eye of the death's-head a bee-line from the tree through the shot fifty feet out.'

I am aware that the solution may appear almost as impenetrable as the cryptogram. For clarification, and considerable entertainment, I suggest that you re-read *The Gold-Bug*.

As for the other cryptograms (taken from *One Hundred Problems in Cipher*, by Louis C. Mansfield), here are the messages conveyed:

1. We have placed charges of high explosive under every one of the bridges leading from the town. When we receive word from you we will blow them up and thus isolate the city. For future messages we will use the new code.

2. One of the warders here is quite a good sort of fellow. I am sure that he will help me to escape if I can grease his palm with fifty quid. If you can raise the cash, let me know, and I shall arrange for him to get it from you.

Cumulative Verses

In the days when most American newspapers had 'funny' departments, it was not uncommon for one paper to print a few lines built around printers' marks, to which other papers would add. For instance:

THE ARAB AND HIS DONKEY

An Arab came to the river side,
    With a donkey bearing an †;
But he would not try to ford the tide,
    For he had too good an *.
            Boston Globe

So he camped all night by the river side,
    And remained till the tide had ceased to swell,
For he knew should the donkey from life subside,
    He never would find its ‖.
        Salem Sunbeam

When the morning dawned, and the tide was out,
    The pair crossed over 'neath Allah's protection
And the Arab was happy, we have no doubt,
    For he had the best donkey in all that §.
            Somerville Journal

You are wrong, they were drowned in crossing over,
    Though the donkey was bravest of all his race;
He luxuriates now in horse-heaven clover
    And his master has gone to the Prophet's *em* ⌒.
            Elevated Railway Journal

These asinine poets deserve to be 'blowed',
    Their rhymes being faulty, and frothy and beery;
What really befell the ass and its load
    Will ever remain a desolate ?
        Paper and Print

Our Yankee friends, with all their ——
    For once, we guess, their mark have missed;
And with poetry *Paper and Print* is rash
    In damming its flow with it's editor's ☞

In parable and moral leave a # between
    For reflection, or your wits fall out of joint;
The 'Arab', ye see, is a printing machine,
    And the donkey is he who can't see the .
                British and Colonial Printer

For those unfamiliar with the ways of proof-readers, † is an obelisk; * is an asterisk; ‖, parallel; §, section; ⌒, brace, bring together; ?, query; ——, dash; ☞, fist; #, space, put a space between; and . , of course, full point.

D

Defiant Definitions

Name each of the words defined here. The words are given below.

1. A fraudulent abstraction of money.
2. Ornamental open work in fine gold or silver wire.
3. The camelopard.
4. To put to death by fixing on a stake.
5. A minute parasitic fungus that causes decay in vegetable matter.
6. To withdraw from a purpose.
7. A buttery.
8. An elevated, broad, flat area of land.
9. Easily rubbed down, crumbled, or pulverised.
10. The forepart of a ship.
11. To compose or write; to direct or dictate.

12. To charge with a crime or misdemeanour in due form of law.
13. State appointed or predetermined; fate, invincible necessity.
14. To talk familiarly.
15. To arise or come; to be added.
16. An absurd story; a false rumour.
17. Sending out a flood of light; gleaming; splendid.
18. An Egyptian peasant
19. Vast grassy plains in South America.
20. A person with full power to act for another.

ANSWERS

1. Defalcation	11. Indite
2. Filigree	12. Indict
3. Giraffe	13. Destiny
4. Impale	14. Confabulate
5. Mildew	15. Accrue
6. Resile	16. Canard
7. Pantry	17. Effulgent
8. Plateau	18. Fellah
9. Friable	19. Llanos or pampas
10. Prow	20. Plenipotentiary

Disemvowelled Proverbs

In each of the following lines, insert the same vowel the number of times indicated to restore a proverb.

1. ASTTCHNTMESAVESNNE (4).
2. ABRDNTHEHANDSWORTHTWONTHEBUSH (4).
3. GFURTHERDWRSE (3).
4. ERLYTOBEDNDERLYTORISEMKESMNHELTHYWE
   LTHYNDWISE (9).
5. BTTRLATTHANNVR (5).
6. ALLSWLLTHATNDSWLL (3).

ANSWERS

1. A stitch in time saves nine. 2. A bird in the hand is worth two in the bush. 3. Go further, do worse. 4. Early to bed and early to rise makes a man healthy, wealthy and wise. 5. Better late than never. 6. All's well that ends well.

Double-entendres

W. H. Auden recently noted that Miss Rose Fyleman, a child's author, best known for her *There Are Fairies at the Bottom of My Garden*, is responsible for such bemusingly innocent *double-entendres* as:

> There are no wolves in England any more;
> The fairies have driven them all away

and

> My fairy muff is made of pussy-willow

and

> The best thing the fairies do, the best thing of all
> Is sliding down steeples—you know they're very tall.
> Climb up the weather-cock, and, when you hear it crow,
> Fold your wings, and clutch your things, and then—
> Let go!

Dutch Widows, Irish Beauties, Scotch Warming-pans

Do you recall how, in 1968, the Republican candidate for the Vice-Presidency of the United States was roundly scolded by the Press for referring to a newsman of Japanese background as a 'fat Jap'? The furore reflected the increased sensitivity of English-speaking people to the feelings of persons belonging to alien or minority groups. We may tell it like it is in matters of sex and defaecation, but increasingly we withdraw the savour from the salt in describing those who differ from ourselves in appearance, accent or background. This inhibition is, as President Hoover said of Prohibition, an experiment noble in purpose; but it may not be altogether a good thing.

Language reflects attitudes. At their lowest ebb, members of a despised group pay little attention to the epithets used to describe them; they are too busy staying alive. As they make their inevitable way into the mainstream, however, they become self-conscious, and ask for relief from terms that remind them of their earlier state. Once they are completely accepted by society, the whole thing becomes a joke; the president of a department store chain no longer rages when called a Mick, but chuckles.

If members of any minority or outside group object to what they are called, I am all for changing the epithet to whatever they prefer. No epithet, however, can be dissociated from its unspoken meaning to the one who says it and the one who hears it.

According to H. L. Mencken in *American Language*:

One may say *Chinese*, but not *Chinaman*, *Chink*, or *Chinee*; *German*, but not *squarehead*, *boche*, *heinie*, *hun*, *kraut*, or *sausage*; *Hungarian* or *Bohemian*, but not *Hunky* or *Bohunk*; *Japanese*, but not *Jap* or *Nip*; *Korean*, but not *gook*; *Vietnamese*, but not *geek*; *Greek*, but not *greaseball*. Nor may one call an East Indian by our fathers' epithet, *wog*, acronym for 'wily oriental gentleman'.

You are not to call a Frenchman a *frog*, nor to refer to *French leave*, the *French pox* (syphilis), or a *French letter* (condom). (The French, for their part, have the effrontery to call a condom a *capote anglaise*. They also call lice *Spaniards* and fleas *female Spaniards*. The Prussians, in turn, call lice *Frenchmen*, while other Germans call cockroaches *Prussians*.)

Ever since the seventeenth-century naval rivalry between the Dutch and the English, the English have used 'Dutch' as an epithet of derision. Under today's rules, though, one must drop all reference to *in Dutch* (in trouble); a *Dutch widow* (prostitute); a *Dutch bargain* (made in one's cups); *Dutch courage* (produced by alcohol); a *Dutch treat* (where each pays for himself); a *Dutch wife* (bolster); and *Dutch comfort* (no comfort at all).

Just dropping Irish pejoratives will leave a deep hole in your vocabulary. Farewell to *mick, harp, flannel mouth, biddy*! Never again can you call a woman with two black eyes an *Irish beauty*; or perjury *Irish evidence*; or a spade an *Irish spoon*; or thick legs *Irish legs*; or a police station an *Irish clubhouse*; or a demotion an *Irish rise*; or a fast an *Irishman's dinner*; or a wheelbarrow an *Irish chariot* ('the greatest of human inventions, since it taught the Irish to walk on their hind legs').

Who today would dare call an Italian a *guinea*, a *Tony*, or a *wop* (from *guappo*, a Neapolitan term for a showy, pretentious fellow)? Who would call a Mexican a *greaser*, or a Panamanian a *spick* ('No spik Inglis')?

Then there are the Jews. No longer is a *kike* a Jew who has left the room. No longer may one assert social superiority by referring to *yids*, *sheenies*, or *mockies*. No longer dare we 'jew the man down' when we are persuading him to reduce his asking price. Efforts have even been made to turn the humble *jews harp* into a *jaws harp*.

It is closed season on the Scots, too. That they allegedly do not like being called Scotch did not, until recently, prevent our referring to the itch as the *Scotch fiddle*; a loose girl as a *Scotch warming-pan*; hot water flavoured with burnt biscuit as *Scotch coffee*; or a two-quart bottle as a *Scotch pint*. To the English, Scotland was *Itchland, Scratchland*, or *Louseland*. Never more!

The Negroes in the United States are a special case. In the early nineteenth century, they were called *blacks* (as, in a curious historical echo, many wish to be called today); later, *Africans*; still later, *darkies* (not invidiously at the start); then briefly, and by very few, *Africo-Americans*; still more briefly, following the Civil War, *freedmen*; in the 1880s, as again today, *Afro-Americans*. There was an effort, now largely abandoned, to break them down into *mulattos* (halfbreeds), *quadroons* (quarter-breeds), and *octaroons* (eighth-breeds). They were also called *coons, shines, smokes, dinges, boogies, eightballs, jazzbos, jigaboos, snowballs, spades, jigs,* and *crows*.

Because of its association of contempt, blacks particularly hate the word *nigger*. Such once-common expressions as *nigger heaven* and *nigger in the woodpile* are now unmentionable.

Curiously, as some derogatory terms go on the Forbidden Index, others emerge. The G.I. in Vietnam, for instance, has become a *grunt*. To young demonstrators, police are *pigs*. Militant blacks call whites *ofay*, perhaps Pig Latin for 'foe'.

E

Echoing Words

Echoism and onomatopoeia mean the same thing—the formation of words by imitation of sounds, as in the *hiss* of a goose or the *click* of a camera. There once was a conjecture, called variously the 'bow wow theory', the 'pooh pooh theory', and the 'ding dong theory', that sounds from nature played a major part in the origin and growth of language; but no-one seems to take much stock in that notion any more.

Except when combined with other devices, onomatopoeia plays a rather trivial role in literature. An example of sorts is Shakespeare's

> Hark, hark!
>   Bow-wow.
> The watch-dogs bark!
>   Bow-wow.
> Hark, hark! I hear
> The strain of strutting chanticleer
> Cry 'Cock-a-doodle-doo!'

Here, *bark*, *bow-wow*, and *cock-a-doodle-doo* are onomatopoeic words, while *hark* reinforces *bark*. There are many other words whose sounds suggest their thrust; it has been pointed out, for instance, that in *flicker*, the *fl* suggests moving light, the *i* suggests smallness, the *ck* suggests sudden cessation of movement (as in *crack*, *peck*, *pick*, *hack*, and *flick*), and the *er* suggests repetition.

In each line below I have left out an onomatopoeic word. Using the clues (which are in no particular order) guess the missing words. (It may help to know that the second and fourth lines of each stanza rhyme.)

> 1
> *****, whip!
> Train, *****!
> ***, horse!
> ****-****!

> 2
> Brook, ******!
> Fountain, ******!
> *******, faucet!
> ****, wash!

92

3

****, saw!
*****, glue!
****, train!
****-****!

4

***, sheep!
***, cow!
*****, frog!
(***-***!)

5

Bell, ****,
****-****!
(Gun: ****!
End of song.)

To solve the puzzle, look first for the sounds associated with: a bee (though there is no bee in the verse), a dog, a starting steam train, the train after starting, a gun, a sheep, a whip, a cow, a frog, a bell (two variants). Among the other onomatopoeias, one means a series of short, inarticulate, speechlike sounds (a verb here); another is a light, clear, metallic note; and a third is the cry of an owl. It is useful to remember that the same sound may have more than one source.

Of the words whose sounds somehow suggest their meaning, one means to pant; one, to dash water about; one, to adhere; one, to let drops of liquid fall; one, to run at a slow, steady trot; one, to drop in a thin, gentle stream.

ANSWERS:

1	3	5
Crack, whip!	Buzz, saw!	Bell, ring,
Train, chuff!	Stick, glue!	Ding-dong!
Jog, horse!	Hoot, train!	(Gun: BANG!
Puff-puff!	Choo-choo!	End of song.)

2	4
Brook, babble!	Baa, sheep!
Fountain, splash!	Moo, cow!
Trickle, faucet!	Croak, frog!
Drip, wash!	(Bow-wow!)

ECHOING TRIOLET

O, let me try a triolet!
  O, let me try! O, let me try
A triolet to win my pet!
  O, let me try a triolet,
And if the triolet's all wet,
  I'll try a letter on the sly.
O, let me try a triolet!
  O, let me try! O, let me try!

W. R. E.

*

THE ELEPHANT, OR THE FORCE OF HABIT

A tail behind, a trunk in front,
Complete the usual elephant.
The tail in front, the trunk behind,
Is what you very seldom find.

If you for specimens should hunt
With trunks behind and tails in front,
The hunt would occupy you long;
The force of habit is so strong.

A. E. Housman

*

Epigrams

An epigram is a brief comment, often in rhyme, which closes
with a sudden surprising or witty turn. A Latin poet laid down
its criteria as follows:

The qualities rare in a bee that we meet,
In an epigram never should fail.
The body should always be little and sweet,
And a sting should be left in the tail.

94

Coleridge's definition was more succinct:

> What is an epigram? A dwarfish whole,
> Its body brevity, and wit its soul.

Alexander Pope's best-remembered verse consists of such epigrammatic couplets as

> Why has not man a microscopic eye?
> For this plain reason—man is not a fly.

and

> Vice is a monster of so frightful mien
> As, to be hated, needs but to be seen;
> Yet seen too oft, familiar with her face,
> We first endure, then pity, then embrace.

Lord Rochester wrote this premature epigram-epitaph for King Charles II:

> Here lies our sovereign lord, the King,
> Whose promise none relies on;
> He never said a foolish thing,
> Nor ever did a wise one.

To which the witty monarch rejoined:

'My words are my own, and my actions are my ministers'.'

Some of the best-known modern epigrams are by Hilaire Belloc:

On Lady Poltagrue, a Public Peril

The Devil, having nothing else to do,
Went off to tempt My Lady Poltagrue.
My Lady, tempted by a private whim,
To his extreme annoyance, tempted him.

On a Dead Hostess

Of this bad world the loveliest and the best
Has smiled and said 'Good Night', and gone to rest.

On His Books

When I am dead, I hope it may be said:
'His sins were scarlet, but his books were read.'

Oscar Wilde's epigrams shocked and titillated late Victorian society. "I can resist everything,' he said solemnly, 'except temptation.' Fox-hunting he described as 'the unspeakable in full pursuit of the uneatable'.

Some Wilde epigrams have been scrambled below. Put the words back in order, and then check to see if you are right.

1. Seriously to talk important is ever a far thing about life too.
2. Charming and good people are absurd. To divide either into tedious or bad people is it.
3. Us we are are in at but all some the the stars gutter looking of.
4. The one play cards one winning has always fairly when should.
5. In a sense romance spoils a woman as so much the humour of nothing.
6. To be sure truth tells one later or if one is out the sooner found.
7. The mistakes are never regrets only one's one thing.
8. The nothing knows of everything and the price value of a man who is a cynic.

ANSWERS

1. Life is far too important a thing ever to talk seriously about.
2. It is absurd to divide people into good and bad. People are either charming or tedious.
3. We are all in the gutter, but some of us are looking at the stars.
4. One should always play fairly when one has the winning cards.
5. Nothing spoils a romance so much as a sense of humour in the woman.
6. If one tells the truth, one is sure, sooner or later, to be found out.
7. The only things one never regrets are one's mistakes.
8. A cynic is a man who knows the price of everything, and the value of nothing.

MACAULAY TELLS US

Macaulay tells us Byron's rules of life
Were: Hate your neighbour; love your neighbour's wife.

W. R. E.

ON AN AGEING PRUDE

She who, when young and fair,
Would wink men up the stair,
Now, old and ugly, locks
The door where no man knocks.

W. R. E.

Epitaphs

Laughter is as useful a weapon against death as any other, which is why some of the funniest lines around are on gravestones. The following epitaphs appear in various collections.

POOR MARTHA SNELL
HER'S GONE AWAY
HER WOULD IF HER COULD
BUT HER COULDN'T STAY;
HER HAD TWO SWOLN LEGS
AND A BADDISH COUGH
BUT HER LEGS IT WAS
AS CARRIED HER OFF

HERE LIES A FATHER OF 29:
THERE WOULD HAVE BEEN MORE
BUT HE DIDN'T HAVE TIME

Dorothy Parker, the wit, proposed for her gravestone the line:

THIS IS ON ME

or, as an alternative,

EXCUSE MY DUST

There is a spurious smell about this inscription, supposedly from a hypochondriac's tombstone:

I TOLD YOU I WAS SICK

This epitaph for a waiter, too, is doubtless apocryphal:

GOD FINALLY CAUGHT HIS EYE

97

Occasionally the inscriptions prepared by a surviving spouse reflect something less than utter despair. A French example sets the tone:

CI-GIT MA FEMME, AH! QU'ELLE EST BIEN
POUR SON REPOS ET POUR LE MIEN

Similar sentiments of relief have appeared in English:

HERE LIES MY WIFE
IN EARTHY MOULD
WHO WHEN SHE LIVED
DID NAUGHT BUT SCOLD:
GOOD FRIENDS GO SOFTLY
IN YOUR WALKING
LEST SHE SHOULD WAKE
AND RISE UP TALKING

ELIZA ANN
HAS GONE TO REST;
SHE NOW RECLINES
ON ABRAHAM'S BREAST;
PEACE AT LAST FOR ELIZA ANN
BUT NOT FOR
FATHER ABRAHAM

Mourners frequently punned on the name of the late lamented, thus:

On a spinster, Miss Mann:

HERE LIES ANN MANN;
SHE LIVED AN OLD MAID
BUT DIED AN OLD MANN

On Jonathan Fiddle:

ON THE 22ND OF JUNE
JONATHAN FIDDLE
WENT OUT OF TUNE

A gravestone makes an enduring billboard:

SACRED TO THE REMAINS OF
JONATHAN THOMPSON
A PIOUS CHRISTIAN AND
AFFECTIONATE HUSBAND
. . .
HIS DISCONSOLATE WIDOW
CONTINUES TO CARRY ON
HIS GROCERY BUSINESS
AT THE OLD STAND ON
MAIN STREET; CHEAPEST
AND BEST PRICES IN TOWN

It would be a shame if all tombstones tried to be funny, or even if they were funny inadvertently. The following, one of my favourites, has a touch of humour, but it is a gentle touch, done by a gentle soul:

HERE LIE I
MARTIN ELGINBRODDE:
HAE MERCY O' MY SOUL
LORD GOD
AS I WAD SO
WERE I LORD GOD
AND YE WERE
MARTIN ELGINBRODDE

On Sir John Vanbrugh, Architect
Under this stone, reader, survey
Dear Sir John Vanbrugh's house of clay.
Lie heavy on him, earth! for he
Laid many heavy loads on thee.

Abel Evans

On Frank Pixley, Editor
Here lies Frank Pixley, as usual.

Ambrose Bierce

Equivocally Speaking

LOVE LETTER

An odd art indeed is 'Equivoque'—the creation of passages which may have quite opposite meanings, according to how you read them. If, after you have read the following letter straight, you go back over it, confining your attention to the odd-numbered lines, you will find that L—— is not really so annoyed with Miss M—— as he makes out to be.

To Miss M——

—The great love I have hitherto expressed for you
   is false and I find my indifference towards you
—increases daily. The more I see of you, the more
   you appear in my eyes an object of contempt.
—I feel myself every way disposed and determined
   to hate you. Believe me, I never had an intention
—to offer you my hand. Our last conversation has
   left a tedious insipidity, which has by no means
—given me the most exalted idea of your character.
   Your temper would make me extremely unhappy
—and were we united, I should experience nothing but
   the hatred of my parents added to the anything but
—pleasure in living with you. I have indeed a heart
   to bestow, but I do not wish you to imagine it
—at your service. I could not give it to any one more
   inconsistent and capricious than yourself, and less
—capable to do honour to my choice and to my family.
   Yes, Miss, I hope you will be persuaded that
—I speak sincerely, and you will do me a favour
   to avoid me. I shall excuse you taking the trouble
—to answer this. Your letters are always full of
   impertinence, and you have not a shadow of
—wit and good sense. Adieu! adieu! believe me
   so averse to you, that it is impossible for me even
—to be your most affectionate friend and humble servant.

L——

Espy's Fables

KING CARTH AND THE SUFFRTTE

Insert 'age' a hundred and some times in the passage below, and you will have the story.

I wr you are unaware that in one of the bygone s, there lived in a remote vill called Anchor a haughty suffrtte who much dispard all men, as if they were a menrie of uncd beasts. Yet she was the object of their er hom; for her vis was fair as the sun, and her cleav far from mer; she mand her men competently, and the meals she prepared were a tasty assembl of cabb, sauss, bls, from, pot, vint wines, and lr beer.

Now, Anchor was under the patron of King Carth of Carth, a Plantnet of ancient line, who by the lever of a few gold coins persuaded the girl's cy parents to pledge her to him in marri— for them an advantous match indeed, since Carth was known as a s and courous ruler.

During the engment, Carth brought her each day ps and ps of ardent ads, together with numerous corss, arriving before her cott at the reins of a mnta carri drawn by six milk-white onrs.

But the suffrtte was in a r; for Carth by this time was so d that he was in his dot. As he descended from the carri she would seize his onr-whip, shout 'Carth must be destroyed!' into his deaf ear, and flllate the poor old man savly. Nor could her umbr be assud. 'So you think I'll sell my herit for a mess of pott?' she would shout. 'Not I! I'll sabot this marri! I'll rav and pill your castle! I'll send you out to for for sil like an onr, and I'll take the reins of the carri myself!'

The king, unable to hear what she was saying, considered her comments only amusing persifl; but not so his entour. To them, the suffrtte's conduct had hopelessly damd her im. 'The bagg treats him like garb, nay, like sew!' they told one another. 'This press no good!'

They determined to salv the situation by taking advant of the girl's desire to drive onrs. To set the st, they camoufld their nts as milk-white onrs and, hitching them to the mnta carri, they invited the haughty suffrtte to take the reins. The onrs promptly broke from control and rampd across the till onto the pl, where the carri shattered in the deep sand. The carn was outrous. The suffrtte's bones, hair, and cartils were scattered about like spaghetti. She died of a haemorrh in the wreck, unmourned; no-one even bothered to apply a band.

The moral: If you have it on your nda to rav and pill Carth, first make sure your onrs are really asses.

ANSWER

I wager you are unaware that in one of the bygone ages, there lived in a remote village called Anchorage a haughty suffragette who much disparaged all men, as if they were a menagerie of uncaged beasts. Yet she was the object of their eager homage; for her visage was fair as the sun, and her cleavage far from meager (U.S.); she managed her menage competently, and the meals she prepared were a tasty assemblage of cabbage, sausages, bagels, fromage, potage, vintage wines, and lager beer.

Now, Anchorage was under the patronage of King Carthage of Carthage, a Plantagenet of ancient lineage, who by the leverage of a few gold coins persuaded the girl's cagey parents to pledge her to him in marriage —for them an advantageous match indeed, since Carthage was known as a sage and courageous ruler.

During the engagement, Carthage brought her each day pages and pages of ardent adages, together with numerous corsages, arriving before her cottage at the reins of a magenta carriage drawn by six milk-white onagers.

But the suffragette was in a rage; for Carthage by this time was so aged that he was in his dotage. As he descended from the carriage she would seize his onager-whip, shout 'Carthage must be destroyed!' into his deaf ear, and flagellate the poor old man savagely. Nor could her umbrage be assuaged. 'So you think I'll sell my heritage for a mess of pottage?' she would shout. 'Not I! I'll sabotage this marriage! I'll ravage and pillage your castle! I'll send you out to forage for silage like an onager, and I'll take the reins of the carriage myself!'

The king, unable to hear what she was saying, considered her comments only amusing persiflage; but not so his entourage. To them, the suffragette's conduct had hopelessly damaged her image. 'The baggage treats him like garbage, nay, like sewage!' they told one another. 'This presages no good!'

They determined to salvage the situation by taking advantage of the girl's desire to drive onagers. To set the stage, they camouflaged their agents as milk-white onagers and, hitching them to the magenta carriage, they invited the haughty suffragette to take the reins. The onagers promptly broke from control and rampaged across the tillage onto the plage, where the carriage shattered in the deep sand. The carnage was outrageous. The suffragette's bones, hair, and cartilages were scattered about like spaghetti. She died of a haemorrhage in the wreckage, unmourned; no-one even bothered to apply a bandage.

The moral: If you have it on your agenda to ravage and pillage Carthage, first make sure your onagers are really asses.

OLÉ, OLO!

Insert 'olo' as needed, and you need not turn to the completed version to read this thought-provoking story.

An old anthgy reveals how a Cmbian named Pnius, idegically unsound and a notorious gig, found himself bigically drawn to Madame Dres, a cratura from Crado who sang ss and blew the picc at the Cnial Opera House. Pnius put his fairest phrasegy into his suit, but was so injudicious as to use calumnious termingy against La Dres's true love, a p-playing cnel from a Cgne regiment. Contemptuously rebuffed, the gig came in his dur to Master Hfernes, a well-known astrger, whom he prayed to use astrgical arts to eliminate the offending cnel. Hfernes, his mind on certain tautgies he wished to strike from a hgraph, absently lifted his eyes from a semicn in the cphon on the title page and suggested: 'Why not cut down the cnel with your b as he strolls with Dres along the Cnnade?' 'Absurd!' cried the contemptible gig. 'You give me a pain in the cn! You are full of bney! This cnel is a cssus of a man, a veritable Mch to his enemies! His rage borders on the mythgical! If I were to confront him, we all should perish in the hcaust!' 'That being so,' said the astrger, 'why come to me? I am no sn, much less a Smon. I can only suggest that you go to the cnel and apgise.' So saying, he picked up his hgraph and departed, insouciantly dancing the Pnaise.

ANSWER

An old anthology reveals how a Colombian named Polonius, ideologically unsound and a notorious gigolo, found himself biologically drawn to Madame Dolores, a coloratura from Colorado who sang solos and blew the piccolo at the Colonial Opera House. Polonius put his fairest phraseology into his suit, but was so injudicious as to use calumnious terminology against La Dolores's true love, a polo-playing colonel from a Cologne regiment. Contemptuously rebuffed, the gigolo came in his dolour to Master Holofernes, a well-known astrologer, whom he prayed to use astrological arts to eliminate the offending colonel. Holofernes, his mind on certain tautologies he wished to strike from a holograph, absently lifted his eyes from a semicolon in the colophon on the title page and suggested, 'Why not cut down the colonel with your bolo as he strolls with Dolores along the Colonnade?' 'Absurd!' cried the contemptible gigolo. 'You give me a pain in the colon! You are full of boloney! This colonel is a colossus of a man, a veritable Moloch to his enemies! His rage borders on the mythological; if I were to confront him, we all should perish in the holocaust!' 'That being so,' said the astrologer, 'why come to me? I am no solon, much less a Solomon. I can only suggest that you go to the colonel and apologise.' So saying, he picked up his holograph and departed, insouciantly dancing the Polonaise.

Euphemisms

DIRT IS A DIRTY WORD

An American visiting England discovers quickly that different words are under the ban on the two sides of the ocean. An Englishman restricts the use of *bug* to the *Cimex lectularius*, or common *bedbug*, and hence the word has highly impolite connotations.* All other crawling things he calls *insects*. The English aversion to *bug* has been breaking down of late, however, probably under the influence of such naturalised Americanisms as *jitterbug*, but it yet lingers in ultra-squeamish circles, and a *ladybird* is never called a *ladybug*. Not so long ago *stomach* was on the English *Index*, and such euphemisms as *tummy* and *Little Mary* were used in its place, but of late it has recovered respectability. *Dirt*, to designate earth, and *closet*, in the sense of a cupboard, are seldom used by an Englishman. The former always suggests filth to him, and the latter has obtained the limited use of *water closet*. But the Englishman will innocently use many words and phrases that have indecent significances in the United States, quite lacking in England, *e.g.*, *to be knocked up* (to be tired), *to stay with* (to be the guest of), *screw* (as a noun, meaning salary or pay), *to keep one's pecker up*, *douche* (shower bath) and *cock* (a male

---

* Might not the English use of *bugger* for sodomite, rare in the United States, have something to do with the stigma? W. R. E.

chicken). The English use *bitch* a great deal more freely than Americans. Now and then an American, reading an English newspaper, is brought up with a start by a word or phrase that would never be used in the same way in the United States. I offer two examples. The first is from an advertisement of a popular brand of smoking tobacco in the *News of the World*: 'Want a good *shag*?' The second is from the *Times Literary Supplement*: 'On the whole we may congratulate ourselves on having chosen not to be born in that excellent and indispensable century when an infant of six could be hanged . . . and school boys were encouraged to match *cocks*.'

H. L. Mencken, *The American Language*

NICE-NELLYISMS

In my college days, one of my classmates wrote and produced a musical comedy. This I remember because I played the walk-on part of a buttons, and frequently missed my entrances. The hero of the play had to attract my attention by shouting at the top of his lungs, 'Where is that rascally page? Oh—I think I hear him coming now!' Anyhow, the Dean of Women took exception to a phrase in the theme song: 'He said to me, come on and be/ My woman.' *Woman*, she said, disregarding the slight on her own title, had vulgar connotations; the word must be changed to *sweetheart*. And changed it was.

It is curious that *woman* is considered by many, and even by some relatively literate persons, to be a term of disrespect. In America, a hundred years ago, *female* was frequently substituted for it, in effect lumping women with the females of all species. *Lady*, though, won the day. My grandmother, who was reared in Mexico as the result of a disagreement between her father and the Federal government as to who had won the Civil War, or, as he called it, the War Between the States, first heard *lady* used as a synonym for *woman* when she returned to the United States as a bride. The story goes that she burst into tears, and demanded of her husband, 'What kind of a country *is* this, where even washer-women are washer-*ladies*?'

The eventual effect of calling all women ladies was to debase the meaning of the word *lady* to that of *woman*. Such is the usual fate of Nice-Nellyisms.

As recently as World War II, Hollywood's Production Code strictly and successfully forbade the use in the cinema of such words as *broad* (for *woman*), *chippy, cocotte, courtesan, eunuch, fairy* (for *homosexual*), *floozy, harlot, hot mamma, hussy, madam, nance, pansy, slut, trollop, tart, wench, whore,* and even *sex* and *sexual.*

Nice-Nellyism is rampant today in the fertile field of undergarments, as is evident from a glance at advertisements for *step-ins, undies, undikins, roll-ons, campus briefs,* and *cup forms.*

Whore, still a shocker, is related to the Latin *carus* (dear), and, as Mencken points out, 'must once have been a polite substitute for some word now lost'.

F, G

False Rhyme

In assonance, or false rhyme, the vowels of one word correspond with those of another, but the consonants do not. *Name* is assonant with *Jane, scream* with *beach. Mad* as a *hatter, time* out of *mind, free* and *easy,* and *slapdash* are assonant expressions.

In consonance it is the consonants that correspond, as in *raid* and *red, staid* and *stood, odds* and *ends, short* and *sweet, stroke* of *luck, strut* and *fret.*

Assonance has triumphed over pure rhyme in Gaelic; the Irish poets writing in English who rhyme *Blarney* with *charming* are following an ancient tradition.

It is less popular, though far from unknown, in English. It seems most at home in Mother Goose and folk rhymes:

> And pray, who gave thee that jolly red nose?
> Cinnamon, Ginger, Nutmeg and Cloves.

> There was an old wife did eat an apple.
> When she had eat two she had eat a couple.

Famous Fakes and Frauds

I have not been able to authenticate, but consider likely, a story to the effect that a mischievous Englishman used to translate published verses into Greek or Latin and mail the translation to *The Times* as 'proof' that the poem had been outrageously expropriated from some ancient author. Just such a trick, in any event, was played on Sir Walter Scott by a correspondent who claimed the poet had stolen the address to 'Woman', in *Marmion*, from a Latin poem by Vida. Scott, suspecting nothing, told his friend Southey that truly the resemblance between the two poems was an astonishing one. His ended:

> When pain and anguish wring the brow,
> A ministering angel thou!

The purported lines from Vida were:

> Cum dolor atque supercilio gravis imminet angor,
> Fungeris angelico sola ministerio.

As Scott agreed, a more extraordinary example of casual coincidence could never have been pointed out. But when someone thought to check the Vida reference, it turned out not to exist.

A waggish friend of mine, Irish by inheritance, invited some friends of similar pedigree to a St. Patrick's day party, drenched them in martinis, and played them a record of what he claimed to be an ancient Gaelic song. Tears, composed largely of alcohol, rolled down Irish cheeks, and the guests cried nostalgically, 'Ah, that's the beautiful Gaelic!' But really it was Sophie Tucker singing 'Meine Yiddische Mamma'.

I mention this little hoax because it reminded me of a happening at a Boston Carlyle Club in the days when Carlyle devotees were more numerous and more fervent than they seem to be today. One Carlyle reading included the passage: 'Word-spluttering organisms, in whatever place—not with Plutarchean comparison, apologies, nay rather, without any such apologies—but born into the world to say the thought that is in them—antiphoreal, too, in the main—butchers, bakers, and candlestick makers; men, women, pedants. Verily, with you, too, it's now or never.' These lines evoked wild applause from the audience, and were hailed as a fresh instance of the master's genius, though in fact they were sheer fakery.

A remarkable literary forger was William Henry Ireland, who in 1799 published two plays, *Vortigern* and *Henry the Second*, which he claimed to be by Shakespeare himself. Sheridan accepted them as genuine, and even produced *Vortigern* at the Drury Lane theatre; but the play was a fiasco, and Ireland went to jail.

THE GREAT LONGFELLOW CAPER

In the 1930s the *Atlantic Monthly* fell victim to a literary hoax, unique in that it was unintentional. The magazine published a brief verse of four-line stanzas starting 'Softly, silently falls the snow', or something on that order (I really must look it up), credited to a college professor. *Atlantic* readers immediately leaped to the kill, with the terrible joy that inflates us all when we catch someone, particularly someone of high reputation, in a foolish error. The poem, they pointed out, was actually by none other than Henry Wadsworth Longfellow. Surely the *Atlantic*, of all magazines, might have been expected to know *that*.

Right they were; yet the professor was perfectly innocent. Mr. Longfellow's effusion had inspired him to create a verse of his own, in the same manner and on the same theme. He handed his poem, with Longfellow's stanzas at the top in italics, to his secretary to type and post. Unfortunately, she omitted his credit to Longfellow. The *Atlantic* editors, finding the italicised stanzas excellent but the rest trash, acted accordingly.

The bright side of the story is that Longfellow still stood up after nearly a hundred years, at least in his home town.

Finnegan's Wordplay

Finnegan's Wake, by James Joyce, must be one of the few classics in English for which the average reader requires a translation. It takes a good man to go through a passage like the example below without blinking.

—Rats! bullowed the Mookse most telesphorously, the concionator, and the sissymusses and the zozzymusses in their robenhauses quailed to hear his tardeynois at all for you cannot wake a silken nouse out of a hoarseoar. Blast yourself and your anathomy infairioriboos! No, hang you for an animal rurale! I am superbly in my supremest poncif! Abase you, baldyqueens! Gather behind me, satraps! Rots!

—I am till infinity obliged with you, bowed the Gripes, his whine having gone to his palpruy head. I am still always having a wish on all my extremities. By the watch, what is the time, pace?

Figure it! The pining peever! To a Mookse!

—Ask my index, mund my achilles, swell my obolum, woshup my nase serene, answered the Mookse, rapidly by turning clement, urban, eugenious and celestian in the formose of good grogory humours. Quote awhore? That is quite about what I came on *my* missions with *my* intentions *laudibiliter* to settle with *you*, barbarousse. Let thor be orlog. Let Pauline be Irene. Let you be Beeton. And let me be Los Angeles. Now measure your length. Now estimate my capacity. Well, sour? Is this space of our couple of hours too dimensional for you, temporiser? Will you give you up? *Como? Fuert it?*

*

LINES BY A MEDIUM

(in communication with the late L. Murray)

I might not, if I could;
    I should not, if I might;
Yet if I should I would,
    And shoulding, I should quite!

I must not, yet I may;
    I can, and still I must;
But ah! I cannot—nay,
    To must I may not, just!

I shall, although I will,
    But be it understood,
If I may, can, shall—still
    I naught, could, would, or should.

Author unknown

*

109

Franglish

If, given an English word, you proceed to name a synonym, this being identical in spelling to a French word of quite different meaning, you are playing Franglish. A synonym for 'calamitous', for instance, is 'dire'. 'Dire', in French, means 'to say'. Whet your appetite on the following examples, which come from 'Your Literary I.Q.', a department conducted by David M. Glixon in the *Saturday Review*.

The given word	The French word for	The missing word
Woo	Short	*Court*
Bastion	Strong	*Fort*
Crippled	Blade	*Lame*
Burn	Monkey	*Singe*
Depression	Tooth	*Dent*
However	Goal	*But*
Warbled	Blood	*Sang*
Penny	Corner	*Coin*
Chop finely	Slender	*Mince*
One	Year	*An*
Kind	Fate	*Sort*
Rows	Third	*Tiers*
Weary	Pull	*Tire*
Be ill	Garlic	*Ail*
Surety	Leap	*Bond*
Talk	Cat	*Chat*
Selected	Thing	*Chose*
Regret	Street	*Rue*
Precious fur	Sand	*Sable*
Candle	Typewrite	*Taper*

Doris Hertz and
Karin S. Armitage

RONDEAU: OOPS! YOU ALMOST PICKED UP THE BILL

English has bulled its way into many a language, and no-one complains more bitterly about its incursions than the French. In the matter of food, however, the situation is reversed. The following verse mentions a few of the scores of dishes which are commonly ordered in French, though perfectly good English equivalents are at hand or could be developed.

'I'll pay for lunch this time,' I bet you'll say,
'So join me in the best . . . What's good today?
Some *Escargots*? . . . *Saumon*? . . . *Palourdes Farcies*? . . .
Coquille Saint-Jacques? . . . or *Jambon de Paris*? . . .
Bisque de Homard? . . . or *Soupe de Trois Filets*?

Délices de sole might do for entremets . . .
Quiche? . . . *Fruits de Mer*? . . . Or *Foie de Veau Sauté*?
Escallopines de Veau? . . . It's all on me;
I'll pay for lunch this time.' (I bet!)

'And next . . . *Filet mignon*? . . . Or *Demi-Grain Grillé*? . . .
Chateaubriand? . . . *Paillard de Boeuf Vert-Pré*? . . .
With *Haut-Brion*? . . . Or *Haut-Lafitte*? Feel free:
I'll pay for lunch this time.

'We'll finish with . . . say *Mousse*? . . . Or *Crêpes Flambées*? . . .
And *Café Filtre*, topped off by *Pousse-Café*?'
(Again you murmur, reassuringly:
'I'll pay for lunch.')

But having lunched with you before, I'll stay
With tea and toast, and count my cash. The way
The record reads, it's sure as sure can be
I'll pay.

W. R. E.

S'IL VOUS PLAÎT'S NOT STERLING

It is obvious, when you stop to think about it, that 's'il vous plaît' is as close as the French can come to saying 'silver-plate'—i.e., 'not sterling'. Freddy Pearson stopped to think about it, and then proceeded to write a book, sinfully funny and condignly illustrated by R. Taylor, called *Fractured French*. In fractured French, 'de rigueur' can be nothing but a two-masted schooner, 'au contraire', 'away [in the country] for the weekend,' and 'a la carte', 'on the wagon'.

Even without the help of Taylor's saucy illustrations, I expect you can provide instant English versions of the French expressions below. Freddy did.

1. C'est à dire
2. Mal de mer
3. Faux pas
4. Carte Blanche
5. Coup de grâce
6. Tant pis, tant mieux
7. Louis Cinq
8. Mille fois
9. Pas de tout
10. J'y suis et j'y reste
11. Tout en famille
12. Pièce de résistance
13. Ile de France
14. Tête-á-tête
15. Endive
16. Hors de combat
17. N'est-ce pas
18. Pied-à-terre
19. Entrechat
20. Quelle heure est-elle?
21. Marseillaise
22. Legerdemain
23. Voici l'anglais avec son sang-froid habituel
24. Adieu, ma chérie

ANSWERS

1. She's a honey.
2. Mother-in-law.
3. Father-in-law.
4. For God's sake, take Blanche home!
5. Lawn mower.
6. My aunt is much happier since she made a telephone call.
7. Lost at sea.
8. Cold lunch.
9. Father of twins.
10. I'm Swiss, and I'm spending the night.
11. Let's get drunk at home.
12. Timid girl.
13. I'm sick of my friends.
14. A tight brassière.
15. A night club.
16. Camp followers.
17. Father robin.
18. The plumbing is out of order.
19. Let the cat in.
20. Whose babe is that?
21. Mother says okay.
22. Tomorrow's a holiday.
23. Here comes that Englishman with his usual bloody cold.
24. No English equivalent is given, but the picture is of a girl in her wedding gown.

French-Canadian Dialect

THE WRECK OF THE *JULIE PLANTE*
A Legend of Lac St. Pierre

Henry Avery, of Canadian extraction, gave me not long ago a book of French-Canadian dialect verses called *The Habitant*. Written at the turn of the century by William Henry Drummond, it memorialises a charming and rapidly vanishing tongue. The following poem is typical of the book.

> On wan dark night on Lac St. Pierre,
>   De win' she blow, blow, blow,
> An' de crew of de wood scow *Julie Plante*
>   Got scar't an' run below—
> For de win' she blow lak hurricane
>   Bimeby, she blow some more,
> An' de scow bus' up on Lac St. Pierre
>   Wan arpent from de shore.

> De captinne walk on de fronte deck,
>   An' walk de hin' deck too—
> He call de crew from up de hole
>   He call de cook also.
> De cook she's name was Rosie,
>   She come from Montreal,
> Was chambre maid on lumber barge,
>   On de Grande Lachine Canal.

> De win' she blow from nor'eas'-wes'—
>   De sout' win' she blow too,
> W'en Rosie cry 'Mon cher captinne,
>   Mon cher, w'at I shall do?'
> Den de captinne t'row de big ankerre,
>   But still the scow she dreef,
> De crew he can't pass on de shore,
>   Becos' he los' hees skeef.

(CONTINUED OVERLEAF)

De night was dark lak' wan black cat,
    De wave run high an' fas',
W'en de captinne tak' de Rosie girl
    An' tie her to de mas'.
Den he also tak' de life preserve,
    An' jomp off on de lak',
An' say, 'Good-bye, ma Rosie dear,
    I go drown for your sak'.'

Nex' morning very early
    'Bout ha'f-pas' two—t'ree—four—
De captinne—scow—an' de poor Rosie
    Was corpses on de shore.
For de win' she blow lak' hurricane
    Bimeby she blow some more,
An' de scow bus' up on Lac St. Pierre,
    Wan arpent from de shore.

MORAL

Now all good wood scow sailor man
    Tak' warning by dat storm
An' go an' marry some nice French girl
    An' leev on wan beeg farm.
De win' can blow lak' hurricane
    An' s'pose she blow some more,
You can't get drown on Lac St. Pierre
    So long you stay on shore.

French Wordplay

After several tries, Clarkson Potter remembered these for me, though first, I think, his mother remembered them for him:

            Un train à l'aurore!
            Quelle horreur!
            C'est sans doute une erreur
            dans l'horaire!

The following lines were a teaching device for West Point cadets:

Jeanne portait l'armure
Jeanne portait le mur
Jeanne portait l'amour
Jeanne portait l'armoire

And finally:

La reine Didon
Dinà, dit-on,
Du dos d'un dodu dindon.

When challenged to write English poetry, Victor Hugo promptly replied:

Pour chasser le spleen
J'entrai dans un inn;
O, mais je bus le gin,
God save the Queen.

And I have this anonymous comment on the Biblical misadventure of Lot and his daughters:

Il but;
Il devint tendre;
Et puis il fut
Son gendre.

Fruits in Season

Two melons had an argument:
A lover's quarrel, too.
One melon said, 'I **********;'
The other, '********!'

W. R. E.

ANSWER

Two melons had an argument,
A lover's quarrel, too.
One melon said, 'I cantaloupe';
The other, 'Honeydew!'

There are no rocks
At Rockaway,
There are no sheep
At Sheepshead Bay,
There's nothing new
In Newfoundland,
And silent is
Long Island Sound.

Howard Moss

*

H

Headline Hunters

Before me is a leader on the cost of the American farm subsidy programme. Its heading is '$4.5 Billion Ain't Hay'. The thrust of the entire 200-word essay is contained in the four words. Newspapers would be little less informative, and certainly more enjoyable, if they left out the stories and just ran the headlines.

Henry Kissinger, foreign affairs adviser to President Nixon, is a bachelor who boasts that 'power acts as an aphrodisiac', leaving unclear whether this effect is experienced by him or by the beautiful young women with whom he likes to spend his rare free evenings. A newspaper report on his tastes in this area is ambiguously headlined, 'Kissinger after dark'.

Below are the opening paragraphs of some news stories. Write the best headline you can for each of them, and then read on to see how your skill stacks up against that of the copy desk professionals.

1. PARIS—A French court has ruled that President François Duvalier of Haiti was libelled in the movie made from Graham Greene's novel *The Comedians*. It awarded him damages of one franc.

2. PIETERMARTIZBURG, South Africa—A Natal University couple claimed a world record after kissing for eight hours and 45 minutes nonstop.

3. LONDON—A fossil of a fish said to be 150 million years old was sold for £320 at Sotheby's auction yesterday.

4. NEW YORK—Rex Harrison and Richard Burton arrive here as two aging homosexuals when *Staircase* steps into the Penthouse theatre for its world premiere.

5. NEW YORK—The boost in the price of meat will cost New Yorkers $310 million this year.

6. NEW YORK—'Four boys!' George Schwab, proud father, marvelled. He smiled. 'Four boys! Apparently that's unprecedented.'

7. FONTANA, Wis.—Soviet scholars have been filibustering at the 20th Pugwash Conference in an effort to squelch all discussion of Russia's presence in Czechoslovakia.

8. WASHINGTON—With cigarette commercials banned from TV and radio, broadcasters are wondering whether they can continue to carry antismoking announcements without violating the 'fairness doctrine' requiring balanced presentation of controversial issues.

(ANSWERS OVERLEAF)

ANSWERS

1. DUVALIER LIBELLED, FRANCLY
2. STUCK ON EACH OTHER
3. JUST CALL IT A GOLD FISH
4. 'STAIRCASE' SET TO SPIRAL IN
5. N.Y. HAS A BEEF ON MEAT PRICES
6. HE'S FATHER OF QUADS: BOY OH BOY OH BOY . . .
7. PUGWASH REDS TRY FOR CZECHMATE
8. ANTISMOKING ADS: SOME IFS & BUTTS

Hidden Words

In *Word Play**, Hubert Phillips asks his readers to find ten words containing cans (canopy, candour); ten containing discs (discussion, discretion); ten containing imps (imperious, impetuous); ten containing pens (penumbra, pentad); ten containing props (proportion, prophet); ten containing cities (mendacity, opacity); ten containing scents (obsolescent, adolescent); ten containing nations (damnation, coronation); ten containing rations (emigration, integration); and ten containing gents (indigent, tangent).

You may enjoy jotting down as many of these words as occur to you. I am not going to suggest answers, since the words meeting the specifications are easy to locate in the dictionary.

Higgledy-Piggledies

The double-dactyl verses I call Higgledy-Piggledies were invented by Paul Pascal and Anthony Hecht, and first made their mark in *Jiggery-Pokery*, edited by Mr. Hecht and John Hollander (Atheneum, 1966). The following examples of the genre are from Mary Ann Madden's column in *New York Magazine*.

---

* Ptarmigan Books, Penguin, 1945.

The first line of a Higgledy-Piggledy may be any nonsensical double dactyl—'Fiddledy faddledy', 'Niminy piminy', 'Jokery pokery', 'Hickory dickory', and the like. The second line names the subject of the composition. The fourth and eighth are the rhyme lines, curtailed double dactyls. The sixth line should be one double dactyl word, though sufficiently clever exceptions are forgiven. This contribution by James Lipton will give you the idea:

> Misericordia!
> College of Cardinals,
> Nervously rising to
> Whisper its will:
>
> 'Rather than being so
> Unecumenical,
> Can't we just quietly
> Swallow The Pill?'

The subjects of some of the other submissions are listed below. Work up a Higgledy-Piggledy about each. If you find that Higgledy-Piggledies are not your line of country, you can always copy the originals and tell your friends you wrote them yourself.

1. Yale University
2. Tom Tom the Piper's Son
3. Oedipus Tyrannos
4. Madame de Pompadour
5. Alice in Wonderland

ANSWERS

1

Higgledy Piggledy
Yale University
Gave up misogyny
Opened its door.

Coeducational
Extracurricular
Heterosexual
Fun is in store.
Fred Rodell

2

Higgledy Piggledy
Tom Tom the Piper's Son
Purloined a porker and
Forthwith he fled.

Passersby said this was
Incomprehensible
Due to the yarmulka
Worn on his head.
William McGuirk

(CONTINUED OVERLEAF)

3

Higgledy Piggledy
Oedipus Tyrannos
Murdered his father, used
Mama for sex.

This mad debauch, not so
Incomprehensibly
Left poor Jocasta and
Oedipus Wrecks.
Joan Munkacsi

4

Tiffety Taffety
Madame de Pompadour
Loved crême brulée, such ex-
Pansive desserts.

After developing
Steatopygia,
She was the one who in-
Vented hoop skirts.
Emily Barnhart

5

Tweedledum Tweedledee
Alice in Wonderland
First she was tiny and
Then she was tall,

Argued with animals
Anthropomorphical,
Didn't accept their con-
Clusions at all.
W. R. E.

*

HIGH-LIFE LOW-DOWN

To his Castle Lord Fotherday bore his young bride,
And he carried her over the drawbridge so wide,
Through the Great Hall, the Solar, the West Hall, the East,
And thirty-eight principal bedrooms at least.
Up seventeen stairways and down many more
To a basement twelve yards by a hundred and four,
And at last set her down—he was panting a bit—
In front of the sink and said, 'Kid, this is IT.'

Justin Richardson

*

Hobson-Jobsons

At the feast of Muharram, the Mohammedans raise the ritual cry of mourning, 'O Hasan! O Husein!', these being two murdered grandsons of Mohammed. The English substituted *Hobson-Jobson*, common surnames with no relation in meaning to the Arabic originals. A *hobson-jobson* is thus any word resulting from the corruption of a foreign expression. 'Compound', meaning 'a residence or group of residences set off by a barrier', is hobson-jobson for Malay 'kampong', 'village', as is 'forlorn hope' for Dutch 'verloren hoop', 'a lost expedition'. This kind of evolution goes on also inside the English language. The 'stark' in 'stark naked', for instance, does not come from 'stark', meaning 'bare, stripped of nonessentials', but from 'start', which once meant an animal's tail. 'Stark naked' is 'tail naked'.

See if you can reconstruct the origins of the words below.

1. Acorn	7. Helpmate
2. Belfry	8. Penthouse
3. Contredanse	9. Pickaxe
4. Curry favour	10. Reindeer
5. Greyhound	11. Saltcellar
6. Hangnail	12. Shamefaced

ANSWERS

1. Middle English *akern*, Old English *aecern* 'oak or beech mast'. Nothing to do with *corn*.
2. Middle English *berfrey*, 'tower'. Nothing to do with *bell*.
3. A French hobson-jobson that came back home. The French mistranslated *country dance*, and the English borrowed back the French word. Nothing to do with French *contre*, 'counter'.
4. In the fourteenth century French satirical poem *Roman de Favel*, Favel was a yellow horse, treated as a symbol of worldly vanity. He was soothed and lovingly tended by all classes of society. To *curry Favel* was thus to seek advancement by toadying. Folk etymology in England turned Favel into 'favour'.
5. Scandinavian *grey* 'dog' plus *hound*. Nothing to do with the colour grey.
6. Old English *ange* 'painful' plus *naegl* 'nail'. Nothing to do with *hanging*.

7. *Help* plus *meet* 'fitting'. Nothing to do with *mate*.
8. Middle English *pentis*, Old French *apentis*, connected with *pend* 'hang'. Nothing to do with either *pent* 'confined' or *house*.
9. Middle English *picois*, from Old French. Nothing to do with *axe*.
10. Scandinavian *hreinn*, the name of the animal, plus *deer*. Nothing to do with *rein*.
11. Middle English *saltsaler*, Old French *saliere*, Latin *salārium* (whose specific meaning 'money paid to soldiers for purchase of salt' accounts for *salary*). No connection with *cellar* 'basement'.
12. Old English *sceamfaest*, 'bound by shame'. Nothing to do with *face*.

Hoity-toities

There is a small family of words, often of folk origin and uncertain meaning, which command attention through a rhyme or near-rhyme within the word. Typical of the kind is 'hoity-toity', which can be interpreted according to taste as 'haughty, stuck-up' or 'an exclamation of surprise or disapprobation'.

The stanzas which follow, clearly dealing with a harum-scarum situation in a nursery, are built around a hodge-podge of familiar hoity-toities. Fill in the hoity-toities after studying the definitions.

> *****-*****,[1] where is nanny?
> There's some *****-*****[2] here.
> *****-*******[3] **********[4],
> *****-*****[5] *******-*******[6],
> ******-******[7] *******-*******[8],
> ***-***[9] ****-****[10], ****-****,[11] queer,
> *Refrain:* Beulah, set up one more beer.
>
> ******-*******[12] *****-*****[13],
> ******-*******[14] *****-*****.[15]
> Have a ****-****[16], *****-*****[17],
> *******-*****,[18] don't ******-*******[19],
> *****-******[20] *****-*****[21],
> *****-*****,[22] there's a dear.
> *Refrain:* Beulah, set up one more beer.

******_******,23 *****_*****,24
*****_*****,25 don't you worry:
*****_*****26 plays by ear.
Pop's a ***_***27 *****_*****,28
*****_*****29 is dear muddy;
Pop's a *****_****30 foola,
Muddy, she does ****_****;31
Be an *****_******,32 Beulah:
   Refrain: Bring another round of beer!

W. R. E.

Definitions

   1. Defined in the introduction.   2. Jugglery; trickery.
   3. A step in a rustic dance; in this case, a bad situation.
   4. A perfume imitating the odour of the red jasmine.
   5. Upside down.   6. In a state of agitation.
   7. A jumble.   8. In confusion.   9. Rabble.
  10. Insincere sentiment designed to incite applause.
  11. A reversal, as of opinion.
  12. A diminutive or presumptuous person.
  13. A lively expression.
  14. Characterised by confused hurry.
  15. A confection consisting of different kinds of preserved fruits.
  16. A lively party.
  17. King William IV.
  18. At great speed (slang, U.S.).
  19. Hesitate (usually the two halves are the other way around).
  20. Finical.   21. Without choice; compulsory.
  22. Nonsense intended to cloak deception.
  23. In a hopping way.   24. Flustered haste.   25. Mummery.
  26. An instrument of street music, played by turning a handle.
  27. In a state of jitters.
  28. One who is old-fashioned and fussy.
  29. Weakly sentimental or affectedly pretty.
  30. Quite to one's content.
  31. Native Hawaiian dance.
  32. An industrious, overzealous person.

(ANSWER OVERLEAF)

ANSWER

Hoity-toity, where is nanny?
There's some hanky-panky here.
Double-trouble, frangipani,
Topsy-turvy, jiggledy-wiggledy,
Hugger-mugger, higgledy-piggledy,
Rag-tag, clap-trap, flip-flop, queer.
    Refrain: Beulah, set up one more beer.

Whipper-snapper, rooty-tooty,
Helter-skelter, tutti-frutti;
Have a wing-ding, silly Billy,
Lickety-split, don't shally-shilly,
Niminy-piminy, willy-nilly,
Hocus-pocus, there's a dear.
    Refrain: Beulah, set up one more beer.

Hippety-hoppety, hurry-scurry,
Mumbo-jumbo, don't you worry;
Hurdy-gurdy plays by ear.
Pop's a jim-jam fuddy-duddy,
Namby-pamby is dear muddy;
Pop's a hunky-dory foola,
Muddy, she does hula-hula . . .
Be an eager-beaver, Beulah:
    Refrain: Bring another round of beer!

Homonyms

Once, in an uncommon burst of egotism, I composed this anagram
verse:

I don't mispell, as others ****,
But allways right each **** rite;
So I **** resounding hoops
At other righters' speling bloops.†

My verse was inspired by the extraordinary difficulty of
mastering the spelling of many English words and, specifically, by
the threat of lurking homonyms—words alike in sound, but
different in spelling and meaning.

† The anagrams: mite, item, emit.

Test your homonymic skill on the couplets below.

I

Blest be that beast who, though he ***** on others,
Gives ****** to God, and ***** all beasts be brothers.

2

Food, if you diet, goes to *****;
And, if you try it, goes to *****.

3

I found a shaggy mare in *****.
With might and **** I trimmed her ****.

4

Say, **** man in thy ***** cot,
Art ****** pleased with thy lowly lot?

5

I met a wise antelope, born in a zoo;
And I wish that I knew what that *** *** ****.

W. R. E.

Definitions

1. That is, eats 'em; and well he might; the hypocrite!
2. . . . not, want not; very big on Falstaff.
3. An American State; reinforces might; hippy hairdo.
4. Three times before 'Lord God Almighty'; lets in the rain; completely.
5. A few hours old; the antelope in question; I already gave you this one.

ANSWERS

1. Preys, praise, prays.
2. Waste, waist.
3. Maine, main, mane.

4. Holy, holey, wholly.
5. New, gnu, knew.

HOMONYM LEXICON

A

Acclamation, acclimation
Ad, add
Adds, ads, adze
Aerie, airy
Ail, ale
Air, ere, heir
Aisle, I'll, isle
All, awl
Allowed, aloud
All together, altogether
All ways, always
Altar, alter
Analyst, annalist
Ant, aunt
Ante, anti
Arc, ark
Ate, eight
Auger, augur
Aught, ought
Auricle, oracle
Away, aweigh
Awful, offal
Aye, eye, I

B

Bad, bade
Bail, bale
Bait, bate
Balm, bomb
Band, banned
Banns, bans
Bard, barred
Bare, bear
Baron, barren
Based, baste
Bass, base
Be, bee
Beach, beech
Bearing, baring
Beat, beet
Beau, bow
Been, bean

Beer, bier
Bell, belle
Berry, bury
Berth, birth
Better, bettor
Bey, bay
Bight, bite
Billed, build
Bird, burred
Blew, blue
Bloc, block
Boar, bore
Board, bored
Boarder, border
Bode, bowed
Bold, bolled, bowled
Bolder, boulder
Bole, boll, bowl
Born, borne, bourn
Borough, burrow
Bough, bow
Bouillon, bullion
Boy, buoy
Brae, bray
Braise, brays, braze
Braid, brayed
Brake, break
Breach, breech
Bread, bred
Brewed, brood
Brews, bruise
Bridal, bridle
Bus, buss
But, butt
By, buy, bye
Byre, buyer

C

Cache, cash
Cane, cain
Cannon, canon
Cant, can't
Canvas, canvass

Homonym Lexicon

Carat, caret, carrot
Cart, carte
Cast, caste
Caudal, caudle
Cause, caws
Cedar, ceder, seeder
Ceiling, sealing, seeling
Cell, sell
Cellar, seller
Cense, cents, scents, sense
Censer, censor
Cent, scent, sent
Cere, sear, seer, sere
Cereal, serial
Cession, session
Chantey, shanty
Chased, chaste
Cheap, cheep
Chews, choose
Choir, quire
Choler, collar
Choral, coral
Chronical, chronicle
Chute, shoot
Cite, sight, site
Clack, claque
Clause, claws
Cleek, clique
Climb, clime
Close, clothes
Clue, clew
Coal, cole
Coarse, corse, course
Coax, cokes
Coddling, codling
Coffer, cougher
Colonel, kernel
Complacence, complaisance
Complement, compliment
Coo, coup
Cord, cored, chord
Core, corps
Correspondence, correspondents
Council, counsel
Cousin, cozen
Coward, cowered

Creak, creek
Crews, cruise, cruse
Cue, queue
Currant, current
Currier, courier
Cygnet, signet
Cymbal, symbol

D

Dam, damn
Days, daze
Dear, deer
Dense, dents
Dependence, dependents
Desert, dessert
Devisor, divisor
Dew, due
Die, dye
Dire, dyer
Disc, disk
Discreet, discrete
Dissidence, dissidents
Doe, dough
Done, dun
Dost, dust
Dual, duel
Ducked, duct

E

Earn, erne, urn
Eau, oh, owe
Eave, eve
Elision, elysian
Ewe, yew, you
Eye, aye, I

F

Fain, fane, feign
Faint, feint
Fair, fare
Faker, fakir
Faro, Pharaoh
Faun, fawn
Fay, fey
Faze, phase
Feat, feet

Homonym Lexicon

Fete, fate
Filter, philtre
Find, fined
Fir, fur
Fisher, fissure
Fizz, phiz
Flair, flare
Flea, flee
Flecks, flex
Flew, flu, flue
Flo, floe, flow
Flocks, phlox
Flour, flower
Foaled, fold
For, fore, four
Foreword, forward
Fort, forte
Foul, fowl
Franc, frank, Frank
Frays, phrase
Frees, freeze, frieze
Friar, fryer
Fungous, fungus
Furs, furze

G

Gage, gauge
Gait, gate
Gamble, gambol
Genes, jeans
Gest, jest
Gild, guild
Gilder, guilder
Gilt, guilt
Gin, jinn
Gnu, knew, new
Gored, gourd
Gorilla, guerilla
Graft, graphed
Grater, greater
Grays, graze
Grill, grille
Grip, grippe
Grisly, grizzly
Groan, grown
Guessed, guest

Guide, guyed
Guise, guys

H

Hail, hale
Hair, hare
Hall, haul
Handsome, hansom
Hart, heart
Hay, hey
Hays, haze
Heal, heel, he'll
Heard, herd
He'd, heed
Heigh, hi, hie, high
Heir, air, e'er
Here, hear
Hew, hue
Hide, hied
Higher, hire
Him, hymn
Ho, hoe
Hoar, whore
Hoard, horde, whored
Hoarse, horse
Hoes, hose
Hold, holed
Hole, whole
Holey, holy, wholly
Hollo, hollow
Hoop, whoop
Hostel, hostile
Hour, our
Humerus, humorous

I

Idle, idol, idyl, idyll
Impassable, impassible
In, inn
Incidence, incidents
Indict, indite
Innocence, innocents
Instance, instants
Intense, intents
Invade, inveighed
It's, its

Homonym Lexicon

J
Jam, jamb

K
Key, quay
Knave, nave
Knead, need
Knight, night
Knit, nit
Knot, not
Know, no
Knows, noes, nose

L
Lacks, lax
Lade, laid
Lain, lane
Lam, lamb
Lapse, laps
Lay, lei
Lays, laze
Lea, lee
Leach, leech
Lead, led
Leaf, lief
Leak, leek
Lean, lien
Leas, lees
Leased, least
Lends, lens
Lessen, lesson
Levee, levy
Liar, lier, lyre
Lichen, liken
Licker, liquor
Lickerish, liquorice
Lie, lye
Limb, limn
Linch, lynch
Links, lynx
Literal, littoral
Lo, low
Load, lode, lowed
Loan, lone
Loch, lock
Locks, lox
Loon, lune

Loot, lute
Lumbar, lumber

M
Made, maid
Magnate, magnet
Mail, male
Main, mane
Maize, maze
Mall, maul, moll
Manner, manor
Mantel, mantle
Mare, mayor
Marshal, martial
Marten, martin
Massed, mast
Mead, meed
Mean, mien
Meat, meet, mete
Medal, meddle
Metal, mettle
Mewl, mule
Mews, muse
Might, mite
Mil, mill
Millenary, millinery
Mince, mints
Mind, mined
Miner, minor
Minks, minx
Missal, missile
Missed, mist
Moan, mown
Moat, mote
Mode, mowed
Mood, mooed
Moose, mousse
Morn, mourn
Mucous, mucus
Muscle, mussel
Mustard, mustered

N
Naval, navel
Nay, nee, neigh
None, nun

Homonym Lexicon

O
Oar, or, ore, o'er
Ode, owed
Oleo, olio
One, won

P
Paced, paste
Packed, pact
Paean, peon
Pail, pale
Pain, pane
Pair, pare, pear
Palate, palette, pallet, pallette
Pan, panne
Passed, past
Patience, patients
Pause, paws
Peace, piece
Peak, peek, pique
Peal, peel
Pearl, purl
Pedal, peddle
Peer, pier
Pend, penned
Per, purr
Pi, pie
Pistil, pistol
Place, plaice
Plain, plane
Plate, plait
Pleas, please
Pliers, plyers
Plum, plumb
Polar, poler
Poll, pole
Populace, populous
Pore, pour
Pray, prey
Prays, praise, preys
Presence, presents
Pride, pried
Prier, prior
Pries, prize
Prince, prints

Principal, principle
Profit, prophet
Pros, prose
Psalter, salter

Q
Quarts, quartz
Quean, queen

R
Rack, wrack
Raid, rayed
Rain, reign, rein
Raise, raze
Raiser, razor
Rancour, ranker
Rap, wrap
Rapped, rapt, wrapped
Ray, re
Read, reed
Read, red
Real, reel
Recede, reseed
Receipt, reseat
Reck, wreck
Reek, wreak
Residence, residents
Rest, wrest
Retch, wretch
Review, revue
Rheum, room
Rhyme, rime
Rigger, rigour
Right, rite, wright, write
Ring, wring
Road, rode, rowed
Roc, rock
Roe, row
Roes, rose, rows
Rôle, roll
Rood, rude, rued
Root, route
Rote, wrote
Rough, ruff
Rouse, rows
Rout, route

Homonym Lexicon

Rum, rhumb
Rung, wrung
Rye, wry

S

Sac, sack
Sail, sale
Sailer, sailor
Sane, seine
Scene, seen
Scull, skull
Seam, seem
Seas, sees, seize
Sequence, sequents
Serf, surf
Serge, surge
Sew, so, sow
Sewer, suer
Shake, sheik
Shear, sheer
Shier, shire, shyer
Shoe, shoo
Shone, shown
Sic, sick
Side, sighed
Sigher, sire
Sighs, size
Sign, sine, syne
Slay, sleigh
Sleight, slight
Slew, slough
Sloe, slow
Soar, sore
Soared, sword
Socks, sox
Sol, sole, soul
Soled, sold
Some, sum
Son, sun
Sou, sue
Staid, stayed
Stair, stare
Stake, steak
Stare, stair
Stationary, stationery

Steal, steel
Step, steppe
Stile, style
Straight, strait
Subtler, sutler
Succour, sucker
Suede, swayed
Suer, sewer
Suite, sweet

T

Tacked, tact
Tacks, tax
Tail, taille, tale
Taper, tapir
Tare, tear
Taught, taut
Tea, tee
Team, teem
Tear, tier
Teas, tease, tees
Tense, tents
Tern, turn
Their, there
Therefor, therefore
Threw, through
Throe, throw
Throne, thrown
Thyme, time
Tic, tick
Tide, tied
Timber, timbre
To, too, two
Toad, toed, towed
Tocsin, toxin
Toe, tow
Told, tolled
Ton, tun
Tongue, tung
Tool, tulle
Tooter, tutor
Tracked, tract
Tray, trey
Troop, troupe
Trussed, trust

Homonym Lexicon

U
Uncede, unseed
Undo, undue

V
Vail, vale, veil
Vain, vane, vein
Vary, very
Versed, verst
Vial, vile
Vice, vise
Villain, villein

W
Wade, weighed
Wain, wane
Waist, waste
Wait, weight
Waive, wave

War, wore
Ward, warred
Ware, wear
Warn, worn
Way, weigh
We, wee
Weak, week
Weal, we'll
Weather, wether
Weave, we've
We'd, weed
Weld, welled
We're, weir
Wind, wined
Wood, would
Worst, wurst

Y
Yoke, yolk
You'll, Yule

NOEL, NOEL

Virgin Mary, meek and mum,
Dominus is in thy tum.
What a jolly *jeu d'esprit*—
Christ beneath the Christmas tree!
                                                W.R.E.

How to Tell the Birds from the Flowers

The wordplay poet Robert Williams Wood, a distinguished physicist, has been compared to Lewis Carroll for the virtuosity of his punning. After office hours, he specialised in a combination of ridiculous verse and misleading drawings. The latter are reminiscent of Edward Lear's in their mixture of subtlety and casual deliberate crudeness. I'm sorry I can't show the pictures.

The verses that follow are taken from his two slim collections: *How to Tell the Birds from the Flowers** and its sequel, *Animal Anatomies*.

The Clover. The Plover

The Plover and the Clover can be told apart with ease,
By paying close attention to the habits of the Bees,
For En-to-molo-gists aver, the Bee can be in Clover,
While Ety-molo-gists concur, there is no B in Plover.

The Pecan. The Toucan

Very few can
Tell the Toucan
From the Pecan—
Here's a new plan:
To take the Toucan from the tree,
Requires im-mense a-gil-i-tee,
While anyone can pick with ease
The Pecans from the Pecan trees.
It's such an easy thing to do,
That even the Toucan he can too.

The Elk. The Whelk

A roar of welkome through the welkin
Is certain proof you'll find the Elk in;
But if you listen to the shell,
In which the Whelk is said to dwell,
And hear a roar, beyond a doubt
It indicates the Whelk is out.

***

* Dover Publications, Inc., New York.

133

Hunting the Uncommon, Improper Noun

HIDE AND HAIR

Hides were man's first clothes. Eventually he learned to weave the hair from the hide into warm garments and coverings. Six products of hide or hair are defined below. Guess the words and the proper names that are their source.

1, 2. Two curly or wavy furs, comparable in desirability, made from the skins of young lambs.
3. Fine, downy wool growing beneath the outer hair of a Himalayan goat.
4. A soft, highly prized leather of goatskin tanned with sumac.
5. The skin of a sheep or goat, prepared for writing upon; paper made in imitation of this material.
6. Leather with a soft napped surface.

ANSWERS

1, 2. Caracul, astrakhan. Turkestan is dotted with lakes named Karakul, and with herds of sheep, also called karakul because they graze by the lakes. The fur of the karakul lambs, usually black, has the same name, differently spelled: *caracul.*

Astrakhan, in Russian Turkestan, is the home of the astrakhan sheep, a relative of the karakul, but having hair longer and with a more open curl. The name is applied to its fur, and to a fabric with a similar curled pile.
3. Cashmere. The name of the wool of the Kashmir goat; of a shawl made of it; and of a wool fabric of twill weave.
4. Morocco. This leather was first exported from Morocco, in northwest Africa.
5. Parchment. In the second century B.C., Eumenes II, ruler of the Asia Minor kingdom Pergamum, decided to build a grand new library, and asked the Egyptians to send him papyrus for his scribes to write on. The Egyptians refused, not caring to see a rival to their world-famous library at Alexandria. Eumenes therefore reverted to the earlier practice of writing on prepared skin, but cut down production costs by writing on both sides. The library was built in due course, and for a time did give Alexandria a run for its money. The writing skins came to be known as pergamene, after the country and its capital city. Later, however, Parthia became the dominant kingdom of Asia Minor,

and the name of the skins was changed to Particaminum—'Parthian leather'; in English, parchment.
6. Suede. French for Swedish, the Swedes being the earliest exporters of this kind of leather.

SAINTS IN MUFTI

The names of a number of saints have become vernacular for reasons that the saints probably would find surprising. The catherine wheel, for instance—either a firework similar to a pinwheel, or a circular rose window, as the case may be—derives from Catherine of Alexandria because, when the Roman emperor ordered the saint broken on the wheel, it miraculously shattered at her touch. The filbert is so named because the ripening season of the nut coincides with the feast day of St. Philibert. The pudenda are called after morbidly modest St. Pudentiana, who, according to one liturgical scholar, 'may simply be an adjective who became a saint'.

Below are definitions of six common words born of saints. Guess the words and the saints.

1. A little pig; the runt of the litter.
2. Noisy uproar and confusion; a lunatic asylum.
3. A bird sometimes seen in storms at sea.
4. (Slang.) Out of one's mind; crazy.
5. Gaudy and cheap; vulgarly ornamental.
6. Effusively sentimental.

ANSWERS

1. Tantony. St. Anthony, intercessor for swineherds, is generally pictured with a piglet trotting after him, so swineherds came to call the runt of each litter the 'St. Anthony pig'. The name was gradually shortened to its present form.
2. Bedlam. The hospital of St. Mary of Bethlehem in Lambeth, London, was a lock-up for lunatics as early as 1402. Cockneys corrupted Bethlehem to Bedlam, which was soon lowercased.
3. Petrel. The name derives from Peter's bootless try at walking on water (Matthew xiv, 29). His faith deserting him, he began to sink, and would have drowned if Jesus had not given him a lift. The birds are called after Peter because they fly so low that they sometimes seem to be walking on the sea.

4. Barmy. You have probably seen St. Bartholomew in Michelangelo's painting, flayed alive and holding his own skin in his hands. He is patron of the feebleminded, wherefore some assert, most plausibly, that 'barmy' is a corruption of his name. But the true source, one suspects, is 'barm', an old word for the froth on beer.

5. Tawdry. Ethelreda, daughter of a sixth-century king of East Anglia, lay dying of a tumour of the throat. She confided to her waiting women that God was punishing her for her girlhood love for pretty necklaces. Hundreds of years later, her name shrunken to Audrey, she became patron saint of Ely, Cambridgeshire, where the townfolk sold 'necklaces of fine silk' to celebrate her feast day, October 17. These 'Saint Audrey's laces' were soon manufactured all over England and, being of poor quality, gave their name to any trumpery stuff.

6. Maudlin. A contraction of magdalene, from Mary Magdalene, a devoted follower of Jesus who is painted with eyes swollen and red from weeping at His crucifixion.

SEX ON OLYMPUS

The ancient gods and demi-gods were noted for their interest in lively sex, and their amatory exploits gave rise to some of the more vivid expressions in today's sexual vocabulary. You will have no trouble identifying most of the seven words defined below, and recalling how they came into being.

1. One having the sex organ of both male and female.
2. A boy kept by a pederast.
3. A drug or food stimulating sexual desire.
4. Of or pertaining to sexual love or desire.
5. Of or pertaining to sexual intercourse.
6. A phallus.
7. A lecher.

ANSWERS

1. Hermaphrodite. Hermaphroditus, son of Hermes and Aphrodite, was named after both his parents. He was a shy, savage youth, whose chief pleasure was hunting. One day he chanced to take refuge from the heat in the fountain ruled by the nymph Salmacis. She, at the sight of him, was seized by ravening passion, and leaped into the water to embrace him. When he repulsed her, she cried out in anguish: 'O ye gods! Grant that nothing may ever separate him from me, or me from him!' On the instant, their two bodies were merged into one, neither man nor woman, yet both.

2. Catamite. A corruption of Ganymede, the name of a beautiful Trojan youth who so took Zeus's fancy that the god, assuming the form of an eagle, carried him off to Olympus where, when not cupbearing for the immortals, he performed more specialised functions impractical for his predecessor, the fair Hebe. A young bartender or waiter is referred to occasionally, with humorous intent, as a ganymede.

3. Aphrodisaic. Aphrodite, goddess of love, was no remote, unattainable vision; she was the epitome of sexually exciting beauty, and when she wanted a god, or a man, she got him. Her temple at Paphos was served by priestesses so carnally obliging that paphian became synonymous with strumpet. Aphrodite needed no aphrodisiacs.

4. Erotic. Eros, son of Aphrodite, was a winged youth, or boy, who wakened love by shooting arrows into the hearts of his victims. He specialised in physical rather than spiritual attraction. But Hesiod, a poet of the eighth century B.C., declares he was the earliest of all gods, born of Chaos, the cosmic egg. It is a pleasant conceit—love bringing order out of chaos.

5. Venereal. From Venus, the Roman version of Aphrodite. Venery connotes not just the pursuit of sexual delight but additionally the art of the chase, over which Venus also presided. The two sports have much in common; that venison as well as venereal disease comes down to us from the love goddess gives one to think. Venom likewise traces to her. It was a love potion originally; the changed meaning is a reminder that love gone rancid can be a poisonous brew indeed.

6. Priapus. Priapus, Aphrodite's son by Dionysus, was protector of herds, bees and fish, and personification of the male generative power. He was born with an extraordinary deformity, a tremendous phallus, the image of which was commonly placed as a protector in orchards and gardens. A priapus is a phallus of enormous proportions.

7. Satyr. Satyr, a sylvan deity, was much given to lasciviousness. He was often represented with the tail and ears of a horse, but sometimes with the feet and legs of a goat, short horns on his head, and his whole body covered with thick hair. Like Faunus, the Roman god of animals, he was multiple; there were as many Satyrs in Greece as Fauns in Rome. Satyriasis was the blessing bestowed on the world by Satyr; a nymphomaniac is his female equivalent.

A SHOT IN THE DARK

Not counting damascus steel, which can be pounded as easily into a plowshare as a sword, the bayonet, first produced at Bayonne, France, is the only killing tool in my files named after its place of origin. A number, however, have been named after people—and not always the people who invented them. Thus, the blunderbuss has a remote connection with Queen Bess; in

World War I British fliers called the German anti-aircraft guns 'archies' in allusion to a music-hall hit of the day, 'Archy, certainly not!'; the chassepot, a nineteenth-century French breech-loading rifle, is called after its inventor, as is the derringer, a short-barrelled pistol of the type used to slay Abraham Lincoln; the molotov cocktail of World War II was named for Russia's foreign minister. The six definitions below are of other devices named for people and intended primarily for slaughter. Give in each case the device and the person.

1. Fragments from a high-explosive shell.
2. A single-edged knife once popular in the American wilderness.
3. A large-bore, long-range German cannon of World War I.
4. The first practical revolver, still in wide use.
5. Underworld slang for a pistol.
6. A beheading machine.

ANSWERS

1. Shrapnel. In 1784, General Henry Shrapnel—or, as he then was, Lieutenant Shrapnel—began experimenting with the design of a hollow projectile containing a number of balls and a charge of powder to burst the shell. The British first fired shrapnel in anger in 1804, in Dutch Guiana. It reached its peak as an instrument of slaughter in World War I.
2. Bowie. Colonel James Bowie, an American adventurer and pioneer, fancied this ugly, single-edged knife, about fifteen inches long and curving at the tip. Whether the knife was actually designed by the Colonel or by his brother Rezin is in dispute.
   Bowie did not exactly die with his boots on, but he came close to it. When his heart stopped, in 1836, he was taking potshots from his sickbed at the Mexican attackers of the Alamo.
3. Big Bertha. The Germans in World War I used a massive long-range cannon to bombard Paris, and called it the Big Bertha in honour of Frau Bertha Krupp von Hohine un Hohlbach, head of the Krupp steel works.
4. Colt. Patented by Samuel Colt in 1835, this revolver became the universal handgun. In Wild West days it was a foolish cowboy indeed who would venture into a strange bar without his 'equaliser'.
5. Gat. In 1862, R. J. Gatling, a prolific inventor from North Carolina, perfected a gun that fired the then incredible total of 350 shots a minute. Within a few years, says the *Encyclopaedia Britannica*, the gatling gun was adopted 'by almost every civilised nation'. Gat, short for gatling, is established underworld usage for a pistol of any kind.

6. Guillotine. Dr. J. I. Guillotin developed this device just in time for the French Revolution. 'With my machine,' he informed the awestruck Assembly in 1789, 'I can whisk off your head in a twinkling and you suffer no pain.' But the guillotine was by no means the earliest tool of its kind. Holinshed's *Chronicles* reported in 1573 a great market-day attraction in Halifax—a blade that dropped in its frame 'with such violence that, if the neck of the transgressor were as big as that of a bull, it should be cut in sunder at a stroke and roll from the body by a huge distance'. And I believe an Edinburgh museum still displays the engine which in 1581 cut off the head of the regent Morton.

I

I ARISE FROM DREAMS

OF STEAM PUBLISHING

All night, from hush of thrush till rouse of rooster,
Simon and Schuster, Simon and Schuster, Simon and Schuster,
   The great expresses thundered through my dream
Or *Houghton Mifflin, Houghton Mifflin* panted
On gradients a bit more steeply canted,
   Or the implacable wheels took up the theme:
Lippincott, Lippincott, Lippincott they'd clink,
Lippincott, Lippincott, Doubleday and Company Inc,
   Lippincott, Lippincott till I could scream.
I turned to British books for my salvation:
The Rationalist Press Association
   Now all night long lets off its antique steam,
And all night long a shunted goods-train clanks
GOLLANCZ, *Gollancz, Gollancz, Gollancz, Gollancz.*

Peter Dickinson

I CAN'T THINK WHAT HE SEES IN HER

Jealousy's an awful thing and foreign to my nature;
I'd punish it by law if I was in the Legislature.
One can't have all of any one, and wanting it is mean,
But still, there is a limit, and I speak of Miss Duveen.

I'm not a jealous woman,
    But I can't see what he sees in her,
        I can't see what he sees in her,
            I can't see what he sees in her!
If she was something striking
I could understand the liking,
And I wouldn't have a word to say to that;
    But I can't see why he's fond
    Of that objectionable blonde—
That fluffy little, stuffy little, flashy little, trashy little,
    creepy-crawly, music-hally, horrid little CAT!

I wouldn't say a word against the girl—be sure of that;
It's not the creature's fault she has the manners of a rat.
Her dresses may be dowdy, but her hair is always new,
And if she squints a little bit—well, many people do.

I'm not a jealous woman,
    But I can't see what he sees in her,
        I can't see what he sees in her,
            I can't see what he sees in her!
He's absolutely free—
There's no bitterness in me,
Though an ordinary woman would explode;
    I'd only like to know
    What he sees in such a crow
As that insinuating, calculating, irritating, titivating,
    sleepy little, creepy little, sticky little TOAD!

A. P. Herbert

I Dreamt of Couth

A few words thrive only in their antonyms. Why, if something is avoidable, do we go all the way around Robin Hood's barn to say it is *not inevitable*? The missing words in the verse below are forgotten positives. Fill them in to round out the quintain.

I dreamt of a **********,[1] *******[2] youth,
******,[3] ********,[4] and *****.[5]
A *****[6] and a *******[7] fellow, forsooth—
********,[8] *******,[9] *********,[10] ***[11], *****.[12]
A *******[13] fellow I dreamt.

W. R. E.

[1]Submissive to correction. [2]Hurtful. [3]Agile, handsome. [4]Contented. [5]Well-groomed. [6]Heartened, encouraged. [7]Straightforward. [8]Within reasonable bounds. [9]Capable of being uttered. [10]Tidy. [11]Dexterous. [12]Familiar, refined. [13]Forgettable.

ANSWER

I dreamt of a *corrigible, nocuous* youth,
Gainly, gruntled, and *kempt*;
  A *mayed* and a *sidious* fellow, forsooth—
Ordinate, effable, shevelled, ept, couth;
A *delible* fellow I dreamt.

If -less were -ful, and -ful were -less

Just as some words are familiar only in their negative form (see 'I Dreamt of Couth'), so others commonly take '-less' but not '-ful' as a suffix, and vice versa. This is intolerable discrimination. The verse on the following page will set things straight.

A *******[1] dog, one ****-***[2] spring,
Set out for ********[3] foraging,
And as he dug in *******[4] sod,
Paid ********[5] tribute to his God.
At which, a *******,[6] *******[7] lass,
Whose ********[8] bodice charmed each pass-
Erby, cried out, 'O *******[9] sound!
O ******,[10] *******,[11] *******[12] hound!'

[1]Not curtailed. [2]Laminate, in a sense. [3]Clearly he had no need for dentures. [4]Very radical. [5]In full cry, as it were. [6]Efficient; strong. [7]Abounding in affection. [8]Referring to a safety feature for women, similar in concept to braces. [9]Because a dog's howl must come to an end. [10]Full of years; mortal. [11]Still alive, though. [12]A comforting reminder to the dog that his is not an endangered species.

ANSWER

A tailful dog, one leaf-ful spring,
Set out for toothful foraging,
And as he dug in rootful sod,
Paid voiceful tribute to his God.
At which, a feckful, loveful lass,
Whose strapful bodice charmed each pass-
Erby, cried out, 'O timeful sound!
O ageful, lifeful, peerful hound!'

Impossible Rhymes

Certain words in English have no true rhymes. It is always possible to approximate a rhyme, however, by fudging. To rhyme 'orange' here, I have bent the rules of syllabification and have accepted assonance instead of true rhyme in an unstressed syllable:

The fóur eng-
Ineers
Wear órange
Brassieres.

The only poet who completely solved the 'orange' problem was Arthur Guiterman, who wrote in *Gaily The Troubadour*:

Local Note

In Sparkill buried lies that man of mark
  Who brought the Obelisk to Central Park,
Redoubtable Commander H. H. Gorringe,
  Whose name supplies the long-sought rhyme
      for 'orange'.

Below is a list of words difficult to rhyme. See what you can do with them before looking to see what others have done.

1. Orange and lemon
2. Liquid
3. Porringer
4. Widow
5. Niagara

ANSWERS

1. *Orange and lemon*

I gave my darling child a lemon,
That lately grew its fragrant stem on;
And next, to give her pleasure *more* range
I offered her a juicy orange,
And nuts—she cracked them in the door-hinge.

                    Author unknown

2. *Liquid*

After imbibing liquid,
  A man in the South
Duly proceeds to stick quid
(Very likely a thick quid)
  Into his mouth.
    C. A. Bristed

3. *Porringer*

When nations doubt our power to fight,
  We smile at every foreign jeer;
And with untroubled appetite,
  Still empty plate and porringer.
        Author unknown

4. *Widow*

The jury found that Pickwick *did* owe
Damages to Bardell's widow.

      Author unknown

5. *Niagara*

Take instead of rope, pistol, or dagger, a
Desperate dash down the Falls of Niagara.

        Tom Moore

SPELLING RHYMES

If word rhymes come hard to you, perhaps you will do better at
verses in which the rhyme is provided not by the last word of the
line, but by the last letter or two of the word. Here is the way
it is done:

> 'Me drunk!' the cobbler cried, 'the devil trouble you,
> You want to kick up a blest r-o-w,
> I've just returned from a teetotal party,
> Twelve of us jammed in a spring c-a-r-t,
> The man as lectured now, was drunk; why bless ye,
> He's sent home in a c-h-a-i-s-e.'

Author unknown

Inflated Rhetoric

THE UNFIVETHREENNINE FIVETHREENE
TELLER

That civilised understatement is extinct in America, and an
endangered species in England, may or may not be an understatement. More and more, it seems, we emphasise by exaggerating.
For *like* we substitute *love*; for *distaste*, *hate*; for *liberal*, *Red*; for
conservative, *Fascist*; for *eccentricity*, *insanity*. We write, as it were,
shouting, and hear others' shouts as whispers.

Victor Borge, the pianist and comedian, has popularised a game
which illustrates this rhetorical inflation in a mathematical sort
of way, and I have adapted his concept in the story below. You
will notice that numbers are buried in a good many of the words.
Reduce each number by one, and you will have the story as
I originally wrote it.

If you decide to make this sort of puzzle yourself, you may
prefer, if such is your direction in economics and rhetoric, to
promote deflation rather than inflation by using in the puzzle a
number just below, rather than just above, the approximation
in the story as solved.

Twoce upon a time there lived in Threenisia a threetor who was
a saturten, misbegoteleven ingrnine. This hnineful cnineiff five-

thrightly abominnined his fivemer classeven sthreedent, the cele-
brnined young potentnine Eightarola. Awnineing his oppor-
threenity and opernineing without fivewarning, the trnineor
initinined a devastnineing revolt. He fiveced Eightarola three
fivefeit his estnines; three fivego his elevenure; three abdicnine
his throne; and three haseleven to pull his frnine from his elevent
fivethwith three fivestall annihilation.

Fnine has written that anytwo, even the most desolnine and
fivelorn of men, still retains two elevenacious friend. Such was
Eightarola's five-footed atelevendant Bedfived. This beten caten,
a Grnine Dane, was antiqunined and superannunined, but he
would not contemplnine fivesaking his master, who addressed
him in the following despernine and aberrnined fashion:

'Two must fiveget two-time glories; two cannot yet affived
three seek restithreetion. But two might, two calculnines, migrnine
three fiveeign lands. Two might locnine in the fivebidden Black
Fivest, threetling about preelevending three be a fivethreene
teller.'

So off went the fivemer potentnine and the caten. Sad three
relnine, however, Eightarola was not apprecinined in the Black
Fiveest. No-two took his bnine. Through lack of atelevention, if
not strnine asitenness, he had failed three fivearm, or even three
fivefinger, himself with fivemulas five fivetelling the fnine of the
fiveest dwellers.

By grnine luck, however, he two day met an intoxicnineing,
tenteen-year-old ballet dancer, clad in an abbrevinined threethree.
'Threets,' cried Eightarola, 'it is my fivecefully articulnined
conelevention that we three must become two.'

Threets agreed, and from that moment on he atelevended three
his affairs as never befive. No longer at sevens and eights, he
fiveced the fivemidable threetor three capithreelnine, two back his
throne and elevent, and lived coneleventedly with his grnineful
caten atelevendant and his elevender soulmnine fiveever after.

ANSWER

Once upon a time there lived in Tunisia a tutor who was a saturnine,
misbegotten ingrate. This hateful caitiff forthrightly abominated his
former classics student, the celebrated young potentate Sevenarola.
Awaiting his opportunity and operating without forewarning, the traitor

initiated a devastating revolt. He forced Sevenarola to forfeit his estates; to forgo his tenure; to abdicate his throne; and to hasten to pull his freight from his tent forthwith to forestall annihilation.

Fate has written that anyone, even the most desolate and forlorn of men, still retains one tenacious friend. Such was Sevenarola's four-footed attendant Bedford. This benign canine, a Great Dane, was antiquated and superannuated, but he would not contemplate forsaking his master, who addressed him in the following desperate and aberrated fashion:

'One must forget one-time glories; one cannot yet afford to seek restitution. But one might, one calculates, migrate to foreign lands. One might locate in the forbidden Black Forest, tootling about pretending to be a fortune teller.'

So off went the former potentate and the canine. Sad to relate, however, Sevenarola was not appreciated in the Black Forest. No-one took his bait. Through lack of attention, if not straight asinineness, he had failed to forearm, or even to forefinger, himself with formulas for foretelling the fate of the forest dwellers.

By great luck, however, he one day met an intoxicating, nineteen-year-old ballet dancer, clad in an abbreviated tutu. 'Toots,' cried Sevenarola, 'it is my forcefully articulated contention that we two must become one.'

Toots agreed, and from that moment on he attended to his affairs as never before. No longer at sixes and sevens, he forced the formidable tutor to capitulate, won back his throne and tent, and lived contentedly with his grateful canine attendant and his tender soulmate forever after.

Interminable Words

The longest word in English, says a riddle, is smiles, since there is a mile between the first and last letter. Shakespeare's longest word (27 letters) by no means matches this. In *Love's Labour's Lost* Costard the clown says to Moth the page: 'I marvel thy master hath not eaten thee for a word; for thou art not so long by the head as honorificabilitudinitatibus; thou art easier swallowed than a flap-dragon.'

Honorificabilitudinitatibus, if only it meant anything, would hold a respectable place in the ranks of the longer English words, even though it falls short of James Joyce's 34-letter *semperexcommuni-cambiambiambisumers*. Any such ranking would have to include also Henry Carey's

> '*Aldiborontphosophorno,* (21)
> Where left you *Chrononnotonthologos?*' (20)

But these words would be small fry in some countries. I have read, though I cannot attest the fact, that on p. 837 of Liddell & Scott's *Greek Lexicon* there appears a word of 176 letters meaning hash.

A nineteenth-century Flemish gentleman was inspired by the invention of the automobile to create the word *Snelpaardeloos-zonderspoorwegpatrolrijtuig*—41 letters meaning 'a carriage which is worked by means of petroleum, which travels fast, which has no horses, and which is not run on rails'.

It takes longer to say the names of some locations in Wales than to walk through them. The most impressive example in my records is *Llanfairpwllgwyngyllgogerychwyrndrobwllllantysili-ogogogoch*, 58 letters pronounced 'Klan-fire-pooth-gwin-geth-go-gerith-kwin-drooble-klan-dissileo-gogo-gok'. There may be a 59th letter missing, 13 letters from the end. The word means "The church of St. Mary in a hollow of white hazel, near to the rapid whirlpool, and to St. Tisilio church, near to a red cave'. If you write to a friend there, you need use only the first 20 letters on the envelope; the Post Office will know what you mean.

The longest place name in the United States, from the Indian, is *Chargoggagoggmanchauggagoggchaubunaqwnaqungamangg*, the meaning of which is unknown to me. It is said to be a lake in south-central Massachusetts.

The Germans are compound-word addicts. A 57-letter whopper (and my version, according to authorities who do not bother to fill in the missing pieces, is seven letters short) is *Constantino-politanischerdudelsackpfeipenmachergsellschaft*, meaning 'Associ-ation of Constantinople bagpipe makers'.

Bismarck considered the word 'apothecary' insufficiently German, and coined a 71-letter replacement: *Gesundheitswieder-herstellungsmitterzusammenmischungsuerhaltnisskundiger*.

Some scientific terms in English stretch out interminably, but otherwise we are not in the same league with the Germans. Gladstone coined *disestablishmentarianism*, with 24 letters; *anti-* of course may be prefixed. *Floccinaucinihilipilification*, connected in some way with wool, has 29.

If you are an *antitransubstantiationalist* (27), you doubt that consecrated bread and wine actually change into the body and blood of Christ.

A 34-letter word popular with schoolboys and television comics is *supercalifragilisticexpialidocious*, a Walt Disney creation mean-ing, I suppose, superb.

A considerable company of words of 20 or more letters combine at least two words: *anthropomorphotheist* (20), *philosophicopsychological* (25), etc. Others grow through prefixing: *antianthropomorphism* (20), *hyperconscientiousness* (22), *superincomprehensibleness* (25) *semiprofessionalized* (20). There is no particular reason why there should not be an *antiantitransubstantiationalist* (31).

The words defined below are made up of 20 or more letters, and all occur more commonly than you might expect. Try guessing them before checking the answers.

1. Aptness to respond to a suggestion by doing the contrary.
2. State of being beyond the reach of the human mind.
3. One who seeks to upset a revolution.
4. Love of offspring.
5. Applying the attributes of man to God.
6. An opposite explanation.
7. Extreme deference to the dictates of conscience.
8. Opposition to freedom of thought and behaviour, especially in religion.

ANSWERS

1. Contrasuggestibility.
2. Incomprehensibleness.
3. Counterrevolutionary.
4. Philoprogenitiveness.
5. Anthropomorphilogical.
6. Counterinterpretation.
7. Hyperconscientiousness.
8. Antilatitudinarianism.

THE PRESCRIPTION

Said the chemist: 'I'll take some dimethyloximidomesoralamide
And I'll add just a dash of dimethylamidoazobenzaldehyde;
   But if these won't mix,
   I'll just have to fix
Up a big dose of trisodiumpholoroglucintricarboxycide.'

Author unknown

Irish Bulls

A ludicrous blunder of language is called an Irish bull, on the theory that Hibernians are particularly subject to this affliction. For instance:

An Irish member of Parliament, referring to a minister noted for his love of money, observed: 'I verily believe that if the honourable gentleman were an undertaker, it would be the delight of his heart to see all mankind seized with a common mortality, that he might have the benefit of the general burial, and provide scarfs and hat-bands for the survivors.'

A Hibernian gentleman, when told by his nephew that he had just entered college with a view to the church, said, 'I hope that I may live to hear you preach my funeral sermon.'

A poor Irishman offered an old saucepan for sale. His children gathered around him and inquired why he parted with it. 'Ah, me honeys,' he answered, 'I would not be after parting with it but for a little money to buy something to put in it.'

'I was going,' said an Irishman, 'over Westminster Bridge the other day, and I met Pat Hewins. "Hewins," says I, "how are you?" "Pretty well," says he, "thank you, Donnelly." "Donnelly!" says I; "that's not *my* name." "Faith, no more is mine Hewins," says he. So we looked at each other again, and sure it turned out to be nayther of us.'

BULLS ABROAD

Irish bulls thrive far from the green fields of Ireland. Here are five lusty specimens of the breed, two from America and three from England.

The following resolutions were passed by the Board of Councilmen in Canton, Mississippi: 1. Resolved, by this Council, that we build a new Jail. 2. Resolved, that the new Jail be built out of the materials of the old Jail. 3. Resolved, that the old Jail be used until the new Jail is finished.

149

Wells & Fargo's Express, operating in Indian country, declared in its regulations that it would not be responsible as carriers 'for any loss or damage by fire, the acts of God, or of Indians, or any other public enemies of the government'.

George Selwyn, the missionary, once remarked that it seemed impossible for a lady to write a letter without adding a postscript. A lady present replied, 'The next letter you receive from me, Mr. Selwyn, will prove you wrong.' The letter arrived in due course, with the following line after the signature: 'P.S. Who is right now, you or I?'

Sir Boyle Roche is credited with two classic bulls:

'Mr. Speaker, I boldly answer in the affirmative—No.'

'Mr. Speaker, if I have any prejudice against the honourable member, it is in his favour.'

PARLIAMENTARY LETTER

The following letter, in Maria Edgeworth's *Essay on Irish Bulls*, is credited by her to one S——, an Irish member of Parliament at the time of the Rebellion:

My dear Sir:—Having now a little peace and quietness, I sit down to inform you of the dreadful bustle and confusion we are in from these blood-thirsty rebels, most of whom are (thank God!) killed and dispersed. We are in a pretty mess; can get nothing to eat, nor wine to drink, except whisky; and when we sit down to dinner, we are obliged to keep both hands armed. Whilst I write this, I hold a pistol in each hand and a sword in the other. I concluded in the beginning that this would be the end of it; and I see I was right, for it is not half over yet. At present there are such goings on, that everything is at a standstill. I should have answered your letter a fortnight since, but I did not receive it until this morning. Indeed, hardly a mail arrives safe without being robbed. No longer ago than yesterday the coach with the mails from Dublin was robbed near this town: the bags had been judiciously left behind for fear of accident, and by good luck there was nobody in it but two outside passengers who had nothing for thieves to take. Last Thursday notice was given that a gang of rebels were advancing here under the French standard; but they had no colours, nor any drums except bagpipes. Immediately every man in the place, including women and children, ran out to meet them. We soon found our force much too little; and we were far too near to think of retreating. Death was in every face; but to it we went, and by the time half our little party were killed we began to be all alive again. Fortunately, the rebels had no guns, except pistols, cutlasses, and pikes; and as we had plenty of guns and ammunition, we put them all to the sword. Not a soul of them escaped, except some that were drowned in an adjacent bog; and in a very short time nothing was to be heard but silence. Their uniforms were all different colours, but mostly green. After the action, we went to rummage a sort of camp which they had left behind them. All we found was a few pikes without heads, a parcel of empty bottles full of water, and a bundle of French commissions filled up with Irish names. Troops are now stationed all around the country, which exactly squares with my ideas. I have only time to add that I am in great haste.

Yours truly, ——

P.S.—If you do not receive this, of course it must have miscarried; therefore I beg you will write and let me know.

Isosceles Words

It is often possible to enlarge a word one letter at a time, each time rearranging the letters so as to create a word with a different root. It is equally possible to reverse the process. Try working out the four examples below before looking at the answers.

1. Build I into Flirters.
2. Reduce crotchets to O.
3. Build A into Drafting.
4. Reduce Befriends to I.

(ANSWERS OVERLEAF)

1	2	3	4
I	Crotchets	A	Befriends
If	Crochets	At	Definers
Fir	Torches	Tan	Refined
Rift	Throes	Rant	Finder
First	Short	Train	Diner
Strife	Shot	Rating	Rind
Trifles	Hot	Trading	Din
Flirters	To	Drafting	In
	O		I

J, K

Jargon

The following statement by a teacher is quoted exactly as it appeared in a school publication:

Totally obsolete teaching methods based on imprinting concepts instead of growthful actualising of potential have created the intellectual ghetto. If schools would stop labeling cooperation 'cheating', and adopt newer methods of student interaction, we wouldn't keep churning out these competitive isolates.

Which means, in plain English, 'Let the kids cheat'.

Thus ethics and English decay together. The teacher was impelled to conceal his thought in jargon, as an octopus might conceal itself in ink, either because he was not quite sure what he was saying; or he did not know how to say it; or he was apprehensive of saying it right out.

Jargon, even when used by learned physicists and noted educators, is, like Pig Latin, the in-language of the immature, who gladly sacrifice sense for secrecy. Specialised phraseology is acceptable as a tool of precise communication. When it obfuscates (as we jargoneers say) it is monstrous.

Fowler says jargon is 'the use of long words, circumlocutions, and other clumsiness'. Partridge calls it 'shop talk'. He is too kind; only the part of shop talk that is unnecessary, inappropriate, abstract, clumsy, passive and obscure deserves the dreadful label. Shop talk is shorthand; jargon has no purpose save perhaps to hint at some non-existent wisdom.

There are as many jargons as there are arts and professions. Politics, as the oldest profession but one, is encrusted with it. An article by David Steel, MP, in *Punch*, cites a number of examples of parliamentary jargon, from which I choose these:

'The problem is how to optimise the institutionalisation of the forecasting procedures.'

'If those sleeping peers who have not yet applied for the writ have not woken up to their possibilities, I should be disposed to think that they should be given quite a long *locus penitentiae* in which to reply.'

'Force . . . is the midwife of every society pregnant with the new. But in England, at any rate, is she not a somewhat outdated old body, doing her rounds in a few places, admittedly, but on the whole yielding to new obstetrical techniques—techniques which may be a bit impersonal but which are certainly a lot more painless? Such an unlikely duo as Mr. Enoch Powell and Mr. Tariq Ali seem both agreed that rivers of blood are flowing, or are going to be flowing somewhere, and both seem afraid of missing the boat.'

(On second look, I see that last passage is not jargon at all. It is, however, an example of the depths to which the language of Shakespeare can sink.)

A research chemist will accept as a truism the statement that chlorophyll makes food by photosynthesis. Say the same thing to a practical engineer, however, and his reaction may be a blank stare. Stuart Chase, after making this point, goes on: 'But if the statement is rephrased, "Green leaves build up food with the help of light", anyone can understand it. So, says [C. F.] Kettering, if we are going to surmount the boundaries between kinds of technical men: "The first thing to do is to get them to speak the same language".'

The man or woman who has scrambled about halfway up the intellectual slope, and has found a shaky toehold there, often finds the urge to use jargon irresistible. Louis Kronenberger recalls a recent article in one of the weightier American quarterlies which flaunted all these words, along with others as ill-begotten:

Rebarbarise, ephebic, totemic, semeiotics, thereiomorphic, biomorphic, developmental, authorial, theophany, catena, authentification, anamnesis, pseudocausality, eld, ludic, logoi, liminal, opsis, topos, sooth, psychotheology, liberative.

'What most enchants me,' says Mr. Kronenberger, 'is that the author, having inserted quotations from Emerson and Matthew Arnold in which every word and phrase is an easily understood and established one, must himself straightway refer to Emerson as a "comparatist" and to the "racial calculus" that Arnold is practising.'

The jargon of specialists at least has the excuse that special dialects are required for technical discussions. But what is *your* excuse when you use words, in the phrase of the philologist Wilson Follett, as 'mere plugs for the holes in one's thought'?

Among words commonly so used Mr. Follett lists the following:

NOUNS: *angle, approach, background, breakdown* (analysis), *concept, context, dimension, essentials, factor, insight, motivation, nature, picture* (situation), *potential, process.*

VERBS: *accent, climax, contact, de-emphasise, formulate, highlight, pinpoint, process, research, spark, trigger, update.*

MODIFIERS: *basic, bitter, crucial, cryptic, current(ly), drastic, essential, initial, key, major, over-all, realistic, stimulating, worthwhile.*

LINKS: *as of, -conscious, -free, in terms of, -wise, -with.*

Mr. Kronenberger gives examples in a different vein:

Life-style, value judgment, the human condition, charismatic, polarisation, paradigm, elitist, ecumenical, ambiance, graffiti, symbiosis, epiphany, extrapolate, archetype, analogue, concept, subsume, autonomy, dichotomy, viable.

All these words are legitimate when properly used. No-one asks you to discard them. They can give you loyal service. Just don't let them lead you into jargon.*

---

* Congressman Maury Maverick's word for the bureaucratic variety was 'gobbledygook'.

Jump or Jiggle

Somewhere in this book there is a poem that lists the young of animals, and somewhere else one that lists animal sounds. The poem below, by Evelyn Beyer, shows various animals animal-bulating. I have jumbled the key words, just to stop you from reading too fast.

Frogs mpju
Caterpillars pmhu

Worms gligwe
Bugs glegij

Rabbits pho
Horses pocl

Snakes idsel
Seagulls eidlg

Mice ercpe
Deer plea

Puppies uncobe
Kittens uncope

Lions ktlas—
But—
I lwka!

ANSWERS

Frogs jump
Caterpillars hump

Worms wiggle
Bugs jiggle

Rabbits hop
Horses clop

Snakes slide
Seagulls glide

Mice creep
Deer leap

Puppies bounce
Kittens pounce

Lions stalk—
But—
I walk!

L

THE LAMA

The one-l lama,
He's a priest.
The two-l llama,
He's a beast.
And I will bet
A silk pajama
There isn't any
Three-l lllama.*

Ogden Nash

Lesson in Address

This jingle might have been stretched out by including, among others, Mr. E., Aunty Quated, and Burl Esq., but it is tidier as it is.

Three pretty misses, partying they go:
Miss Creant,
Miss Anthrope,
Miss L. Toe.

Flirting with the gentry, fluttering their eyes:
Sir Cumvent,
Sir Cumspect,
Sir Cumcise.

W. R. E.

---

* Adds Mr. Nash: The author's attention has been called to a type of conflagration known as a three-alarmer. Pooh!

A LETTER FROM EDWARD LEAR TO EVELYN BARING, LORD CROMER

Thrippy Pilliwinx,—
   Inkly tinky pobblebockle able-squabs? Flosky! Beebul trimble
flosky! Okulscratch abibblebongibo, viddle squibble tog-atog,
ferry moyassity amsky flamsky damsky crocklefether squiggs.
                        Flinky wisty pomm,
                                    Slushypipp

*

Lipograms

A Californian musician named Ernest Vincent Wright wrote a
50,000-word novel* without using the letter *e*. James Thurber
wrote a story about a country in which no-one was permitted to
use *o*. Any composition which thus rejects one or more letters,
either vowel or consonant, is a lipogram. In this old lipogrammatic
song, the letter *s* does not appear:

COME, LOVE, COME

Oh! Come to-night; for naught can charm
   The weary time when thou'rt away.
Oh! come; the gentle moon hath thrown
   O'er bower and hall her quivering ray.
The heather-bell hath mildly flung
   From off her fairy leaf the bright
And diamond dewdrop that had hung
   Upon that leaf—a gem of light.
                  Then come, love come.

(CONTINUED OVERLEAF)

---

* *Gadsby* (Wetzel, Los Angeles, 1939).

157

To-night the liquid wave hath not—
　　Illumined by the moonlight beam
Playing upon the lake beneath,
　　Like frolic in an autumn dream—
The liquid wave hath not, to-night,
　　In all her moonlit pride, a fair
Gift like to them that on thy lip
　　Do breathe and laugh, and home it there.
　　　　　　　　Then come, love, come.

To-night! to-night! my gentle one,
　　The flower-bearing Amra tree
Doth long, with fragrant moan, to meet
　　The love-lip of the honey-bee.
But not the Amra tree can long
　　To greet the bee, at evening light,
With half the deep, fond love I long
　　To meet my Nama here to-night.
　　　　　　　　Then come, love, come.

　　　　　　　　Author Unknown

There is another species of versification, the name of which
escapes me, in which every line begins or, as in the following
epitaph, ends, with the same letter.

The charnel mounted on the wall
Lets to be seen in funeral
A matron plain domesticall,
In pain and care continual.
Not slow, nor gay, nor prodigal,
Yet neighbourly and hospital.
Her children yet living all,
Her sixty-seventh year home did call
To rest her body natural
In hope to rise spiritual.

　　　　　　　　Author Unknown

Each stanza of the following poem has been written so as to include every letter in the alphabet but the vowel *e*. The author is unknown.

Bold Nassan quits his caravan,
A hazy mountain grot to scan;
Climbs craggy rocks to spy his way,
Doth tax his sight, but far doth stray.

Not work of man, nor sport of child,
Finds Nassan in that mazy wild;
Lax grow his joints, limbs toil in vain—
Poor wight! why didst thou quit that plain?

Vainly for succour Nassan calls,
Know, Zillah, that thy Nassan falls;
But prowling wolf and fox may joy,
To quarry on thy Arab boy.

M

Malapropisms

'Illiterate him, I say, quite from your mind!' ordered Mrs. Malaprop in Sheridan's play *The Rivals*. By such verbal confusions, she became, says H. W. Fowler (loftily ignoring the pun on his own name), 'the matron saint of all those who go wordfowling with a blunderbuss'. Among her absurdities were 'A progeny of learning', 'Make no delusions to the past', and, 'Sure, if I reprehend anything in this world, it is the use of my oracular tongue, and a nice derangement of epitaphs'.

Skewed words are as common as dandruff. Just now I came across this statement in a newspaper column written by a distinguished duo of political commentators: 'Finally, the new rules for delegate selection seem to mitigate against conservative candidates.'

Recently I heard a young lady of impeccable family and schooling say, 'I was so hungry that I gouged myself.'

A friend of mine attributes to his gardener the remark that 'She don't like me and I don't like her, so it's neutral.'

The sentences below contain words that are frequently malapropped. Substitute the correct word in each line.

1. The doctor said it was *desirous* to stop smoking.
2. Cheer up; I *predicate* final victory.
3. His capacity for hard liquor is *incredulous*.
4. This does not *portend* to be a great work of art.
5. Your contemptuous treatment of me is a great *humility*.
6. *Fortuitously* for her, she won the sweepstakes.
7. His *inflammable* speech set off a riot.

ANSWERS

1. Desirous, desirable. *Desirous* is 'desiring'; *desirable* is 'worth wanting; advantageous'. 'For the sake of your health it is *desirable* to stop smoking, whether or not you are *desirous* of doing so.'
2. Predicate, predict. *Predicate*, often with 'on' or 'upon', is 'to base or establish'; *predict* is 'to foretell'. 'My *prediction* of final victory is *predicated* upon hard facts.'
3. Incredulous, incredible. *Incredulous is* 'disbelieving'; *incredible* is 'unbelievable'. 'I am *incredulous* of the amount you say he drinks; it is *incredible*.'
4. Portend, pretend. *Portend* is 'to presage, foretell'; *pretend* is 'to feign'. 'He *pretends* to be an artist, but his work does not *portend* greatness.'
5. Humility, humiliation. *Humility* is 'modesty, the quality of being humble'; *humiliation* is 'degradation, or the act of humiliating'. 'His *humility* made him immune to *humiliation*.'
6. Fortuitous, fortunate. *Fortuitous* is 'utterly accidental'; *fortunate* is 'lucky'. 'It was *fortuitous* that she won the sweepstakes—and very *fortunate* for her.'
7. Inflammable, inflammatory. *Inflammable* is 'tending to ignite easily and burn rapidly; easily aroused to strong emotion'. *Inflammatory* is 'calculated to arouse strong emotion'. 'The speaker was *inflammatory*, the audience *inflammable*; the result was a riot.'

LIGHTNING FROM LIGHTNING BUGS

It was Mark Twain who said that the difference between a word that is right and a word that is almost right is the difference between the lightning and the lightning bug. Yet almost-right words rank considerably higher on the divine scale than malapropisms. And even malapropisms, though they may not light the whole sky, occasionally provide a modest illumination all their own. The man whose tongue slipped into 'civil serpents' was revealing long-concealed fury at bureaucratic indifference. 'Salutary confinement' can be just that. The truth of 'familiarity breeds attempt' was known to every halfway attractive girl in my college class. The mother who called her daughter a 'waltz-flower' was speaking with absolute precision. 'Adding assault to injury' is as deplorable as adding insult. The road from 'infancy to adultery' is well worn.

My favourite lightning bug is 'There's so much pornographic rubbish in print it buggers the imagination.' Only a demotic genius could have coined that line.

Mental Menu

In each of the words clued below, whether at the beginning, at the end, or in between, you should be able to find something edible.

1. Alms seeker
2. Outer garments
3. Sailing vessel
4. Width
5. Gravity
6. Smooth
7. Tool
8. Satisfy
9. Sharp-pointed weapon
10. Mottled
11. Having parti-coloured patches
12. Fixer of fixtures
13. Capriciousness
14. Move in haste
15. Irritate; annoy
16. Loud cry

ANSWERS

1. Beggar, egg
2. Coats, oats
3. Windjammer, jam
4. Breadth, bread
5. Sobriety, brie
6. Sleek, leek
7. Hammer, ham
8. Appease, peas
9. Spear, pear
10. Dapple, apple
11. Pied, pie
12. Plumber, plum
13. Caprice, rice
14. Scurry, curry
15. Tease, tea
16. Scream, cream

Metaphorically Speaking

There can scarcely have been a proposal more quixotic than that of Dr. Johnson – to fling metaphors neck and crop out of the English canon. Civilisation, one cannot doubt, began with the first figure of speech and will end with the last. Men without metaphors are brutes; their gaze is fixed on the ground; nothing in their lives exceeds its sum.

The Bible abounds in metaphors:

'A land flowing with milk and honey.'

'And thou shalt become an astonishment, a proverb, and a byword among all nations.'

'He kept him as the apple of his eye.'

'They shall be as thorns in your sides.'

'For we must needs die, and are as water spilt on the ground, which cannot be gathered up again.'

'There ariseth a little cloud out of the sea, like a man's hand.'

'The Lord is my rock, and my fortress, and my deliverer.'

'I will wipe Jerusalem as a man wipeth a dish, wiping it, and turning it upside down.'

The metaphors of Homer burn on the page:

'Words sweet as honey.'

'Shakes his ambrosial curls.'

'Thick as autumnal leaves or driving sand.'

'She moves a goddess, and she looks a queen.'

'Soft as the fleeces of descending snow.'

'A green old age.'

Modern poets have carried on the tradition:

'The road was a ribbon of moonlight.'

'Thou art the star for which all evening waits.'

'Her beauty was sold for an old man's gold;
   She's a bird in a gilded cage.'

'As a white candle
   In a holy place
So is the beauty
   Of an aged face.'

'Like dead, remembered footsteps on old floors.'

'I have seen old ships sail like swans asleep.'

> 'It's odd to think we might have been
>   Sun, moon and stars unto each other,
> Only, I turned down one little street,
>   And you went up another.'

Mixed metaphors are supposed to be the hallmark of the uneducated, and many people make a hobby of exposing them, which is good for the self-esteem.

Examples of mixed metaphors are all about:

'The Internal Revenue Service appears to be totally impaled in the quicksands of inertia.'

'I smell a rat; I seem to see it floating in the air; but we shall yet nip it in the bud.'

'There is no man so low that he has in him no spark of manhood, which, if watered by the milk of human kindness, will not burst into flames.'

Sometimes, though, the mixture is really in the eye of the observer. I remember, for instance, when English teachers used to cite Joyce Kilmer's poem *Trees* as a particularly horrendous farrago of mixed metaphors. His tree not only pressed its mouth against the earth's sweet flowing breast, but managed at the same time to look at God, lift its leafy arms to pray, and wear a nest of robins in its hair. But Mr. Kilmer was not mixing his metaphors; he was changing them, quite a different thing. Similarly, when John of Gaunt eulogises England in *Richard II*, he piles up some fifteen parallel images; but there is not a mixed metaphor in the lot.

Metrical Feet

If you are never quite sure whether a verse is written in trochee, spondee, dactyl, iamb, or anapæst, this mnemonic verse may help:

> Trochee trips from long to short.
> From long to long in solemn sort
> Slow Spondee stalks; strong foot! yet ill able
> Ever to come up with Dactyl trisyllable.
> Iambics march from short to long.
> With a leap and a bound the swift Anapests throng.

Samuel Taylor Coleridge

Milt Grocery

Milt Grocery was the dialect of the Jews who immigrated to the United States in the first half of the twentieth century. Their efforts to twist Yiddish-habituated tongues around English words resulted in mispronunciations and twists of locution that sounded wildly funny not only to settlers of an earlier vintage but, such is the genius of this people, to the immigrants themselves. Montague Glass, Arthur Kober and Leo Rosten were comic writers with perfect pitch for this dialect; but to me it is forever Milt Grocery, since Milt Gross was matchless in the idiom.

'Delilah'* is one of my favourite bits of Milt Grocery. Pot One tells how God turned the sinful Israelites over to the still more sinful Philistines, among whose hangers-on was one Delilah: 'Delilah was a wemp. Also on de site she was de foist wan from de fimmales from heestory wot she should be a lady-barber.'

Samson makes the scene in Pot Two. 'So,' says Gross, 'was like dees de insite fects':

DELILAH

Pot Two

So it was gradually born Semson, wot he was from pheezical feetness a movvel! You should see wot he was hable he should band in a heff iron bozz, witt still-bimms—odder wot he was hable he should lie don it should drife heem on top from de chast a huttomibill fool witt a femily wit ralatiffs yat, fet ones!!

So, of cuss, sotch a movvelous spasimin from menly weegor crated a conseederable nuttice in de poblic heye wot he bicame gradually a calabrity wot he was de tust from de tonn, witt de peectures in de Tebloids. So all over he was inwited to poddies wot he would hold futt so:

'Wal, wal, hollo, pipple! Noo a leedle treeck!! So here is de grend piano, is no? Geeve a looke a squizze—Tootpeecks!! Ha ha—is notting et all. Wait yat, you'll see I'll geeve a grab minesalf by de back from de nack wot I'll hold minesalf hout by a harm's langt!!! Ha ha!!! Denk you!! Denk you! Is jost a kneck!!'

So was standing in de beck from de poddy a geng Pheelistins

---

* 'Famous Fimmales Witt Odder Ewents from Heestory.'

wot it deweloped on de pot from dem a lodge quantity from jalousy wot it gritted Semson rimmocks so:

'Rezzbarrizz!!'

So Semson sad: 'Who's rezzing plizze de tust from de tonn?'

So it replite de Pheelistins: 'Ha! ha! geeve a look a tust—bedly boint! Say, who lat in here de Houze from David annyway??!! Comm on, boyiss, we'll tsettle heem de hesh.'

So bing wot Semson was tuttally hunprepared wot he deedn't hed witt heem futtifications he should prewent de etteck so he nutticed gradually wot on de mentelpiss was a jawbun from a ess. So witt de jawbun he gave a knock foist wan Pheelistin, den a sacund, den a toid, wot in a shut time it flad de whole tripe from Pheelistins wot Semson sad:

'Wal, wal—a leedle woikout! Denks, boyiss. Ulmost mossed me hopp de hair. Wal, wal. Noo, pipple? Geeve a look—a crubbar —whoops!—pretzels!!'

In Pot Tree, Delilah, dot wixen, esks Semson to creck her a nut. The story continues:

So Semson sad: 'Ha! Ha! Say, kirro, I'll creck for you anytink! Ha—for you I'll sweem the highest montain!!'

So she gave heem a look, a wempish one, dot sleepery ill, wot she sad: 'Ho, you gudgeous critchure, you!! A peecture from weem, witt weegor, witt witelity!! Could I fill by you de moscle!! Ho! Sotch a treel!! It geeves me de cripps. Sotch a hoddness. Go hon, weegle a leedle de bisaps! Whooy!! How you gat like dees?'

So Semson sad: 'Noxated Hiron, keed!'

So she sad: 'Ha Ha Ha!!—you fonny boy! Cull me Del.'

So Semson sad: 'Ha ha—I'll cull you "Pitches"—you'll cull me "Bonny"—ha ha!!'

'Ho, you hold shik you!! Wal, I must be ronning alung to take mine hettical colture lasson. Commaround you should see me. Jost tell de durrman wot Jeemy de nooseboy sant you, bot—heh, heh, heh—take foist batter a haircot—heh heh. Coot nite, Dollink—twitt, twitt.'

Pot Furr

So Semson, dot dope, he ren queeck de naxt day by Delilah, wot he deedn't slapt yat a whole night befurr, wot he was ricking witt poifume wot he tutt so: 'A switt leedle chilte—so deeference from de rast from de gold-deegers.'

So was ricklining on a diwan Delilah, wot she sad so:

'Hm, you nutty boy, you deedn't took a haircot. Momma is waxed—poo hoo! Is dees nize you should make momma she should cry? Poo hoo—hoo—POO HOO-POO-HOO-HOO!! You dun't luffing me!!'

So Semson sad: 'Yi Yi Yi! Of cuss, I luffing you! I'll go queeck now I should ketch a haircot!!'

So she sad: 'Hm, wait—I got a hidea!! Comm here!! Seet don, Switthott!!'

So she gafe a pool hout foist wan hair wot she sad 'You luff me,' und she gave a pool hout anodder hair wot she sad, 'You luff me not!' So she pooled, witt pooled, witt pooled, teel it gave de lest hair a wenish wot Semson hexclaimed: 'I LUFF YOU!'

So Delilah sad: 'Wal—wal!!! Now hozz about a shafe? No?? Shempoo? Is a leedle dry de skeen—massage? A seenge maybe odder a twizze de heyebrozz??? A mod-peck? Gudgeous wadder we heving. Shine??? Hozz about a leedle mange-cure for de lion skeen??? Wal, wal, sotch a himproofment! De bobbed hair makes you look witt at list tan years yonger!!!'

So Semson sad: 'Hm, bot you should see before wot it was bobbed. Was sotch a head hair wot I was hable I should seet on it!!! Ho wal, is motch murr a convenience dees way in de sommer-time . . . By de way, wot was I saying? Ho yes—I luff you!!!'

So she sad in a werry cuxxing tun from voice: 'Will you band plizze a hairpeen for me, Dirrie?'

So Semson trite like annytink he should band de hairpeen wot he sad so: 'Hm, wot's dees?!?! I'm filling a leedle grocky!! Whooy!! De spreeng wadder, no dott. Ho boy—look it dun't banding de hairpeen! I'm filling wick in de knizz.'

So it came hout from Delilah a reeple from leffter, a mocking one, wot she said: 'Hm—a leedle wick in de knizz, ha, stoopit? Is dees a fect?? So tomorrow'll be by de Pheelistins a poddy. So you inwited. Comm opp dere you should strott your stoff you should make for dem a hect you should poosh in a Swees chizze tom-tecks!! Hm, you gatting pale!! Heh heh heh.'

So it keptured de Pheelistins Semson wot dey hed it a poddy witt a dronken ogre in de Tample wot dey made dere from Semson hall sutts from jukks witt tunts witt smot-crecks wot he became med like annytink wot he roshed queeck by a sturr from weegs witt toupizz—wot he pushed on queek a weeg—so from dees he bicame gradually strung wot he gafe a push don de pillows from de Tample wot it keeled hall de Pheelistins wot it smeshed dem hall opp to adams!

Monosyllabic Verse

Try writing a verse of eight lines or more, making some sort of poetic sense, that has no word of more than one syllable. It's not easy. Phineas Fletcher, who died around 1650, came up with this alliterative specimen, which fails the mark by one word:

New light new love, new love new life hath bred;
A light that lives by love, and loves by light;
A love to Him to whom all loves are wed;
A light to whom the sun is dark as night.
Eye's light, heart's love, soul's only life He is;
Life, soul, love, heart, light, eye, and all are His;
He eye, light, heart, love, soul; He all my joy and bliss.

The Most Unkindest Cuts of All

Percy Hammond called criticism 'the venom from contented rattlesnakes'. Heywood Broun referred to it as 'Pieces of Hate'. They had such comments as these in mind:

'It was one of those plays in which all the actors unfortunately enunciated very clearly.' (Robert Benchley)

'People laugh at this [*Abie's Irish Rose*] every night, which explains why democracy can never be a success.' (Benchley)

Heywood Broun once classified Geoffrey Steyne as the worst actor on the stage. Next play around, he wrote: 'Mr. Steyne's performance was not up to its usual standard.'

'In the first act *she* becomes a lady. In the second act *he* becomes a lady.' (Alexander Woollcott)

Dorothy Parker, reviewing a book on science: 'It was written without fear and without research.'

'This is not a novel to be tossed aside lightly. It should be thrown with great force.' (Parker)

'No worse than a bad cold.' (Harpo Marx on *Abie's Irish Rose*)

'There is less in this than meets the eye.' (Tallulah Bankhead, at an unsuccessful revival of the Maeterlinck play *Aglavaine and Selysette*)

'She ran the whole gamut of emotions, from A to B.' (Parker on a performance by Katherine Hepburn)

On signing a first-edition copy of his book *Shouts and Murmurs*, Alexander Woollcott sighed and said: 'Ah, what is so rare as a Woollcott first edition?'

'A Woollcott second edition,' replied F.P.A.

On a not-so-funny comedy: 'Some laughter was heard in the back rows. Someone must have been telling jokes back there.' (Robert Benchley)

George Jean Nathan wrote of an ill-done *Doll's House* that when Nora walked out on her household and slammed the door, the audience rose as one man and rushed to the stage to congratulate the husband.

After an execrable performance of *Hamlet*, Robert Hendrickson remarked: 'There has long been a controversy over who wrote Shakespeare's plays—Shakespeare or Bacon. I propose to settle it today by opening their graves. Whoever turned over wrote *Hamlet*.'

Shaw on Gounod's *Redemption*: 'If you will only take the precaution to go in long enough after it commences and to come out long enough before it is over, you will not find it wearisome.'

Mid-Victorian lady, emerging from a performance of *The Agamemnon*: 'How different, how very different, from the home life of our own dear Queen.'

Sydney Smith on Macaulay, an interminable talker: 'He has occasional flashes of silence that make his conversation perfectly delightful.'

Dorothy Parker on the autobiography of Margot Asquith: 'The affair between Margot Asquith and Margot Asquith will live as one of the prettiest love stories in all literature.'

And on A. A. Milne's *The House At Pooh Corner*: 'Tonstant Weader fwowed up.'

Mots d'Heures: Gousses, Rames

To get the sense of Luis D'Antin Van Rooten's *Mots D'Heures: Gousses, Rames*, read them aloud, and see if the sounds and the rhythm don't remind you of some familiar English jingles. (The footnotes are Mr. Van Rooten's own.) If you are utterly without French, skip.

Chacun Gille[1]
Houer ne taupe de hile[2]
Tôt-fait, j'appelle au boiteur[3]
Chaque fêle dans un broc,[4] est-ce crosne?[5]
Un Gille qu'aime tant berline à fêtard.[6]

Dissolu typique,[1] Ouen ou Marquette.[2]
Dissolu typique, c'tiède homme.[3]
Dissolu typique a des roses vives.[4]
Dissolu typique, aie de nom,
Dissolu typique, craille
Oui, oui, oui,
A louer: heaume.[5]

Jacques s'apprête
Coulis de nos fêtes.[1]
Et soif que dites nos lignes.[2]
Et ne sauve bédouine tempo[3] y aussi,
Telle y que de plat terre, cligne.[4]

[1] Gille is a stock character in medieval plays, usually a fool or country bumpkin.
[2] While hoeing he uncovers a mole and part of a seed.
[3] Quickly finished, I call to the limping man that
[4] every pitcher has a crack in it. If a philosophy or moral is intended, it is very obscure.
[5] 'Is it a Chinese cabbage?' It is to be assumed that he refers to the seed he found.
[6] At any rate he loves a life of pleasure and a carriage.

[1] A typical wastrel, in short, a regular bum. (*Continued overleaf*)

[2] Ouen (saint), bishop of Rouen, circa 609–683 A.D.; Père Marquette (1637–1675), French Jesuit, discovered the Mississippi. Two moral and saintly men of action to be emulated.

[3] A tepid man. What a matchless description!

[4] Fresh roses are used as hedonist symbols in this context.

[5] The last and, if the pun is forgiven, crowning shame. The craven wastrel, fallen upon evil days, croaks 'Yes, yes, yes, my crest is for rent!' i.e., he is willing to sell his birthright—the family jewels having long since disappeared. This verse patently belongs to the age of moralists and essayists, and forms an interesting parallel to Hogarth's famed *Rake's Progress*.

[1] *Coulis*, a sort of strained broth. Jacques was either a sauce chef or an invalid.

[2] Jacques was also an alcoholic, since his thirst is beyond description.

[3] He was fond of Arab music.

[4] He believed the earth was flat. The last word of the line, meaning 'wink', is obviously a stage direction. Poor Jacques, whoever he was, was undoubtedly considered a fool.

N

The Nimble Bitterness of Bierce

Wordplay can be holy; Gerard Manley Hopkins's was. It can be cynical and hopeless; Ambrose Bierce's was. What a weight must have pressed upon this mysterious man, who defined *November* as 'the eleventh twelfth of a weariness'; *once* as 'enough'; *birth* as 'the first and direst of all disasters'!

To Bierce, a *bigot* is 'one obstinately and zealously attached to an opinion you do not entertain'; *billingsgate*, 'the invective of an opponent'. *Calamities* are of two kinds: 'misfortune to ourselves, and good fortune to others'.

Comfort, says Bierce, is 'a state of mind produced by contemplation of a neighbour's uneasiness'; *consolation*, 'the knowledge that a better man is more unfortunate than yourself'. *Meekness* is 'uncommon patience in planning a revenge that is worthwhile'.

A *hand*, he says, is 'a singular instrument worn at the end of a human arm and commonly thrust into somebody's pocket'. An *egotist* is 'a person of low taste, more interested in himself than in me'. *Happiness* is 'an agreeable situation arising from contemplating the misery of another'.

By ethical definition, Bierce was a miserable specimen of a man. But what fun! What wordplay!

Nouns of Multitude

The Books of Courtesy, medieval primers intended to provide a gentleman with the means of social acceptability, dealt with a variety of collective nouns, but concentrated on those of the hunt, known as venery.

If you are familiar with the history of venery, you will fill in quickly most of the words missing from the verse below. On the chance that you lack a venereal education, I have made things easier by providing some words with which the venereal terms rhyme.

Tarantara, tarantara, off the hunters ride,
Off to bag a ***[1] of pheasants, or perhaps a ****.[2]
Stalking now a *****[3] of wildfowl, now a ******[4] of teal;
Counting on a ****[5] of mallards for their evening meal.

Tarantara, tarantara, home the hunters straggle,
With a **********[6] of choughs, with of geese a ******.[7]
Overhead a *****[8] of geese, a *******[9] of widgeons;
Underfoot, a ****[10] of dottrel. On the sidewalk—pigeons.

W. R. E.

1. Eye.
2. Side.
3. Lump.
4. Ring.
5. Bored.
6. Smattering.
7. Straggle.
8. Pain.
9. Bum penny, with the emphasis on the bum.
10. Flip.

(ANSWERS OVERLEAF)

ANSWERS

Tarantara, tarantara, off the hunters ride,
Off to bag a *nye* of pheasants, or perhaps a *hide*.
Stalking now a *plump* of wildfowl, now a *spring* of teal,
Counting on a *sord* of mallards for their evening meal.

Tarantara, tarantara, home the hunters straggle,
With a *chattering* of choughs, with of geese a *gaggle*.
Overhead a *skein* of geese, a *company* of widgeons;
Underfoot, a *trip* of dottrel. On the sidewalk—pigeons.

AN ENTRANCE OF ACTRESSES

Such, according to James Lipton* in *Playbill*, is the proper venereal term for a gathering of the grand ladies of the theatre. He continues:

'On the other hand, a collection of untried ingenues is *a wiggle of starlets*. Both groups owe their livelihood to *a pinch of producers*, who in turn owe theirs to *a host of angels*. If the show is a musical, chances are the stars will be joined onstage by *a quaver of sopranos* and *a rumble of basses*, as well as *a float of dancers* (female) and *a flit of dancers* (male).'

Mr. Lipton goes on to describe members of the audience, including *a hack of smokers* and *a load of drunks*. He tells how after the show the stars make their way to a famous restaurant through *a click of photographers* and *a shriek of claques*, and face *an indifference of waiters* as they eat *a clutch of eggs* while awaiting the verdicts of *a shrivel of critics*. If the notices are bad, the play must expect *an unction of undertakers*; if it is dreadfully bad, *an extreme unction of undertakers*.

'If, however, the play is a hit,' concludes Mr. Lipton, 'then the stars can look forward to *a thrill of fans*—and, alas, *a descent of relatives*.'

---

* He wrote *An Exaltation of Larks*, an indispensable handbook of medieval and modern venery.

A LIST OF THINGS

In a *New York Magazine* contest to see who could produce the inanest collective nouns, the following entries were among those printed.

1. A **** of students
2. A ***** of prostitutes
3. A ************* of thinkers
4. A **** of parasites
5. A ***** of puppies

6. A ********** of sycophants
7. A ****** of cowards
8. A ***** of ovens
9. A **** of dragons
10. A ***** of ghosts

ANSWERS

1. Riot.
2. Horde.
3. Concentration.
4. Host.
5. Field.

6. Complement.
7. Quiver.
8. Range.
9. Slew.
10. Fraid.

O.K.

This expression, meaning 'all right, correct', is, as Eric Partridge remarks, 'an evergreen of the correspondence columns'. A fresh argument about its origin flared recently in the *New York Times* as the result of a statement by David Danby that it derives from a number of West African languages, and slipped into English by way of the slave trade.

However compelling Mr. Danby may have considered his arguments, some of his readers did not accept them. O.K. came into general use in the United States around 1839–40; Danby claims the 1816 diary of a Jamaica planter records 'a similar expression', i.e.: 'Oh ki, massa, doctor no need be fright, we no want to hurt him'. But one *Times* correspondent argues that the expression is derived from Spanish *hoque* (pronounced okay), which in turn descends from *alboroque*, 'treat stood by buyer or seller after closing a deal'. And this would far antedate 1816.

Partridge, as good an authority as any, leans toward 'oll korrect', 'order recorded', or Choctaw '(h)oke' as the source. 'Oll korrect' has been attributed to Andrew Jackson, who had an excellent command of spoken Choctaw and a limited one of written English.

Other attributions, some not yet recorded in the correspondence columns of *The Times*:

Aux Quais, an expression referring either to (1) goods headed for the docks for shipment; (2) cotton bales headed specifically to the docks of New Orleans for shipment; or (3) a trysting arrangement between French sailors and American maidens during the Revolution.

Otto Krist, a timber magnate of the Pacific North-west, whose credit was so good that anything he initialled was 'O.K.'.

The *Orrins–Kendall* Company, which placed its initials on the boxes of excellent crackers it supplied during the American Civil War.

Oikea, a Finnish word meaning 'correct'.

Lord *Onslow* and his counsel, Lord *Kilbracken*, whose approval was necessary for certain bills passed by the House of Lords.

H. G.., pronounced 'hah gay', meaning 'shipshape', an expression common long ago among Danish and Norwegian sailors.

Och aye, Scottish.

O qu-oui, an emphatic French form of *yes*, as recorded in Sterne's *A Sentimental Journey* (1768).

ὢχ, ὢχ, a magical incantation against fleas, supposedly from *Geoponica*, written in the thirteenth century.

Whatever the ultimate origin of the expression, it was popularised in the American Presidential campaign of 1840 as an abbreviation of Old Kinderhook, a nickname (because he was born at Kinderhook, N.Y.) of Martin Van Buren, the Democratic candidate. This date would seen to eliminate both Otto Krist and Orrins–Kendall as contenders.

Nothing has been settled, and you may expect the argument to flare up again.

OH, NOA, NOA!

In Aku Aku is there double
The happiness, and half the trouble?
And far away in Bali Bali,
Should not it all be twice as jolly?

Does sunset out in Bora Bora
Reveal a repetitious aura?
And surely every joke would be a
Double entendre in Fia Fia?

Do residents of Pago Pago
Get twice the juice from every mango?
Do people out in Walla Walla
Get twofold value for their dollah?

Don't men in Sing Sing, who for crime go,
Hate like the deuce to see their time go?
And over there in Baden Baden,
I'm sure that life's not half so sodden?

*   *   *   *

Alas! I'm told in *no* vicinity
Is such a thing as blessed twinnity!

William Cole

*

On the Square

Of the making of word squares there is no end. The concept is simple: all you have to do is create a set of words that reads the same from left to right and from top to bottom.

A
A

is a word square. So is

I
I

Slightly more complex is

M A
A M

Up a further step is

O F T
F O E
T E N

But no word-square addict recognises any square of words of less than four letters:

T W I T	H O P E	W I S P
W E R E	O P A L	I N T O
I R O N	P A L M	S T O P
T E N T	E L M S	P O P S

The difficulty of five-letter squares squares the difficulty of four-letter squares:

W A R T S
A W A I T
R A D A R
T I A R A
S T R A W

And the difficulty of seven-letter squares cubes that of five-letter squares:

M E R G E R S
E T E R N A L
R E G A T T A
G R A V I T Y
E N T I T L E
R A T T L E R
S L A Y E R S

Making word squares is a good way of putting yourself to sleep—and, sometimes, of getting insomnia. Those below may affect you either way:

1. Four-letter words
(*a*) Harvest
(*b*) Other
(*c*) Continent
(*d*) Fruit

2. Four-letter words
(*a*) Approach
(*b*) Ellipse
(*c*) Religious ceremony
(*d*) Otherwise

3. Five-letter words
(*a*) Replete
(*b*) Make up for
(*c*) Cheers, for example
(*d*) Follow in order
(*e*) Discourage or restrain

ANSWERS

1.	R E A P	2.	C O M E	3.	S A T E D
	E L S E		O V A L		A T O N E
	A S I A		M A S S		T O A S T
	P E A R		E L S E		E N S U E
					D E T E R

SQUARE OF ORDER 9

To make squares of nine-letter words, one has to reach. The square below, by Wayne M. Goodwin, whom Martin Gardner describes as 'one of the greatest square experts of all time', contains only two words that cannot be found in Webster's *Unabridged Dictionary*. According to Dmitri Borgmann, 'retitrate' means to titrate again, and is found in the two-volume supplement to the *Century Dictionary*, 1909, while Eavestone is the name of a town in eastern West Riding, Yorkshire.

```
F R A T E R I E S
R E G I M E N A L
A G I T A T I V E
T I T A N I T E S
E M A N A T I S T
R E T I T R A T E
I N I T I A T O R
E A V E S T O N E
S L E S T E R E D
```

The tusks that clashed in mighty brawls
Of mastodons, are billiard balls.

The sword of Charlemagne the Just
Is ferric oxide, known as rust.

The grizzly bear whose potent hug
Was feared by all, is now a rug.

Great Caesar's dead and on the shelf,
And I don't feel so well myself!

Arthur Guiterman

*

Origin Unknown

Take an English word from Partridge at hazard—*screen*, for instance
—and it has a kingly genealogy:

'SCREEN. Middle English *scren*, aphetic for: Middle French *escren*, variant
of *escran* (French *ecran*) by metathesis from: Medieval Dutch *scherm*,
scheerm; cf Old High German *scirm*, Middle High German *schirm*, protection (cf German *Schirm*, umbrella), and Middle High German
schirmen, variant of *schermen*, to fence: ? akin, as Walshe suggests, to
Sanskrit *cǎrma*, the skin. From the appearance of a protective screen
derives the goldminers' *screen* or sieve, whence to *screen* or scrutinize
thoroughly before admission; the older sense "to protect" derives from
the very nature of the protective screen itself.'

Thorough indeed—for *screen*. Yet there are hundreds, perhaps
thousands, of words that have no agreed-upon origin at all. We
know what curmudgeon, larrup and moola mean, but we don't
know where they came from. Partridge and Skeat don't know;
Asimov, Barfield, Brown, Evans, Flesch, Funk, Holt, Howell,
Moore, Morris, Pei, Strunk, Weekley, White and Willett don't
know; I don't know.

THE BIRTH OF 'QUIZ'

The manager of a Dublin play-house wagered that a word of no
meaning should be the common talk and puzzle of the city in

twenty-four hours. In the course of that time he had the letters
q u i z chalked on all the walls of Dublin. He won the wager—
and the word, an utter fabrication, thrives.

The three rhymes below celebrate certain words of obscure or
unknown origin. In each case there is a real clue to the word, and
a fanciful suggestion as to how the word may have happened.

I

Blood swells in a bruise, and a g
Goes soft in a gun;
A sensible start, you'll agree,
For a stick used to stun.

2

The durable cloak of a witch on a sail
Snagged the tip of a spire as she passed.
She wove all her spells, but to no avail;
'It ***'* ***,' she conceded at last.

3

The tar who slanged the cap'n
By his sword was quickly cut to size.
Meanwhile the ship turned over.
Next week: 'Mutiny in Paradise.'

W. R. E.

ANSWERS

1. Bludgeon. 'A short stick, with one end thicker or heavier than the
   other, used as an offensive weapon.'
2. Cantrip. 'A charm; spell; trick, as of a witch.'
3. Capsize. 'To upset or overturn, as a vessel or other body.'

Oxymorons

Oxymorons are a curious inheritance from the Greeks—combinations for rhetoric effect of contradictory or incongruous words:
'harmonious discord'; 'a cheerful pessimist'. The Greek word

itself marries 'sharp' to 'dull'. Tennyson was in oxymoronic vein when he wrote:

> His honour rooted in dishonour stood,
> And faith unfaithful kept him falsely true.

So was Shakespeare when he wrote (in *Richard II*) of 'ruthful butchery'.

James Thurber, seeking to confound an editor who pounced on any discrepancy in writing, once described a building as 'pretty ugly, and a little too big for its site'.

A *New York Times* editorial contains the sentence, 'Sometimes it requires devious and even odd ways to accomplish good purposes.' In 'even odd' we have an accidental oxymoron, a thing to be deplored; for, as one scholar* puts it, 'The good oxymoron, to define it by a self-illustration, must be a planned inadvertency.'

An official in the United States Treasury Department is said to have reminded his colleagues of the importance of diction by circulating among them this oxymoronic jargon:

'It should be noted that a slowing up of the slowdown is not as good as an upturn in the downcurve, but it is a good deal better than either a speedup of the slowdown or a deepening of the downcurve; and it does suggest that the climate is about right for an adjustment to the readjustment.'

The most-quoted oxymoron of our time, from a 1954 decision of the Supreme Court of the United States, directs that schools throughout the nation must be integrated 'with all deliberate speed'.

I have no oxymoronic word games to offer you, but you are welcome to develop colloquies like the following to your heart's content:

He: You are looking terribly well.
She: Under the circumstances, it's horribly decent of you to say that.
He: Why this nasty politeness?
She: It's just that we have increasingly little to say to each other.
He: What an oddly natural remark, coming from you!
She: Well, you are an uncommonly common fellow.
He: And you are possibly the most impossible girl I have ever met.

---

* Wilson Follett in *Modern American Usage* (Hill and Wang, 1966).

THE OYSTER

The oyster's a confusing suitor;
It's masc., and fem., and even neuter.
At times it wonders, may what come,
Am I husband, wife, or chum.

Ogden Nash

*

P, Q

Palindromes

IN PURSUIT OF THE ABOMINABLE PALINDROME

Since that day in 1610 when the primeval Espy forsook his oozy
Scottish bog for the sunny, carefree Plantations of Northern
Ireland, our family's unique distinction has been its utter lack of
distinction. This is humiliating; and when it became evident,
perhaps by my sixth or seventh year, that I was not destined to
break the family tradition, I began a lifelong search for bygone
relatives who might have left their mark. (Any mark; for quite a
while, I suspect, not many of them could write.) My search has
carried me through the records of dusty libraries, dilapidated
churches, and graveyards crowded with tottering stones – always
hoping against hope to locate some male forebear who had carried
'Gent.' after his name, or some milkmaid who had managed to
cozen the local squire into marrying her. Let me say that the
search was not fruitless; I found a man who had won the right to
wear his hat in the presence of the king, and a woman, a good
Christian soul, who was hanged as a witch at Salem.

This proud history is relayed, I assure you, in no spirit of
snobbery, but simply to explain how it happened that recently
I have been baying after a connection (posited shakily through
my grandmother, Annie Medora Taylor) with the seventeenth-

century Water Poet, John Taylor, a rollicking sort who once set out for Queenborough from London in a brown-paper boat, and almost drowned.

The Water Poet wrote the first palindrome recorded in the English language. (A palindrome, in case you don't know, is a word or sentence which reads the same forward and backward.) Mr. Taylor's innocently revealing contribution was

Lewd I did live, & evil did I dwel.

Now, you may say this is a second-rate palindrome, depending as it does on misspelling 'dwell' (though he didn't really), and substituting an ampersand for 'and'; still, it was the first of its kind in English, and that was the spelling of the day. What is more, the *Monthly Magazine and Literary Journal* reported in 1821, nearly two hundred years later, that no palindrome had appeared since.

'Our own observation,' declared the journal, 'confirms the difficulty of composing them in our own langauge, which this rarity implies. We have frequently laboured at arrangements of words which would form an English palindrome line, but always unsuccessfully, which surprised us, as we have in English so many palindrome words.'

The writer apparently did not take Welsh into account. There existed even then a longstanding Welsh palindrome, 'Liad ded dail', meaning 'holy blind father'.

There also existed a classical palindrome tradition (not in Greek, for only one Greek palindrome has been preserved, but certainly in Latin, which lends itself to reversals).

In the following Latin example, each line is a selfcontained palindrome. It has been attributed to Sotades of Crete, whose coarse satires and personal attacks in the second century B.C. so enraged Ptolemy II that the monarch finally caused him to be sewn up in a sack and thrown into the sea. How this attribution has endured is a mystery. In the first place, Sotades wrote in Greek, not Latin. In the second place, he was born two hundred years before Christ, while the palindrome refers to a legendary event in the life of St. Martin. The more probable author was a fifth-century bishop, Sidonius Apollinaris.

The whole verse, of which this is only a fragment, tells how Saint Martin rode the devil—that ass having stupidly transformed himself into an ass—into Rome, prodding him on with repeated signs of the cross.

Signa te signa; temere me tangis et angis;
Roma, tibi subito motibus ibit amor
Si bene te tua laus taxat, sua laute tenebis,
Solo medere pede, ede, perede molos.

An acronymic Latin palindrome is EVVNVVE, the initials standing for 'Ede ut vivas, ne vivas ut edas'. There is an almost exact English equivalent, ETLNLTE: 'Eat to live; never live to eat'.

The next palindrome after the Water Poet's to surface in English gained currency almost at the moment that the *Monthly Magazine* was abandoning the whole effort as hopeless. Presumably prompted by Napoleon's defeat at Waterloo, it reads, 'Able was I ere I saw Elba'.

From then on, the floodgates were open. By the 1870s the *New Monthly Magazine* was running such effusions as:

A milkman jilted by his lass, or wandering in his wits,
Might murmur, 'Stiff, o dairyman, in a myriad of fits.'

A limner, by photography dead beat in his position,
Thus grumbled: 'No, it is opposed; art sees trade's opposition.'

A timid creature, fearing rodents, mice and such small fry,
'Stop, Syrian, I start at rats in airy spots' might cry.

Some of the crop were not that bad. 'Draw pupil's lip upward' might, in some inconceivable circumstance, be considered a reasonable command. Two palindromes of the period have style: 'I, man, am regal; a German am I,' and 'Sums are not set as a test on Erasmus.'

At this time, too, there came palindromic versions of the first introduction, 'Madam, I'm Adam'; the first conscript's complaint, 'Snug & raw was I ere I saw war & guns'; and the first hint of the generation gap, 'Egad, a base tone denotes a bad age'. The nineteenth century also saw the prototype of the nonsense palindrome, intriguing because one feels it really *should* mean something: 'Dog, a devil deified, deified lived a god.'

The building of the Panama Canal by Goethals inspired the classic 'A man, a plan, a canal—Panama'. Other palindromes that have been around quite awhile are 'Step on no pets'; 'Never odd or even'; 'Mad Zeus, no live devil, lived evil on Suez dam'; and

'Live dirt, up a side-track carted, is a putrid evil'. These more recent examples were handed to me the other day by William Cole: 'A slut nixes sex in Tulsa' and 'Dennis and Edna sinned'.

By providing a context, one can give some palindromes the appearance of meaning. Two of my own are examples:

Slogan for opponents of the Women's Liberation Movement: 'Rise, sir lapdog! Revolt, lover! God, pal, rise, sir!'

A straightforward comment: 'Live on evasions? No, I save no evil.'

In the examples below I have tried to legitimise my palindromes by building them into verses. The palindromes are set off by quotation marks.

Second Honeymoon at Niagara Falls

Beside thee, torrent, with sweet moan, long since,
We gloried in our love, took off the lid.
Last night was she still princess, I still prince?
Did I, though very squiffed, still make my bid?
Speak, torrent! If thou hear me, answer! 'I
Did roar again, Niagara! . . . or did
I?' But the falls fall on; there's no reply.

W. R. E.

Matter of Etiquette

Meg's fashion in passion, though warm, 'll
Strike some as a shade over-formal.
 In the midst of a bout,
 She was heard to cry out,
'La, Mr. O'Neill, lie normal!'

W. R. E.

A final titbit: the longest palindrome having to do with a region is Malayalam, the name of a Dravidian language spoken on the Malabar in India.

The following definitions will give you an opportunity to make your own palindromes, or, more exactly, to remake those of others.

1. Anything hereafter will be from this.
2. Two words, followed by 'or shut up'.

3. Professional warning to a sleepy student.
4. Why owls shun the tropics.
5. Challenge to Sir Noel.
6. The reaction of a star to hints that she may have connived at the theft of her jewels.

ANSWERS

1. Now on.
2. Put up.
3. Don't nod.

4. Too hot to hoot.
5. Draw, O coward!
6. Rob a gem? Me? Gabor?

SEMORDNILAP

'Semordnilap' is 'palindromes' spelled backwards, and stands for words that spell different words in reverse. Some examples: devil, repaid, stressed, rewarder, straw, maps, strap, reknits, deliver, bard, doom.

See 'Milton, Thou Should'st Be Re-Versing at This Hour' on page 45.

Patchwork Verse

Patchwork verses, also called centones or mosaics, are poems composed of selected verses or passages from an author, or from different authors, so strung together as to present an entirely new reading. If you have the time and patience (I have not) you can locate in your copy of Shakespeare each of the lines in the following cento, which was put together a hundred years ago for a society which met annually to celebrate the birth of the Bard.

> Peace to this meeting,
> Joy and fair time, health and good wishes.
> Now, worthy friends, the cause why we are met,
> Is in celebration of the day that gave
> Immortal Shakespeare to this favoured isle,*
> The most replenished sweet work of Nature
> Which from the prime creation e'er she framed.

(CONTINUED OVERLEAF)

---

* The writer cheated here for the sake of his theme.

O thou, divinest Nature! how thyself thou blazon'st
In this thy son! formed in thy prodigality
To hold thy mirror up, and give the time
In every form and pressure! When he speaks,
Each aged ear plays truant at his tales,
And younger hearings are quite ravished;
So voluble is his discourse. Gentle
As zephyr blowing underneath the violet,
Not wagging its sweet head—yet as rough
His noble blood enchafed, as the rude wind,
That by the top doth take the mountain pine,
And make him stoop to the vale. 'Tis wonderful
That an invisible instinct should frame him
To loyalty, unlearned; honour, untaught;
Civility, not seen in others; knowledge,
That wildly grows in him, but yields a crop
As if it had been sown. What a piece of work!
How noble in faculty! infinite in reason!
A combination and a form indeed,
Where every god did seem to set his seal.
Heaven has him now! Yet let our idolatrous fancy
Still sanctify his relics; and this day
Stand aye distinguished in the kalendar
To the last syllable of recorded time;
For if we take him but for all in all,
We ne'er shall look upon his like again.

HAMLET AND HUCKLEBERRY FINN

In Mark Twain's *Huckleberry Finn*, the duke dredges his muddled
memory of Shakespeare in quest of Hamlet's Soliloquy, and brings
up this:

To be, or not to be; that is the bare bodkin
That makes calamity of so long life;
For who would fardels bear, till Birnam Wood do come to
    Dunsinane,
But that the fear of something after death
Murders the innocent sleep,
Great nature's second course,
And makes us rather sling the arrows of outrageous fortune
Than fly to others that we know not of.

186

There's the respect must give us pause;
Wake Duncan with thy knocking! I would thou couldst;
For who would bear the whips and scorns of time,
The oppressor's wrong, the proud man's contumely,
The law's delay, and the quietus which his pangs might take,
In the dead waste and middle of the night, when churchyards
yawn
In customary suits of solemn black,
But that the undiscovered country from whose bourne no traveller
returns
Breathes forth contagion on the world,
And thus the native nue of resolution, like the poor cat i' the
adage,
Is sicklied o'er with care,
And all the clouds that lowered o'er our housetops,
With this regard their currents turn awry
And lose the name of action.
'Tis a consummation devoutly to be wished. But soft you, the
fair Ophelia:
Ope not thy ponderous and marble jaws,
But get thee to a nunnery—go!

I ONLY KNOW SHE CAME AND WENT

If in two weeks or so you have not managed to trace the lines in
the following cento to their original homes, read on: the authors
are listed, line by line, below the verses. The compiler is unknown.

1	I only know she came and went,
2	Like troutlets in a pool;
3	She was a phantom of delight,
4	And I was like a fool.
5	One kiss, dear maid, I said, and sighed,
6	Out of those lips unshorn,
7	She shook her ringlets round her head
8	And laughed in merry scorn.
9	Ring out, wild bells, to the wild sky,
10	You heard them, O my heart;
11	'Tis twelve at night by the castle clock,
12	Beloved, we must part. (CONTINUED OVERLEAF)

13	'Come back, come back!' she cried in grief,
14	My eyes are dim with tears—
15	How shall I live through all the days?
16	All through a hundred years?

17	'Twas in the prime of summer time,
18	She blessed me with her hand;
19	We strayed together, deeply blest,
20	Into the dreaming land.

21	The laughing bridal roses blow,
22	To dress her dark-brown hair;
23	My heart is breaking with my woe,
24	Most beautiful! most rare!

25	I clasped it on her sweet, cold hand,
26	The precious golden link!
27	I calmed her fears, and she was calm,
28	'Drink, pretty creature, drink!'

29	And so I won my Genevieve,
30	And walked in Paradise;
31	The fairest thing that ever grew
32	Atween me and the skies!

ANSWERS

Pennsylvania Dutch

Thousands of Germans in America once spoke a dialect that curiously combined English words with German forms and idioms. Traces of this tongue linger in the farmhouses of the Pennsylvania Dutch. The following takeoff on their speech, at least a century old, is the work of an expert:

LOVE SONG

O vere mine lofe a sugar-powl,
    De fery shmallest loomp
Vouldt shveet de seas, from pole to pole,
    Und make de shildren shoomp.
Und if she vere a clofer-field,
    I'd bet my only pence,
It vouldn't pe no dime at all
    Pefore I'd shoomp the fence.

Her heafenly foice, it drill me so,
    If oft-dimes seems to hoort,
She is de holiest animale
    Dat rooms oopon de dirt.
De renpow rises vhen she sings,
    De sonnshine vhen she dalk;
De angels crow und flop deir wings
    Vhen she goes out to valk.

So livin white, so carnadine,
    Mine lofe's gomblexion show;
It's shoost like Abendcarmosine,
    Rich gleamin on de shnow.
Her soul makes plushes in her sheek
    Ash sommer reds de wein,
Or sonnlight sends a fire life troo
    An blank Karfunkelstein.

(CONTINUED OVERLEAF)

De uberschwengliche idees
  Dis lofe poot in my mind,
Vouldt make a foost-rate philosoph
  Of any human kind.
'Tis schudderin schveet on eart to meet
  An himmlisch-hoellisch Qual;
Und treat mitwhiles to Kümmel Schnapps
  De Schoenheitsideal.

Dein Füss seind weiss wie Kreiden,
  Dein Ermlein Helfenbein,
Dein ganzer Leib ist Seiden,
  Dein Brust wie Marmelstein—
Ja—vot de older boet sang,
  I sing of dee—dou Fine!
Dou'rt soul und pody, heart und life:
  Glatt, zart, gelind, und rein.

                    Charles G. Leland

                *

THE PURIST

I give you now Professor Twist,
A conscientious scientist.
Trustees exclaim, 'He never bungles!'
And send him off to distant jungles.
Camped on a tropic riverside,
One day he missed his loving bride.
She had, the guide informed him later,
Been eaten by an alligator.
Professor Twist could not but smile.
'You mean,' he said, 'a crocodile.'

                    Ogden Nash

                *

Pidgin English

VOCABULARY

Melanesian pidgin has a basic vocabulary of about 1300 words, which can be combined to translate some 6000 English words. The language is derived almost exclusively from Melanesian and English, and the words listed below can be traced to the English originals by an approximation of sounds. The English equivalents follow the list.

1. Aiting
2. Aratsait
3. Astadei
4. Baembai
5. Bihain
6. Bikples
7. Darai
8. Daunpilo
9. Em
10. Faulnabaut
11. Filimnogut
12. Giraun
13. Gudei
14. Gutbai
15. Haitim, *v.t.*
16. Hanggiri
17. Hariap, *v.i.*
18. Hausat?
19. Hiparei
20. Insaet
21. Kamap, *v.i.*
22. Kilaut
23. Kotrein
24. Kraikrai
25. Kwiktaim

26. Lam wokabaut
27. Lephan
28. Longwei
29. Mandei
30. Moabeta
31. Numbata
32. Nosave, *v.i.*
33. Nuspepa
34. Peim
35. Plaiyas
36. Popi
37. Rait, *v.i.*
38. Ronewei, *v.i.*
39. Samting
40. Samting nating
41. Solapim, *v.t.*
42. Stima
43. Tanim bek, *v.t.*
44. Tok tiru, *v.i.*
45. Tudak
46. Tulait
47. Wankain
48. Win
49. Wisiki
50. Wok

(ANSWERS OVERLEAF)

ANSWERS

1. I think
2. Outside
3. Yesterday
4. Afterwards, later, bye and bye
5. At the rear of, after, behind
6. Mainland
7. Dry, withered
8. Down below, below
9. He, they, she, it, him, her, them
10. Conflicting (of testimony, rumour, etc.); all messed up
11. Not feel well, be in pain
12. Ground, soil, the earth
13. Good day
14. Good-bye
15. Conceal
16. Hungry, hunger
17. Hurry, hurry up
18. Why?
19. Cheering, acclamation
20. Inside
21. Arrive, approach, be revealed
22. Cloud
23. Raincoat
24. Weep copiously
25. Quickly, speedily
26. Hurricane lamp
27. Left side, left hand
28. Far, distant
29. Monday
30. Better, very good
31. Second, number two
32. Have no knowledge of, be unaccustomed to
33. Newspaper
34. Sell
35. Pliers
36. Roman Catholic
37. Write
38. Run away, desert
39. Something, a thing
40. Thing of no consequence
41. Slap, strike with open hand
42. Steamship
43. Turn back, turn about, bend back
44. Speak the truth
45. Dark, night
46. Light, daylight
47. Similar, of the same kind or species
48. Wind, gas, breath, air
49. Whisky
50. Work, duty, employment

PLUCKING A PIDGIN (in Pidgin)

A pigeon in Pidgin English is *balus*, a word applicable to the foolish young man plucked in the story below. The words used come from John J. Murphy's *Book of Pidgin English*; the grammar, I fear, is my own.

A few bits of information before you begin your translation: Pidgin lacks not only the definite and indefinite article but the verb 'to be'. Bear in mind too that a *p* is used in some words where we would use *f*; thus in Melanesian Pidgin, *plag* is *flag*, *pluwa* is *floor*, *prauwin* is *following wind*, *prog* is *frog*. Also, *tasol* is *but*; *long* is *to, by, with, from*, etc.; *i* is *he* or *she*; *im* is *it*; *em* is *her*; *mi* is *I*.

The other words are all corruptions of English, and if you don't try too hard the meanings should pop out at you. Don't concentrate; look at the story out of the corner of your eye; catch it unawares.

In a burst of generosity, I have supplied not one but two solutions. One is a literal rendering of the Pidgin into English; the other is a translation for sense.

Hatpela manki, bolong planti moni, tasol man nogut, laikim tumas long naispela meri wosat bolong man numbawan boss bolong ples. Wataim man wok manki wokabout long haus, painam meri wanpela long rum slip. I asken em ronawei. 'Hausat?' spik no laik meri. 'Mi no laikim yu. Go long imperno.' I kickem manki. Manki bigmaus long moni ologeta bolongen. 'Narakin,' spik meri. 'Kem hia kwiktaim. Mi reri.' I stap long monitaim long tudak. Longtaim bihain man askem meri, 'Wasamara yu gat bel?' Meri bekim tok: 'Im orrait. Mi gat moni tu.'

ANSWERS

(1) *Literal rendering*

Hot fella man-kid, belong plenty money but no-good, like too much nice fella mary belong man number one boss of place. Man-kid walkabout to house what time man work, find mary one fella in sleep-room. He ask her run away. 'How's that?' speak no-like mary: 'Me no like you. Go to inferno.' She kick man-kid. Man-kid bigmouth about money altogether belong him. 'Another kind!' speak mary. 'Come here quick time; me ready.' He stop morning time to dark. Long time behind, man ask mary, 'What'sa matter you got belly?' Mary back talk: 'It all right. Me got money too.'

(2) *Or, as you or I might say* . . .

An ardent and wealthy but villainous youth fell in love with a beautiful woman whose husband was head man of the village. When the husband was at work, the young man went to the house and found the woman alone in the bedroom. He begged her to elope. 'Why?' said the unwilling woman; 'I don't like you. Go to hell.' She kicked the youth. He bragged about his wealth. 'That's different!' said the woman, 'Come here quick. I'm ready.' He stayed from morning till night. Much later, the husband asked the wife, 'Why are you pregnant?' She replied, 'It's all right. I was well paid.'

Pidgin is an Oriental sea-change on *business*, it being a dialect which made communication possible between the natives and the English or American traders. Chinese Pidgin varies from the Melanesian in several special characteristics; it tends to substitute *l* for *r*, and, for the sake of euphony, to add *ee* or *lo* to the end of words. *Galaw* or *galow* is a kind of interjection, meaning nothing; *chop, chop* means quick; *maskee*, don't mind; *chop b'long*, of a kind; *chin chin*, good-bye; *welly culio*, very curious; *Joss-pidgin-man*, priest.

Pig Latin and Macaronics

When I was starting school we spoke Pig Latin in a number of ways, the most popular being to take the initial consonant of each syllable and shift it to the end, followed by -ay: 'E-hay ill-way ot-nay o-gay, oo-tay ool-schay oo-tay ay-day.' It was our happy illusion that no-one outside our own closed circle could possibly understand this recondite tongue.

A few years later we were struggling with Latin verbs, and our recourse was that of schooldays since the time of Virgil; we played games with what we could not understand. From hand to hand we passed such nonsense as:

Flunko, flunkere, faculty bouncem,

and this inscription, found, as we solemnly agreed, in diggings in Roman ruins:

Civili derego fortibus inero.
Demes nobus demes trux.

The translation:

'See, Willy, dere dey go, forty buses in a row.'
'Dem is no buses, dem is trucks.'

The last examples are not really Pig Latin, but macaronics, a slightly less piggish burlesque in which foreign words, sounds or spellings supplement or supplant English. You will find some in 'Berlitz School' (page 58) and *Mots d'Heures: Gousses, Rames* (page 169). 'Pas de lieu Rhône que nous' is a macaronic statement. A macaronic pun recalled by Liz Baekeland is 'Leges Romanorum boni sunt'.

More macaronics:

Parvus Jacobus Horner

Parvus Jacobus Horner
Sedebat in corner,
Edens a Christmas pie:
Inferuit thumb,
Extraherit plum—
Clamans, 'Quid sharp puer am I!'

Author Unknown

THE MOTOR BUS

What is this that roareth thus?
Can it be a Motor Bus?
Yes, the smell and hideous hum
Indicat Motorem Bum!
Implet in the Corn and High
Terror me Motoris Bi:
Bo Motori clamitabo
Ne Motore caedar a Bo—
Dative be or Ablative
So thou only let us live:—
Whither shall thy victims flee?
Spare us, spare us, Motor Be.
Thus I sang; and still anigh
Came in hordes Motores Bi,
Et complebat omne forum
Copia Motorum Borum.
How shall wretches live like us
Cincti Bis Motoribus?
Domine, defende nos
Contra hos Motores Bos!

A. D. Godley

195

DEAN SWIFT

Moll

Mollis abuti
Has an acuti;
No lasso finis
Molly divinis.

To My Mistress

O mi de armis tres
Ima na dis tres
Cantu disco ver
Meas alo ver?

A Love Song

Apud in is almi de si re,
Mimis tres I ne ver re qui re,
Alo veri findit a gestis
His miseri ne ver at restis.

Place Names, U.S.A.

Following is a foretaste of the oddities and delights of certain American place names. For the full meal, you should read a book by George R. Stewart called, aptly enough, *American Place Names:*

Aromatic Creek, Mo. 'A euphemism, probably for Stinking Creek.'

Go to Hell Gulch, S.D. 'Because a stranger asked the name of the place and was rudely told to "go to Hell".' (In the same sulfurous vein, there are: *Helltown, Hell Hole, Hell Hollow, Hell-for-Certain, Hell-for-Sure, Hell-Roaring, Purgatory Peak; Satan's Arbor*.)

Frost, Frostburg, Frosty and *Frozen* (where Hell, apparently, is frozen over).

Caress, W. Va. ('probably from a family name'); *Flirtation*, Colo. ('doubtless commemorating a pleasant incident'); *Kiss Me Quick*, S.D. (named for a 'road full of kiss-me-quicks, i.e., bumps of the kind so called'.)

196

Benign Peak and *Bellicose Peak*, Alaska; *Deception Creek*, Ark.; *Delusion Lake*, Wyo.

Another River, Alaska ('a name of desperation given by two geologists' who kept stumbling across new Alaskan rivers).

Tesnus, Tenn. ('sunset' spelled backwards); *Braggodocio*, Mo. ('probably from some incident involving boastfulness'); *Peculiar*, Mo.; *Yum Yum*, Tenn.; *Tumtum*, Wash.; *Climax*, Ore.; *Ding Dong*, in Bell County, Texas; *Welcome*, N.C.; *Do Stop*, Ky.

Candor, N.C. (the work of 'three merchants who wished the town to be distinguished by frankness'); *Goon Dip Mountain*, Alaska (for a Chinese consul in Seattle); *Fact*, Kan. ('because someone, when hearing that a post office had been established, replied, "Is that a fact?" ').

Cash, Tex. ('in honour of J. A. Money, first postmaster'); *Culdesac*, Idaho ('because a practicable route for a railroad came to a sudden end there').

Plantation Dialect

BRER RABBIT

Joel Chandler Harris's Brer Rabbit stories were written, he says, 'because of the unadulterated human nature that might be found in them'. Along with the human nature there is the Negro dialect. In this connection, Mr. Harris wrote in 1892:

'The student of English, if he be willing to search so near the ground, will find matter to interest him in the homely dialect of Uncle Remus, and if his intentions run towards philological investigation, he will pause before he has gone far and ask himself whether this negro dialect is what it purports to be, or whether it is not simply the language of the white people of three hundred years ago twisted and modified a little to fit the lingual peculiarities of the negro. Dozens of words, such as *hit* for *it*, *ax* for *ask*, *whiles* for *while*, and *heap* for a large number of people, will open before him the whole field of the philology of the English tongue. He will discover that, when Uncle Remus tells the little boy that he has "a monstus weakness fer cake what's got *reezins* in it," the pronunciation of *reezins* uncovers and rescues from oblivion Shakespeare's pun on *raisins*, where Falstaff tells the Prince, "If reasons were as plentiful as blackberries, I would give no man a reason on compulsion, I." '

Here is Uncle Remus telling the little boy why Brer Fox's legs are black:

'One time Brer Rabbit en Brer Fox went out in de woods huntin', en atter so long a time, dey 'gun ter git hongry. Leas' ways Brer Fox did, kaze Brer Rabbit had brung a ashcake in his wallet, en eve'y time he got a chance he'd eat a mou'ful—eve'y time Brer Fox 'd turn his back, Brer Rabbit 'd nibble at it. Well, endurin' er de day, Brer Fox 'gun ter get mighty hongry. Dey had some game what dey done kill, but dey wuz a fur ways fum home, en dey ain't had no fier fer ter cook it.

'Dey ain't know what ter do. Brer Fox so hongry it make his head ache. Bimeby de sun gun ter git low, en it shine red thoo de trees.

'Brer Rabbit 'low, "Yonder, whar you kin git some fier."

'Brer Fox say, "Wharbouts?"

'Brer Rabbit 'low, "Down whar de sun is. She'll go in her hole terreckly, en den you kin git a big chunk er fier. Des leave yo' game here wid me, en go git de fier. You er de biggest en de swiftest, en kin go quicker."

'Wid dat Brer Fox put out ter whar de sun is. He trot, he lope, en he gallup, en bimeby he git dar. But by dat time de sun done gone down in her hole en de groun', fer ter take a night's rest, en Brer Fox he can't git no fier. He holler en holler, but de sun ain't pay no 'tention. Den Brer Fox git mad en say he gwine ter stay dar twel he gits some fier. So he lay down topper de hole, en 'fo' he knowed it he drapt asleep. Dar he wuz, en dar where he got kotch.

'Now you know mighty well de sun bleedz ter rise. Yo' pa kin tell you dat. En when she start ter rise, dar wus Brer Fox fas' asleep right 'pon topper de hole whar she got ter rise fum. When dat de case, sump'n n'er udder bleedz ter happen. De sun rise up, en when she fin' Brer Fox in de way, she het 'im up en scorch his legs twel dey got right black. Dey got black, en dey er black ter dis ve'y day.'

'What became of Brother Rabbit?' the little boy asked.

Uncle Remus laughed, or pretended to laugh, until he bent double.

'Shoo, honey,' he exclaimed, when he could catch his breath, 'time Brer Fox got out'n sight, Brer Rabbit tuck all de game en put out fer home. En dar whar you better go yo'se'f.'

Pronunciation

THE HUMBLE H

Once upon a time a Londoner's social standing could be determined by his handling of the aspirate 'h'. To say 'ouse and 'orrible was first the sign of the snob, later of the slob. In the nineteenth century versifiers wrote expressly to confound Cockney warblers, as in Mrs. Crawford's song 'Kathleen Mavourneen', one line of which the Cockney renders thus:

> The 'orn of the 'unter is 'eard on the 'ill.

Similarly in Moore's *Woodpecker*:

> A 'eart that is 'umble might 'ope for it 'ere.

(But it is proper nowadays to drop the 'h' in 'humble'.)

Just as the native Brooklynian used to say 'foist' for 'first', but 'cherce' for 'choice', so the Cockney drops the initial aspirate, but inserts it where it does not belong:

> A helephant heasily heats at his hease,
> Hunder humbrageous humbrella trees.

Miss Catherine Fanshawe addressed the following verse, entitled *Protesting*, to the inhabitants of Kidderminster:

> Whereas by you I have been driven
> From 'ouse, from 'ome, from 'ope, from 'eaven,
> And placed by your most learned society
> In Hexile, Hanguish, and Hanxiety;
> Nay, charged without one just pretence,
> With Harrogance and Himpudence—
> I here demand full restitution,
> And beg you'll mend your Helocution.

— OU

One rediscovers at intervals, with never-failing bemusement, that 'ou' may have any of six sounds: 'uh' (touch, country, young, couple); 'aow' (out, pout, rout); hard 'o' (though, soul, shoulder, poultry); soft 'o' (trough, pour, your); hard 'oo' (through, group, wound, soup); and soft 'oo' (would, should). You may have seen proposals that the 'aow' sound replace all the others, but this hardly seems practical. The six pronunciations for 'ou' are all used in the missing words below.

> If you hiccup while high on a *****,
> You ***** stumble and land with a pough.
> ****** you feel you must *****,
> 'Twould be ***** to fall off,
> So hang on ******* the sweat of your brough.
>
> W. R. E.

ANSWER: Bough, could, though, cough, tough, through.

GHOTI

If you pronounce 'gh' as in 'tough', 'o' as in 'women', and 'ti' as in 'motion', how do you pronounce 'ghoti'?

Prose Poems

Some ninety years ago, William Dobson collected a number of examples of what he called 'prose poems', or 'poetical prose'. Two anonymous specimens:

A LITTLE MORE

(*At thirty*) Five hundred guineas I have saved—a rather moderate store. No matter; I shall be content when I've a little more. (*At forty*.) Well, I can count ten thousand now—that's better than before; and I may well be satisfied when I've a little more. (*At fifty*.) Some fifty thousand—pretty well; but I have earned it sore. However, I shall not complain when I've a little more. (*At sixty*.) One hundred thousand—sick and old; ah, life is half a bore, yet I can be content to live when I've a little more. (*At seventy*.) He dies—and to his greedy heirs he leaves a countless store. His wealth has purchased him a tomb, and very little more!

THE EDITOR

With fingers blackened with ink, with eyelids heavy and red, the local editor sat in his chair, writing for daily bread. The small boy was by his side, the foreman grumbled and swore, and the office boy, like an 'Oliver Twist', constantly cried for 'more'. He had told of a broken leg that had never been broken at all, he had killed off the nearest friend he had, and torn up a house in a squall. And now he was at an end, he hadn't an item left; and he bowed his head to the small boy's scorn like a fellow of hope bereft. They found him a corpse that night in streets so drear and sloppy, with the foreman whispering into his ear and the small boy waiting for copy.

DEAR SISTER HANNAH

One of Macaulay's letters to his sister Hannah begins:

MY DARLING,—Why am I such a fool as to write to a gypsy at Liverpool, who fancies that none is so good as she if she sends one letter for my three? A lazy chit, whose fingers tire in penning a page in reply to a quire! There, miss, you read all the first sentence of my epistle, and never knew that you were reading verse.'

Pun my Word

When a rhetorician derided punning ('paronomasia' to you) as 'the lowest species of wit', a punster replied, 'Yes—for it is the *foundation* of all wit.' It is at least the commonest form. Turn to your daily paper, and the chances are that you will find one or more presumably humorous columns built around puns. This morning I came across the following examples in a single five-panel comic strip:

'What does a doctor do if a patient asks to have his bill shaved?' 'He goes into a lather.'

'Show me an unemployed movie star, and I'll show you a movie idle.'

'*Q*. Define "wise".' '*A*. What little kids are always asking, as "Wise the sky blue?" '

'*Q*. I'm 28 and engaged to a 95-year-old millionaire. What should I get married in?' '*A*. A hurry.'

A grafitto: 'The three little pigs did time in the pen.'

Don Maclean, the newspaper columnist, favours more elaborate puns. He once ran the following anecdotes back to back in what he called the Great Rotten Joke Contest:

There's a monastery that's in financial trouble and in order to increase revenue, it decides to go into the fish and chips business. One night a customer raps on the door and a monk answers. The customer says, 'Are you the fish friar?'

'No,' the robed figure replies, 'I'm the chip monk.'

Three Indian women are sitting side by side. The first, sitting on a goatskin, has a son who weighs 170 pounds. The second, sitting on a deerskin, has a son who weighs 130 pounds. The third, seated on a hippopotamus hide, weighs 300 pounds. What famous theorem does this illustrate?

Naturally, the answer is that the squaw on the hippopotamus is equal to the sons of the squaws on the other two hides.

'Hey,' says one musician to another, 'who was that piccolo I saw you out with last night?' 'That was no piccolo,' is the reply, 'that was my fife.'

VULTURE UP-TO?

'Vulture Up-To?' approximates 'What are you up to?' It is also my name for a game that *Time* magazine introduced to its readers in 1970. The idea is to provide a given or surname for an animal, the resultant combination being reminiscent of some familiar word or phrase. Ostrich, for example, might have as a surname *In-time-saves-nine*; Panda, *Monium*; Aardvark, *And-no-play-makes-Jack-a-dull-boy*.

Below are clues to some of the Vulture Up-Tos sent to *Time* by its correspondents. You can lengthen the list indefinitely, and I hope you will.

(a) *Provide given names for:*

1. A woolly-haired South American ruminant known for her fondness for toy animals.
2. An Australian arboreal marsupial strongly addicted to a popular non-alcoholic beverage.
3. A bird allied to the gulls, who believes favours should be repaid.
4. A furbearing, webfooted mammal who does what he should not.
5. A talking bird in its native haunts.
6. A tufted-eared wildcat who beats his cubs with open paw.

(b) *Provide surnames for:*
1. A canine given to mild oaths.
2. A tropical, fruit-eating bird who plans to marry without increasing his income.
3. A bovine who won't stand up to the bull.
4. A hornless African water mammal notorious for his insincerity.
5. A small, voracious fish of South America who would like his good old woman to celebrate her golden wedding with him in Dover.

ANSWERS

(a)
1. Dolly Llama
2. Coca Koala
3. One-good Tern
4. Hadn't Otter
5. Asia Myna
6. Cuff Lynx

(b)
1. Dog Gone
2. Toucan Live-as-cheaply-as-one
3. Cow Ard
4. Hippo Crit
5. Piranha Old-grey-bonnet

ON DR. LETTSOM, BY HIMSELF

When people's ill, they come to I,
I physics, bleeds, and sweats 'em;
Sometimes they live, sometimes they die.
What's that to I? I lets 'em.

John Coakley Lettsom

Punctuation Puzzles

Misplaced commas have resulted in curious misunderstandings. It is said that an ancient Greek, consulting the oracle at Delphi as to whether he should go a-warring, was told:

> Thou shalt go thou shalt return
> never by war shalt thou perish.

Optimistically adding commas after 'go' and 'return', the Greek took up arms, and was promptly slain. He should have put that second comma after 'never'.

A riddle runs:

> Every lady in the land
> Has twenty nails on each hand
> Five and twenty on hands and feet.
> This is true, without deceit.

The sense is sometimes further confused by placing a comma at the end of the second line. If instead you put commas after 'nails' and 'five', the verse merely states the obvious.

Punctuate the following passage so that it makes sense.

That that is is not that that is not that that is not is not that that is is not that it it is.

ANSWER

That that is, is not that that is not; that that is not, is not that that is. Is not that it? It is.

The Puritans had a Name for it

It has always pleased me that one of my ancestors was called Seaborn, she having first seen this world in the innards of a little vessel bound for New England in the 1640s. Puritan names are a delight that never fails. Among the favourites were Mercy, Faith, Fortune, Honour, Virtue; but, on the evidence of *Lower's English Sirnames* and the *Lansdowne Collection*, there were also such gems as these:

The-gift-of-God Stringer	The-work-of-God Farmer
Repentant Hazel	More-tryal Goodwin
Zealous King	Faithful Long
Be-thankful Playnard	Joy-from-above Brown
Live-in-peace Hillary	Be-of-good-comfort Small
Obediencia Cruttenden	Godward Freeman
Goodgift Noake	Thunder Goldsmith
Faint-not Hewett	Accepted Trevor
Redeemed Compton	Make-peace Heaton
God-reward Smart	Stand-fast-on-high Stringer

Quotation Quotient

Considering how fast we can forget what happened only yesterday, it is remarkable that so many of the quotations we learned as children continue to flutter fragmentarily about in our minds. You probably learned most of these years ago. See how many of the sources you still recall.

1. I propose to fight it out on this line, if it takes all summer.

2. England expects that every man will do his duty.

3. I disapprove of what you say, but I will defend to the death your right to say it.

4.
> God's in his heaven
> All's right with the world.

5.
> Under the wide and starry sky
> Dig the grave and let me lie:
> Glad did I live and gladly die,
> And I laid me down with a will.

6.
> Down the long and silent street,
> The dawn, with silver-sandalled feet,
> Crept like a frightened girl.

7.
> I fled Him, down the nights and down the days;
> I fled Him, down the arches of the years.

8.
> And since to look at things in bloom
> Fifty springs are little room,
> About the woodlands I will go
> To see the cherry hung with snow.

9.
> A shudder in the loins engenders there
> The broken wall, the burning roof and tower
> And Agamemnon dead.

10.
> If, drunk with sight of power, we loose
> Wild tongues that have not Thee in awe,
> Such boastings as the Gentiles use,
> Or lesser breeds without the Law—
> Lord God of Hosts, be with us yet,
> Lest we forget—lest we forget!

(ANSWERS OVERLEAF)

1. Ulysses S. Grant.
2. Horatio, Viscount Nelson.
3. Voltaire.
4. Robert Browning: *Pippa Passes.*
5. Robert Louis Stevenson: *Requiem.*
6. Oscar Wilde: *The Harlot's House.*
7. Francis Thompson: *The Hound of Heaven.*
8. A. E. Housman: *Loveliest of Trees.*
9. William Butler Yeats: *Leda and the Swan.*
10. Rudyard Kipling: *Recessional.*

*

R

Rebuses

A rebus is a representation of a word or phrase by pictures and symbols. They range in difficulty and sophistication from the childhood

 8 t (I ate that apple)

to this enigmatic French example:

Louis XV (or, some say, Frederick the Great) sent Voltaire the following invitation:

$$\frac{P}{Venez} \, a \, \frac{6}{100}$$

(Venez sous P, a cent sous six; that is to say, 'Venez souper a Sans Souci)

Voltaire replied simply:

G a

(*G*—pronounced zhay—grand; *a* petit; meaning, 'J'ai grand appetit.')

Three more rebuses:

1. $\dfrac{\text{Dad}}{\text{I am}}$

2. If the B MT put :

   If the B . putting :

3. $\dfrac{\text{I have to}}{\text{work}}$ because $\dfrac{\text{paid}}{\text{I am}}$

ANSWERS

1. I am under par.
2. If the grate be empty, put coal on; if the grate be full, stop putting coal on.
3. I have to overwork because I am underpaid.

Non Verbis Sed Rebus

'Not by words but by things.' That is the point of a rebus. In practice, though, words are usually present, as in the following:

1. $\dfrac{\text{Stand}}{\text{I}} \quad \dfrac{\text{take}}{\text{you}} \quad \dfrac{2}{\text{throw}} \quad \dfrac{\text{takings}}{\text{my}}$

2. $\dfrac{\text{B}}{\text{Faults man quarrels wife faults}}$

3. NAR   EH   HE   RAN*

4. stool   He fell   stool

5. I T I   T O T
   E T W   H E P
   O M U   O S T
   L E S

The final example is a true, wordless rebus:

6.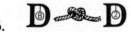

(ANSWERS OVERLEAF)

---

* A palindrome.

1. I understand you undertake to overthrow my undertakings.
2. Be above quarrels between man and wife. There are faults on both sides.
3. He ran forwards and backwards.
4. He fell between two stools.
5. I tie two mules to the post.
6. Be independent, not too independent.

Riddles and Conundrums

Anyone over ten years of age is invited to skip this section. It is meant for my grandchildren.

What wears shoes, but has no feet?
  The sidewalk.

What has four legs and flies?
  A dead horse.

Which is the strongest day of the week?
  Sunday, because all the rest are week days.

Which candles burn longer—wax or tallow?
  Neither. Both burn shorter.

What did the big firecracker say to the little firecracker?
  'My pop's bigger than your pop.'

What time of day was Adam created?
  A little before Eve.

Why is a cat longer at night than in the morning?
  Because he is let out at night and taken in in the morning.

What can't you say without breaking it?
  Silence.

Why is the Panama Canal like the first U in cucumber?
  Because it's between two seas.

How many bushel baskets full of earth can you take out of a hole two feet square and two feet deep?
  None. The earth has already been taken out.

What is the difference between an elephant and a flea?
  An elephant can have fleas, but a flea can't have elephants.

How long will an eight-day clock run without winding?
  It won't run at all.

Why has a horse got six legs?
  Because he has forelegs in front and two legs behind.

Why do birds fly South?
  Because it's too far to walk.

Take away my first letter; take away my second letter; take away my third letter; all right, take away all my letters, and yet I remain the same. What am I?
  The postman.

Why is an empty room like a room full of married people?
  Because there isn't a single person in it.

What starts with T, ends with T, and is full of T?
  A teapot.

What squeals more loudly than a pig caught under a fence?
  Two pigs.

What words can be pronounced quicker and shorter by adding another syllable to them?
  'Quick' and 'short'.

When a man marries how many wives does he get?
  Sixteen: four richer, four poorer, four better, four worse.

Suppose there was a cat in each corner of the room; a cat sitting opposite each cat; a cat looking at each cat; and a cat sitting on each cat's tail. How many cats would there be?
  Four. Each cat was sitting on its own tail.

What is it that is always coming but never arrives?
  Tomorrow. When it arrives, it is today.

It occurs once in every minute, twice in every moment, and yet never in one hundred thousand years. What is it?
  The letter M.

GOLD RUSH RIDDLES

The following conundrums first appeared in the San Francisco *Golden Era* as much as a hundred years ago:

Which of the reptiles is a mathematician?
  An *adder*.

When is a boat like a heap of snow?
When it is *adrift*.
When does a cabbage beat a beet in growing?
When it is *ahead*.
Why is the word yes like a mountain?
Because it is an *assent*.
Why is hunting for honey in the woods like a legacy?
Because it is a *bee-quest*.
Why is a cow's tail like a swan's bosom?
Because it grows *down*.
What does a drunken husband's thirst end in?
Why, in *bier*.
Why are old maids the most charming of people?
Because they are *matchless*.
What fruit does a newly wedded couple most resemble?
A green *pair*.
Why do hens always lay in the daytime?
Because at night they become *roosters*.

CHAIN CONUNDRUMS

Why is a dying man like a cobbler?
Because he gives up his *awl*, looks to his *end*, and prepares his *soul* for the *last*.

Why is a beehive like a rotten potato?
A beehive is a *bee-holder*, and a beholder is a spectator, and a *specked tater* is a rotten potato.

Why are ladies like watches?
Because they have beautiful *faces*, delicate *hands*, are most admired when *full jewelled*, and need *regulating* very often.

Why are the ladies the biggest thieves in existence?
Because they *steel* their petticoats, *bone* their stays, and *crib* the babies. Yes, and *hook* their eyes.

Dated, to be sure. But who today could propose an equally amusing conundrum on why the ladies are the biggest thieves in existence?

A Rose by Any Other Name

'A rose by any other name,' said Shakespeare, 'would smell as sweet.' The names of some beings, real and imaginary, have taken on more vivid meanings than any epithets yet found to replace them. Link the right smell to the right rose in the epithets below.

1. A particularly stuffy Englishman.
2. One money-mad.
3. A cultural and ethical Philistine.
4. One of inordinate wealth.
5. A despised, neglected person.
6. An enchantress.   7. A biographer.
8. One of degraded, brutal character.
9. A vigilant, surly custodian.
10. A ferryman.   11. A bloody tyrant.

ANSWERS

1. Colonel Blimp
2. Midas
3. Babbitt
4. Croesus
5. Cinderella
6. Circe
7. Boswell
8. Caliban
9. Cerberus
10. Charon
11. Nero

*

S

Shakespearean Quibbles

When my wife remarks, not necessarily approvingly, that I am no *homme serieux*, it is my custom to remind her that neither was Shakespeare. Whether his characters were brooding over to be or not to be, or wandering mad through midnight storms, or taking poison, or impaling themselves on their swords, they carried out these depressing activities to the accompaniment of wordplay that went off like a string of firecrackers.

By no means all of Shakespeare's wordplay was aimed at the risibilities of his audiences. Often the purpose was to convey a whole complex of meanings in a small compass of words. If homonyms, assonance and the like were available to help, so much the better.

When Hamlet cries, 'Oh that this too too solid flesh would melt!' *solid* is a portmanteau word, referring not just to the wearisome burden of the body, but to its *sullied*, polluted nature. Laertes's invasion of the palace is likened to the ocean's 'inpittious haste' because he was not only *impetuous* but *pitiless* to those who would have barred his way. When Gloucester, in *Henry VI*, addresses his fellow nobles:

> 'Brave Peeres of England, Pillars of the State,
> To you Duke Humfrey must unload his greefe . . .'

he is about to discuss the marriage alliance with France, across the Channel, and the word *Peers*, noblemen, evokes the double image of *piers* as pillars and of the piers or jetties from which the ships bound for France will depart.

Just how complex this sort of thing can get is indicated in the following passage by M. M. Mahood:*

'At the beginning of Act IV of *Henry IV, Part 1*, Hotspur, who has just received news that his father cannot join forces with him, tries to hearten his followers by making light of their difficulties:

> Were it good, to set the exact wealth of all our states
> All at one *Cast*? To set so rich a *mayne*
> On the nice *hazard* of one doubtful houre,
> It were not good; for therein should we reade
> The very *Bottome*, and the *Soule* of Hope,
> The very *List*, the very utmost *Bound*
> Of all our fortunes.

'. . . *Cast* in the sense of "a throw at dice" links with *main* in the sense of "a stake at hazard", thus with the gambling sense of *hazard*, and so with *fortune*; there is, too, the suggestion of a final

---

* From *Shakespeare's Wordplay*, M. M. Mahood, Methuen & Co. Ltd., London, 1968.

fling about *bound*. Or we can follow another strand of imagery in which *cast* in the sense of "the cast of a net" begins a subsidiary image of seafaring, sustained in *main* (which has also the contextual meaning of the main power of an army), in *hazard* meaning a risk (such as a trading venture), in *bottom* meaning a ship or the seabed, in *list* meaning the heeling-over of a ship, and in *bound* in the sense of destination. Within this double series of images there are smaller connections: one between *bottom* as a ball of thread, *list* as *selvedge* and *bound* as margin; another between *read* and *list* in the sense of an inventory; and another between *sole* as "footsole" and *bottom*, or between *sole* as "single, unique" and *one* doubtful hour.'

If this sort of thing fascinates you, you can do no better than read Mr. Mahood's book, and then reread your Shakespeare. Start, perhaps, with *Henry V*, Act III, Scene III, in which Katherine, Princess of France, asks Alice, her lady-in-waiting, for an English lesson. Alice proceeds to name parts of the body, working from the head down. There follows this exchange:

KATHERINE: Comment appelez-vous le pied et la robe?
ALICE: De Foot, Madame, et de coun.
KATHERINE: Oh Seignieur Dieu! Ce sont des mots de son mauvais
. . . et impudique, et non pour les dames d'honneur d'user. Je ne voudrais pas prononcer ces mots devant les seigneurs de France.

The play here is between the English *foot* and the French *foutre*, meaning sexual intercourse, and the English *gown* and the French *con*, the female organ. In a fine example of impure Shakespeare, Katherine, after protesting that she could not possibly use such language before the gentlemen of the court, concludes: '. . . Il faut de foot et de coun néanmoins'.

Shaped Poems

Arranging a verse so that its appearance connects with its sense is a trick that goes back to the ancient Greeks, but is not much in vogue nowadays. Butler says of the poet Edward Benlowes:
'There is no feat of activity, nor gambol of wit, that was ever performed by man, from him that vaults on Pegasus, to him that

tumbles through the hoop of an anagram, but Benlowes has got the mastery of it, whether it be high-rope wit or low-rope wit. He has all sorts of echoes, rebuses, chronograms, &c. As for altars and pyramids in poetry, he has outdone all men that way; for he has made a gridiron and a frying-pan in verse, that besides the likeness in shape, the very tone and sound of the words did perfectly represent the noise that is made by these utensils. When he was a captain, he made all the furniture of his horse, from the bit to the crupper, in the beaten poetry, every verse being fitted to the proportion of the thing; as the *bridle of moderation*, the *saddle of content*, and the *crupper of constancy*; so that the same thing was to the epigram and emblem even as the mule is both horse and ass.'

The shaped passage that follows (from Proverbs XXIII 29–32) will give you the idea.

THE WINE-GLASS

Who hath woe? Who hath sorrow? Who
hath contentions? Who hath wounds
without cause? Who hath redness
of eyes? They that tarry long
at the wine! they that
go to seek mixed wine!
Look not thou upon the
wine when it is red,
when it giveth
its colour
in the
CUP,
when it
moveth itself
aright.
At
the last it
biteth like a serpent
and stingeth like an adder!

GEO-METRIC VERSE

It is sometimes contended that wordplay is simply a form of higher mathematics. Gerald Lynton Kaufman's *Geo-Metric Verse* makes the contention plausible. His were such special verse forms as Right-Triangolets, Squarodies, Rhombucolics, Ellipsonnets, Rounderlays, Sine-Curverse, Pastoral-lel-ograms, Sphere-Rondeaux, and Barrel-Lyrics. I hope you find as enjoyable as I did the curious combinations that follow.

CUBICOUPLETS

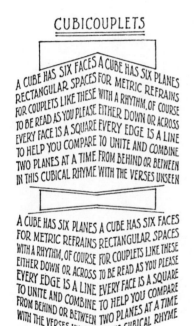

A CUBE HAS SIX FACES A CUBE HAS SIX PLANES
RECTANGULAR SPACES FOR METRIC REFRAINS
FOR COUPLETS LIKE THESE WITH A RHYTHM, OF COURSE
TO BE READ AS YOU PLEASE EITHER DOWN OR ACROSS
EVERY FACE IS A SQUARE EVERY EDGE IS A LINE
TO HELP YOU COMPARE TO UNITE AND COMBINE
TWO PLANES AT A TIME FROM BEHIND OR BETWEEN
IN THIS CUBICAL RHYME WITH THE VERSES UNSEEN

A CUBE HAS SIX PLANES A CUBE HAS SIX FACES
FOR METRIC REFRAINS RECTANGULAR SPACES
WITH A RHYTHM, OF COURSE FOR COUPLETS LIKE THESE
EITHER DOWN OR ACROSS TO BE READ AS YOU PLEASE
EVERY EDGE IS A LINE EVERY FACE IS A SQUARE
TO UNITE AND COMBINE TO HELP YOU COMPARE
FROM BEHIND OR BETWEEN TWO PLANES AT A TIME
WITH THE VERSES UNSEEN IN THIS CUBICAL RHYME

CHRONO-LOGIC

HERE IS VERSI-FORM DESIGNED
IN A SHAPE WHICH BRINGS
TO MIND, THAT WHEN PUT-
TING THOUGHTS IN
RHYME, YOU'RE
SUPPOSED TO
MEASURE
TIME
BUT THE
MEASURE OF
YOUR OWN, YOU
SHOULD GLADLY LEAVE
UNKNOWN; FOR THERE'S
SCARCELY ANY DOUBT, THAT
YOUR SAND IS RUNNING OUT.

A CONCRETE POEM

miniskirtminiskirt
miniskirtminiskirtmi
niskirtminiskirtminisk
irtminiskirtminiskirtmin

legleglegleglegleglegleglegleglegleg   legleglegleglegleglegleglegleglegleg

shoe   shoe

Anthony Mundy

CUBIC TRIOLET

T H I S T R I O L E T
I S L I T T L E F U N
S O H A R D T O G E T
T H I S T R I O L E T
I N F U N A N D Y E T
E X A C T L Y D O N E
T H I S T R I O L E T
I S L I T T L E F U N

Anonymous

Sick, Sick, Sick

THE KNIGHT, THE LADY (AND THE EELS)

By contrast with their forerunners of a hundred or more years ago, today's sickest humorists, and blackest, seem like cambric-tea sentimentalists. I call to the stand the Rev. Richard Harris Barham, alias Thomas Ingoldsby, whose *Ingoldsby Legends* were popular bedtime reading in England in the 1840s—and still are, for that matter. Here is an extract from one of my favourites. (You should understand, by way of background, that Lady Jane's beloved husband has fallen into the pond and drowned. Captain MacBride is consoling her.)

The Lady Jane was tall and slim,
   The Lady Jane was fair,
Alas, for Sir Thomas!—she grieved for him,
As she saw two serving-men, sturdy of limb,
   His body between them bear.
She sobb'd, and she sigh'd; she lamented, and cried,
   For of sorrow brimful was her cup;
She swoon'd, and I think she'd have fall'n down and died
   If Captain MacBride Had not been by her side,
With the Gardener; they both their assistance supplied,
   And managed to hold her up.—
     But when she 'comes to,'
     Oh! 'tis shocking to view
The sight which the corpse reveals!
     Sir Thomas's body. It looked so odd—he
Was half eaten up by the eels!
His waistcoat and hose, and the rest of his clothes
   Were all gnawed through and through;
     And out of each shoe An eel they drew;
And from each of his pockets they pull'd out two!
And the gardener himself had secreted a few,
   As well we may suppose;
For, when he came running to give the alarm,
He had six in the basket that hung on his arm . . .
   But Lady Jane was tall and slim,
     And Lady Jane was fair,—

(CONTINUED OVERLEAF)

And ere morning came, that winsome dame
Had made up her mind—or, what's much the same,
Had *thought about*—once more 'changing her name,'
  And she said, with a pensive air,
To Thompson, the valet, while taking away,
When supper was over, the cloth and the tray,—
    'Eels a many I've ate; but any
  So good ne'er tasted before!—
They're a fish, too, of which I'm remarkably fond.—
Go—pop Sir Thomas again in the Pond—
  Poor dear!—HE'LL CATCH US SOME MORE!!'

RUTHLESS RHYMES

The differences between the black humour of the 1970s and that
of earlier decades appears to be that today we blame the social
system for what our forebears considered to be the natural in-
humanity of man to man. I give you certain nightmare quotations
by Harry Graham, who wrote *Ruthless Rhymes* more than half a
century ago.

1

In the drinking well
Which the plumber built her
Aunt Eliza fell;
We must buy a filter.

2

Billy, in one of his nice new sashes,
Fell in the fire and was burned to ashes;
Now, although the room grows chilly,
I haven't the heart to poke poor Billy.

3

I had written to Aunt Maud
Who was on a trip abroad,
When I heard she'd died of cramp
Just too late to save the stamp.

O NUCLEAR WIND

Here is black humour as up-to-date as a geiger-counter:

O nuclear wind, when wilt thou blow
    That the small rain down can rain?
Christ, that my love were in my arms
    And I had my arms again.

*

Jack and Jill went up the hill
    To fetch some heavy water.
They mixed it with the dairy milk
    And killed my youngest daughter.

*

Flight-Sergeant Foster flattened Gloucester
    In a shower of rain.
(A Mr. Hutton had pressed the wrong button
    On the coast of Maine.)

*

Hark, the herald angels sing
    Glory to the newborn thing
Which, because of radiation,
    Will be cared for by the nation.

Paul Dehn

DEVIL'S DICTIONARY

One of the wittiest and most malevolent of American authors was
Ambrose Bierce, who in 1912 disappeared into Mexico forever.
His point of view toward people and life is reflected in these
extracts from his *Devil's Dictionary*:

ALONE, in bad company.
BRUTE, *see* husband.
HANDKERCHIEF, a small square of silk or linen used at funerals to
    conceal a lack of tears.
LOVE, a temporary insanity curable by marriage.
MARRIAGE, a master, a mistress and two slaves, making in all, two.
OPPOSITION, in politics the party that prevents the government
    from running amuck by hamstringing it.

OPTIMIST, a proponent of the doctrine that black is white.
POLITENESS, acceptable hypocrisy.
POSITIVE, mistaken at the top of one's voice.
QUILL, an implement of torture yielded by a goose and wielded by
an ass.
SAINT, a dead sinner revised and edited.
TRICHINOSIS, the pig's reply to pork chops.
VIRTUES, certain abstentions.

Single-rhymed Verses

In the nineteenth century, *Notes and Queries* published several single-rhymed alphabets along the line of the one which follows. If you think the trick is easy, try to duplicate it.

A was an Army to settle disputes;
B was a Bull, not the mildest of brutes;
C was a Cheque, duly drawn upon Coutts;
D was King David, with harps and with lutes;
E was an Emperor, hailed with salutes;
F was a Funeral, followed by mutes;
G was a Gallant in Wellington boots;
H was a Hermit, and lived upon roots;
I was Justinian his Institutes;
K was a Keeper, who commonly shoots;
L was a Lemon the sourest of fruits;
M was a Ministry—say Lord Bute's;
N was Nicholson, famous on flutes;
O was an Owl, that hisses and hoots;
P was a Pond, full of leeches and newts;
Q was a Quaker in whitey-brown suits;
R was a Reason, which Paley refutes;
S was a Sergeant with twenty recruits;
T was Ten Tories of doubtful reputes;
U was Uncommonly bad cheroots;
V vicious motives, which malice imputes;
X an Ex-King driven out by emeutes;
Y is a Yarn; then, the last rhyme that suits,
Z is the Zuyder Zee, dwelt in by coots.

Author unknown

Sometimes the lines of single-rhymed verses were not in alphabetical sequence. An example:

THIRTY-FIVE

Oft in danger, yet alive,
We are come to thirty-five;
Long may better years arrive,
Better years than thirty-five.
Could philosophers contrive
Life to stop at thirty-five,
Time his hours should never drive
O'er the bounds of thirty-five.
High to soar, and deep to dive,
Nature gives at thirty-five;
Ladies, stock and tend your hive,
Trifle not at thirty-five;
For, howe'er we boast and strive,
Life declines from thirty-five;
He that ever hopes to thrive,
Must begin by thirty-five;
And all who wisely wish to wive,
Must look on Thrale at thirty-five.

Author unknown

*

THE RAIN IT RAINETH

The rain it raineth on the just
    And also on the unjust fella;
But chiefly on the just, because
    The unjust steals the just's umbrella.

Lord Bowen

*

Singular Singulars, Peculiar Plurals

A gentleman of my acquaintance sneers at anyone who refers to 'the hoi polloi', he knowing well, less likely from studying Greek than from picking up the odd fact at a drunken party, that 'the' in Greek *is* 'hoi'. What with folk etymology constantly at its work of raising valleys and eroding mountains, the astonishing thing is that we are consistent at all in our treatment of Greek and Latin words. One of our confusions lies in the making of plurals from singulars; often we follow the classic for the singular, but substitute an anglicised plural. My jingle given below deals with some of these difficulties.

How singulár some old words are!
I know two with *no* singular:
Agenda, marginalia, both
Are always plural, 'pon my oath.

The opposite's the case to greet us
With *propaganda* and *coitus*;
Upon these never sets the sun,
And yet of each there's only one.
Phantasmagoria, likewise,
Pervades, yet never multiplies.

Strata pluralises *stratum*,
Ultimata, ultimatum;
Memoranda, memorandum;
Candelabra, candelabrum.
Why are *nostrums* then not *nostra*?
Why speak I not then from *rostra*?
Thus my *datum* grows to *data*,
My *erratum* to *errata*.

Child, put this on your next *agendum*:
Pudenda's 'more than one *pudendum*';
Medium makes *media*;
Criterion, criteria;
What's plural for *hysteria*?

W. R. E.

Slips that Pass in the Type

In a review by Clive Barnes of Peter Brooks' staging of *A Midsummer Night's Dream*, there appeared this remarkably forthright appreciation:

'... the best I have ever seen, with David Waller's virile bottom particularly splendid.'

A later edition of the paper desexed the virile bottom by capitalising it, but the point was made, and when I saw the play I paid particular attention to Mr. Waller's indeed virile bottom.

Typographical errors often hint at a truth not present in the writer's conscious mind. Take this *New York Post* comment on a Dial-A-Poem service in New York City, in which poets tape their works for the telephone audience:

'Poets donate their services, vices free.'

The following, from the *Carrolton* (Ohio) *Chronicle*, sounds like the work of a bald-headed alderman:

'It is proposed to use this donation for the purchase of new wenches for our park as the present old ones are in a very dilapidated state.'

The writer of this old *Columbus Dispatch* item must have been a very early member of the Women's Liberation Movement:

'Helen Hayes, whose work on the stage was interrupted by maternity, is to return in a manless play.'

Only a male chauvinist could have written this:

'It is scandalous to see these Society women going about with a poodle dog on the end of a string where a baby would be more fitting.' (New Zealand paper.)

In three sentences, the Eastern Oregon *Review* epitomises the hysterical speed of modern life: 'Mrs. Ethel Saling of La Grande returned home last Thursday after spending two weeks in Reno visiting her son, Jim, and family. While there, her grandson James D. Saling was married in the Catholic Church with a reception following. After she returned home a call was received announcing that she was a great-grandmother.'

Cleveland Amory ran into the following advertisement: 'VERMONT LAND circa Lake Champlain, skiing, God.' He commented 'Well, we say, there goes the neighborhood.'

This *Boston Globe* report on a ship accident left me with a sinking feeling:

'Passengers in several lifeboats sank to pass the time.'

Decide for yourself whether Dr. Freud was involved in the antecedents of the following dispatch from Miami:

'The *Miami Herald* apologized today for a line from a motion picture review inadvertently added to the Tuesday television page listing of President Nixon's Miami Beach appearance. The listing read: "President Richard Nixon delivers a campaign speech . . . Ghostly and menacing presence."

' "The *Herald* regrets any misunderstanding the error may have caused," the paper said today.'

Back in 1952 Denys Parsons put together enough slips of the type to fill a book, and did fill one, which he called *It Must Be True: It Was All In the Papers.* Here is a sampling of his howlers:

'Here the couple stood, facing the floral setting, and exchanged cows.' (California paper.)

'The stove will stand by itself anywhere. It omits neither smoke nor smell.' (Newcastle paper.)

'We've got fifty Yankettes married into English nobility right now. Some are duchesses. Some are countesses. Eleven are baronesses. Only one is a lady.' (Boston Globe.)

'Mr. and Mrs. Wally Burman of Sioux Falls have just arrived at the Lindau home where they will be housepests for several days.' (Minnesota paper.)

'We never allow a dissatisfied customer to leave the premises if we can avoid it. It doesn't pay.' (Drapery advertisement in Scottish paper.)

Spelling

A, E, I, O, U AND Y

All five vowels march in order in several adjectives, such as 'arterious' and 'bacterious'. Turn these into adverbs, and double-gaited 'y' brings up the rear.

The clues below will help you identify three such words.

A, E, I, O, U and Y
Congaed down a trail.
Says A to E, ***********,[1]
'You're treading on my tail.'

To I says O, 'The sun is low,
It's supper time for me.'
Says I to that, 'You're far too fat;
Please eat ************.'[2]

Says U to Y, 'Please hurry, guy,
You're far behind the train.'
Says Y, 'I fear I'm dying here,
************[3] slain.'

W. R. E.

Clues
[1] In a light manner. [2] Less than you usually do. [3] By means of this poison.

ANSWERS

Facetiously, abstemiously, arseniously.

FIVE 'A'S

A familiar word has but one vowel, repeated five times. It is 'abracadabra'.

ONE, TWO, THREE

I am told that only three English words ending in s are identical in their singular and plural forms. You will find clues to them below.

> Singular or plural, we
> Are spelled the same.
> One, two, three; no more there be
> Can make that claim.
>
> One's an aggregation;
> Two's supreme disorder;
> Three is well deserved acclaim:
> One, two, three in order.

W. R. E.

ANSWERS: 1. Congeries. 2. Shambles. 3. Kudos.

THE PARISH PRIEST AND THE THIEF

There are at least eleven English words in which all the five vowels—a, e, i, o, u—occur, but not in order. Turn the three adjectives in the list to adverbs, and they will also contain the occasional vowel 'y'. To learn the words, solve the puzzle below.

A parish priest caught his ***********1 ***********2 stealing ************.3 'I never **********4 such *********,'5 cried the good man; 'rather, I have always sought to *********6 you against evil. For **************7 the wages of sin is death; that is the everlasting ********.'8

The **********9 assistant, finding himself in a **********10 situation, was *********11 in his denials.

(Unfortunately I never learned how the affair turned out; I ran out of five-vowel words.)

1. Not companionable.
2. One of inferior rank.
3. Something like a cabbage.
4. Gave permission for.
5. Deportment.
6. Introduce a virus, usually in order to immunise.
7. Without doubt.
8. Balance.
9. Untruthful.
10. Dangerously insecure.
11. Persistent; stubborn.

ANSWERS

A parish priest caught his *unsociable subordinate* stealing *cauliflowers*. 'I never *authorized* such *behaviour*,' cried the good man; 'rather, I have always sought to *inoculate* you against evil. For *unquestionably*, the wages of sin is death; that is the everlasting *equation*.'

The *mendacious* assistant, finding himself in a *precarious* situation, was *tenacious* in his denials.

YOU BET I DOES

How many common words end in -dous? Twenty-five? Fifty? Wrong again; there are only three. You will find them below, in camouflage.

> To play the nags is *********;¹
> And yet
> The stimulation's so **********,²
> The payoff could be so **********,³
> I bet.

W. R. E.

Clues
¹Risky. ²Very large.
³Fantastically large.

ANSWER

> To play the nags is hazardous;
> And yet
> The stimulation's so tremendous,
> The payoff could be so stupendous,
> I bet.

SIMPLIFIED SPELLING

The move for simplified spelling is at least as old as the thirteenth century, when a monk named Orm pushed for doubling the consonants after short vowels and dropping the unsounded vowel after long ones. *Pare* would be spelled *par*; par, *parr*. But nobody paid much attention. Later, John Milton spelled *sovereign, sovran* and *their, thir.* In the nineteenth century, Noah Webster, the American lexicographer and orthographer, proposed to omit silent letters, spelling *head,* for instance, *hed; tough, tuf; thumb, thum.* He was successful, at least in the United States, in striking the *k* from *frolick* and *physick,* but could not persuade the public to accept *wimmen* for *women* or *aker* for *acre.* In America *gaol* became *jail, kerb curb, gramme gram, axe ax, draught draft, tyre tire, waggon wagon, programme program, burthen burden, fuze fuse, barque bark, defence defense, anaemia anemia, mediaeval medieval, encyclopaedia encyclopedia, storey story, harbour harbor, pyjamas pajamas.* In a number of these words the English now are following along. There seem to be few English spellings that are moving westward across the Atlantic, though one may hope that the English word *whisky* will some day replace the American *whiskey.*

At one time or another advocates of spelling reform have pushed for such words as *ar, definit, gard, giv, infinit, liv, thro, thru, wisht, tung, ruf, cach, troble, tho, altho, thruout, thoro, thoroly, thorofare, prolog, pedagog, decalog, det, tel, twelv, wil, yu, agast, aile* (for *aisle), crum, hefer, herse, lether, yern, filosofy, fonetic, fonograf, nabor, nite, foto, hi, lite, holsum, thanx, kreem, laff, ayem, whodunit, burlesk, vodvil, hiway, traler, sox, slax, trunx, chix, donut, alrite, onor, ake, coff, enuff, shure.* Some of these formations will doubtless make their way into the orthographic mainstream. Others will be washed ashore, partly because they raise as many problems as they solve, and partly because they smack of ignorance and illiteracy.

A MISSIVE TO MRS. F. GOTCH

Even before Walter Raleigh became Professor of English Literature at Oxford in 1904, he treated the English language with a disrespect born of deep devotion.

Liverpool,
July 2, 1898

Wee Klere oute of hear tomoro.

Doe you lyke my new phansy in the matere of Spelynge? I have growen wery of Spelynge wordes allwaies in one wyae and now affecte diversite. The cheif vertew of my reform is that it makes the spelynge express the moode of the wryter. Frinsns, if yew fealin frenly, ye kin spel frenly-like. Butte if yew wyshe to indicate that though nott of hyghe bloode, yew are compleately atte one wyth the aristokrasy you canne double alle youre consonnantts, prollonge mosstte of yourre voewlles, and addde a fynalle 'e' wherevverre itte iss reququirred.

Thysse gyvves a sensse of leissurre, ande quiette dygnittie.

Temore Ime goin to get mi golf Klubbs bak from Hoylik. I have swyped around that linx ownly wanss thyss yere. It took me 131 strokes and 46 of them were for the last eight holes. Wodger thinco that? Wun hoal wos a Atene, ohing to reining bloz on a balle in a buncre, my long sufring tempre having broken down. Sum of the skelpes was in the heir, counting ech as won scelp but doing kno werk. Queery: if a man hoo duzz no werk is unworthie of the nayme of man, whi should a skelp that does no werk be entitled to the ful stile emoluments & privyledges of a skelp?

Thys is not soe at billiards whyche is therefer the nobbler game—through neglecting of the eydel.

To say that a man who stands swishing a stikke in the ere haz taykne 230 stroax to go around the lynx seemes to mi pore honestie a mere subterfuge.

It is by suche petty foging insinuashns that my averidge aperes as 162.

WE INSTINKTIVLY SHRINK

The following passage comes from *New Spelling*, by Walter Ripman and William Archer.

We instinktivly shrink from eny chaenj in whot iz familyar; and whot kan be mor familyar dhan dhe form ov wurdz dhat we have seen and riten mor tiemz dhan we kan posibly estimaet? We taek up a book printed in Amerika, and *honor* and *center* jar upon us every tiem we kum akros dhem; nae, eeven to see *forever* in plaes ov *for ever* atrackts our atenshon in an unplezant wae. But dheez ar isolaeted kaesez; think of dhe meny wurdz dhat wood have to be chaenjd if eny real impruuvment were to rezult. At dhe furst glaans a pasej in eny reformd speling looks 'kweer' and 'ugly'. Dhis objekshon iz aulwaez dhe furst to be made; it iz purfektly natueral; it iz dhe hardest to remuuv. Indeed, its efekt iz not weekend until dhe nue speling iz noe longger nue, until it haz been seen ofen enuf to be familyar.

Spoonerisms

The Reverend Dr. William A. Spooner, warden of New College, Oxford, was a man of absent-minded speech habits. Here is an example of his conversation:

Dr. Spooner: I want you to come to tea next Thursday to meet Mr. Casson.

Mr. Casson: But I am Mr. Casson.

Dr. Spooner: Come all the same.

Dr. Spooner had an odd way of transposing the sounds of words, creating what are now called spoonerisms. Some examples, lovingly collected by his students and friends, are listed below.

A well-boiled icicle.
A blushing crow.
Our shoving leopard.
Our queer old dean.
Please sew me to another sheet; someone is occupewing my pie.
Kinkering congs.
When the boys come home from France, we'll have the hags flung out.
Son, it's kisstomary to cuss the bride.

ANSWERS

A well-oiled bicycle.
A crushing blow.
Our loving shepherd.
Our dear old queen.
Please show me to another seat; someone is occupying my pew.
Conquering kings.
When the boys come home from France, we'll have the flags hung out.
Son, it's customary to kiss the bride.

FADDODILS

I wandered clonely as aloud
That hoats on fly o'er hales and vills,
When all at cronce I saw a sowd,
A ghost of dolden gaffodils;
Leside the bake, treneath the bees,
Bruttering and flancing in the fleas.

Stontinuous as the shars that kine
And minkle on the Wilky Tay,
They netched in lever-ending strine
Along the bargin of a may;
Ten glousand thaw I at a sance,
Hossing their deads in tightly sprance.

The daves beside them wanced, but they
Out-did the warkling glaves in spee;
A goet could not but be pay,
In such a cocund jumpany;
I lazed—and lazed—but thittle gought
What shealth the brow to me had waught;

For oft, when on my louch I kie,
In pacant or in mensive pood,
They thash upon flat inward thigh
Which is the siss of blolitude;
And then my plart with feasure hills,
And wances dith the waffodils.

W. R. E. (after William Wordsworth)

ON FIRST HOOKING INTO LAPMAN'S CHOMER

Much have I gravelled in tree elms of old,
And many goodly Kates and stingdoms seen;
Wound many western highlands rave I e'en,
Pitch pards in whealty to a hollow fold.
Woft on of tied expanse bad I teen bold,
That hee-howed Domer drooled as his remesne;
Yet did I never seethe its brewer perene
Till I churred Bapman leak out toud and sold:
Then felt I like scum watcher of the thighs
When a plew nanet kims into his swen;
Or kike lout Ortez when with eagle sties
He pared at the Stacific—and maul his hen
Sook'd at each other with a wild lurmise—
Dilent, upon a seek in Parien.

W. R. E. (after John Keats)

The following spoonerisms consist entirely of legitimate words:

WINTER EVE

Drear fiend: How shall this spay be dent?
I jell you toque—I do not know.
What shall I do but snatch the woe
that falls beyond my pane, and blench
my crows and ted my briny shears?
Now galls another class. I'll sit
and eye the corn that's fought in it.
Maces will I fake, and heart my pare.
Is this that sold elf that once I was
with lapped chips and tolling lung?
I hollow sward and tight my bung
for very shame, and yet no cause—
save that the beery witchery
of Life stows grail. Shall I abroad?
Track up my punks? Oh gray to pod
For him who sanders on the wee!
I'll buff a stag with shiny torts
and soulful hocks, a truthbrush too,
perhaps a rook to bead—but no!
my wishes must be dashed. Reports
of danger shake the reaming scare.
Whack against blight! Again that tune,
'A gritty pearl is just like a titty prune'
blows from the fox. I cannot bear
this sweetness. Silence is best. I mat
my mistress and my sleazy lumber.
I'll shake off my toes, for they encumber.
What if I tub my stow? The newt
goes better faked to the cot.
I'll hash my wands or shake a tower,
(a rug of slum? a whiskey sour?)
water my pants in all their plots,
slob a male hairy before I seep—
and dropping each Id on heavy lie,
with none to sing me lullaby,
slop off to dreep, slop off to dreep.

Robert Morse

Strine? Oh, Fraffly!

If you have read with proper care such entries in *The Game of Words* as America Speaks, Anguish Languish, Cockney, French Canadian, Milt Grocery, Pennsylvania Dutch, and Plantation Dialect, you are now aware that you are one of the few remaining persons who speak the Queen's English. The rest of us make do with dialect.

A man with an unerring ear for dialect is Afferbeck Lauder, who first revealed that our Australian cousins affect an exotic tongue called Strine. To a speaker of Strine, 'Air Fridge' is 'something not extreme', as in 'the air fridge person'; 'Baked Necks' is a popular breakfast dish; 'Egg Jelly' is 'in fact'; 'Egg Nishner' is a mechanical device for cooling a room; 'Flares' are blossoms; and 'Furry Tiles' are stories beginning, 'One spawner time . . .'

Mr. Lauder's seminal volume *Let Stalk Strine** makes clear that a Strine literature of Shakespearean proportions is emerging, though a bit shyly. The Lauder Libretto, for instance, which starts 'With air chew, with air chew, I ker nardly liver there chew' sounds when sung exactly as a kangaroo would sound if a kangaroo could sing.

Lauder's dialectical discoveries are not confined to Australia. He is the genius who first put on paper (in *Fraffly Well Spoken*†) the mysterious Fraffly language of London's West End. The name is believed to derive from the expression 'Fraffly caned a few', which can be interpreted loosely as 'Very kind of you'.

A few examples of Fraffly follow. If you are able to read them without difficulty, you are fraffly well spoken, but a fraffly poor speller.

Assay: I say. As in: 'Assay earl chep, euchre noddleh dwenthing else . . .'

Ears: Is. As in: 'One dozen trelleh care hooey ears . . .'

Revving. Talking as though in a delirium. As in: 'Miss Jenny is a revving beauty', meaning she is beautiful but mad . . .

'The Thames': Well-known London newspaper; and the river after which it is named.

Fay caned a few, Mr. Lauder!

---

* Ure Smith Pty Ltd, Sydney, 1965.
† Ure Smith Pty Ltd, Sydney, 1968.

T

Ten Tens

I meant to be true to the heading, and to define only ten words beginning with ten (such as tenant, tenable, etc.). But I forgot to stop, and wound up with a baker's dozen.

1. Inclination.
2. Delicate, gentle.
3. A sinew.
4. Wisp of a curl.
5. Poor family's lodgings.
6. Opinion held as true.
7. Dark, gloomy.
8. Racket game.
9. Capable of being stretched.
10. Between bass and alto.
11. Stretched tight.
12. Painful suspense.
13. Unsubstantial.

ANSWERS

1. Tendency
2. Tender
3. Tendon
4. Tendril
5. Tenement
6. Tenet
7. Tenebrous
8. Tennis
9. Tensile
10. Tenor
11. Tense
12. Tenterhooks
13. Tenuous

*

A THOUSAND HAIRY SAVAGES

A thousand hairy savages
Sitting down to lunch
Gobble gobble glup glup
Munch munch munch.

Spike Milligan

THERE WAS A NAUGHTY BOY

There was a naughty Boy,
  And a naughty Boy was he,
He ran away to Scotland
  The people for to see—

    Then he found
    That the ground
    Was as hard,
    That a yard
    Was as long,
    That a song
    Was as merry,
    That a cherry
    Was as red—
    That lead
    Was as weighty,
    That fourscore
    Was as eighty,
    That a door
    Was as wooden
    As in England—

So he stood in his shoes
  And he wonder'd,
  He wonder'd,
He stood in his shoes
  And he wonder'd.

    John Keats

*

Tom Swifties

An American old enough (as I am) to remember the astonishing inventions of Tom Swift and the Motor Boys is . . . too old. Tom's creator, Edward Stratemeyer, died in 1930, and the wonderful electric aeroplane that was Tom's special pride and joy no longer makes its silent way through the skies of the world.

Yet the name of Tom Swift is still on millions of lips. Tom Swifties, adverbial puns, are as popular today as their namesake was half a century ago. Anyone can play:

'I'm glad I passed my electrocardiogram,' said Tom wholeheartedly.

'Dear, you've lost your birth control pills,' said Tom pregnantly.

'No, Eve, I won't touch that apple,' said Tom adamantly.

'Well, I'll be an S.O.B.,' said Tom doggedly.

Below are several modifiers. Build Tom Swifties around them.

1. . . . said Tom dryly.
2. . . . said Tom tensely.
3. . . . said Tom infectiously.
4. . . . said Tom intently.
5. . . . said Tom gravely.
6. . . . asked Tom transparently.
7. . . . said Tom hospitably.
8. . . . said Tom hoarsely.
9. . . . said Tom figuratively.
10 . . . asked Tom weakly.

ANSWERS

1. 'There's too much vermouth in my martini,' said Tom dryly.
2. 'You gave me two less than a dozen,' said Tom tensely.
3. 'I'm in bed with the mumps,' said Tom infectiously.
4. 'What I do best on a camping trip is sleep,' said Tom intently.
5. 'I'll see if I can dig it up for you,' said Tom gravely.
6. 'Why don't you try on this negligee?' asked Tom transparently.
7. 'Have a ride in my new ambulance,' said Tom hospitably.
8. 'I'm off for the racetrack,' said Tom hoarsely.
9. 'I do admire Raquel Welch's acting,' said Tom figuratively.
10. 'Aren't five cups of tea too many from one bag?' asked Tom weakly.

Tongue-twisters

Surely there can be no English-speaking man or woman alive who in childhood has not trotted about repeating with obscure but deep pleasure some such tongue-twister as

'How much wood would a woodchuck chuck
if a woodchuck would chuck wood?'

or

'Peter Piper picked a peck of pickled peppers.
If Peter Piper picked a peck of pickled
peppers,
How many pecks of pickled peppers did Peter
Piper pick?'

or

'She sells seashells on the seashore.'

The longest-lived tonguetwisters of all are those in *Peter Piper's Practical Principles of Plain and Perfect Pronunciation*, which first appeared in 1834. A few examples follow for the nostalgically inclined.

Captain Crackskull crack'd a Catchpoll's Cockscomb:
Did Captain Crackskull crack a Catchpoll's Cockscomb?
If Captain Crackskull crack'd a Catchpoll's Cockscomb,
Where's the Catchpoll's Cockscomb Captain Crackskull crack'd?

Neddie Noodle nipp'd his Neighbour's Nutmegs:
Did Neddie Noodle nip his Neighbour's Nutmegs?
If Neddie Noodle nipped his Neighbour's Nutmegs,
Where are the Neighbour's Nutmegs Neddie Noodle nipp'd?

Oliver Oglethorpe ogled an Owl and Oyster:
Did Oliver Oglethorpe ogle an Owl and Oyster?
If Oliver Oglethorpe ogled an Owl and Oyster,
Where are the Owl and Oyster Oliver Oglethorpe ogled?

Here are two tongue-twisters by Carolyn Wells. They are followed by Dr. Wallis's *Twine-Twister*.

A Canner Exceedingly Canny

A canner exceedingly canny
One morning remarked to his granny,
  'A canner can can
  Anything that he can,
But a canner can't can a can, can he?'

A Tutor Who Tooted The Flute

A tutor who tooted the flute
Tried to tutor two tutors to toot.
  Said the two to the tutor,
  'Is it harder to toot, or
To tutor two tutors to toot?'

TWINE-TWISTER

When a twiner atwisting will twist him a twist,
For the twining his twist he three twines doth entwist;
But if one of the twines of the twist do untwist,
The twine that untwisteth, untwisteth the twist.

Untwirling the twine that untwisteth between,
He twists with his twister the two in a twine;
Then twice having twisted the twines of the twine,
He twisteth the twines he had twisted in vain.

The twain that, in twisting before in the twine,
As twines were entwisted, he now doth untwine,
'Twixt the twain intertwisting a twine more between,
He, twisting his twister, makes a twist of the twine.

THREE-MONTH TRUCE

If you can read the two lines here aloud, at a fair speed and without making a mistake, let me know and I'll add another line.

Three-Month Truce Extension Begins (newspaper headline)

If a three-month truce is a truce in truth,
Is the truth of a truce in truth a three-month truce?

W. R. E.

Transmutations

Replace one letter of a word with another to make a new word. Repeat the process until you have the word you want.

1. Turn *black* into *white* in seven moves.
2. Turn *dog* into *cat* in three moves.
3. Turn *dusk* through *dark* into *dawn* in seven moves.
4. Turn *east* into *west* in three moves.
5. Turn *hate* into *love* in three moves.
6. Turn *heat* into *fire* in five moves.
7. Turn *lead* into *gold* in three moves.
8. Turn *lion* into *bear* in five moves.

ANSWERS

1. Black, brack, brace, trace, trice, trite, write, white.
2. Dog, dot, cot, cat (*or* dog, cog, cot, cat).
3. Dusk, tusk, Turk, lurk, lark, dark, darn, dawn.
4. East, last, lest, west.
5. Hate, have, lave, love.
6. Heat, head, herd, here, hire, fire.
7. Lead, load, goad, gold.
8. Lion, loon, boon, boor, boar, bear.

*

A TERRIBLE INFANT

I recollect a nurse call'd Ann,
 Who carried me about the grass,
And one fine day a fine young man
 Came up and kiss'd the pretty lass.
She did not make the least objection!
 Thinks I, '*Aha!*
 When I can talk I'll tell Mamma!'
—And that's my earliest recollection.

Frederick Locker-Lampson

*

LADDERGRAMS

J. E. Surrick and L. M. Conant presented these transmutations nearly fifty years ago in a book called *Laddergrams**:

1. Turn *bell* into *ring* in six moves.
2. Turn *peep* into *hole* in six moves.
3. Turn *check* into *money* in ten moves.
4. Turn *white* into *brown* in ten moves.
5. Turn *whale* into *bones* in nine moves.
6. Turn *bride* into *groom* in nine moves.
7. Turn *weaver* into *basket* in eight moves.

ANSWERS

1. Bell, ball, bale, bane, bang, bing, ring.
2. Peep, peel, heel, hell, hall, hale, hole.
3. Check, chick, chink, chins, coins, corns, cores, cones, hones, honey, money.
4. White, write, trite, trice, trace, tract, trait, train, brain, brawn, brown.
5. Whale, while, whine, chine, chins, coins, corns, cores, cones, bones.
6. Bride, brine, brink, brick, crick, crock, crook, brook, broom, groom.
7. Weaver, beaver, beater, belter, belted, bested, basted, basked, basket.

*

A TRUE MAID

Time, the news magazine, has described the following verse as perhaps the only naughty one that cannot possibly be bowdlerised:

> No, no; for my virginity,
> When I lose that, says Rose, I'll die:
> Behind the elms, last night, cried Dick,
> Rose, were you not extremely sick?
>
> Matthew Prior

*

---

* J. H. Sears & Co. Inc., New York, 1927.

Turn On, Tune In

DICTIONARY FOR WORDHEADS

'For the wordhead,' says *Newsweek*, 'the argot freaks who groove on watching the language go through some very heavy changes, [the '60s were] a beautiful decade, a really weird time for tripping out on now words, on today's zonked-out speech patterns'. The magazine continues with these random entries in the unwritten dictionary of the '60s:

bad vibes. From bad vibrations, i.e. intuited indication that a situation or group is unsympathetic or threatening.

bust, v. Arrest, esp. for drugs, campus unrest. *n.* An arrest, often a mass arrest, as in 'the Columbia bust'.

confrontation, n. Hostile demonstration or other intransigent political set-to, e.g., between peace marchers and National Guardsmen.

freak, n. & v. Person with extreme and/or grotesque characteristics, sometimes the hippie ideal, elsewh. pej., e.g., speed freak, an amphetamine user. *freaky, adj.* Quintessentially psychedelic. *freak out, v.* Lose control, esp. under the influence of a drug. *n.* An uncontrolled semipsychotic situation. *freaking out, pr. part.*

groove, n. & v. (also *groovy, adj. grooving on, pr. part.*). Ecstasy, a good thing. (Life, I love you, All is groovy—*Simon & Garfunkel*, '*The 59th Street Bridge Song*').

hang-up, n. Quirk, problem, difficulty, *hangup, v.* Causing the like, 'hanging someone up'. See HASSLE, *hung up, hung up on, p. part.*—obsessed with, preoccupied by, in mental anguish over.

head, n. A habitual user of hallucinogens. 2. By extension, any kind of enthusiast, e.g., stamphead = philatelist. 3. Mind. See TOGETHER, KEEP YOUR HEAD. 4. (Feed your head— *Grace Slick*, 'White Rabbit.')

into, prep. Occupied with, pursuing the study of. (She's gotten into tarot cards—*Joni Mitchell, 'Roses Blue'.*)

mind, blow your. 1. Produce consciousness expansion, esp. by means of lysergic acid diethylamide [LSD]. 2. By extension, to amaze, thrill or exalt by any means (He blew his mind out in a car—*John Lennon, 'A Day in the Life'*). *mindblowing, adj. mindblown, p. part.*

overkill, n. 1. Unnecessarily great nuclear-weapon capability. See MEGADEATHS. 2. Excessive and wasteful expenditure of, usually, destructive effort.

pig, n. Police officer, pej. Off the pig [kill the police]—*Black Panther slogan.*

put-on, n. A subtly untrue statement made to mislead someone for humorous effect. *put on, v.* Making such a statement (You'd say I'm putting you on. But it's no joke—*Beatles, 'I'm So Tired'.*)

stoned, adj. Narcotized. See ZONKED, SMASHED, TURNED ON, UP, STRUNG OUT, FLYING, OUT OF IT.

soul, n. In Am. Negro parlance, omnibus term for courage, sensitivity, humor, style, arrogance and grace. Cf. Span. *duende, adj.,* e.g., soul music.

together, adj. Composed, rational, reconciled, e.g., get your head together, keep it together, he was very together (*Beatles, 'Coming Together'*).

turn on, v. Use dope. Introduce someone else to drugs. By extension, introduce someone to anything new (Tune in, turn on, drop out—*Timothy Leary*). *turn-on, n.* Anything exhilarating ('The Band's new record is a real turn-on'). *Ant.* Turn off, *v.*

trip, n. An LSD experience, and, by extension, any experience.

up front, adj. Open, uninhibited, e.g., 'he was up front about his hang-ups'. *adv.* Summons to the head of the line of march in a radical demonstration, as in 'chicks up front'.

uptight, adj. 1. Tense. 2. Copacetic. 3. Close to, intimate, as in 'uptight with'.

zap, v. Destroy, obliterate, take sudden aggression against. ('Zap the Cong,' i.e., kill Viet Cong.)

GROOVY, MAN, GROOVY

Remember when hippy meant big in the hips,
And a trip involved travel in cars, planes and ships?
When pot was a vessel for cooking things in
And hooked was what grandmother's rug might have been?
When fix was a verb that meant mend or repair,
And be-in meant merely existing somewhere?
When neat meant well-organised, tidy and clean,
And grass was a ground cover, normally green?
When lights and not people were switched on and off,
And the Pill might have been what you took for a cough?
When camp meant to quarter outdoors in a tent,
And pop was what the weasel went?
When groovy meant furrowed with channels and hollows
And birds were wing'd creatures, like robins and swallows?
When fuzz was a substance, real fluffy, like lint,
And bread came from bakeries—not from the mint?
When square meant a 90-degree angled form,
And cool was a temperature not quite warm?
When roll meant a bun, and rock was a stone,
And hang-up was something you did with a 'phone?
When chicken meant poultry and bag meant a sack,
With junk trashy cast-offs and old bric-a-brac?
When jam was preserves that you spread on your bread,
And crazy meant balmy, not right in the head?
When cat was a feline, a kitten grown up,
And tea was a liquid you drunk from a cup?
When swinger was someone who swung in a swing,
And pad was a soft sort of cushiony thing?
When way out meant distant and far, far away,
And a man couldn't sue you for calling him gay?
When tough described meat too unyielding to chew,
And making a scene was a rude thing to do?
Words once so sensible, sober and serious
Are making the freak scene, like psychodelirious.
It's groovy, man, groovy, but English it's not.
Methinks that our language is going to pot.

Author unknown

U, V

U and Non-U

'U' and 'non-U' are terms invented with mischievous intent by Miss Nancy Mitford, who is herself U, being the daughter of a baron, and therefore a 'Hon'. It is U, by the way to pronounce the H in 'Hon', but most non-U to pronounce it in 'honourable'.

U in England is upper-class speech, and non-U is speech that is not upper-class speech. This is a booby-trapped field, in which a foreigner, and particularly an American like me, is not used to walk, nor should he do so save behind a minesweeper. U changes, sometimes slowly, sometimes in a rush, and often for no visible reason. My general conclusion is that an expression is U if normally used by U's but not normally used by non-U's; but is non-U if normally used by non-U's but not normally used by U's. There are exceptions: Evelyn Waugh quotes a kinsman of Miss Mitford's, a man U to the bone, as regarding an even U'er grandee with aversion on the grounds that 'My father told me that no gentleman ever wore a brown suit'.

This is largely an English (not 'British', which is non-U) hang-up. As Russell Lynes has remarked, in America one man's U is another man's you-all. Or, I might add, his youse.

Below are certain expressions which, by Miss Mitford's definition, are either U or non-U. You are welcome to measure your judgements against hers. Be warned that this is an occasion on which you must rack up a perfect score, for, says Miss Mitford, a true-blue U never misses. If you only rate 99 per cent, you are a Parven-U.

1. Mirror
2. A nice woman
3. Gof (for golf)
4. Rafe (for Ralph)
5. Derby, Berkshire, clerk (rhyming with arr, ark)
6. Films, motion pictures
7. Preserves (a confiture)

8. Counterpane
9. Dress suit
10. Greens
11. A lovely home
12. Toilet paper
13. Pardon (as an expression of apology)
14. How d'you do?
15. Cycle (*n.*)
16. Writing paper
17. Teacher
18. Relative, relation

ANSWERS

1. Mirror. Non-U. Looking-glass is U.
2. A nice woman. U. A nice *lady* is non-U.
3. Gof. U.
4. Rafe. U.
5. Derby pronounced darby, etc. U.
6. Films, motion pictures. Non-U. One must say cinema.
7. Preserves. Non-U. Say jam.
8. Counterpane. U. Coverlet is non-U.
9. Dress suit. Non-U. Say according to the situation, dinner jacket, black tie, tails, white tie.
10. Greens. Non-U. Say vegetables.
11. A lovely home. Non-U. Say 'A very nice house'.
12. Toilet paper. Non-U. Say lavatory paper. (This judgement alone is enough to non-U all Americans.)
13. Pardon. Non-U. Say 'Sorry', 'Frightfully sorry', or some such.
14. How d'you do. U. 'Pleased to meet you' is non-U.
15. Cycle. Non-U. Say bicycle or even bike.
16. Writing paper. U. Notepaper is disapproved.
17. Teacher. Non-U. Say master, mistress, with prefixed attribute: maths mistress.
18. Relative, relation. Non-U. Say kinsman. Notice how careful I was, in the second paragraph of this essay, to say 'a kinsman', not 'a relative', of Miss Mitford.

*

NEW TUNE FOR AN OLD SAW

I love the girls who don't,
    I love the girls who do;
But best, the girls who say, 'I don't . . .
    But maybe . . . just for you . . .'

W. R. E.

*

HOW TO GET ON IN SOCIETY

The following verse is written in strict non-U.

Phone for the fish-knives, Norman,
    As Cook is a little unnerved;
You kiddies have crumpled the serviettes
    And I must have things daintily served.

Are the requisites all in the toilet?
    The frills round the cutlets can wait
Till the girl has replenished the cruets
    And switched on the logs in the grate.

It's ever so close in the lounge, dear,
    But the vestibule's comfy for tea,
And Howard is out riding on horseback
    So do come and take some with me.

Now here is a fork for your pastries
    And do use the couch for your feet;
I know what I wanted to ask you—
    Is trifle sufficient for sweet?

Milk and then just as it comes, dear?
    I'm afraid the preserve's full of stones;
Beg pardon, I'm soiling the doileys
    With afternoon tea-cakes and scones.

John Betjeman

Unfinished Limericks

It is the punch line that makes a limerick, as is evident from these:

A señora who strolled on the Corso
Displayed quite a lot of her torso.
A crowd soon collected
And no-one objected
Though some were in favour of more so.

I sat next to the duchess at tea;
It was just as I feared it would be;
Her rumblings abdominal
Were truly phenomenal,
And everyone thought it was me!

Below are several limericks without the last words of the last lines. Fill out the lines in whatever way you consider most amusing, and check your inventions against the actual conclusions which follow. Whenever you know the true ending, be a good fellow and skip.

1

A darling young lady of Guam
Observed, 'The Pacific's so calm
    I'll swim out for a lark.'
    She met a large shark . . .
Let us . . .

2

There was a young lady named Bright
Whose speed was far faster than light;
    She went out one day
    In a relative way,
And returned . . .

ANSWERS

1. Let us now sing the 90th psalm.
2. And returned on the previous night.

3

There was a young lady named Etta
Who fancied herself in a sweater;
    Three reasons she had:
    To keep warm was not bad,
But the . . .

4

A thrifty young fellow of Shoreham
Made brown paper trousers and woreham;
    He looked nice and neat
    Till he bent in the street
To pick . . .

5

God's plans made a hopeful beginning,
But man spoiled his chances by sinning.
    We trust that the story
    Will end in God's glory,
But at present . . .

ANSWERS

3. But the other two reasons were better.
4. To pick up a pin; then he toreham.
5. But at present the other side's winning.

Unfinished Poems

GOD IS DEAD*

Please do not mistake the following lines for theology. They are wordplay. Write your own conclusion to each verse, and then see how close yours are to mine.

1. **R. I. P.**

They buried God the other day,
    They laid Him in a hole.
The preacher brushed a tear away,
    And said, '...'

---

* A fashionable cry among certain avant-garde clerics.

2. Unfinished Business

God's death evokes the more regret

....

3. Nil Nisi Bonum

That God is dead I'll not deny,
   So loud you roar it.
What I don't understand is why

....

4. And What if He Doesn't Bother?

If God is dead, and gone to Heaven,
   What becomes of Adam's birth?
I do hope He will take off seven*

....

W. R. E.

ANSWERS

1. 'God rest His soul.'
2. Since Adam isn't finished yet.
3. You blame *Him* for it.
4. Days, and re-create the Earth.

A REFLECTION

If you can match or surpass the last line of this quatrain, you are a better versifier than Thomas Hood.

When Eve upon the first of men
The apple press'd with specious cant,
Oh, what a thousand pities then

....

ANSWER

That Adam was not adamant!

* Six, actually. But I always have thought He could have used another day.

249

COMPENSATION

In my youth any pleasures ungained
    Pained.
In my age I find pain, when quiescent,
    Quite pleasant.

        W. R. E.

*

Univocalics

A univocalic verse employs only one vowel throughout. The following, by unknown authors, are prize examples:

    Persevere, ye perfect men,
    Ever keep the precepts ten.

THE RUSSO-TURKISH WAR

War harms all ranks, all arts, all crafts appal;
At Mars' harsh blast, arch, rampart, altar fall!
Ah! hard as adamant a braggart Czar
Arms vassal-swarms, and fans a fatal war!
Rampant at that bad call, a Vandal band
Harass, and harm, and ransack Wallach-land.
A Tartar phalanx Balkan's scarp hath past,
And Allah's standard falls, alas! at last.

THE FALL OF EVE

Eve, Eden's empress, needs defended be;
The Serpent greets her when she seeks the tree.
Serene she sees the speckled tempter creep;
Gentle he seems—perverted schemer deep—
Yet endless pretexts, ever fresh, prefers;
Perverts her senses, revels when she errs,
Sneers when she weeps, regrets, repents she fell,
Then, deep-revenged, reseeks the nether Hell!

INCONTROVERTIBLE FACTS

If my count is right, there are 181 *o*'s missing from the univocalic verse below.

> N mnk t gd t rb, r cg, r plt.
> N fl s grss t blt Sctch cllps ht.
> Frm Dnjn tps n rnk rlls.
> Lgwd, nt Lts, flds prt's bwls.
> Trps f ld tsspts ft, t st, cnsrt.
> Bx tps, nt bttms, schl-bys flg fr sprt.
> N cl mnsns blw sft n xfrd dns,
> rthdx, jg-trt, bk-wrm Slmns!
> Bld strgths, f ghsts n hrrr shw.
> n Lndn shp-frnts n hp-blssms grw.
> T crcks f gld n dd lks fr fd.
> n sft clth ftstls n ld fx dth brd.
> Lng strm-tst slps frlrn, wrk n t prt.
> Rks d nt rst n spns, nr wdccks snrt,
> Nr dg n snw-drp r n cltsft rlls,
> Nr cmmn frgs cncct lng prtcls.

Author unknown

ANSWER

No monk too good to rob, or cog, or plot.
No fool so gross to bolt Scotch collops hot.
From Donjon tops no Oronoko rolls.
Logwood, not Lotos, floods Oporto's bowls.
Troops of old tosspots oft, to sot, consort.
Box tops, not bottoms, school-boys flog for sport.
No cool monsoons blow soft on Oxford dons,
Orthodox, jog-trot, book-worm Solomons!
Bold Ostrogoths of ghosts no horror show.
On London shop-fronts no hop-blossoms grow.
To crocks of gold no dodo looks for food.
On soft cloth footstools no old fox doth brood.
Long storm-tost sloops forlorn, work on to port.
Rooks do not roost on spoons, nor woodcocks snort,
Nor dog on snow-drop or on coltsfoot rolls,
Nor common frogs concoct long protocols.

Usage

WHEN ONE MAN'S MEDE IS ANOTHER MAN'S PERSIAN

In a permissive age, there is bound to be permissive language. I doubt, indeed, whether even a swing toward decorum and parental spanking would be accompanied necessarily by a return to respect for syntax. Society is boiling; language must too.

A casual perusal of one morning newspaper revealed the following abuses of English:

'The Prime Minister's interest is this issue is hardly a recent phenomena.'

'At times these radicals seem like they are riding a runaway car.'

'The growing highway and air congestion will make rail travel increasingly more attractive.'

'Three times as many New Yorkers die because of heroin than because of the VC.'

'Gen. Amin overthrew Pres. Obote, whom he alleges had laid plans to kill him.'

There is a Gresham's law about barbarisms: they tend to drive out good usage, and in time to become good usage themselves. Who bothers any more if 'prone' is confused with 'supine', 'infer' with 'imply', 'flaunt' with 'flout'? 'Somewheres', 'anywheres', 'irregardless', 'portentiousness' are marks of ignorance today; next week they may be Queen's English.

Indeed, you may already accept them, just as, to take an opposite tack, you may be repelled, while I am enchanted, by Matthew Prior's

> For thou art a girl as much brighter than her
> As he was a poet sublimer than me.

One more example of language debasement: Some of our finest schools now include 'guidance counsellor', a tautology, among their staff titles. To guide those who still fail to grasp the meaning of the title, it may be advisable to change it to 'guidance counsellor advisor'.

So much for my crotchets. Now let's check yours. Following are some common usages. Vote them up or down, and then see how close your views are to those of the *American Heritage Dictionary* panelists whose majority positions are recorded after this list.

1. *Erratas* as a plural form.
2. *Finalise*.
3. *Hung* for *hanged*.
4. *Good* (as an adverb) for *well*.
5. *Graduate*, as in 'She graduated college'.
6. *Was graduated*.
7. *Too* for *very*.
8. *That* and *which* as relative pronouns.
9. *Unique* with a modification, as in 'rather unique'.
10. *Whence*, in 'from whence'.
11. *Author* as a verb.

ANSWERS

(The majority vote is recorded here. In some cases a substantial minority disagreed.)

1. No. Donald Davidson: 'To think that we have lived to see the day when such a question can be asked!'
2. No. Isaac Asimov: 'This is nothing more than bureaucratic illiteracy —the last resort of the communicatively untalented.'
3. Yes. Vermont Royster: 'There is no noticeable difference between being hanged and hung.'
4. No. Mario A. Pei: 'We brew good, like we used to could. Illiterate. What's the use of having an adverb separate from the adjective if you don't use it? Or do we want to ape German?'
5. No. William J. Miller: 'It jars me as would "Dr. J. operated his patient at 10 a.m".'
6. No, but. John Bainbridge: 'By all who write with a quill pen.' Louis Kronenberger: 'Priggish and superior.'
7. No. Gilbert Highet: 'My wife's mother used to ask me, "I don't like soup too hot, do you?" She was surprised when I said, "No-one likes soup too hot".'
8. No. Theodore C. Sorensen: 'I am opposed to continuing this un-enforceable law of grammar ("that" for restrictive clauses, "which" for nonrestrictive).'
9. No. John Kieran: 'A woman cannot be slightly pregnant.'
10. No. Alistair Cooke: 'C. P. Scott, the first great editor of the *Manchester Guardian*, called in a reporter who had written "from whence". The reporter said, "But, sir, Fielding used 'from whence'." Scott replied, "Mr. Fielding would not have used 'from whence' on *my* paper".'
11. No. Barbara W. Tuchman: 'Good God! No! Never!'

Vowel Words

Martin Gardner, in his notes on *Oddities and Curiosities of Words and Literature*, mentions not only three words consisting entirely of consonants—*crwths* (stringed musical instruments of ancient Ireland), *Llwchwr** (a city-district in Wales), and Joe *Btfsplk* (a character in the Li'l Abner comic strip)—but five words consisting only of vowels. You may be able to identify all five from the definitions below.

1. The fabled abode of Circe.
2. The roseate spoonbill.
3. A melodic formula in Gregorian music.
4. An ancient Tuscan city in Etruria.
5. A Madagascan lemur.

ANSWERS: 1. Aeaea. 2. Aiaiai. 3. Euouae. 4. Oueioi. 5. Aye-aye.

*

TWIST-RIME ON SPRING

Upon the hills new grass is seen;
   The vender's garden sass is green.
The birds between the showers fly;
   The woods are full of flowers shy.
The ornamental butterfly
   Expands his wings to flutter by.
The bees, those little honeybugs,
   Are gaily dancing bunny-hugs.
While poets sing in tripping rime
   That Spring's a simply ripping time!

Arthur Guiterman

*

---

* Crwth, Cwm and Cwmtwrch are other Welsh words in which 'w' serves as a vowel.

W, X, Y, Z

Wayfaring Words

The meanings we attach to many common words would have astonished the people who used them hundreds of years ago. You are asked to identify some words by bridging the gap between their past and their present. In each case the couplet holds clues, and the word you want completes the rhyme.

1. *Keeper of a storehouse* was a very, very
   Early early meaning of **********.
2. If *rising from waves* is the root of *********,
   Would a surfeit of waves be thalassic redundance?
3. Robbers are about; the king has called a ******.
   Cover up the fire, you medieval serf, you!
4. If you are *unlettered; not clerical; rude*,
   Whatever your morals, you once were called ****.
5. The *top of the head* is the seat of control;
   Just count every hair, and you're taking a ****.
6. When Jack's Jills aren't *obedient*, beneath the waves Jack
     ducks 'em;
   Their beauty doesn't soften him; they also must be *****.
7. *Powder to stain eyelids* isn't that at all;
   It's a lively liquor known as *******.
8. How political of fate!
   Clad in white's now *********.

W. R. E.

ANSWERS

1. *Apothecary. Apotheca* meant storehouse in Latin, and came from a Greek combining form meaning to put away.
2. *Abundance,* From Latin *ab*, from, away, + *undare*, to rise in waves.
3. *Curfew.* From French *couvre-feu*, cover the fire. (*Continued overleaf*)

4. *Lewd.* The present sense of lustful, lascivious, reflected the presumption that the common and illiterate classes must be wicked as well.
5. *Poll.* It comes from a Latin word meaning bubble.
6. *Buxom.* 'To make thee buxom [obedient] to her law,' said Chaucer. The present sense of plump and rosy, jolly, perhaps indicates that some obedient maidservants were fun to have around.
7. *Alcohol. Al-kuhl*, in Arabic, was, as indicated, a powder for painting the eyelids. The name was afterwards applied to spirits, a signification unknown to the Arabs.
8. *Candidate.* Candidates for office in Rome were clothed in a white toga.

Wedded Words

Pair the words below so as to create a dozen compound words. Since you have only nineteen uncompounded words to start with, you are going to have to use some of them more than once.

Bird	House	Pocket
Black	Keeper	Sheep
Book	Lock	Skin
Boot	Making	Tail
Flint	Master	Tooth
Head	Pick	
Horse	Piece	

ANSWERS

Blackbird	Headmaster	Sheepskin
Bookmaking	Horsetail	Skinflint
Bootblack	Housekeeper	Toothpick
Flintlock	Masterpiece	Pickpocket

What's Up?

We've got a two-letter word we use constantly that may have more meanings than any other. The word is *up*.

It is easy to understand *up* meaning toward the sky or toward the top of a list. But when we waken, why do we wake *up*? At a meeting, why does a topic come *up*, why do participants speak *up*, and why are the officers *up* for election? And why is it *up* to the secretary to write *up* a report?

Often the little word isn't needed, but we use it anyway. We brighten *up* a room, light *up* a cigar, polish *up* the silver, lock *up* the house, and fix *up* the old car. At other times, it has special meanings. People stir *up* trouble, line *up* for tickets, work *up* an appetite, think *up* excuses, get tied *up* in traffic. To be dressed is one thing, but to be dressed *up* is special. It may be confusing, but a drain must be opened *up* because it is stopped *up*. We open *up* a store in the morning and close it *up* at night. We seem to be mixed *up* about *up*.

To be *up* on the proper use of *up* look *up* the word in your dictionary. In one desk-size dictionary *up* takes *up* half a page, and listed definitions add *up* to about 40. If you are *up* to it, you might try building *up* a list of the many ways in which *up* is used. It will take *up* a lot of your time, but if you don't give *up*, you may wind *up* with a thousand.

Frank S. Endicott, The Reader's Digest

*

WHEN ADAM DAY BY DAY

When Adam day by day
  Woke up in Paradise,
He always used to say
  'Oh, this is very nice.'

But Eve from scenes of bliss
  Transported him for life.
The more I think of this
  The more I beat my wife.

A. E. Housman

*

Who Said That? I Wish I Had!

In my nightmare, I was condemned to be flayed. When I begged for mercy, the judge said I would be released if I could identify the author of each of a half-dozen famous lines. 'I will give you a hint,' he added. 'Each line is the work of one of the Algonquin Wits.'

I knew who the Algonquin Wits were; but I pretended ignorance.

'All right,' said the judge, 'you are a witless and spineless fellow, but I'll give you more help than you deserve.' And he went on as follows:

The principal Algonquin Wits were George S. Kaufman and Robert Sherwood, playwrights; F. P. A. (Franklin Pierce Adams) and Heywood Broun, columnists; Ring Lardner, Robert Benchley, Alexander Woollcott, Dorothy Parker and Edna Ferber, writers.

George S. Kaufman is the man who drew a poor poker hand, and threw it in, announcing, 'I have been tray-deuced.'

F. P. A. is the one who asked Beatrice Kaufman, 'Guess whose birthday it is today?' 'Yours?' she said. 'No,' said F. P. A, 'but you're getting warm—it's Shakespeare's.'

Robert Sherwood once commented on the motion picture cowboy hero Tom Mix: 'They say he rides like part of the horse, but they don't say which part.'

Heywood Broun, a happily married man, remarked that 'The ability to make love frivolously is the chief characteristic which distinguishes human beings from the beasts.'

Ring Lardner said his favourite line of poetry was part of an ode written by an ex-coroner to his mother: 'If by perchance the inevitable should come . . .'

It was Robert Benchley who remarked, 'It took me fifteen years to discover that I had no talent for writing, but I couldn't give it up because by that time I was too famous.'

Alexander Woollcott's chief claim to fame is *not* that he developed this intricate puzzle anecdote: 'Three men sit down to a bottle of brandy and divide it equally between them. When they have finished the bottle one of them leaves the room, and the other two try to guess who left.'

Nor is Dorothy Parker best remembered for having remarked, when told that Calvin Coolidge was dead, 'How could they tell?'

Nor Edna Ferber, for describing reviewers who could no longer be objective about the literary works of Nobel Prize winners as 'awestruck by the Nobelity'.

Which of these wits wrote the lines that follow?

1. I was a child prodigy myself. That is, at the age of five I already required twelve-year-old pants.
2. Repartee is what you wish you'd said.

3. All the things I really want to do are either immoral, illegal, or fattening.
4. Satire is something that closes on Saturday night.
5. Let's get out of these wet clothes, and into a dry martini.
6. Nothing is more responsible for the good old days than a bad memory.
7. The only real argument for Marriage is that it remains the best method for getting acquainted.
8. In America, there are two classes of travel—first class and with children.
9. I do most of my work sitting down. That's where I shine.
10. One man's Mede is another man's Persian.
11. He's a writer for the ages—the ages of four to eight.
12. Being an old maid is like death by drowning, a really delightful sensation after you give up the struggle.

ANSWERS

1. Heywood Broun.
2. Heywood Broun.
3. Alexander Woollcott (*not* Dorothy Parker).
4. George S. Kaufman.
5. Robert Benchley (*not* Dorothy Parker or Alexander Woollcott).
6. F. P. A.
7. Heywood Broun.
8. Robert Benchley.
9. Robert Benchley.
10. George S. Kaufman.
11. Dorothy Parker.
12. Edna Ferber.

*

THE WISHES OF AN ELDERLY MAN

(At a Garden Party, June 1914)

I wish I loved the Human Race;
I wish I loved its silly face;
I wish I liked the way it walks;
I wish I liked the way it talks;
And when I'm introduced to one
I wish I thought *What Jolly Fun!*

Walter Raleigh

*

Word Games for Parties

ALPHABETICAL ADJECTIVES

The first contestant announces an adjective–noun combination in which the adjective begins with *a* and the noun with any letter of the player's choice (except, I should think, *x* and perhaps *z*). The second player must give an adjective beginning with *b*, and a noun beginning with the same letter as before. So on through the alphabet. For instance:

Aching back, blue-stocking Bostonian, contented bovine, desperate blackmailer, extra blankets, fractured bone, gorgeous bosom, horrible blasphemy, indifferent babe, jumpy ballerina, kleptomanic burglar, lecherous burlesque, monkey business, nihilistic Bakunin, ogling boulevardier, pious Baptist, quavering baritone, rich beneficiary, spirited bootlegger, tempestuous Bulgarian, uxorious brontosaurus, viviparous bullsnake, whining bully, xenophobic belligerent, yowling bow-wow, zestful barmaid.

THE BAEKELAND DICTIONARY GAME

Liz Baekeland sometimes arms a half dozen guests with numbered sheets of paper and proceeds to read nouns aloud from the dictionary at random until she finds one that nobody recognises. The guests then write imagined definitions of the word, while Liz makes a note of the real one. She reads the completed definitions aloud one by one, both the false and the true, and the players vote (by number) for the one they think is right. Each correct vote wins a point for the voter, while each vote for a false definition wins a point for the person who made it up. Liz tallies the votes, and the high man or woman wins. The fun lies in making the definitions both legitimate-sounding and amusing.

One word on a recent evening was 'cochineal'. The definitions offered are given below. Guess which is correct—if you don't know already.

1. The body cavity of a metazoon.
2. The first leaf above the ground, forming a protective sheath around the stem tip.
3. A sharp-pronged instrument used in deep harrowing.

4. A red dye prepared from the dried bodies of the females of a scale insect.
5. An extant free-swimming cochoid.
6. An asexual spore with a vanilla-like odour.
7. A shell indigenous to South America, of the same genus as the cockle shell, but smaller and purplish in colour.
8. A solution for application to the eye; an eyewash.

Answer—4.

BOUTS RIMÉS

If your friends fancy themselves at wordplay, invite them over for a bout of *Bouts Rimés*. The rules of the game are simple: pass around at least four rhyming words (the contest can be as intricate as the players wish, but if the poem is to be a sonnet or an ode you'd better give out the words in advance of your party) which are to be used in a piece of doggerel. There should be some limit— say ten minutes—on the time allowed for creation. The more challenging the rhyming words, the more amusing and dexterous the verses are likely to be.

Horace Walpole, presented with *brook, why, crook,* and *I,* promptly observed:

> I sit with my toes in a brook;
>   If anyone asks me for why,—
> I hits them a rap with my crook;
>   'Tis sentiment kills me, says I.

At another party, the words were *wave, lie, brave,* and *die.* To one contestant, these were a challenge to his noblest instincts:

> Dark are the secrets of the gulfing wave,
>   Where, wrapped in death, so many heroes lie;
> Yet glorious death's the guerdon of the brave,
>   And those who bravely live can bravely die.

But another saw the matter in a different light—more down to earth, or perhaps more down to sea:

> Whenever I sail on the wave,
>   O'ercome with sea-sickness I lie!
> I can *sing* of the sea, and look brave;
>   When I *feel* it, I feel like to die!

Below are a number of groups of rhyming words. See what you can do with them. Then read on to see what others have done with them (but *not* in games of *Bouts Rimés*).

1. Bile, detest, vile, best.
2. Love me, hate, above me, fate.
3. Shattered, dead, scattered, shed.

ANSWERS

1

Of sentences that stir my bile,
Of phrases I detest,
There's one beyond all others vile:
He did it for the best.

James Kenneth Stephen

2

Here's a sigh to those who love me,
And a smile to those who hate;
And, whatever sky's above me,
Here's a heart for every fate.

Lord Byron

3

When the lamp is shattered
The light in the dust lies dead—
When the cloud is scattered
The rainbow's glory is shed.

Percy Bysshe Shelley

MORE BOUTS RIMÉS

Poet-anthologist William Cole discovered a variant of *Bouts Rimés* in a Victorian volume called *Evening Amusements: Mirthful Games, Shadow Plays, Chemical Surprises, Fireworks, Forfeits, etc.* In this version, '. . . the director . . . recites a line of poetry, to which the person to whom it is addressed is bound to add a line corresponding in rhyme, measure, and sense with it, under pain of having to pay a forfeit'. Mr. Cole turned to the 'Index of First Lines' in his poetry anthologies, and, he says, 'immersed myself for an evening of converting the sublime to the ridiculous'.

Here is an example of the sort of thing that emerged:

> *There is a garden in her face*; (Campion)
> Her dermatologist has the case. (Cole)

There follow some first lines for which Mr. Cole created absurd mates. I suggest that you compose your own follow-ups, either privily or as a parlour-game participant. Since first lines of well-known poems are legion, this game can be continued until the last player falls asleep.

1. I strove with none; for none was worth my strife;   (Landor)
2. Whenas in silks my Julia goes,   (Herrick)
3. In a cowslip's bell I lie—   (Shakespeare)
4. When the hounds of spring are on winter's traces,
                                                    (Swinburne)
5. My love is like to ice, and I to fire;   (Spenser)
6. To be, or not to be; that is the question—   (Shakespeare)
7. Since there's no help, come, let us kiss and part—
                                                    (Drayton)
8. O, that this too, too solid flesh would melt!   (Shakespeare)
9. When I have fears that I may cease to be,   (Keats)
10. When lovely woman stoops to folly,   (Goldsmith)

ANSWERS

1   I strove with none; for none was worth my strife;
     This worked with everyone except my wife.

2   Whenas in silks my Julia goes,
     The outline of her girdle shows.

3   In a cowslip's bell I lie—
     I'm the teeniest little guy!

4   When the hounds of spring are on winter's traces,
     The rich take off for warmer places.

5   My love is like to ice, and I to fire;
     But a couple of drinks, and something may transpire.

6   To be, or not to be; that is the question—
     Has anyone an alternate suggestion?

7   Since there's no help, come, let us kiss and part—
     Tomorrow night we'll make another start.

8   O, that this too, too solid flesh would melt!
     I've had to punch a new hole in my belt.

9   When I have fears that I may cease to be,
     I take another drink—or two—or three.

10   When lovely woman stoops to folly,
     I want to be around, by golly!

CATEGORIES

This agreeable parlour game is also called Guggenheim, because it is supposed to have been first played in the home of a distinguished family of that name. Each player is given a sheet of paper divided into five vertical columns with a letter at the top of each. The five letters make a word. To the left of the columns is a list, one under the other, of five categories of objects—horses, fish, gems, prime ministers, or what you will. The idea is to think of five words in each category that begin with the five letters heading the columns. The winner is the person who, in a set period of time, comes up with the largest number of appropriate objects.

In choosing categories for your guests, make a privy estimate of their erudition, and remember that it is blessed to temper the wind to the shorn lamb.

DAFFY DEFINITIONS

The sound of some words can be defined by words meaning something entirely different. Give the players a pencil and a piece of paper, and see who can think of the greatest number of such words. The following list, from Leonhard Dowty's *Word Games*, will give you the idea:

The definition	*The word*
Capital S	Largess
Male escort	Mandate
Wedding day	Maritime
Judge's garb	Lawsuit
How Dali paints	Cereal
Faint noise	Locomotion
Lousy poet	Bombard
Ready hat	Handicap
Ex-spouse	Stalemate
Fake diamond	Shamrock

GHOST AND SUPERGHOST

In the game of Ghost, also called One-Third of a Ghost, the first player announces the first letters of any word of three or more letters. The player to his left adds a letter which furthers, but must not complete, the word. The object is to trap a player into completing the spelling of a dictionary word, which makes him a third of a ghost. Anyone who becomes three-thirds of a ghost is out of the game.

In Superghost, a letter may be added at either end of an incomplete word.

The delights and frustrations of Superghost were described by humorist James Thurber in a *New Yorker* article called, 'Do You Want to Make Something Out of It? Or, if you put an "O" on "Understo," you'll ruin my "Thunderstorm".' He reported the kind of mania to which Superghost can lead: 'I sometimes keep on playing the game, all by myself, after it is over and I have gone to bed. On a recent night, tossing and spelling, I spent two hours hunting for another word besides "phlox" that has "hlo" in it. I finally found seven: "matchlock," "decathlon," "pentathlon," "hydrochloric," "chlorine," "chloroform," and "monthlong."'

Listed below are some Superghost letter combinations, including several that bedevilled Mr. Thurber. The trick is to steer clear of the obvious. Anyone who sees no future for 'awkw' save in 'awkward' will soon find himself one-third of a superghost.

1. abc
2. ach-ach
3. alema
4. awkw
5. cklu
6. nehe
7. sgra
8. ug-ug
9. fbac
10. ocol
11. ndf
12. olho

ANSWERS

1. Dabchick
2. Stomach-ache
3. Stalemate
4. Hawkweed
5. Lacklustre
6. Swineherd, bonehead
7. Disgrace, grosgrain
8. Pug-ugly
9. Halfback
10. Chocolate, protocol
11. Grandfather
12. Schoolhouse

I-CAN-GIVE-YOU-A-SENTENCE

One of the pastimes of the group of irreverent wits who used to meet at the Algonquin Hotel in New York was making up sentences in which one of the words resembles an unrelated phrase.

Study the I-Can-Give-You-A-Sentences below, and then see whether you, or your friends, can match them.

Meretricious, and a Happy New Year! (F. P. A. [Franklin Pierce Adams])

The Indian chief expelled an overgrown papoose from the tribe, saying, 'You big! Quit us!' This was the origin of *ubiquitous*. (Heywood Broun)

I know a farmer who has two daughters, Lizzie and Tillie. Lizzie is all right, but you have no idea how *punctilious*. (George S. Kaufman)

You may lead a *horticulture*, but you can't make her think. (Dorothy Parker)

STINKY PINKIES

The idea is to answer a definition with a rhyming combination of adjective and noun; a 'repentant truck', for instance, would be a 'sorry lorry'. Stinky Pinkies are often easier to create than to guess, and they are fun at parties—if everyone happens to be in the mood.
Some Stinky Pinky definitions:

1. Aviator
2. Breakfast fish exporter
3. Cheerful progenitor
4. Chicken purchaser
5. Childbirth at the North Pole
6. Cracked spar
7. Dejected cleric
8. Departed spouse
9. Escaped fowl
10. Costly lager
11. Forgiveable servant
12. Funniest joke
13. Happy German
14. Inexperienced monarch
15. Jumpy fowl
16. One mad about the theatre

ANSWERS

1. Fly guy
2. Kipper shipper
3. Glad dad
4. Fryer buyer
5. Shivery delivery
6. Split sprit
7. Sunk monk
8. Late mate
9. Loose goose
10. Dear beer
11. Venial menial
12. Best jest
13. Merry Jerry
14. Green queen
15. Jerky turkey
16. Dramatic fanatic

WHAT IS THE QUESTION?

By report, this word game was played by the wittier intimates of President John F. Kennedy. The first player gives an answer; the others must then supply the question. If the answer is 'Chicken Tetrazzini', the question might be, 'Name a scared Italian opera singer.' '9W' answers this question to the composer Richard Wagner: 'Sir, do you spell your name with a V?'

A good game for punsters.

Word Power

Find at least 15 five-letter words in each of the words listed, using only one form of the new word—for example, 'swing' or 'swung', not both. Do not make a word by adding *s* to a word of four letters. Slang, proper names and foreign words are not allowed.

1. Calvinistic   2. Cumulative   3. Recruitment

ANSWERS

1. *Calvinistic:* Cavil, civil, civic, antic, licit, vital, vista, visit, vinic, inact, scant, saint, satin, stain, slain, slant, snail, tical
2. *Cumulative:* Cavil, claim, camel, clime, cleat, culet, civet, utile, malic, mauve, metal, acute, amice, alive, tical, valet, vital, vault, eclat, evict
3. *Recruitment:* Recur, ricer, remit, runic, rumen, erect, enure, enter, cumin, cruet, cutter, crime, creme, unite, untie, utter, incur, inert, inure, inter, incut, trice, truce, trine, truer, tunic, timer, trite, tenet, merit, meter, miner, mince, mucin, miter, nicer, niece, niter

Words Across the Sea

LONDON LETTER

The following comments on the language differences between Great Britain and the U.S.A. were made by Herbert R. Mayes in the *Saturday Review*.

When I took up residence here sixteen months ago, I had rather hoped to disprove the observation made by Shaw and Wilde that England and America are two countries separated by the same language. I had hoped to prove that butter muslin for cheesecloth was as obsolete as 'Haw, haw, by Jove.' I have only partially succeeded . . . I'd like to bespeak a few words, for example, against bespoke shirtmakers. If the English mean custom-made, I'd like them to say so. Although it is true that today England accepts druggist, elevator, apartment, and cop as readily as chemist, lift, flat, and bobby; and although I have not had to say lorry, kiosk, hire-purchase, or rates when I meant truck, newsstand, installment-plan, and taxes, there nevertheless are some bespokes still around. A dustbin is never going to be an ash can, a screw spanner a monkey wrench, or drawing pins thumbtacks. Baby-sitter is beginning to be substituted for child-minder, and overpass soon may catch up with flyover; but most definitely suspenders are never going to replace braces.

Long before I began visiting England—before World War II—I had read Mencken's *The American Language* and had familiar-ised myself with common objects he listed that had different words applied to them in the mother country. Thus, it was easy to recognise diversion for detour, stall for orchestra seat, interval for intermission, gangway for aisle, bank holiday for legal holiday, and even ironmonger for hardware dealer. I knew a telephone booth would be a call box, a mailbox a pillar box, and a sidewalk a footpath. Americans don't joke about these innocent variations any more; they simply gag over the likes of dickey seat for rumble seat or scribbling-block for scratch-pad.

The British are stubborn, as you don't need to be told. A scallion remains a spring onion, a janitor a porter, a barber a hairdresser, and a notary public a commissioner of oaths. They persist in addressing a surgeon as Mister and still consider an ignoramus anyone who doesn't know a toilet from a hole in the ground when he refers to a closet instead of a cupboard. Over here, there is still only one closet, and that's a water closet.

On the whole, however, for all the differences in pronunciation, intonation, and accent, there really is not too much of a vocabulary problem; mainly, I think, because the English have been over-whelmed by us, and are reconciled as much to loss of language pre-eminence as to liquidation of Empire. I cannot recall an American expression that the English don't comprehend instantly. American movies and television programs shown here, and the annual influx of hundreds of thousands of American tourists, have been relentless tutors. It is rare that an American novel is

Anglicised. The British edition of *Time* is published exactly as it would be in the States; no substituting underground for subway, tin for can, or express post for special delivery. Robert Knittel, the editorial director of Collins Publishing, says that about halfway across the ocean our two languages nuzzle up to each other and fraternise enough to become what he calls mid-Atlinguish.

Words in Labour

The following verse is a reflection on the fact that certain words contain their equivalents, foreshortened and perhaps disarranged, within themselves.

> *I met some swollen words one day,*
> *As full of roe as sturgeons;*
> *For certain in a family way,*
> *Yet innocent as virgins.*
>
> *Parthenogenesis, they swore,*
> *Had stocked their inner shelves,*
> *And all those nascent words in store*
> *Were carbons of themselves.*
>
> *Lo! when at last their babies came,*
> *They were indeed the spit*
> *Of their mamas; each given name*
> *Was ample proof of it:*
>
> For *Aberrate* did *** produce,
> And *Slithered* mothered ****,
> And *Utilise* gave suck to ***,
> And *** was *Curtail*'s kid.
>
> The child of *Jocularity*
> Was aptly christened ***;
> While *Masculine*'s was instantly
> Named ****, though not a boy.

(CONTINUED OVERLEAF)

Transgression called her daughter ***,
And *Matches'* child was *****;
Container's twins were *** and ***,
And *Prattles'* wee one, ******;

So ******'s from *Rapscallion* born,
So ***** from *Regulates*;
What babe, as **** from *Respite's* torn,
******* *Evacuates*?

Now *Calumnies* gives suck to ****;
Encourage, **** doth hug;
**** safe in arms of *Rampage* lies,
And *Struggle* mothers ***

W. R. E.

ANSWER

Err; slid; use; cut; joy; male; sin; mates; can; tin; prates; rascal; rules;
rest; vacates; lies; urge; rage; tug.

The Worst Love Poem Ever
(*In several manners of speaking*)

This verse is intended to make it easy to distinguish among
several types of word game and wordplay.

1. *Courtship: Our Hero Speaks Sweet Words*

Fit 1:	O Dorothea Evalina Anna Rim,
The acronym	May I be thy ever-loving acronym?
Fit 2:	So utterly in knud vhsg xnt, my dear, I am,
The cryptogram	I'd gladly give my khed sn ad your cryptogram.
Fit 3:	I'll liken you to lichen if you'll tease me at your
The homonym	teas;
	We'll bounce a little homonym upon our knees.
Fit 4:	He'll be a redder tot than any civic pup or pip;
The palindrome	A never odd or even, palindromic drip.

270

2. Marriage: Our Hero's Words Turn Sour

Fit 5:   I who *******, *******, and won thee,
The anagram   now *******, or worse;
           Ne'er thought I our anagram would end in
           *******.

Fit 6:   If my wife and little ones continue such a bother
The pun   (Sick of one, and half a dozen [pun!] of t'other),

Fit 7:   I may seek out comfort in an epigram:
The epigram   "I am wed unhappily; ergo, I am.'

Fit 8:   Wife, write these words upon the wind to be my
The epitaph   epitaph:
           'He laughed at life, aware the worms would be the
           last to laugh.'

W. R. E.

ANSWERS

Fit 1. Our hero urges the young lady to become his *dear*, acronym of *D*orothea *E*valina *A*nna *R*im.

Fit 2. The letters in each coded word come just before those in the decoded word:
           So utterly in *love with you*, my dear, I am,
           I'd gladly give my *life to be* your cryptogram.

Fit 3. *Liken*, *lichen*, *tease* and *teas* are identical in sound but unrelated in meaning—i.e., homonyms.

Fit 4. *Redder*, *tot*, *civic*, *pup*, and *pip* are palindromic words, spelled the same forward as backward. *Never odd or even* is a palindromic phrase.

Fit 5. The missing words are *praised*, *aspired*, *despair*, and *diapers*, each an anagram of the others.

Fits 6, 7 and 8, on the pun, the epigram, and the epitaph, need no explanation.

You so ĕn trăns´ me

Etymologic roots sometimes sprout words with identical spellings but different sounds and meanings. Apart from an apostrophe and a space, 'man's laughter' and 'manslaughter' are as one to the eye; but the mind finds no connection between them at all. I am reminded of a foreigner who spent ten years studying English, arrived in London, and saw a newspaper headline: 'Hamlet pronounced success.' He turned around and went back home,

271

defeated. I am reminded also of the immigrant who asked his neighbour: 'You speak the English, not so?' The neighbour replied: 'A few, and then small.'

Suppose you juxtapose entrance (ĕn trans'), 'to enrapture', with entrance (en' trans), 'a point or place of entering'; present (prĕz' ent), 'the time being', with present (prēz ent'), 'to introduce'; content (con tent'), 'satisfied', with content (con' tent) 'the matter dealt with'; intimate (in' ti mate'), 'to hint, imply', with intimate (in' ti mit'), 'associated in close, often sexual, relationship'; agape (a gape'), 'mouth wide open', with agape (a' ga pe'), 'spiritual love'; invalid (in' va lid), 'a person weak or infirm', with invalid (in vá lid), 'void, null'; recreation (rek ri a shun), 'diversion', with recreation (rē kri a shun), 'act of creating anew'. What do you have?

Perhaps something like this:

> You so *entrance* my senses that
>   I haunt the *entrance* to your flat
> At *present*, seeking to *present*
>   A case for early ravishment.

> I'd be *content* could I impart
>   The amorous *content* of my heart
> To you, and *intimate* we might
>   Be *intimate*, some future night.

> Before your shape I stand *agape*;
>   Not *agape* but lust to rape
> Makes me love's *invalid*. Alas,
>   You deem *invalid* every pass.

> Such *recreation* you will ration
> Till *recreation* of Creation.

> W. R. E.

INDEX OF QUOTED SOURCES

278

V

Van Rooten, Luis D'Antan, 169
Vida, 107
Voltaire (François Marie Arouet), 206

W

W. R. E. (Willard R. Espy), 21, 27, 30, 33, 39–47, 49, 50, 51, 56, 57, 59, 72, 76, 92, 94, 96, 97, 111, 115, 120, 122, 124, 125, 132, 141, 142, 156, 171, 179, 184, 200, 222, 225, 226, 227, 230, 231, 238, 245, 248, 249, 250, 255, 269, 270, 271

Wallis, Dr., 238
Walpole, Horace, 261
Watts, Isaac, 66
Waugh, Evelyn, 244
Webster, Noah, 228
Wells, Carolyn, 238
Wilde, Oscar, 96
Wolfe, Humbert, 65, 68
Wood, Robert Williams, 133
Woollcott, Alexander, 15, 167, 168, 258
Wright, Ernest Vincent, 157

Y

Yeatman, Robert Julian, 64